# FIRST AID

D0315270

# USMLE
# STEP 1
# 2010

## 20th Anniversary Edition

**TAO LE, MD, MHS**

Assistant Clinical Professor of Medicine and Pediatrics
Chief, Section of Allergy and Immunology
Department of Medicine
University of Louisville

**VIKAS BHUSHAN, MD**

Diagnostic Radiologist
Los Angeles

**NEIL VASAN**

Medical Scientist Training Program
Yale University

**JULIANA TOLLES**

Yale University
Class of 2011

 **Medical**

New York / Chicago / San Francisco / Lisbon / London / Madrid / Mexico City
Milan / New Delhi / San Juan / Seoul / Singapore / Sydney / Toronto

**First Aid for the® USMLE Step 1 2010: A Student-to-Student Guide**

1 2 3 4 5 6 7 8 9 0    WDQ/WDQ    14 13 12 11 10 9

ISBN 978-0-07-163340-6
MHID 0-07-163340-5
ISSN 1532-6020

---

### Notice

Medicine is an ever-changing science. As new research and clinical experience broaden our knowledge, changes in treatment and drug therapy are required. The authors and the publisher of this work have checked with sources believed to be reliable in their efforts to provide information that is complete and generally in accord with the standards accepted at the time of publication. However, in view of the possibility of human error or changes in medical sciences, neither the authors nor the publisher nor any other party who has been involved in the preparation or publication of this work warrants that the information contained herein is in every respect accurate or complete, and they disclaim all responsibility for any errors or omissions or for the results obtained from use of the information contained in this work. Readers are encouraged to confirm the information contained herein with other sources. For example and in particular, readers are advised to check the product information sheet included in the package of each drug they plan to administer to be certain that the information contained in this work is accurate and that changes have not been made in the recommended dose or in the contraindications for administration. This recommendation is of particular importance in connection with new or infrequently used drugs.

---

This book was set in Electra LH by Rainbow Graphics.
The editor was Catherine A. Johnson.
Project management was provided by Rainbow Graphics.
The production supervisor was Phil Galea.
The designer was Marsha Cohen/Parallelogram.
Worldcolor Dubuque was printer and binder.

This book is printed on acid-free paper.

McGraw-Hill books are available at special quantity discounts to use as premiums and sales promotions, or for use in corporate training programs. To contact a representative please e-mail us at bulksales@mcgraw-hill.com.

To the contributors to this and past editions, who took time to share their knowledge, insight, and humor for the benefit of students.

*and*

To Dr. William Ganong, a beloved teacher and an early believer in the power of *First Aid*.

# CONTENTS

# CONTRIBUTING AUTHORS

**FERAS AKBIK**

Medical Scientist Training Program
Yale University

**PANOS CHRISTAKIS**

Yale University
Class of 2011

**LILANGI EDIRIWICKREMA**

Yale University
Class of 2011

**AARON FEINSTEIN**

Yale University
Class of 2011

**PETER M. GAYED**

Yale University
Class of 2011

**GWENDOLYN J. GODFREY, DO, MPH**

Resident
Department of Pathology and Laboratory Medicine
University of Louisville

**GUSON KANG**

Yale University
Class of 2011

**ANDREW KOBETS**

Yale University
Class of 2011

**BADRI MODI**

Yale University
Class of 2011

**JOSHUA MOTELOW**

Medical Scientist Training Program
Yale University

**MONA SADEGHPOUR**

Yale University
Class of 2011

# WEB AND IMAGE CONTRIBUTORS

**MARK D. SUGI**

University of California, Los Angeles
Class of 2011

**DANIEL J. DURAND, MD**

Senior Resident in Radiology
The Johns Hopkins University School of Medicine

**RAVISH AMIN**

University of Medicine and Dentistry of New Jersey
Class of 2010

**JAYSSON BROOKS**

Loma Linda University
Class of 2011

**KEVIN DAY**

Northwestern University
Class of 2011

**ANDREW DEGNAN**

George Washington University
Class of 2011

**SWAPNA GHANTA**

University of Medicine and Dentistry of New Jersey
Class of 2010

**SUMEET K. GOEL**

Edward Via Virginia College of Osteopathic Medicine
Class of 2010

**JOSEPH A. SANFORD, JR.**

College of Medicine
University of Arkansas for Medical Sciences
Class of 2010

**MICHAEL L. STERN**

Albany Medical Center
Class of 2011

# FACULTY REVIEWERS

**DIANA M. ANTONIUCCI, MD, MAS**

Assistant Professor of Medicine, Division of Endocrinology
University of California, San Francisco

**SUSAN BASERGA, MD, PhD**

Professor of Molecular Biophysics and Biochemistry, Genetics, and
    Therapeutic Radiology
Yale University

**LINDA S. COSTANZO, PhD**

Professor of Physiology
Virginia Commonwealth University

**JANINE EVANS, MD**

Associate Professor of Medicine
Program Director, Rheumatology Fellowship Program
Yale University

**STUART D. FLYNN, MD**

Associate Dean, Academic Affairs
Professor, Departments of Pathology and Basic Medical Sciences
University of Arizona

**FRED GORELICK, MD**

Professor of Medicine and Cell Biology
Yale University and VAMC West Haven

**RAJESH JARI, MD, MSC**

Resident in Physical Medicine and Rehabilitation
Johns Hopkins University

**SHANTA KAPADIA, MD**

Lecturer, Surgical Anatomy and Experimental Surgery
Yale University

**BERTRAM KATZUNG, MD, PhD**

Professor of Pharmacology
University of California, San Francisco

**WARREN LEVINSON, MD, PhD**

Professor of Microbiology and Immunology
University of California, San Francisco

**PETER MARKS, MD, PhD**

Associate Professor of Hematology
Yale University

**CHRISTIAN MERLO, MD, MPH**

Instructor, Medicine
Division of Pulmonary and Critical Care Medicine
Johns Hopkins University

**DANIEL MUNDY, MD**

Assistant Professor of Psychiatry
New York Medical College

**DHASAKUMAR S. NAVARATNAM, PhD**

Assistant Professor of Neurology and Neurobiology
Yale University

**ANDREA OECKINGHAUS, PhD**

Postdoctoral Fellow
Columbia University

**SANJIV J. SHAH, MD**

Assistant Professor of Medicine
Division of Cardiology, Department of Medicine
Northwestern University

**STEPHEN F. THUNG, MD**

Assistant Professor, Department of Obstetrics and Gynecology
Yale University

**ADAM WEINSTEIN, MD**

Department of Pediatrics/Pediatric Nephrology
Dartmouth Hitchcock Medical Center

# TWENTIETH ANNIVERSARY FOREWORD

It feels oddly premature to be writing a 20th-edition foreword given how vivid preparing for the exam remains in our minds. In 1989, our original idea was to cobble together a "quick and dirty" study guide so that we would never again have to deal with the USMLE Step 1. We passed, but in a Faustian twist, we now relive the exam yearly while preparing each new edition.

Like all students before us, we noticed that certain topics tended to appear frequently on examinations. So we compulsively bought and rated review books and pored through a mind-numbing number of "recall" questions, distilling each into short facts. We had a love-hate relationship with mnemonics. They went against our purist desires for conceptual knowledge, but remained the best way to absorb the vocabulary and near-random associations that unlocked questions and eponyms.

To pull it all together, we used a then–"state-of-the-art" computer database (Paradox/MS DOS 4) that fortuitously limited our entries to 256 characters. That single constraint mandated brevity, while the three-column layout created structure—and this was the blueprint upon which *First Aid* was founded.

The printed, three-column database was first distributed in 1989 at the University of California, San Francisco. The next year, the official first edition was self-published under the title *High-Yield Basic Science Boards Review: A Student-to-Student Guide*. The following year, our publisher dismissed the *High-Yield* title as too confusing and came up with *First Aid for the Boards*. We thought the name was a bit cheesy, but it proved memorable. Interestingly, our "High-Yield" name resurfaced years later as the title of a competing board review series.

We lived in San Francisco and Los Angeles during medical school and residency. It was before the Web, and before med students could afford cell phones and laptops, so we relied on AOL e-mail and bulky desktops. One of us would drive down to the other person's place for multiple weekends of frenetic revisions fueled by triple-Swiss white chocolate lattes from the Coffee Bean & Tea Leaf, with R.E.M. and the Nusrat Fateh Ali Khan playing in the background. Everything was marked up on 11- by 17-inch "tearsheets," and at the end of the marathon weekend we would converge on the local 24-hour Kinko's followed by the FedEx box near LAX (10 years before these two great institutions merged). These days we work with Adobe Acrobat, iPhones, and ubiquitous broadband Internet, and sadly, we rarely get to see each other.

What hasn't changed, however, is the collaborative nature of the book. Hundreds of authors, editors, and contributors have enriched our lives and made this book possible. Most helped for a year or two and moved on, but a few, like Ted Hon, Chirag Amin, and Andi Fellows, made long-lasting contributions. Like the very first edition, the team is always led by student authors who live and breathe (and fear) the exam, not professors years away from that reality.

We're proud of the precedent that *First Aid* set for the many excellent student-to-student publications that followed. More importantly, *First Aid* itself owes its success to the global community of medical students and international medical graduates (IMGs) who each year contribute ideas, suggestions, and new content. In the early days, we used book coupons and tear-out business-reply mail forms. These days, we get more than 2,000 contributions each year via blog, e-mail, and Facebook.

At the end of the day, we don't take any of this for granted. There are big changes in store for the USMLE, and a bigger job ahead of us to try to keep *First Aid* indispensable to students and IMGs. We want and need your participation in the *First Aid* community. (See How to Contribute, p. xvii.) With your help, we are hoping editing *First Aid* for the next 20 years will be just as fun and rewarding as the past 20 years have been.

|  |  |
|---|---|
| *Louisville* | Tao Le |
| *Los Angeles* | Vikas Bhushan |

*First Aid for the* USMLE *Step 1* Through the Years

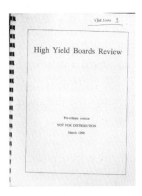
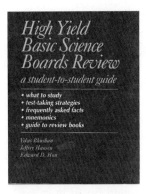
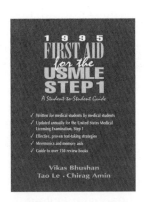

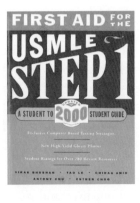
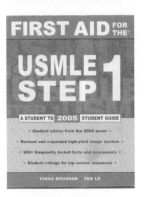
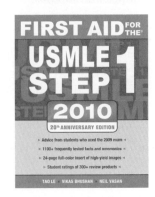

With the 20th anniversary 2010 edition of *First Aid for the USMLE Step 1*, we continue our commitment to providing students with the most useful and up-to-date preparation guide for the USMLE Step 1. This edition represents a major revision in many ways and includes:

- A revised and updated exam preparation guide for the USMLE Step 1. Includes detailed analysis as well as study and test-taking strategies for the new FRED v2 format.
- Revisions and new material based on student experience with the 2009 administrations of the computerized USMLE Step 1.
- Revised USMLE advice for international medical graduates, osteopathic medical students, podiatry students, and students with disabilities.
- More than 1100 frequently tested facts and useful mnemonics, including hundreds of new or revised entries in reorganized sections.
- A high-yield collection of nearly 200 glossy photos similar to those appearing on the USMLE Step 1 exam.
- An updated guide to hundreds of recommended USMLE Step 1 review resources based on a nationwide survey of randomly selected third-year medical students.
- Bonus Step 1 high-yield facts, cases, video lectures, corrections, and updates exclusively at our blog at **www.firstaidteam.com**.

The 20th anniversary 2010 edition would not have been possible without the help of the hundreds of students and faculty members who contributed their feedback and suggestions. We invite students and faculty to continue sharing their thoughts and ideas to help us improve *First Aid for the USMLE Step 1*. (See How to Contribute, p. xvii.)

| | |
|---|---|
| *Louisville* | Tao Le |
| *Los Angeles* | Vikas Bhushan |
| *New Haven* | Neil Vasan |
| *New Haven* | Juliana Tolles |

# ACKNOWLEDGMENTS

This has been a collaborative project from the start. We gratefully acknowledge the thoughtful comments, corrections, and advice of the many hundreds of medical students, international medical graduates, and faculty who have supported the authors in the continuing development of *First Aid for the USMLE Step 1*.

For support and encouragement throughout the process, we are grateful to Thao Pham and Jonathan Kirsch, Esq. Thanks to Selina Franklin and Louise Petersen for organizing and supporting the project.

Thanks to our publisher, McGraw-Hill, for the valuable assistance of its staff. For enthusiasm, support, and commitment for this ongoing and ever-challenging project, thanks to our editor, Catherine Johnson. For editorial support, an enormous thanks to Andrea Fellows. A special thanks to Rainbow Graphics, especially David Hommel and Susan Cooper, for remarkable editorial and production work.

For submitting contributions and corrections, thanks to Bibhav Acharya, Elizabeth Ames, Jodie Bachman, Megan Baker, Craig Baribault, Andrea Benton, Ryan Blum, Jessica Dara Bod, Katherine Bohnert, Carolyn Botros, Cari Brown, Brent Bushman, Elizabeth Butler, Yu Kwan Chan, Janet Chiang, Betty Chung, Kristina C. Coale, Reid Collins, Natalie Cosgrove, Andrew Degnan, Ashley E. Delgaudio, Stacey Elcik, Maxwell Elia, Toks Famakinwa, Chesney Fowler, Regan Gage, Anish Ghodadra, Amy Heinzen, Anneka Hooft, Bridget L. Hopewell, Elizabeth Horn, Kimberly Houck, Ryan Jacobson, Jenifer Jarrell, Rula Kanj, Karen Kaplan, Vishwala Kasbekar, Staci D. King, Sophia Kogan, Rory Kretzmer, Shelby Kunishima, Ian Joseph Lalich, Ashley Larrimore, Heather Laughridge, Joan Lee, Young Lee, Joshua Lennon, Anna Lim, William Lin, Sara Mansfield, Sarah Martin, Kathleen McKeegan, Nadia Merchant, Jill Moes, Ryan Montoya, Michelle Morales, Lance Needham, Kim Nguyen, Nina Ni, Amy Ondeyka, Katrina Pack, Shravani Pasupneti, Ankita Patel, Patricia Peter, Mary Linton Peters, Carolyn Pierce, Salman A. Raheem, Frederik Rebling, Jeff C. Riddell, Birju Ringwala, Robert Ross, Jeremy Rubinstein, Maribeth Ruiz, Deniz Sarhaddi, Clara Savage, Michael Schiraldi, Noah Schmuckler, Jennifer Scholwin, Nat Schuster, Neal Shah, Lovy Shukla, Kristi Stanley, Kathryn Storck, Christopher Struble, Laneshia Thomas, Frank Tsai, Kristin Walsh, Rachel Wang, Ruth Wangondu, Michael Westrol, Carmen Wolfe, Dongqi Xing, Jina Youn, Mary Yu, and Theresa Zaleski.

Thanks to Kristopher Jones, Kristina Panizzi, and Peter Anderson of the Department of Pathology, University of Alabama at Birmingham, for use of images from the Pathology Education Instructional Resource Digital Library (http://peir.net), and to Vishal Pall, Vipal Soni, and Dhanashree Rajderkar for their contributions to the High-Yield Image section.

Finally, thanks to Ted Hon, one of the founding authors of this book, for his vision in developing this guide on the computer, and to Chirag Amin for his enormous contributions as an editor and author over many editions.

| | |
|---|---|
| *Louisville* | Tao Le |
| *Los Angeles* | Vikas Bhushan |
| *New Haven* | Neil Vasan |
| *New Haven* | Juliana Tolles |

# HOW TO CONTRIBUTE

This version of *First Aid for the USMLE Step 1* incorporates hundreds of contributions and changes suggested by faculty and student reviewers. We invite you to participate in this process. We also offer **paid internships** in medical education and publishing ranging from three months to one year. Please send us your suggestions for:

- Study and test-taking strategies for the new computerized USMLE Step 1
- New facts, mnemonics, diagrams, and illustrations
- High-yield topics that may reappear on future Step 1 exams
- Personal ratings and comments on review books that you have examined

For each entry incorporated into the next edition, you will receive a **$10 gift certificate** per entry from the author group, as well as personal acknowledgment in the next edition. Diagrams, tables, partial entries, updates, corrections, and study hints are also appreciated, and significant contributions will be compensated at the discretion of the authors. Also let us know about material in this edition that you feel is low yield and should be deleted.

The preferred way to submit entries, suggestions, or corrections is via our blog:

### www.firstaidteam.com

Otherwise, please send entries, neatly written or typed or on disk (Microsoft Word), to:

**First Aid Team**
**914 N. Dixie Avenue**
**Suite 100**
**Elizabethtown, KY 42701**

Contributions received by June 15, 2010, receive priority consideration for the 2011 edition of *First Aid for the USMLE Step 1*.

## NOTE TO CONTRIBUTORS

All contributions become property of the authors and are subject to editing and reviewing. Please verify all data and spellings carefully. In the event that similar or duplicate entries are received, only the first entry received will be used. Include a reference to a standard textbook to facilitate verification of the fact. Please follow the style, punctuation, and format of this edition if possible.

The author team of Bhushan and Le is pleased to offer part-time and full-time paid internships in medical education and publishing to motivated medical students and physicians. Internships may range from three months (e.g., a summer) up to a full year. Participants will have an opportunity to author, edit, and earn academic credit on a wide variety of projects, including the popular *First Aid* series. English writing/editing experience, familiarity with Microsoft Word, and Internet access are required. Go to our blog at www.firstaidteam.com to apply for an internship. A sample of your work or a proposal of a specific project is helpful.

# HOW TO USE THIS BOOK

Medical students who have used previous editions of this guide have given us feedback on how best to make use of the book.

**It is recommended that you begin using this book as early as possible** when learning the basic medical sciences. You can use Section IV to select first-year course review books and Internet resources and then use those books for review while taking your medical school classes.

**Use different parts of the book at different stages in your preparation for the USMLE Step 1.** Before you begin to study for the USMLE Step 1, we suggest that you read Section I: Guide to Efficient Exam Preparation and Section IV: Top-Rated Review Resources. **If you are an international medical graduate student, an osteopathic medical student, a podiatry student, or a student with a disability,** refer to the appropriate Section I supplement for additional advice. Devise a study plan and decide what resources to buy. We strongly recommend that you invest in at least one or two top-rated review books in each subject. *First Aid* is not a comprehensive review book, and it is not a panacea that can compensate for not studying during the first two years of medical school. Scanning Sections II and III will give you an initial idea of the diverse range of topics covered on the USMLE Step 1.

As you study each discipline, **use the corresponding high-yield-fact section in *First Aid for the USMLE Step 1* as a means of consolidating the material and testing yourself** to see if you have covered some of the frequently tested items. Work with the book to integrate important facts into your fund of knowledge. Using *First Aid for the USMLE Step 1* as a review can serve as both a self-test of your knowledge and a repetition of important facts to learn. High-yield topics and vignettes are abstracted from recent exams to help guide your preparation.

**Return to Sections II and III frequently during your preparation and fill your short-term memory with remaining high-yield facts a few days before the USMLE Step 1.** The book can serve as a useful way of retaining key associations and keeping high-yield facts fresh in your memory just prior to the examination.

Reviewing the book immediately after the exam is probably the best way to **help us improve the book in the next edition.** Decide what was truly high and low yield and **send in your comments or your entire annotated book.**

# First Aid Checklist for the USMLE Step 1

This is an example of how you might use the information in Section I to prepare for the USMLE Step 1. Refer to corresponding topics in Section I for more details.

## Years Prior
☐ Select top-rated review books as study guides for first-year medical school courses.

## Months Prior
☐ Review computer test format and registration information.
☐ Register six months in advance. Carefully verify name and address printed on scheduling permit. Call Prometric for test date ASAP.
☐ Define goals for the USMLE Step 1 (e.g., comfortably pass, beat the mean, ace the test).
☐ Set up a realistic timeline for study. Cover less crammable subjects first. Review subject-by-subject emphasis and clinical vignette format.
☐ Simulate the USMLE Step 1 to pinpoint strengths and weaknesses in knowledge and test-taking skills.
☐ Evaluate and choose study methods and materials (e.g., review books, practice tests, software).
☐ Ask advice from those who have recently taken the USMLE Step 1.

## Weeks Prior
☐ Simulate the USMLE Step 1 again. Assess how close you are to your goal.
☐ Pinpoint remaining weaknesses. Stay healthy (exercise, sleep).
☐ Verify information on admission ticket (e.g., location, date).

## One Week Prior
☐ Remember comfort measures (loose clothing, earplugs, etc.).
☐ Work out test site logistics such as location, transportation, parking, and lunch.
☐ Call Prometric and confirm your exam appointment.

## One Day Prior
☐ Relax.
☐ Lightly review short-term material if necessary. Skim high-yield facts.
☐ Get a good night's sleep.
☐ Make sure the name printed on your photo ID appears EXACTLY the same as the name printed on your scheduling permit.

## Day of Exam
☐ Relax. Eat breakfast. Minimize bathroom breaks during the exam by avoiding excessive morning caffeine.
☐ Analyze and make adjustments in test-taking technique. You are allowed to review notes/study material during breaks on exam day.

## After the Exam
☐ Celebrate, regardless.
☐ Send feedback to us on our blog at **www.firstaidteam.com**.

# Guide to Efficient Exam Preparation

Relax.

This section is intended to make your exam preparation easier, not harder. Our goal is to reduce your level of anxiety and help you make the most of your efforts by helping you understand more about the United States Medical Licensing Examination, Step 1 (USMLE Step 1). As a medical student, you are no doubt familiar with taking standardized examinations and quickly absorbing large amounts of material. When you first confront the USMLE Step 1, however, you may find it all too easy to become sidetracked and not achieve your goal of studying with maximal effectiveness. Common mistakes that students make when studying for Step 1 include the following:

- Not understanding how scoring is performed or what your score means
- Starting *First Aid* too late
- Starting to study too late
- Using inefficient or inappropriate study methods
- Buying the wrong books or buying more books than you can ever use
- Buying only one publisher's review series for all subjects
- Not using practice examinations to maximum benefit
- Not using review books along with your classes
- Not analyzing and improving your test-taking strategies
- Getting bogged down by reviewing difficult topics excessively
- Studying material that is rarely tested on the USMLE Step 1
- Failing to master certain high-yield subjects owing to overconfidence
- Using *First Aid* as your sole study resource

In this section, we offer advice to help you avoid these pitfalls and be more productive in your studies.

### ▶ USMLE STEP 1—THE BASICS

The USMLE Step 1 is the first of three examinations that you must pass in order to become a licensed physician in the United States. The USMLE is a joint endeavor of the National Board of Medical Examiners (NBME) and the Federation of State Medical Boards (FSMB). The USMLE serves as the single examination system for U.S. medical students and international medical graduates (IMGs) seeking medical licensure in the United States.

*The CBT format of Step 1 is simply a computerized version of the former paper exam.*

### How Is the Computer-Based Test (CBT) Structured?

The CBT Step 1 exam consists of seven question "blocks" of 48 questions each (see Figure 1) for a total of 336 questions, timed at 60 minutes per block. A short 11-question survey follows the last question block. The computer begins the survey with a prompt to proceed to the next block of questions. Don't be fooled! "Block 8" is the NBME survey.

**FIGURE 1. Schematic of CBT Exam.**

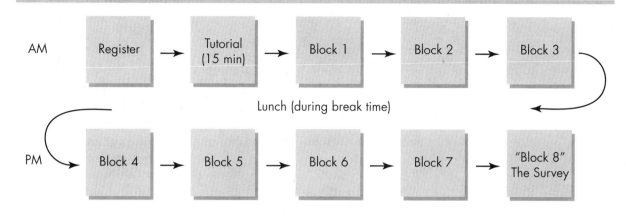

AM: Register → Tutorial (15 min) → Block 1 → Block 2 → Block 3

Lunch (during break time)

PM: Block 4 → Block 5 → Block 6 → Block 7 → "Block 8" The Survey

Once an examinee finishes a particular question block on the CBT, he or she must click on a screen icon to continue to the next block. Examinees **cannot** go back and change their answers to questions from any previously completed block. However, changing answers is allowed **within** a block of questions as long as time permits—**unless** the questions are part of a sequential-item test set (see What Is the CBT Like?).

*Don't be fooled! After the last question block comes the NBME survey ("Block 8").*

## What Is the CBT Like?

Given the unique environment of the CBT, it's important that you become familiar ahead of time with what your test-day conditions will be like. In fact, familiarizing yourself with the testing interface before the exam can add 15 minutes to your break time! This is because the 15-minute tutorial offered on exam day may be skipped if you are already familiar with the exam procedures and the testing interface. The 15 minutes is then added to your allotted break time (should you choose to skip the tutorial). Examinees may familiarize themselves with the CBT format by taking the 150 practice questions available online or by signing up for a practice session at a test center (for details, see What Does the CBT Format Mean to Me?).

*Skip the tutorial and add 15 minutes to your break time!*

For security reasons, examinees are not allowed to bring any personal electronic equipment into the testing area. This includes both digital and analog watches, cellular telephones, and electronic paging devices. Food and beverages are also prohibited. The testing centers are monitored by audio and video surveillance equipment. However, most testing centers allot each examinee a small locker outside the testing area in which he or she can store snacks, beverages, and personal items.

In May 2009, the USMLE began transitioning from the FRED v1 computer-based format to FRED v2. FRED v2 is similar to FRED v1 but has several additional features. These include highlight and strikeout functions for text, searchable lab values, and a calculator function. The USMLE advises examinees to familiarize themselves with both versions, information on which can be downloaded from www.usmle.org.

*Test illustrations include:*

- *Gross photos*
- *Histology slides*
- *Radiographs*
- *EMs*
- *Line drawings*

*Familiarize yourself with the commonly tested normal laboratory values.*

*Ctrl-Alt-Delete are the keys of death during the exam. Don't touch them!*

The typical question screen in FRED consists of a question followed by a number of choices on which an examinee can click, together with several navigational buttons on the top of the screen. There is a countdown timer on the upper left-hand corner of the screen as well. There is also a button that allows the examinee to mark a question for review. If a given question happens to be longer than the screen (which occurs very rarely), a scroll bar will appear on the right, allowing the examinee to see the rest of the question. Regardless of whether the examinee clicks on the answer or leaves it blank, he or she must click the "Next" button to advance to the next question.

In May 2008, the USMLE began to add a small number of media clips to the exam in the form of audio and/or video. No more than five media questions will be found on any given examination, and the USMLE orientation materials now include several practice questions in these new formats.

In 2009, USMLE introduced a sequential-item test format for some questions. This format will be indicated in the numbering of questions at the left-hand side of the screen. Questions in a sequential set must be completed in order. After an examinee answers the first question, he or she will be given the option to proceed to the next item but will be warned that his or her answer to the first question will be locked. **After proceeding, examinees will not be able to change the answer selected for that question.** The question stem and the answer chosen will be available to the examinee as he or she answers the next question in the sequence. No more than five sets of sequential questions will be found in any given examination.

Some Step 1 questions may also contain figures or color illustrations. These are typically situated to the right of the question. Although the contrast and brightness of the screen can be adjusted, there are no other ways to manipulate the picture (e.g., there is no zooming or panning). During the exam tutorial, however, examinees are given an opportunity to ensure that both the audio headphones and the volume are functioning properly.

The examinee can call up a window displaying normal lab values. In order to do so, he or she must click the "Lab" icon on the top part of the screen. Afterward, the examinee will have the option to choose between "Blood," "Cerebrospinal," "Hematologic," or "Sweat and Urine." The normal-values screen may obscure the question if it is expanded. The examinee may have to scroll down to search for the needed laboratory values.

FRED allows the examinee to see a running list of questions on the left part of the screen at all times. The new software also permits examinees to highlight or cross out information by using their mouse. Finally, there is an "Annotate" icon on the top part of the screen that allows students to write notes to themselves for review at a later time. Examinees need to be careful with all of these new features, because failure to do so can cost valuable time!

## What Does the CBT Format Mean to Me?

The significance of the CBT to you depends on the requirements of your school and your level of computer knowledge. If you hate computers and freak out at the mere sight of one, you might want to confront your fears as soon as possible. Spend some time playing with a Windows-based system and pointing and clicking icons or buttons with a mouse. These are the absolute basics, and you won't want to waste valuable exam time figuring them out on test day. Your test taking will proceed by pointing and clicking, essentially without the use of the keyboard.

For those who feel they might benefit, the USMLE offers an opportunity to take a simulated test, or "CBT Practice Session at a Prometric center." Students are eligible to register for this three-and-one-half-hour practice session after they have received their scheduling permit.

The same USMLE Step 1 sample test items (150 questions) available on the USMLE Web site, www.usmle.org, are used at these sessions. **No new items will be presented.** The session is divided into three one-hour blocks of 50 test items each and costs about $42. Students receive a printed percent-correct score after completing the session. No explanations of questions are provided.

You may register for a practice session online at www.usmle.org. A separate scheduling permit is issued for the practice session. Students should allow two weeks for receipt of this permit.

## How Do I Register to Take the Exam?

Prometric test centers offer Step 1 on a year-round basis, except for the first two weeks in January and major holidays. The exam is given every day except Sunday at most centers. Some schools administer the exam on their own campuses.

You can apply for Step 1 at the NBME Web site. This application allows applicants to select one of 12 overlapping three-month blocks in which to be tested (e.g., April–May–June, June–July–August). The application also includes a photo ID form that must be certified by an official at your medical school to verify your enrollment. After the NBME processes your application, it will send you a scheduling permit.

The scheduling permit you receive from the NBME will contain your USMLE identification number, the eligibility period in which you may take the exam, and two additional numbers. The first of these is known as your "scheduling number." You must have this number in order to make your exam appointment with Prometric. The second number is known as the "candidate identification number," or CIN. Examinees must enter their CINs at the Prometric workstation in order to access their exams. Prometric has no access to the codes. **Do not lose your permit!** You will not be allowed to take the boards unless you present this permit along with an unexpired, government-issued photo identification that includes your signature (such as a

*Keyboard shortcuts:*
*A–E–Letter choices.*
*Enter or spacebar–Move to*
*next question.*
*Esc–Exit pop-up Lab and*
*Exhibit windows.*
*Alt-T–Countdown timers for*
*current session and overall*
*test.*

*Test scheduling is done on a*
*"first-come, first-served" basis.*
*It's important to call and*
*schedule an exam date as*
*soon as you receive your*
*scheduling permit.*

*Testing centers are closed on*
*major holidays and during the*
*first two weeks of January.*

driver's license or passport). Make sure the name on your photo ID exactly matches the name that appears on your scheduling permit.

Once you receive your scheduling permit, you may call Prometric's toll-free number to arrange a time to take the exam. Although requests for taking the exam may be completed more than six months before the test date, examinees will not receive their scheduling permits earlier than six months before the eligibility period. The eligibility period is the three-month period you have chosen to take the exam. Most medical students choose the April–June or June–August period. Because exams are scheduled on a "first-come, first-served" basis, it is recommended that you telephone Prometric as soon as you receive your permit. After you've scheduled your exam, it's a good idea to confirm your exam appointment with Prometric at least one week before your test date. Prometric does not provide written confirmation of exam date, time, or location. Be sure to read the *2010 USMLE Bulletin of Information* for further details.

### What If I Need to Reschedule the Exam?

You can change your test date and/or center by contacting Prometric at 1-800-MED-EXAM (1-800-633-3926) or www.prometric.com. Make sure to have your CIN when rescheduling. If you are rescheduling by phone, you must speak with a Prometric representative; leaving a voice-mail message will not suffice. To avoid a rescheduling fee, you will need to request a change before noon EST at least five business days before your appointment. Please note that your rescheduled test date must fall within your assigned three-month eligibility period.

### When Should I Register for the Exam?

Although there are no deadlines for registering for Step 1, you should plan to register at least six months ahead of your desired test date. This will guarantee that you will get either your test center of choice or one within a 50-mile radius of your first choice. For most U.S. medical students, the desired testing window is in June, since most medical school curricula for the second year end in May or June. Thus, U.S. medical students should plan to register before January in anticipation of a June test date. The timing of the exam is more flexible for IMGs, as it is related only to when they finish exam preparation.

*Register six months in advance for seating and scheduling preference.*

Choose your three-month eligibility period wisely. If you need to reschedule outside your initial three-month period, you must submit a new application along with another application fee.

### Where Can I Take the Exam?

Your testing location is arranged with Prometric when you call for your test date (after you receive your scheduling permit). For a list of Prometric locations nearest you, visit www.prometric.com.

## How Long Will I Have to Wait Before I Get My Scores?

The USMLE reports scores three to six weeks after the examinee's test date. Examinees will be notified via e-mail when their scores are available. By following the online instructions, examinees will be able to view, download, and print their score report. Additional information about score timetables and accessibility is available on the official USMLE Web site.

## What About Time?

Time is of special interest on the CBT exam. Here's a breakdown of the exam schedule:

| | |
|---|---|
| 15 minutes | Tutorial (skip if familiar) |
| 7 hours | 60-minute question blocks |
| 45 minutes | Break time (includes time for lunch) |

*Be careful to watch the clock on your break time.*

The computer will keep track of how much time has elapsed on the exam. However, the computer will show you only how much time you have remaining in a given block. Therefore, it is up to you to determine if you are pacing yourself properly (at a rate of approximately one question per 75 seconds).

The computer will **not** warn you if you are spending more than your allotted time for a break. You should therefore budget your time so that you can take a short break when you need one and have time to eat. You must be especially careful not to spend too much time in between blocks (you should keep track of how much time elapses from the time you finish a block of questions to the time you start the next block). After you finish one question block, you'll need to click the mouse to proceed to the next block of questions.

*Gain extra break time by skipping the tutorial or finishing a block early.*

Forty-five minutes is the minimum break time for the day. You can gain extra break time (but not time for the question blocks) by skipping the tutorial or by finishing a block ahead of the allotted time.

## If I Freak Out and Leave, What Happens to My Score?

Your scheduling permit shows a CIN that you will enter onto your computer screen to start your exam. Entering the CIN is the same as breaking the seal on a test book, and you are considered to have started the exam when you do so. However, no score will be reported if you do not complete the exam. In fact, if you leave at any time from the start of the test to the last block, no score will be reported. The fact that you started but did not complete the exam, however, will appear on your USMLE score transcript.

The exam ends when all question blocks have been completed or when their time has expired. As you leave the testing center, you will receive a printed test-completion notice to document your completion of the exam. To receive an official score, you must finish the entire exam.

*Nearly three-fourths of Step 1 questions begin with a description of a patient.*

*The mean Step 1 score for U.S. medical students rose from 200 in 1991 to 222 in 2009.*

## What Types of Questions Are Asked?

**One-best-answer items** are the only multiple-choice format on the exam. Most questions consist of a clinical scenario or a direct question followed by a list of five or more options. You are required to select the one best answer among the options given. There are no "except," "not," or matching questions on the exam. A number of options may be partially correct, in which case you must select the option that best answers the question or completes the statement. Additionally, keep in mind that experimental questions may appear on the exam (see Difficult Questions, p. 20).

## How Is the Test Scored?

Each Step 1 examinee receives an electronic score report that includes the examinee's pass/fail status, two test scores, and a graphic depiction of the examinee's performance by discipline and organ system or subject area. The actual organ system profiles reported may depend on the statistical characteristics of a given administration of the examination.

The NBME provides two overall test scores based on the total number of items answered correctly on the examination (see Figure 2). The first score, the three-digit score, is reported as a scaled score in which the mean is 222 and the standard deviation is approximately 22. The second score scale, the two-digit score, defines 75 as the minimum passing score (equivalent to a score of 185 on the first scale). A score of 82 is equivalent to a score of 200 on the first score scale. To minimize confusion, we refer to scores using the three-digit scale.

**FIGURE 2.  2009 Scoring Scales for the USMLE Step 1.**

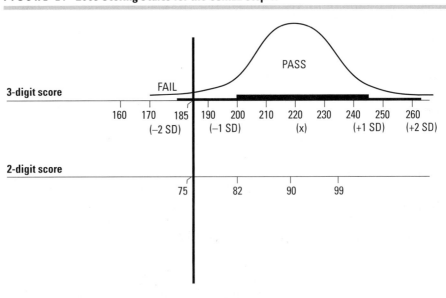

A score of **185** or higher is required to pass Step 1 as of 2009. Passing Step 1 is estimated to correspond to answering 60–70% of questions correctly. The NBME may adjust the minimum passing score for 2010, so please check the USMLE Web site or Firstaidteam.com for updates (see Table 1).

According to the USMLE, medical schools receive a listing of total scores and pass/fail results plus group summaries by discipline and organ system. Students can withhold their scores from their medical school if they wish. Official USMLE transcripts, which can be sent on request to residency programs, include only total scores, not performance profiles.

*Passing the CBT Step 1 is estimated to correspond to answering 60–70% of the questions correctly.*

Consult the USMLE Web site or your medical school for the most current and accurate information regarding the examination.

### What Does My Score Mean?

For students, the most important point with the Step 1 score is passing versus failing. Passing essentially means, "Hey, you're on your way to becoming a fully licensed doc."

Beyond that, the main point of having a quantitative score is to give you a sense of how you've done aside from the fact that you've passed the exam.

**TABLE 1. Passing Rates for the 2007–2008 USMLE Step 1.**

|  | 2007 | | 2008 | |
|---|---|---|---|---|
|  | No. Tested | % Passing | No. Tested | % Passing |
| Allopathic 1st takers | 17,028 | 95% | 17,494 | 94% |
| Repeaters | 1,190 | 65% | 1,361 | 61% |
| Allopathic total | 18,218 | 93% | 18,855 | 92% |
| Osteopathic 1st takers | 1,411 | 82% | 1,605 | 81% |
| Repeaters | 59 | 49% | 56 | 46% |
| Osteopathic total | 1,470 | 81% | 1,661 | 80% |
| **Total U.S./Canadian** | **19,688** | **92%** | **20,516** | **91%** |
| IMG 1st takers | 15,762 | 70% | 14,889 | 73% |
| Repeaters | 6,126 | 37% | 5,534 | 37% |
| IMG total | 21,888 | 61% | 20,423 | 63% |
| **Total Step 1 examinees** | **41,576** | **76%** | **40,939** | **77%** |

The two-digit or three-digit score gauges how well you have performed with respect to the content of the exam.

Since the content of the exam is what drives the score, the profile of the exam is what remains relatively constant over the years. That is to say that each exam profile includes a certain number of "very hard" questions along with "medium" and "easy" ones. The questions vary, but the profile of the exam doesn't change substantially. This ensures that someone who scored 200 on the boards yesterday has achieved a level of knowledge comparable to that of a person who scored 200 four years ago.

## Official NBME/USMLE Resources

We strongly encourage students to use the free materials provided by the testing agencies (see p. 22) and to study in detail the following NBME resources, all of which are available at the USMLE Web site, www.usmle.org:

*Practice questions may be easier than the actual exam.*

- *USMLE Step 1 2010 Computer-based Content and Sample Test Questions* (information given free to all examinees)
- *2010 USMLE Bulletin of Information* (information given free to all examinees)
- Comprehensive Basic Science Self-Assessment

The *USMLE Step 1 2010 Computer-based Content and Sample Test Questions* contains approximately 150 questions that are similar in format and content to the questions on the actual USMLE Step 1 exam. This practice test offers one of the best means of assessing your test-taking skills. However, it does not contain enough questions to simulate the full length of the examination, and its content represents a limited sampling of the basic science material that may be covered on Step 1. Moreover, most students felt that the questions on the actual 2009 exam were more challenging than those contained in that year's sample questions. Others, however, reported that they had encountered a few near-duplicates of these sample questions on the actual Step 1 exam. Presumably, these are "experimental" questions, but who knows? So the bottom line is, know these questions!

The extremely detailed *Step 1 Content Outline* provided by the USMLE has not proved useful for students studying for the exam. The USMLE even states that ". . . the content outline is not intended as a guide for curriculum development or as a study guide." [1] We concur with this assessment.

The *2010 USMLE Bulletin of Information* contains detailed procedural and policy information regarding the CBT, including descriptions of all three Steps, scoring of the exams, reporting of scores to medical schools and residency programs, procedures for score rechecks and other inquiries, policies for irregular behavior, and test dates.

The NBME also offers the Comprehensive Basic Science Self-Assessment (CBSSA), which tests users on topics covered during basic science courses in a format similar to that of the USMLE Step 1 examination. Students who prepared for the examination using this Web-based tool reported that they found the format and content highly indicative of questions tested on the Step 1 examination. In addition, the CBSSA is a fair predictor of USMLE performance (see Table 2).

The CBSSA exists in two forms: a standard-paced and a self-paced format, both of which consist of four sections of 50 questions each (for a total of 200 multiple-choice items). The standard-paced format allows the user up to one hour to complete each section, reflecting the time limits of the actual exam. By contrast, the self-paced format places a four-hour time limit on answering the multiple-choice questions. Keep in mind that this bank of questions is available only on the Web. The NBME requires that users log on, register, and start the test within 30 days of registration. Once the assessment has begun, users are required to complete the sections within 20 days. Following completion of the questions, the CBSSA will provide a performance profile indicating each user's relative strengths and weaknesses, much like the report profile for the USMLE Step 1 exam. However, keep in mind that this self-assessment does **not** provide the user with a list of correct answers. Table 2 provides an approximate correlation of scores between the CBSSA and the USMLE. Feedback from the self-assessment takes the form of a performance profile and nothing more. The NBME charges $45 for this service, which is payable by credit card or money order. For more information regarding the CBSSA, please visit the NBME's Web site at www.nbme.org and click on the link labeled "NBME Self-Assessment Services."

### ▶ DEFINING YOUR GOAL

It is useful to define your own personal performance goal when approaching the USMLE Step 1. Your style and intensity of preparation can then be matched to your goal. Your goal may depend on your school's requirements, your specialty choice, your grades to date, and your personal assessment of the test's importance. Do your best to define your goals early so that you can prepare accordingly.

Certain highly competitive residency programs, such as those in plastic surgery and orthopedic surgery, have acknowledged their use of Step 1 scores in the selection process. In such residency programs, greater emphasis may be placed on attaining a high score, so students who seek to enter these programs may wish to consider aiming for a very high score on the Step 1 exam (see Figure 3). At the same time, your Step 1 score is only one of a number of factors that are assessed when you apply for residency. Indeed, many residency programs value other criteria more highly than a high score on Step 1. Fourth-year medical students who have recently completed the residency application process can be a valuable resource in this regard.

**TABLE 2. CBSSA to USMLE Score Comparison.**

| CBSSA SCORE | APPROXIMATE USMLE STEP 1 SCORE |
|---|---|
| 200 | < 136 |
| 250 | 148 |
| 300 | 163 |
| 350 | 178 |
| 400 | 192 |
| 450 | 206 |
| 500 | 219 |
| 550 | 230 |
| 600 | 240 |
| 650 | 248 |
| 700 | 256 |
| 750 | 261 |
| 800 | > 265 |

*Fourth-year medical students have the best feel for how Step 1 scores factor into the residency application process.*

*Some competitive residency programs place more weight on Step 1 scores in their selection process.*

**FIGURE 3.** Median USMLE Step 1 Score for Matched U.S. Seniors.[a]

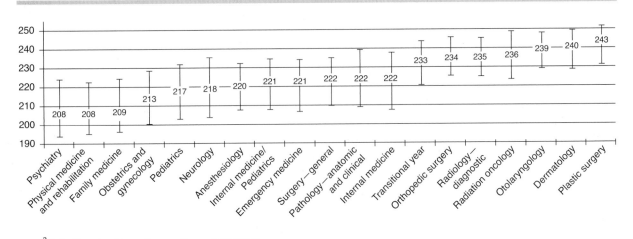

[a] Vertical lines show interquartile range. Source: www.nrmp.org.

### Make a Schedule

After you have defined your goals, map out a study schedule that is consistent with your objectives, your vacation time, and the difficulty of your ongoing coursework (see Figure 4). Determine whether you want to spread out your study time or concentrate it into 14-hour study days in the final weeks. Then factor in your own history in preparing for standardized examinations (e.g., SAT, MCAT).

*Time management is key. Customize your schedule to your goals and available time.*

Typically, students allot between five and seven weeks to prepare for Step 1. Some students reserve about a week at the end of their study period for final review; others save just a few days. When you have scheduled your exam date, do your best to adhere to it. Recent studies show that a later testing date does not translate into a higher score, so avoid pushing back your test date.[2]

Another important consideration is when you will study each subject. Some subjects lend themselves to cramming, whereas others demand a substantial long-term commitment. The "crammable" subjects for Step 1 are those for which concise yet relatively complete review books are available. (See Section IV for highly rated review and sample examination materials.) Behavioral science and physiology are two subjects with concise review books. Three subjects with longer but quite comprehensive review books are microbiology, pharmacology, and biochemistry. Thus, these subjects could be covered toward the end of your schedule, whereas other subjects (anatomy and pathology) require a longer time commitment and could be studied earlier. Many students prefer using a "systems-based" approach (e.g., GI, renal, cardiovascular) to integrate the material across basic science subjects. See Section III to study anatomy, pathology, physiology, and pharmacology facts by organ system.

**FIGURE 4.** Typical Timeline for the USMLE Step 1.

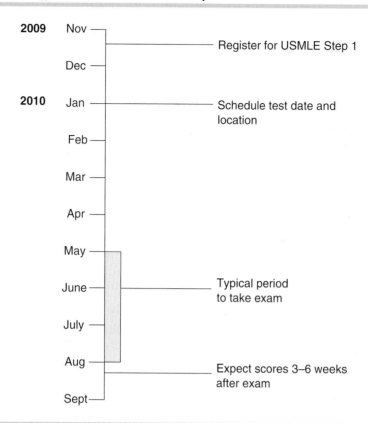

Make your schedule realistic, and set achievable goals. Many students make the mistake of studying at a level of detail that requires too much time for a comprehensive review—reading *Gray's Anatomy* in a couple of days is not a realistic goal! Revise your schedule regularly on the basis of your actual progress. Be careful not to lose focus. Beware of feelings of inadequacy when comparing study schedules and progress with your peers. **Avoid students who stress you out.** Focus on a few top-rated resources that suit your learning style—not on some obscure books your friends may pass down to you. Accept the fact that you cannot learn it all.

*"Crammable" subjects should be covered later and less crammable subjects earlier.*

You will need time for uninterrupted and focused study. Plan your personal affairs to minimize crisis situations near the date of the test. Allot an adequate number of breaks in your study schedule to avoid burnout. Maintain a healthy lifestyle with proper diet, exercise, and sleep.

*Avoid burnout. Maintain proper diet, exercise, and sleep habits.*

## Year(s) Prior

The NBME asserts that the best preparation for the USMLE Step 1 resides in "broadly based learning that establishes a strong general foundation of understanding of concepts and principles in basic sciences."[3] We agree. Although you may be tempted to rely solely on cramming in the weeks and months before the test, you should not have to do so. The knowledge you gained during your first two years of medical school and even during your undergraduate years should provide the groundwork on which to base your test preparation. Student scores on NBME subject tests (commonly known as "shelf exams") have been shown to be highly correlated with subsequent Step 1 scores.[4] Moreover, undergraduate science GPAs as well as MCAT scores are strong predictors of performance on the Step 1 exam.[5]

*Buy review books early (first year) and use while studying for courses.*

We also recommend that you buy highly rated review books early in your first year of medical school and use them as you study throughout the two years. When Step 1 comes along, these books will be familiar and personalized to the way in which you learn. It is risky and intimidating to use unfamiliar review books in the final two or three weeks preceding the exam.

## Months Prior

Review test dates and the application procedure. In 2009, testing for the USMLE Step 1 continued on a year-round basis (see Table 3). If you have any disabilities or "special circumstances," contact the NBME as early as possible to discuss test accommodations (see p. 46, First Aid for the Student with a Disability).

*Simulate the USMLE Step 1 under "real" conditions before beginning your studies.*

Before you begin to study earnestly, simulate the USMLE Step 1 under "real" conditions to pinpoint strengths and weaknesses in your knowledge and test-taking skills. Be sure that you are well informed about the examination and that you have planned your strategy for studying. Consider what study methods you will use, the study materials you will need, and how you will obtain your materials. Plan ahead. Get advice from third- and fourth-year medical students who have recently taken the USMLE Step 1. There might be strengths and weaknesses in your school's curriculum that you should take into account in deciding where to focus your efforts. You might also choose to share books, notes, and study hints with classmates. That is how this book began.

## Three Weeks Prior

Two to four weeks before the examination is a good time to resimulate the USMLE Step 1. You may want to do this earlier depending on the progress of

**TABLE 3. 2009 USMLE Exams.**

| STEP | FOCUS | NO. OF QUESTIONS/ NO. OF BLOCKS | TEST SCHEDULE/ LENGTH OF CBT EXAM | PASSING SCORE |
|---|---|---|---|---|
| Step 1 | Basic mechanisms and principles | 336/7 | One day (eight hours) | 185 |
| Step 2 CK | Clinical diagnosis and disease pathogenesis | 368/8 | One day (nine hours) | 184 |
| Step 3 | Clinical management | 480/11 | Two days (16 hours) | 187 |

your review, but be sure not to do it later, when there will be little time to remedy defects in your knowledge or test-taking skills. Make use of remaining good-quality sample USMLE test questions, and try to simulate the computerized test conditions so that you can adequately assess your test performance. Recognize, too, that time pressure is increasing as more and more questions are framed as clinical vignettes. Most sample exam questions are shorter than the real thing. Focus on reviewing the high-yield facts, your own notes, clinical images, and very short review books.

*In the final two weeks, focus on review and endurance. Avoid unfamiliar material. Stay confident!*

## One Week Prior

Make sure you have your CIN (found on your scheduling permit) as well as other items necessary for the day of the examination, including a driver's license or another form of photo identification with your signature (make sure the name on your ID **exactly** matches that on your scheduling permit). Confirm the Prometric testing center location and test time. Work out how you will get to the testing center and what parking and traffic problems you might encounter. If possible, visit the testing site to get a better idea of the testing conditions you will face. Determine what you will do for lunch. Make sure you have everything you need to ensure that you will be comfortable and alert at the test site.

*Confirm your testing date at least one week in advance.*

## One Day Prior

Try your best to relax and rest the night before the test. Double-check your admissions and test-taking materials as well as the comfort measures discussed earlier so that you will not have to deal with such details on the morning of the exam. Do not study any new material. If you do feel compelled to study, quickly review short-term-memory material (e.g., Rapid Review) before going to sleep. However, do not quiz yourself, as you may risk becoming flustered and confused. Remember that regardless of how hard you have studied, you cannot know everything. There will be things on the exam that you have never even seen before, so do not panic. Do not underestimate your abilities.

Many students report difficulty sleeping the night prior to the exam. This is often exacerbated by going to bed much earlier than usual. Do whatever it takes to ensure a good night's sleep (e.g., massage, exercise, warm milk). Do not change your daily routine prior to the exam. Exam day is not the day for a caffeine-withdrawal headache.

*No notes, books, calculators, pagers, recording devices, or watches of any kind are allowed in the testing area.*

## Morning of the Exam

On the morning of the Step 1 exam, wake up at your regular time and eat a normal breakfast. Make sure you have your scheduling permit admission ticket, test-taking materials, and comfort measures as discussed earlier. Wear loose, comfortable clothing. Plan for a variable temperature in the testing center. Arrive at the test site 30 minutes before the time designated on the admission

*Arrive at the testing center 30 minutes before your scheduled exam time. If you arrive more than half an hour late, you will not be allowed to take the test.*

*Some students recommend reviewing certain "theme" topics that tend to recur throughout the exam.*

*If you pass Step 1, you are not allowed to retake the exam in an attempt to raise your score.*

ticket; however, do not come too early, as doing so may intensify your anxiety. When you arrive at the test site, the proctor should give you a USMLE information sheet that will explain critical factors such as the proper use of break time. Seating may be assigned, but ask to be reseated if necessary; you need to be seated in an area that will allow you to remain comfortable and to concentrate. Get to know your testing station, especially if you have never been in a Prometric testing center before. Listen to your proctors regarding any changes in instructions or testing procedures that may apply to your test site.

Starting in July 2009, the USMLE began using the Biometric Identity Management System (BIMS) at some test center locations. BIMS converts a fingerprint, taken on test day, to a digital image used for identification of examinees during the testing process.

Finally, remember that it is natural (and even beneficial) to be a little nervous. Focus on being mentally clear and alert. Avoid panic. Avoid panic. Avoid panic. When you are asked to begin the exam, take a deep breath, focus on the screen, and then begin. Keep an eye on the timer. Take advantage of breaks between blocks to stretch and relax for a moment.

## After the Test

After you have completed the exam, be sure to have fun and relax regardless of how you may feel. Taking the test is an achievement in itself. Remember, you are much more likely to have passed than not. Enjoy the free time you have before your clerkships. Expect to experience some "reentry" phenomena as you try to regain a real life. Once you have recovered sufficiently from the test (or from partying), we invite you to send us your feedback, corrections, and suggestions for entries, facts, mnemonics, strategies, resource ratings, and the like (see p. xvii, How to Contribute). Sharing your experience will benefit fellow medical students and IMGs.

### ▶ IF YOU THINK YOU FAILED

After the test, many examinees feel that they have failed, and most are at the very least unsure of their pass/fail status. There are several sensible steps you can take to plan for the future in the event that you do not achieve a passing score. First, save and organize all your study materials, including review books, practice tests, and notes. Familiarize yourself with the reapplication procedures for Step 1, including application deadlines and upcoming test dates. The CBT format allows an examinee who has failed the exam to retake it no earlier than the first day of the month after 60 days have elapsed since the last test date. Examinees will, however, be allowed to take the exam no more than three times within a 12-month period should they repeatedly fail.

The performance profiles on the back of the USMLE Step 1 score report provide valuable feedback concerning your relative strengths and weaknesses. Study these profiles closely. Set up a study timeline to strengthen gaps in your knowledge as well as to maintain and improve what you already know. Do not neglect high-yield subjects. It is normal to feel somewhat anxious about retaking the test—but if anxiety becomes a problem, seek appropriate counseling.

Fifty-two percent of the NBME-registered first-time takers who failed the June 1998 Step 1 repeated the exam in October 1998. The overall pass rate for that group in October was 60%. Eighty-five percent of those scoring near the old pass/fail mark of 176 (173–176) in June 1998 passed in October. However, 1999 pass rates varied widely depending on initial score (see Table 4, which reflects the most current data available at the time of publishing).

Although the NBME allows an unlimited number of attempts to pass Step 1, both the NBME and the FSMB recommend that licensing authorities allow a minimum of three and a maximum of six attempts for each Step examination.[6] Again, review your school's policy regarding retakes.

**TABLE 4. Pass Rates for USMLE Step 1 Repeaters, 1999.**

| INITIAL SCORE | % PASS |
| --- | --- |
| 176–178 | 83 |
| 173–175 | 74 |
| 170–172 | 71 |
| 165–169 | 64 |
| 160–164 | 54 |
| 150–159 | 31 |
| < 150 | 0 |
| **Overall** | **67** |

## ▶ IF YOU FAILED

Even if you came out of the exam room feeling that you failed, seeing that failing grade can be traumatic, and it is natural to feel upset. Different people react in different ways: For some it is a stimulus to buckle down and study harder; for others it may "take the wind out of their sails" for a few days; and for still others it may lead to a reassessment of individual goals and abilities. In some instances, however, failure may trigger weeks or months of sadness, feelings of hopelessness, social withdrawal, and inability to concentrate—in other words, true clinical depression. If you think you are depressed, please seek help.

*Near the failure threshold, each three-digit scale point is equivalent to about 1.5 questions answered correctly.[7]*

## ▶ STUDY MATERIALS

### Quality and Cost Considerations

Although an ever-increasing number of review books and software are now available on the market, the quality of such material is highly variable. Some common problems are as follows:

- Certain review books are too detailed to allow for review in a reasonable amount of time or cover subtopics that are not emphasized on the exam.
- Many sample question books were originally written years ago and have not been adequately updated to reflect recent trends.
- Many sample question books use poorly written questions or contain factual errors in their explanations.
- Explanations for sample questions vary in quality.

### Basic Science Review Books

In selecting review books, be sure to weigh different opinions against each other, read the reviews and ratings in Section IV of this guide, examine the books closely in the bookstore, and choose carefully. You are investing not only money but also your limited study time. Do not worry about finding the "perfect" book, as many subjects simply do not have one, and different students prefer different styles.

*If a given review book is not working for you, stop using it no matter how highly rated it may be or how much it costs.*

There are two types of review books: those that are stand-alone titles and those that are part of a series. Books in a series generally have the same style, and you must decide if that style works for you. However, a given style is not optimal for every subject. For example, charts and diagrams may be the best approach for physiology and biochemistry, whereas tables and outlines may be preferable for microbiology.

You should also find out which books are up to date. Some new editions represent major improvements, whereas others contain only cursory changes. Take into consideration how a book reflects the format of the USMLE Step 1.

### Practice Tests

Taking practice tests provides valuable information about potential strengths and weaknesses in your fund of knowledge and test-taking skills. Some students use practice examinations simply as a means of breaking up the monotony of studying and adding variety to their study schedule, whereas other students rely almost solely on practice tests. Your best preview of the computerized exam can be found in the practice exams on the USMLE Web site. Some students also recommend using computerized test simulation programs. In addition, students report that many current practice-exam books have questions that are, on average, shorter and less clinically oriented than those on the current USMLE Step 1.

*Most practice exams are shorter and less clinical than the real thing.*

After taking a practice test, try to identify concepts and areas of weakness, not just the facts that you missed. Do not panic if you miss a lot of questions on a practice examination; instead, use the experience you have gained to motivate your study and prioritize those areas in which you need the most work. Use quality practice examinations to improve your test-taking skills. Analyze your ability to pace yourself.

*Use practice tests to identify concepts and areas of weakness, not just facts that you missed.*

### Clinical Review Books

Keep your eye out for more clinically oriented review books; purchase them early and begin to use them. A number of students are turning to Step 2 books, pathophysiology books, and case-based reviews to prepare for the clinical vignettes. Examples of such books include:

- *First Aid for the Wards* (McGraw-Hill)
- *First Aid Clerkship* series (McGraw-Hill)

- *Blueprints* clinical series (Lippincott Williams & Wilkins)
- *PreTest Physical Diagnosis* (McGraw-Hill)
- *Washington Manual* (Lippincott Williams & Wilkins)
- Various USMLE Step 2 review books

## Texts, Syllabi, and Notes

Limit your use of texts and syllabi for Step 1 review. Many textbooks are too detailed for high-yield review and include material that is generally not tested on the USMLE Step 1 (e.g., drug dosages, complex chemical structures). Syllabi, although familiar, are inconsistent and frequently reflect the emphasis of individual faculty, which often does not correspond to that of the USMLE Step 1. Syllabi also tend to be less organized than top-rated books and generally contain fewer diagrams and study questions.

## ▶ TEST-TAKING STRATEGIES

Your test performance will be influenced by both your fund of knowledge and your test-taking skills. You can strengthen your performance by considering each of these factors. Test-taking skills and strategies should be developed and perfected well in advance of the test date so that you can concentrate on the test itself. We suggest that you try the following strategies to see if they might work for you.

*Practice and perfect test-taking skills and strategies well before the test date.*

## Pacing

You have seven hours to complete 336 questions. Note that each one-hour block contains 48 questions. This works out to about 75 seconds per question. NBME officials note that time was not an issue for most takers of the CBT field test. However, pacing errors have in the past been detrimental to the performance of even highly prepared examinees. The bottom line is to keep one eye on the clock at all times!

*Time management is an important skill for exam success.*

## Dealing with Each Question

There are several established techniques for efficiently approaching multiple-choice questions; see what works for you. One technique begins with identifying each question as easy, workable, or impossible. Your goal should be to answer all easy questions, resolve all workable questions in a reasonable amount of time, and make quick and intelligent guesses on all impossible questions. Most students read the stem, think of the answer, and turn immediately to the choices. A second technique is to first skim the answer choices and the last sentence of the question and then read through the passage quickly, extracting only relevant information to answer the question. Try a variety of techniques on practice exams and see what works best for you.

## Difficult Questions

*Do not dwell excessively on questions that you are on the verge of "figuring out." Make your best guess and move on.*

Because of the exam's clinical emphasis, you may find that many of the questions on the Step 1 exam appear workable but take more time than is available to you. It can be tempting to dwell on such questions because you feel you are on the verge of "figuring it out," but resist this temptation and budget your time. Answer difficult questions with your best guess, mark them for review, and come back to them only if you have time after you have completed the rest of the questions in the block. This will keep you from inadvertently leaving any questions blank in your efforts to "beat the clock."

Another reason for not dwelling too long on any one question is that certain questions may be **experimental** or may be **incorrectly phrased**. Moreover, not all questions are scored. Some questions serve as "embedded pretest items" that do not count toward your overall score. In fact, anywhere from 10% to 20% of exam questions have been designated as experimental on past exams.

*Remember that some questions may be experimental.*

## Guessing

There is **no penalty** for wrong answers. Thus, no test block should be left with unanswered questions. A hunch is probably better than a random guess. If you have to guess, we suggest selecting an answer you recognize over one with which you are totally unfamiliar.

## Changing Your Answer

*Your first hunch is not always correct.*

The conventional wisdom is not to change answers that you have already marked unless there is a convincing and logical reason to do so—in other words, go with your "first hunch." However, studies show that if you change your answer, you are twice as likely to change it from an incorrect answer to a correct one than vice versa. So if you have a strong "second hunch," go for it!

## Fourth-Quarter Effect (Avoiding Burnout)

*Do not terminate a question block too early. Carefully review your answers if possible.*

Pacing and endurance are important. Practice helps develop both. Fewer and fewer examinees are leaving the examination session early. Use any extra time you might have at the end of each block to return to marked questions or to recheck your answers; you cannot add the extra time to any remaining blocks of questions or to your break time. Do not be too casual in your review or you may overlook serious mistakes. Remember your goals, and keep in mind the effort you have devoted to studying compared with the small additional effort you will need to maintain focus and concentration throughout the examination. Never give up. If you begin to feel frustrated, try taking a 30-second breather.

In recent years, the USMLE Step 1 has become increasingly clinically oriented. Students polled from 2003 exams reported that nearly 80% of the questions were presented as clinical vignettes. This change mirrors the trend in medical education toward introducing students to clinical problem solving during the basic science years. The increasing clinical emphasis on Step 1 may be challenging to those students who attend schools with a more traditional curriculum.

*Be prepared to read fast and think on your feet!*

## What Is a Clinical Vignette?

A clinical vignette is a short (usually paragraph-long) description of a patient, including demographics, presenting symptoms, signs, and other information concerning the patient. Sometimes this paragraph is followed by a brief listing of important physical findings and/or laboratory results. The task of assimilating all this information and answering the associated question in the span of one minute can be intimidating. So be prepared to read quickly and think on your feet. Remember that the question is often indirectly asking something you already know.

*Practice questions that include case histories or descriptive vignettes are critical for Step 1 preparation.*

## Strategy

Remember that Step 1 vignettes usually describe diseases or disorders in their most classic presentation. So look for buzzwords or cardinal signs (e.g., malar rash for SLE or nuchal rigidity for meningitis) in the narrative history. Be aware, however, that the question may contain classic signs and symptoms instead of mere buzzwords. Sometimes the data from labs and the physical exam will help you confirm or reject possible diagnoses, thereby helping you rule answer choices in or out. In some cases, they will be a dead giveaway for the diagnosis.

*Step 1 vignettes usually describe diseases or disorders in their most classic presentation.*

Making a diagnosis from the history and data is often not the final answer. Not infrequently, the diagnosis is divulged at the end of the vignette, after you have just struggled through the narrative to come up with a diagnosis of your own. The question might then ask about a related aspect of the diagnosed disease.

*Sometimes making a diagnosis is not necessary at all.*

One strategy that many students suggest is to skim the questions and answer choices before reading a vignette, especially if the vignette is lengthy. This focuses your attention on the relevant information and reduces the time spent on that vignette. Sometimes you may not need much of the information in the vignette to answer the question.

- **National Board of Medical Examiners (NBME)**
  Department of Licensing Examination Services
  3750 Market Street
  Philadelphia, PA 19104-3102
  (215) 590-9700
  Fax: (215) 590-9457
  E-mail: webmail@nbme.org
  www.nbme.org

- **Educational Commission for Foreign Medical Graduates (ECFMG)**
  3624 Market Street
  Philadelphia, PA 19104-2685
  (215) 386-5900
  Fax: (215) 386-9196
  E-mail: info@ecfmg.org
  www.ecfmg.org

- **Federation of State Medical Boards (FSMB)**
  P.O. Box 619850
  Dallas, TX 75261-9850
  (817) 868-4000
  Fax: (817) 868-4099
  E-mail: usmle@fsmb.org
  www.fsmb.org

- **USMLE Secretariat**
  3750 Market Street
  Philadelphia, PA 19104-3190
  (215) 590-9700
  E-mail: webmail@nbme.org
  www.usmle.org

► **REFERENCES**

1. Federation of State Medical Boards and National Board of Medical Examiners, *USMLE: 1993 Step 1 General Instructions, Content Outline, and Sample Items*, Philadelphia, 1992.

2. Pohl, Charles A., Robeson, Mary R., Hojat, Mohammadreza, and Veloski, J. Jon, "Sooner or Later? USMLE Step 1 Performance and Test Administration Date at the End of the Second Year," *Academic Medicine*, 2002, Vol. 77, No. 10, pp. S17–S19.

3. Case, Susan M., and Swanson, David B., "Validity of NBME Part I and Part II Scores for Selection of Residents in Orthopaedic Surgery, Dermatology, and Preventive Medicine," *Academic Medicine*, February Supplement 1993, Vol. 68, No. 2, pp. S51–S56.

4. Holtman, Matthew C., Swanson, David B., Ripkey, Douglas R., and Case, Susan M., "Using Basic Science Subject Tests to Identify Students at Risk for Failing Step 1," *Academic Medicine*, 2001, Vol. 76, No. 10, pp. S48–S51.

5. Basco, William T., Jr., Way, David P., Gilbert, Gregory E., and Hudson, Andy, "Undergraduate Institutional MCAT Scores as Predictors of USMLE Step 1 Performance," *Academic Medicine*, 2002, Vol. 77, No. 10, pp. S13–S16.

6. "Report on 1995 Examinations," *National Board Examiner*, Winter 1997, Vol. 44, No. 1, pp. 1–4.

7. O'Donnell, M. J., Obenshain, S. Scott, and Erdmann, James B., "I: Background Essential to the Proper Use of Results of Step 1 and Step 2 of the USMLE," *Academic Medicine*, October 1993, Vol. 68, No. 10, pp. 734–739.

# Special Situations

"International medical graduate" (IMG) is the term now used to describe any student or graduate of a non-U.S., non-Canadian, non–Puerto Rican medical school, regardless of whether he or she is a U.S. citizen. The old term "foreign medical graduate" (FMG) was replaced because it was misleading when applied to U.S. citizens attending medical schools outside the United States.

### The IMG's Steps to Licensure in the United States

If you are an IMG, you must go through the following steps (not necessarily in this order) to become licensed to practice in the United States. You must complete these steps even if you are already a practicing physician and have completed a residency program in your own country.

- Complete the basic sciences program of your medical school (equivalent to the first two years of U.S. medical school).
- Take the USMLE Step 1. You can do this while still in school or after graduating, but in either case your medical school must certify that you completed the basic sciences portion of your school's curriculum before taking the USMLE Step 1.
- Complete the clinical clerkship program of your medical school (equivalent to the third and fourth years of U.S. medical school).
- Take the USMLE Step 2 Clinical Knowledge (CK) exam. If you are still in medical school, you must have completed two years of school.
- Take the Step 2 Clinical Skills (CS) exam.
- Graduate with your medical degree.
- Then, send the ECFMG a copy of your degree and transcript, which will be verified with your medical school.
- Obtain an ECFMG certificate. To do this, candidates must accomplish the following:
  - Graduate from a medical school that is listed in the International Medical Education Directory (IMED). The list can be accessed at www.ecfmg.org.
  - Pass Step 1, the Step 2 CK, and the Step 2 CS within a seven-year period.
  - Have your medical credentials verified by the ECFMG.
- The standard certificate is usually sent two weeks after all the above requirements have been fulfilled. You must have a valid certificate before entering an accredited residency program, although you may begin the application process before you receive your certification.
- Apply for residency positions in your field of interest, either directly or through the Electronic Residency Application Service (ERAS) and the National Residency Matching Program, or NRMP ("the Match"). To be entered into the Match, you need to have passed all the examinations necessary for ECFMG certification (i.e., Step 1, the Step 2 CK, and the Step 2 CS) by the rank order list deadline (usually in late February before the Match). If you do not pass these exams by the deadline, you will be withdrawn from the Match.

*More detailed information can be found in the 2010 edition of the ECFMG Information Booklet, available at www.ecfmg.org/ pubshome.html.*

*Applicants may apply online for the USMLE Step 2 CK or Step 2 CS or request an extension of the USMLE eligibility period at www.ecfmg.org/usmle/ index.html or www.ecfmg.org/usmle/ step2cs/index.html.*

- Obtain a visa that will allow you to enter and work in the United States if you are not already a U.S. citizen or a green-card holder (permanent resident).

- If required for IMGs by the state in which your residency is located, obtain an educational/training/limited medical license. Your residency program may assist you with this application. Note that medical licensing is the prerogative of each individual state, not of the federal government, and that states vary with respect to their laws about licensing (although all 50 states recognize the USMLE).

- In order to begin your residency program, make sure your scores are valid.

- Once you have the ECFMG certification, take the USMLE Step 3 during your residency, and then obtain a full medical license. Once you have a license in any state, you are permitted to practice in federal institutions such as VA hospitals and Indian Health Service facilities in any state. This can open the door to "moonlighting" opportunities and possibilities for an H1B visa application. For details on individual state rules, write to the licensing board in the state in question or contact the FSMB.

- Complete your residency and then take the appropriate specialty board exams in order to become board certified (e.g., in internal medicine or surgery). If you already have a specialty certification in your home country (e.g., in surgery or cardiology), some specialty boards may grant you six months' or one year's credit toward your total residency time.

- Currently, many residency programs are accepting applications through ERAS. For more information, see *First Aid for the Match* or contact:

  **ECFMG/ERAS Program**
  P.O. Box 11746
  Philadelphia, PA 19101-0746
  (215) 386-5900
  e-mail: eras-support@ecfmg.org
  www.ecfmg.org/eras

### The USMLE and the IMG

The USMLE is a series of standardized exams that give IMGs a level playing field. It is the same exam series taken by U.S. graduates even though it is administered by the ECFMG rather than by the NBME. This means that passing marks for IMGs for Step 1, the Step 2 CK, and the Step 2 CS are determined by a statistical process that is based on the scores of U.S. medical students. For example, to pass Step 1, you will probably have to score higher than the bottom 8–10% of U.S. and Canadian graduates.

### Timing of the USMLE

For an IMG, the timing of a complete application is critical. It is extremely important that you send in your application early if you are to garner the maximum number of interview calls. A rough guide would be to complete all exam requirements by August of the year in which you wish to apply. This would translate into sending both your score sheets and your ECFMG certificate with your application.

In terms of USMLE exam order, arguments can be made for taking the Step 1 or the Step 2 CK exam first. For example, you may consider taking the Step 2 CK exam first if you have just graduated from medical school and the clinical topics are still fresh in your mind. However, keep in mind that there is substantial overlap between Step 1 and Step 2 CK topics in areas such as pharmacology, pathophysiology, and biostatistics. You might therefore consider taking the Step 1 and Step 2 CK exams close together to take advantage of this overlap in your test preparation.

### USMLE Step 1 and the IMG

**What Is the USMLE Step 1?** It is a computerized test of the basic medical sciences that consists of 336 multiple-choice questions divided into seven blocks.

**Content.** Step 1 includes test items in the following content areas:

- Anatomy
- Behavioral sciences
- Biochemistry
- Microbiology and immunology
- Pathology
- Pharmacology
- Physiology
- Interdisciplinary topics such as nutrition, genetics, and aging

**Significance of the Test.** Step 1 is required for the ECFMG certificate as well as for registration for the Step 2 CS. Since most U.S. graduates apply to residency with their Step 1 scores only, it may be the only objective tool available with which to compare IMGs with U.S. graduates.

**Official Web Sites.** www.usmle.org and www.ecfmg.org/usmle.

**Eligibility.** Both students and graduates from medical schools that are listed in IMED are eligible to take the test. Students must have completed at least two years of medical school by the beginning of the eligibility period selected.

**Eligibility Period.** A three-month period of your choice.

**Fee.** The fee for Step 1 is $710 plus an international test delivery surcharge (if you choose a testing region other than the United States or Canada).

**Retaking the Exam.** In the event that you failed the test, you can apply to retake the exam. You cannot take the same Step more than three times in any 12-month period. You cannot retake the exam if you passed. The minimum score to pass the exam is 75 on a two-digit scale. To pass, you must answer roughly 60–70% of the questions correctly.

**Statistics.** In 2007, only 70% of ECFMG candidates passed Step 1 on their first attempt, compared with 95% of U.S. and Canadian medical students and graduates. Of note, 1994–1995 data showed that USFMGs (U.S. citizens attending non-U.S. medical schools) performed 0.4 SD lower than IMGs (non-U.S. citizens attending non-U.S. medical schools). Although their overall scores were lower, USFMGs performed better than IMGs on behavioral sciences. In general, students from non-U.S. medical schools perform worst in behavioral science and biochemistry (1.9 and 1.5 SDs below U.S. students) and comparatively better in gross anatomy and pathology (0.7 and 0.9 SD below U.S. students). Although derived from data collected in 1994–1995, these data may help you focus your studying efforts.

**Tips.** Although few if any students feel totally prepared to take Step 1, IMGs in particular require serious study and preparation in order to reach their full potential on this exam. It is also imperative that IMGs do their best on Step 1, as a poor score on Step 1 is a distinct disadvantage in applying for most residencies. Remember that if you pass Step 1, you cannot retake it in an attempt to improve your score. Your goal should thus be to beat the mean, because you can then assert with confidence that you have done better than average for U.S. students. Good Step 1 scores will also lend credibility to your residency application and help you get into highly competitive specialties such as radiology, orthopedics, and dermatology.

**Commercial Review Courses.** Do commercial review courses help improve your scores? Reports vary, and such courses can be expensive. Many IMGs decide to try Step 1 on their own and then consider a review course only if they fail. Just keep in mind that many states require that you pass Step 1 within three attempts. (For more information on review courses, see Section IV.)

## USMLE Step 2 CK and the IMG

**What Is the Step 2 CK?** It is a computerized test of the clinical sciences consisting of 368 multiple-choice questions divided into eight blocks. It can be taken at Prometric centers in the United States and several other countries.

**Content.** The Step 2 CK includes test items in the following content areas:

- Internal medicine
- Obstetrics and gynecology
- Pediatrics
- Preventive medicine
- Psychiatry
- Surgery
- Other areas relevant to the provision of care under supervision

**Significance of the Test.** The Step 2 CK is required for the ECFMG certificate. It reflects the level of clinical knowledge of the applicant. It tests clinical subjects, primarily internal medicine. Other areas that are tested are surgery, obstetrics and gynecology, pediatrics, orthopedics, psychiatry, ENT, ophthalmology, and medical ethics.

**Official Web Sites.** www.usmle.org and www.ecfmg.org/usmle.

**Eligibility.** Students and graduates from medical schools that are listed in IMED are eligible to take the Step 2 CK. Students must have completed at least two years of medical school. This means that students must have completed the basic medical science component of the medical school curriculum by the beginning of the eligibility period selected.

**Eligibility Period.** A three-month period of your choice.

**Fee.** The fee for the Step 2 CK is $710 plus an international test delivery surcharge (if you choose a testing region other than the United States or Canada).

**Retaking the Exam.** In the event that you fail the Step 2 CK, you can apply to take the exam again. You cannot take the same Step more than three times in any 12-month period. You cannot retake the exam if you passed.

**Statistics.** In 2006–2007, 79% of ECFMG candidates passed the Step 2 CK on their first attempt, compared with 96% of U.S. and Canadian candidates.

**Tips.** It's better to take the Step 2 CK after your internal medicine rotation because most of the questions on the exam give clinical scenarios and ask you to make medical diagnoses and clinical decisions. In addition, because this is a clinical sciences exam, cultural and geographic considerations play a greater role than is the case with Step 1. For example, if your medical education gave you ample exposure to malaria, brucellosis, and malnutrition but little to alcohol withdrawal, child abuse, and cholesterol screening, you must work to familiarize yourself with topics that are more heavily emphasized in U.S. medicine. You must also have a basic understanding of the legal and social aspects of U.S. medicine, because you will be asked questions about communicating with and advising patients.

### USMLE Step 2 CS and the IMG

**What Is the Step 2 CS?** The Step 2 CS is a test of clinical and communication skills administered as a one-day, eight-hour exam. It includes 10 to 12 encounters with standardized patients (15 minutes each, with 10 minutes to write a note after each encounter). Test results are valid indefinitely.

**Content.** The Step 2 CS tests the ability to communicate in English as well as interpersonal skills, data-gathering skills, the ability to perform a physical exam, and the ability to formulate a brief note, a differential diagnosis, and a list of diagnostic tests. The areas that are covered in the exam are as follows:

- Internal medicine
- Surgery
- Obstetrics and gynecology
- Pediatrics
- Psychiatry
- Family medicine

Unlike the USMLE Step 1, Step 2 CK, or Step 3, there are no numerical grades for the Step 2 CS—it's simply either a "pass" or a "fail." To pass, a candidate must attain a passing performance in **each** of the following three components:

- Integrated Clinical Encounter (ICE): includes Data Gathering, Physical Exam, and the Patient Note
- Spoken English Proficiency (SEP)
- Communication and Interpersonal Skills (CIS)

According to the NBME, the most common component that IMGs fail on the Step 2 CS is the CIS component.

**Significance of the Test.** The Step 2 CS is required for the ECFMG certificate. It has eliminated the Test of English as a Foreign Language (TOEFL) as a requirement for ECFMG certification.

**Official Web Site.** www.ecfmg.org/usmle/step2cs.

**Eligibility.** Students must have completed at least two years of medical school in order to take the test. That means students must have completed the basic medical science component of the medical school curriculum at the time they apply for the exam.

**Fee.** The fee for the Step 2 CS is $1200.

**Scheduling.** You must schedule the Step 2 CS within **four months** of the date indicated on your notification of registration. You must take the exam within 12 months of the date indicated on your notification of registration. It is generally advisable to take the Step 2 CS as soon as possible in the year before your Match, as often the results either come in late or arrive too late to allow you to retake the test and pass it before the Match.

**Retaking the Exam.** There is no limit to the number of attempts you can make to pass the Step 2 CS. However, you cannot take the exam more than three times in a 12-month period.

**Test Site Locations.** The Step 2 CS is currently administered at the following five locations:

- Philadelphia, PA
- Atlanta, GA
- Los Angeles, CA
- Chicago, IL
- Houston, TX

For more information about the Step 2 CS exam, please refer to *First Aid for the Step 2 CS.*

### USMLE Step 3 and the IMG

**What Is the USMLE Step 3?** It is a two-day computerized test in clinical medicine consisting of 480 multiple-choice questions and nine computer-based case simulations (CCS). The exam aims at testing your knowledge and its application to patient care and clinical decision making (i.e., this exam tests if you can safely practice medicine independently and without supervision).

**Significance of the Test.** Taking Step 3 before residency is critical for IMGs seeking an H1B visa and is also a bonus that can be added to the residency application. Step 3 is also required to obtain a full medical license in the United States and can be taken during residency for this purpose.

**Official Web Site.** www.usmle.org.

**Fee.** The fee for Step 3 is $690 (the total application fee can vary among states).

**Eligibility.** Most states require that applicants have completed one, two, or three years of postgraduate training (residency) before they apply for Step 3 and permanent state licensure. The exceptions are the 13 states mentioned below, which allow IMGs to take Step 3 at the beginning of or even before residency. So if you don't fulfill the prerequisites to taking Step 3 in your state of choice, simply use the name of one of the 13 states in your Step 3 application. You can take the exam in any state you choose regardless of the state that you mentioned on your application. Once you pass Step 3, it will be recognized by all states. Basic eligibility requirements for the USMLE Step 3 are as follows:

- Obtaining an MD or DO degree (or its equivalent) by the application deadline.
- Obtaining an ECFMG certificate if you are a graduate of a foreign medical school or are successfully completing a "fifth pathway" program (at a date no later than the application deadline).
- Meeting the requirements imposed by the individual state licensing authority to which you are applying to take Step 3. Please refer to www.fsmb.org for more information.

The following states do not have postgraduate training as an eligibility requirement to apply for Step 3:

- Arkansas
- California
- Connecticut
- Florida
- Louisiana
- Maryland
- Nebraska*
- New York
- South Dakota
- Texas
- Utah*
- Washington
- West Virginia

* Requires that IMGs obtain a "valid indefinite" ECFMG certificate.

The Step 3 exam is not available outside the United States. Applications can be found online at www.fsmb.org and must be submitted to the FSMB.

## Residencies and the IMG

In the residency Match, the number of U.S.-citizen IMG applications has grown for the past few years, while the percentage accepted has been stable (see Table 5). More information about residency programs can be obtained at www.ama-assn.org.

## The Match and the IMG

Given the growing number of IMG candidates with strong applications, you should bear in mind that good USMLE scores are not the only way to gain a

**TABLE 5. IMGs in the Match.**

| APPLICANTS | 2006 | 2007 | 2008 |
|---|---|---|---|
| U.S.-citizen IMGs | 2,435 | 2,694 | 2,969 |
| % U.S.-citizen IMGs accepted | 51 | 50 | 52 |
| Non-U.S.-citizen IMGs | 6,442 | 6,992 | 7,335 |
| % non-U.S.-citizen IMGs accepted | 49 | 46 | 42 |
| U.S. graduates (non-IMGs) | 15,008 | 15,206 | 15,242 |
| % U.S. graduates accepted | 94 | 93 | 94 |

competitive edge. However, USMLE Step 1 and Step 2 CK scores continue to be used as the initial screening mechanism when candidates are being considered for interviews.

Based on accumulated IMG Match experiences over recent years, here are a few pointers to help IMGs maximize their chances for a residency interview:

- **Apply early.** Programs offer a limited number of interviews and often select candidates on a first-come, first-served basis. Because of this, you should aim to complete the entire process of applying for the ERAS token, registering with the Association of American Medical Colleges (AAMC), mailing necessary documents to ERAS, and completing the ERAS application before September (see Figure 5). Community programs usually send out interview offers earlier than do university and university-affiliated programs.

- **U.S. clinical experience helps.** Externships and observerships in a U.S. hospital setting have emerged as an important credential on an IMG application. Externships are like short-term medical school internships and offer hands-on clinical experience. Observerships, also called "shadowing," involve following a physician and observing how he or she manages patients. Externships are considered superior to observerships, but having

**FIGURE 5.** **IMG Timeline for Application.**

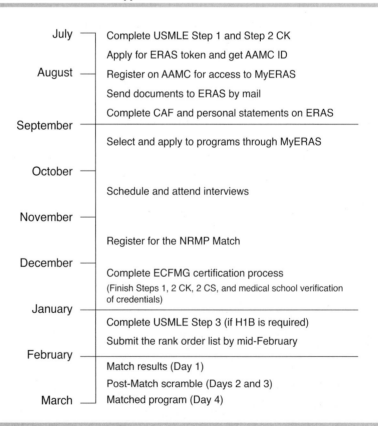

either of them is always better than having none. Some programs require students to have participated in an externship or observership before applying. It is best to gain such an experience before or at the time you apply to various programs so that you can mention it on your ERAS application. If such an experience or opportunity comes up after you apply, be sure to inform the programs accordingly.

- **Clinical research helps.** University programs are attracted to candidates who show a strong interest in clinical research and academics. They may even relax their application criteria for individuals with unique backgrounds and strong research experience. Publications in well-known journals are an added bonus.

- **Time the Step 2 CS well.** ECFMG has published the new Step 2 CS score-reporting schedule for the years 2009–2010 at http://ecfmg.org/announce.htm#reportsched. Most program directors would like to see a passing score on the Step 1, Step 2 CK, and Step 2 CS exams before they rank an IMG on their rank order list in mid-February. There have been too many instances in which candidates have relinquished a position on the rank order list—and have thus lost a potential match—either because of delayed CS results or because they have been unable to retake the exam on time following a failure. It is difficult to predict a result on the Step 2 CS, since the grading process is not very transparent. Therefore, it is advisable to take the Step 2 CS as early as possible in the application year.

- **U.S. letters of recommendation help.** Letters of recommendation from clinicians practicing in the United States carry more weight than recommendations from home countries.

- **Step up the Step 3.** If H1B visa sponsorship is desired, aim to have Step 3 results by January of the Match year. In addition to the visa advantage you will gain, an early and good Step 3 score may benefit IMGs who have been away from clinical medicine for a while as well as those who have low scores on Step 1 and the Step 2 CK.

- **Verify medical credentials in a timely manner.** Do not overlook the medical school credential verification process. The ECFMG certificate arrives only after credentials have been verified and after you have passed Step 1, the Step 2 CK, and the Step 2 CS, so you should keep track of the process and check with the ECFMG from time to time about your status.

- **Schedule interviews with pre-Matches in mind.** Schedule interviews with your favorite programs first. This will leave you better prepared to make a decision in the event that you are offered a pre-Match position.

### Resources for the IMG

- **ECFMG**
  3624 Market Street
  Philadelphia, PA 19104-2685
  (215) 386-5900
  Fax: (215) 386-9196
  www.ecfmg.org

The ECFMG telephone number is answered only between 9:00 A.M. and 12:30 P.M. and between 1:30 P.M. and 5:00 P.M. Monday through Friday EST. The ECFMG often takes a long time to answer the phone, which is frequently busy at peak times of the year, and then gives you a long voice-mail message—so it is better to write or fax early than to rely on a last-minute phone call. Do not contact the NBME, as all IMG exam matters are conducted by the ECFMG. The ECFMG also publishes an information booklet on ECFMG certification and the USMLE program, which gives details on the dates and locations of forthcoming USMLE and English tests for IMGs together with application forms. It is free of charge and is also available from the public affairs offices of U.S. embassies and consulates worldwide as well as from Overseas Educational Advisory Centers. You may order single copies of the handbook by calling (215) 386-5900, preferably on weekends or between 6 P.M. and 6 A.M. Philadelphia time, or by faxing to (215) 386-9196. Requests for multiple copies must be made by fax or mail on organizational letterhead. The full text of the booklet is also available on the ECFMG's Web site at www.ecfmg.org.

- **FSMB**
  P.O. Box 619850
  Dallas, TX 75261-9850
  (817) 868-4000
  Fax: (817) 868-4099
  www.fsmb.org

  The FSMB has a number of publications available, including the *FSMB Handbook*, for $15. In addition, a number of policy documents are available for free. To obtain these publications, print and mail the order form on the Web site listed above. Payment options include Visa or Master-Card. Alternatively, write to Federation Publications at the above address. All orders must be prepaid with a personal check drawn on a U.S. bank, a cashier's check, or a money order payable to the FSMB. Foreign orders must be accompanied by an international money order or the equivalent, payable in U.S. dollars through a U.S. bank or a U.S. affiliate of a foreign bank. For Step 3 inquiries, the telephone number is (817) 868-4041. You may e-mail the FSMB at usmle@fsmb.org or write to Examination Services at the address above.

- The AMA has dedicated a portion of its Web site to information on IMG demographics, residencies, immigration, and the like. This information can be found at www.ama-assn.org/ama/pub/about-ama/our-people/member-groups-sections/international-medical-graduates.shtml.

- *First Aid for the International Medical Graduate*, 2nd ed., by Keshav Chander (2002; 295 pages; ISBN 9780071385329), is an excellent resource written by a successful IMG. The book includes interviews with successful IMGs and students gearing up for the USMLE, complete "getting settled" information for new residents, and tips for dealing with possible social and cultural transition difficulties. The book provides useful advice on the U.S. curriculum, the health care delivery system, and ethical issues—and the differences IMGs should expect. Dr. Chander points out the weaknesses IMGs often face and suggests ways they can improve their performance on standardized tests as well as on academic and clinical evaluations. As a bonus, the guide contains information on how to get good fellowships after residency. The bottom line is that this is a reassuring guide that can help IMGs boost their confidence and proficiency. A great "first of its kind" that will empower IMGs with information that they need to succeed.

Other books that may be useful and of interest to IMGs are as follows:

- *International Medical Graduates in U.S. Hospitals: A Guide for Directors and Applicants,* by Faroque A. Khan and Lawrence G. Smith (1995; ISBN 9780943126418).
- *Insider's Guide for the International Medical Graduate to Obtain a Medical Residency in the U.S.A.,* by Ahmad Hakemi (1999; ISBN 9781929803002).

## What Is the COMLEX-USA Level 1?

In 1995, the National Board of Osteopathic Medical Examiners (NBOME) introduced a new assessment tool called the Comprehensive Osteopathic Medical Licensing Examination, or COMLEX-USA. As with the former NBOME examination series, the COMLEX-USA is administered over three levels. In 1995, only Level 3 was administered, but by 1998 all three levels had been implemented. The COMLEX-USA is now the only exam offered to osteopathic students. One goal of this changeover is to have all 50 states recognize this examination as equivalent to the USMLE. Currently, the COMLEX-USA exam sequence is accepted for licensure in all 50 states.

The COMLEX-USA series assesses osteopathic medical knowledge and clinical skills using clinical presentations and physician tasks. A description of the COMLEX-USA Written Examination Blueprints for each level, which outline the various clinical presentations and physician tasks that examinees will encounter, is given on the NBOME Web site. Another stated goal of the COMLEX-USA Level 1 is to create a more primary care–oriented exam that integrates osteopathic principles into clinical situations. As of July 1, 2004, the NBOME has initiated the administration of a Performance Evaluation/Clinical Skills component of the COMLEX-USA, designated Level 2-PE, that candidates must pass in order to be eligible for the COMLEX Level 3.

To be eligible to take the COMLEX-USA Level 1, you must have satisfactorily completed at least one-half of your sophomore year in an American Osteopathic Association (AOA)–approved medical school. In addition, you must obtain verification that you are in good standing at your medical school via approval of your dean. Applications may be downloaded from the NBOME Web site.

For all three levels of the COMLEX-USA, raw scores are converted to a percentile score and a score ranging from 5 to 800. For Levels 1 and 2, a score of 400 is required to pass; for Level 3, a score of 350 is needed. COMLEX-USA scores are usually mailed eight weeks after the test date. The mean score is always 500. From 2002 through October 2005, the standard deviation for Level 1 was 79.

If you pass a COMLEX-USA examination, you are not allowed to retake it to improve your grade. If you fail, there is no specific limit to the number of times you can retake it in order to pass. Level 2 and 3 exams must be passed in sequential order within seven years of passing Level 1.

## What Is the Structure of the COMLEX-USA Level 1?

The final paper-and-pencil COMLEX-USA Level 1 examination was administered on October 11–12, 2005. In 2006, the NBOME began delivering the COMLEX-USA Level 1 by computer. This conversion to a computer-based examination reduced the test duration from two days to one day, decreased the total number of questions from about 800 to 400, and decreased the total testing time from 16 hours to 8 hours.

The computer-based COMLEX-USA Level 1 examination consists of multiple-choice questions in the same format as that of the old paper-and-pencil COMLEX-USA Level 1 examination. Most of the questions are in one-best-answer format, but a small number are matching-type questions. Some one-best-answer questions are bundled together around a common question stem that usually takes the form of a clinical scenario. New question formats may gradually be introduced, but candidates will be notified if this occurs.

Questions are grouped into six sections of 50 questions each in a manner similar to the USMLE. Reviewing and changing answers may be done only in the current section. A "review page" is presented for each block in order to advise test takers of questions completed, questions marked for further review, and incomplete questions for which no answer has been given.

Students are allowed to take a 10-minute break at the end of two sections. Students who do not take this 10-minute break and continue to section 3 can apply the 10 minutes toward their test time. Similarly, after section 4, students are given a 40-minute lunch break and another 10-minute break after section 6. More information about the computer-based COMLEX-USA examinations can be obtained from www.nbome.org.

## What Is the Difference Between the USMLE and the COMLEX-USA?

According to the NBOME, the COMLEX-USA Level 1 exam focuses broadly on the following categories, with osteopathic principles and practices integrated into each section:

- Health promotion and disease prevention
- The history and physical
- Diagnostic technologies
- Management
- Scientific understanding of mechanisms
- Health care delivery

Although the COMLEX-USA and the USMLE are similar in scope, content, and emphasis, some differences are worth noting. For example, the COMLEX-USA Level 1 tests osteopathic principles in addition to basic science materials but does not emphasize lab techniques. In addition, although both exams often require that you apply and integrate knowledge over several areas of basic science to answer a given question, many students who took both tests in 2004 reported that the questions differed somewhat in style. Students reported, for example, that USMLE questions generally required that the test taker reason and draw from the information given (often a two-step process), whereas those on the COMLEX-USA exam tended to be more straightforward. Furthermore, USMLE questions were on average found to be considerably longer than those on the COMLEX-USA.

Students also commented that the COMLEX-USA utilized "buzzwords," although limited in their use (e.g., "rose spots" in typhoid fever), whereas the USMLE avoided buzzwords in favor of descriptions of clinical findings or symptoms (e.g., rose-colored papules on the abdomen rather than rose spots). Finally, the 2004 USMLE had many more photographs than did the COMLEX-USA. In general, the overall impression was that the USMLE was a more "thought-provoking" exam, while the COMLEX-USA was more of a "knowledge-based" exam.

### Who Should Take Both the USMLE and the COMLEX-USA?

Aside from facing the COMLEX-USA Level 1, you must decide if you will also take the USMLE Step 1. We recommend that you consider taking both the USMLE and the COMLEX-USA under the following circumstances:

- **If you are applying to allopathic residencies.** Although there is growing acceptance of COMLEX-USA certification on the part of allopathic residencies, some allopathic programs prefer or even require passage of the USMLE Step 1. These include many academic programs, programs in competitive specialties (e.g., orthopedics, ophthalmology, or dermatology), and programs in competitive geographic areas (such as California). Fourth-year doctor of osteopathy (DO) students who have already matched may be a good source of information about which programs and specialties look for USMLE scores. It is also a good idea to contact program directors at the institutions you are interested in to ask about their policy regarding the COMLEX-USA versus the USMLE.
- **If you are unsure about your postgraduate training plans.** Successful passage of both the COMLEX-USA Level 1 and the USMLE Step 1 is certain to provide you with the greatest possible range of options when you are applying for internship and residency training.

The clinical coursework that some DO students receive during the summer of their third year (as opposed to their starting clerkships) is considered helpful in integrating basic science knowledge for the COMLEX-USA or the USMLE.

In addition, the COMLEX-USA Level 1 exam has in recent years placed increasing emphasis on questions related to primary care medicine and prevention. Having a strong background in family or primary care medicine can help test takers when they face questions on prevention.

### How Do I Prepare for the COMLEX-USA Level 1?

Student experience suggests that you should start studying for the COMLEX-USA four to six months before the test is given, as an early start will allow you to spend up to a month on each subject. The recommendations made in Section I regarding study and testing methods, strategies, and resources, as well as the books suggested in Section IV for the USMLE Step 1, hold true for the COMLEX-USA as well.

Another important source of information is in the *Examination Guidelines and Sample Exam*, a booklet that discusses the breakdown of each subject while also providing sample questions and corresponding answers. Many students, however, felt that this breakdown provided only a general guideline and was not representative of the level of difficulty of the actual COMLEX-USA. The sample questions did not provide examples of clinical vignettes, which made up approximately 25% of the exam. You will receive this publication with registration materials for the COMLEX-USA Level 1 exam, but you can also receive a copy and additional information by writing:

**NBOME**
8765 W. Higgins Road, Suite 200
Chicago, IL 60631-4174
(773) 714-0622
Fax: (773) 714-0631

or by visiting the NBOME Web page at www.nbome.org.

The NBOME developed the Comprehensive Osteopathic Medical Self-Assessment Examination (COMSAE) series to fill the need for self-assessment on the part of osteopathic medical students. Many students take the COMSAE exam before the COMLEX-USA in addition to using test-bank questions and board review books. Students can purchase a copy of this exam at www.nbome.org/comsae.asp.

The 2009 COMLEX-USA exam consisted of 50 questions per section. There were eight sections, with one hour dedicated to each section for an examination total of eight hours. Each multiple-choice question accompanied a small case (about one to two sentences long).

In recent years, students have reported an emphasis in certain areas. For example:

- There was an increased emphasis on upper limb anatomy/brachial plexus.
- Specific topics were repeatedly tested on the exam. These included cardiovascular physiology and pathology, acid-base physiology, diabetes, benign prostatic hyperplasia, sexually transmitted diseases, measles, and rubella. Thyroid and adrenal function, neurology (head injury), specific drug treatments for bacterial infection, migraines/cluster headaches, and drug mechanisms also received heavy emphasis.
- Behavioral science questions were based on psychiatry.
- High-yield osteopathic manipulative technique (OMT) topics on the 2007 exam included an extremely heavy emphasis on the sympathetic and parasympathetic innervations of viscera and nerve roots, rib mechanics/diagnosis, and basic craniosacral theory. Students who spend time reviewing basic anatomy, studying nerve and dermatome innervations, and understanding how to perform basic OMT techniques (e.g., muscle energy or counterstrain) can improve their scores.

Starting in 2009, the COMLEX-USA Level 1 exam will also include multi-media-based questions. Such questions test the student's ability to perform a good physical exam and to elicit various physical diagnostic signs (e.g., Murphy's sign).

Since topics that were repeatedly tested appeared in all four booklets, students found it useful to review them in between the two test days. It is important to understand that the topics emphasized on the 2008 exam may not be stressed on the 2009 exam. However, some topics are heavily tested each year, so it may be beneficial to have a solid foundation in the above-mentioned topics.

The National Board of Podiatric Medical Examiners (NBPME) tests are designed to assess whether a candidate possesses the knowledge required to practice as a minimally competent entry-level podiatrist. The NBPME examinations are used as part of the licensing process governing the practice of podiatric medicine. The NBPME exam is recognized by all 50 states and the District of Columbia, the U.S. Army, the U.S. Navy, and the Canadian provinces of Alberta, British Columbia, and Ontario. Individual states use the examination scores differently; therefore, doctor of podiatric medicine (DPM) candidates should refer to the *NBPME Bulletin of Information: 2009 Examinations.*

The NBPME Part I is generally taken after the completion of the second year of podiatric medical education. Unlike the USMLE Step 1, there is no behavioral science section, nor is biomechanics tested. The exam samples seven basic science disciplines: general anatomy (10%); lower extremity anatomy (22%); biochemistry (10%); physiology (12%); medical microbiology and immunology (15%); pathology (15%); and pharmacology (16%). A detailed outline of topics and subtopics covered on the exam can be found in the *NBPME Bulletin of Information,* available on the NBPME Web site.

## Your NBPME Appointment

In early spring, your college registrar will have you fill out an application for the NBPME Part I. After your application and registration fees are received, you will be mailed the *NBPME Bulletin of Information: 2009 Examinations.* The exam will be offered at an independent location in each city with a podiatric medical school (New York, Philadelphia, Miami, Cleveland, Chicago, Des Moines, Phoenix, and San Francisco). You may take the exam at any of these locations regardless of which school you attend. However, you must designate on your application which testing location you desire. Specific instructions about exam dates and registration deadlines can be found in the *NBPME Bulletin.*

## Exam Format

The NBPME Part I is a written exam consisting of 205 questions. The test consists entirely of multiple-choice questions with four answer choices. Examinees have three hours in which to take the exam and are given scratch paper and a calculator, both of which must be turned in at the end of the exam. Some questions on the exam will be "trial questions." These questions are evaluated as future board questions but are not counted in your score.

## Interpreting Your Score

Three to four weeks following the exam date, test takers will receive their scores by mail. NBPME scores are reported as pass/fail, with a scaled score of at least 75 needed to pass. Eighty-five percent of first-time test takers pass the

NBPME Part I. Failing candidates receive a report with one score between 55 and 74 in addition to diagnostic messages intended to help identify strengths or weaknesses in specific content areas. If you fail the NBPME Part I, you must retake the entire examination at a later date. There is no limit to the number of times you can retake the exam.

## Preparation for the NBPME Part I

Students suggest that you begin studying for the NBPME Part I at least three months prior to the test date. The suggestions made in Section I regarding study and testing methods for the USMLE Step 1 can be applied to the NBPME as well. This book should, however, be used as a supplement and not as the sole source of information. Keep in mind that you need only a passing score. Neither you nor your school or future residency will ever see your actual numerical score. Competing with colleagues should not be an issue, and study groups are beneficial to many.

A potential study method that helps many students is to copy the outline of the material to be tested from the *NBPME Bulletin*. Check off each topic during your study, because doing so will ensure that you have engaged each topic. If you are pressed for time, prioritize subjects on the basis of their weight on the exam. Approximately 22% of the NBPME Part I focuses on lower extremity anatomy. In this area, students should rely on the notes and material that they received from their class. Remember, lower extremity anatomy is the podiatric physician's specialty—so everything about it is important. Do not forget to study osteology. Keep your old tests and look through old lower extremity class exams, since each of the podiatric colleges submits questions from its own exams. This strategy will give you an understanding of the types of questions that may be asked. On the NBPME Part I, you will see some of the same classic lower extremity anatomy questions you were tested on in school.

The NBPME, like the USMLE, requires that you apply and integrate knowledge over several areas of basic science in order to answer exam questions. Students report that many questions emphasize clinical presentations; however, the facts in this book are very useful in helping students recall the various diseases and organisms. DPM candidates should expand on the high-yield pharmacology section and study antifungal drugs and treatments for *Pseudomonas*, methicillin-resistant *S. aureus*, candidiasis, and erythrasma. The high-yield section focusing on pathology is very useful; however, additional emphasis on diabetes mellitus and all its secondary manifestations, particularly peripheral neuropathy, should not be overlooked. Students should also focus on renal physiology and drug elimination, the biochemistry of gout, and neurophysiology, all of which have been noted to be important topics on the NBPME Part I exam.

A sample set of questions is found in the *NBPME Bulletin of Information: 2009 Examinations*. These samples are similar in difficulty to actual board questions. If you do not receive an *NBPME Bulletin* or if you have any questions regarding registration, fees, test centers, authorization forms, or score reports, please contact your college registrar or:

**NBPME**
P.O. Box 510
Bellefonte, PA 16823
(814) 357-0487
E-mail: NBPMEOfc@aol.com

or visit the NBPME Web page at www.nbpme.info.

The USMLE provides accommodations for students with documented disabilities. The basis for such accommodations is the Americans with Disabilities Act (ADA) of 1990. The ADA defines a disability as "a significant limitation in one or more major life activities." This includes both "observable/physical" disabilities (e.g., blindness, hearing loss, narcolepsy) and "hidden/mental disabilities" (e.g., attention-deficit hyperactivity disorder, chronic fatigue syndrome, learning disabilities).

To provide appropriate support, the administrators of the USMLE must be informed of both the nature and the severity of an examinee's disability. Such documentation is required for an examinee to receive testing accommodations. Accommodations include extra time on tests, low-stimulation environments, extra or extended breaks, and zoom text.

### Who Can Apply for Accommodations?

Students or graduates of a school in the United States or Canada that is accredited by the Liaison Committee on Medical Education (LCME) or the AOA may apply for test accommodations directly from the NBME. Requests are granted only if they meet the ADA definition of a disability. If you are a disabled student or a disabled graduate of a foreign medical school, you must contact the ECFMG (see below).

### Who Is Not Eligible for Accommodations?

Individuals who do not meet the ADA definition of disabled are not eligible for test accommodations. Difficulties not eligible for test accommodations include test anxiety, slow reading without an identified underlying cognitive deficit, English as a second language, and learning difficulties that have not been diagnosed as a medically recognized disability.

### Understanding the Need for Documentation

Although most learning-disabled medical students are all too familiar with the often exhausting process of providing documentation of their disability, you should realize that **applying for USMLE accommodation is different from these previous experiences.** This is because the NBME determines whether an individual is disabled solely on the basis of the guidelines set by the ADA. Previous accommodation does not in itself justify provision of an accommodation, so be sure to review the NBME guidelines carefully.

## Getting the Information

The first step in applying for USMLE special accommodations is to contact the NBME and obtain a guidelines and questionnaire booklet. This can be obtained by calling or writing to:

**Testing Coordinator**
Office of Test Accommodations
National Board of Medical Examiners
3750 Market Street
Philadelphia, PA 19104-3102
(215) 590-9509

Internet access to this information is also available at www.nbme.org. This information is also relevant for IMGs, since the information is the same as that sent by the ECFMG.

Foreign graduates should contact the ECFMG to obtain information on special accommodations by calling or writing to:

**ECFMG**
3624 Market Street
Philadelphia, PA 19104-2685
(215) 386-5900

When you get this information, take some time to read it carefully. The guidelines are clear and explicit about what you need to do to obtain accommodations.

NOTES

# High-Yield General Principles

*"There comes a time when for every addition of knowledge you forget something that you knew before. It is of the highest importance, therefore, not to have useless facts elbowing out the useful ones."*
— Sir Arthur Conan Doyle, A *Study in Scarlet*

*"Never regard study as a duty, but as the enviable opportunity to learn."*
—Albert Einstein

*"Live as if you were to die tomorrow. Learn as if you were to live forever."*
—Gandhi

▶ Behavioral Science

▶ Biochemistry

▶ Embryology

▶ Microbiology

▶ Immunology

▶ Pathology

▶ Pharmacology

The 2010 edition of *First Aid for the USMLE Step 1* contains a revised and expanded database of basic science material that student authors and faculty have identified as high yield for board reviews. The information is presented in a partially organ-based format. Hence, Section II is devoted to pathology, the foundational principles of behavioral science, biochemistry, embryology, microbiology and immunology, and pharmacology. Section III focuses on organ systems, with subsections covering the embryology, anatomy and histology, physiology, pathology, and pharmacology relevant to each. Each subsection is then divided into smaller topic areas containing related facts. Individual facts are generally presented in a three-column format, with the **Title** of the fact in the first column, the **Description** of the fact in the second column, and the **Mnemonic** or **Special Note** in the third column. Some facts do not have a mnemonic and are presented in a two-column format. Others are presented in list or tabular form in order to emphasize key associations.

The database structure used in Sections II and III is useful for reviewing material already learned. These sections are **not** ideal for learning complex or highly conceptual material for the first time. At the beginning of each subsection, we list supplementary high-yield clinical vignettes and topics that have appeared on recent exams in order to help focus your review.

The database of high-yield facts is not comprehensive. Use it to complement your core study material and not as your primary study source. The facts and notes have been condensed and edited to emphasize the essential material, and as a result each entry is "incomplete." Work with the material, add your own notes and mnemonics, and recognize that not all memory techniques work for all students.

We update the database of high-yield facts annually to keep current with new trends in boards content as well as to expand our database of information. However, we must note that inevitably many other very high yield entries and topics are not yet included in our database.

We actively encourage medical students and faculty to submit entries and mnemonics so that we may enhance the database for future students. We also solicit recommendations of alternate tools for study that may be useful in preparing for the examination, such as diagrams, charts, and computer-based tutorials (see How to Contribute, p. xvii).

### Disclaimer

The entries in this section reflect student opinions of what is high yield. Owing to the diverse sources of material, no attempt has been made to trace or reference the origins of entries individually. We have regarded mnemonics as essentially in the public domain. All errors and omissions will gladly be corrected if brought to the attention of the authors, either through the publisher or directly by e-mail.

# Behavioral Science

*"It's psychosomatic. You need a lobotomy. I'll get a saw."*
—Calvin, "Calvin & Hobbes"

A heterogeneous mix of epidemiology, biostatistics, ethics, psychology, sociology, and more falls under the heading of behavioral science. Many medical students do not study this discipline diligently because the material is felt to be easy or a matter of common sense. In our opinion, this is a missed opportunity.

Behavioral science questions may seem less concrete than questions from other disciplines, requiring an awareness of the social aspects of medicine. For example: If a patient does or says something, what should you do or say in response? These so-called "quote" questions now constitute much of the behavioral science section. Medical ethics and medical law are also appearing with increasing frequency. In addition, the key aspects of the doctor-patient relationship (e.g., communication skills, open-ended questions, facilitation, silence) are high yield, as are biostatistics and epidemiology. Make sure you can apply biostatistical concepts such as specificity and predictive values in a problem-solving format.

▶ Epidemiology/ Biostatistics

▶ Ethics

▶ Development

▶ Physiology

## Types of studies

| Study type | Design | Measures/example |
|---|---|---|
| **Case-control study**<br>Observational and retrospective | Compares a group of people with disease to a group without.<br>Asks, "What happened?" | **Odds ratio** (OR).<br>"Patients with COPD had higher odds of a history of smoking than those without COPD." |
| **Cohort study**<br>Observational and prospective | Compares a group with a given risk factor to a group without to assess whether the risk factor ↑ the likelihood of disease.<br>Asks, "What will happen?" | **Relative risk** (RR).<br>"Smokers had a higher risk of developing COPD than did nonsmokers." |
| **Cross-sectional study**<br>Observational | Collects data from a group of people to assess frequency of disease (and related risk factors) at a particular point in time.<br>Asks, "What is happening?" | **Disease prevalence.**<br>Can show risk factor association with disease, but does not establish causality. |

```
            Case control          Cohort

        ◄──────────────────┼──────────────────►

                      Cross-sectional
```

| | | |
|---|---|---|
| **Twin concordance study** | Compares the frequency with which both monozygotic twins or both dizygotic twins develop a disease. | Measures heritability. |
| **Adoption study** | Compares siblings raised by biologic vs. adoptive parents. | Measures heritability and influence of environmental factors. |

---

| **Clinical trial** | Experimental study involving humans. Compares therapeutic benefits of 2 or more treatments, or of treatment and placebo. Highest-quality study when randomized, controlled, and double-blinded. |  |
|---|---|---|
| | **Study sample** | **Purpose** |
| Phase I | Small number of patients, usually healthy volunteers. | Assesses safety, toxicity, and pharmacokinetics. |
| Phase II | Small number of patients with disease of interest. | Assesses treatment efficacy, optimal dosing, and adverse effects. |
| Phase III | Large number of patients randomly assigned either to the treatment under investigation or to the best available treatment (or placebo). | Compares the new treatment to the current standard of care. Is more convincing if double-blinded (i.e., neither patient nor doctor knows if the patient is in the treatment or control group). |

---

| **Meta-analysis** | Pools data from several studies to come to an overall conclusion. Achieves greater statistical power and integrates results of similar studies. Highest echelon of clinical evidence. | May be limited by quality of individual studies or bias in study selection. |
|---|---|---|

---

| **Evaluation of diagnostic tests** | Uses 2 × 2 table comparing test results with the actual presence of disease. TP = true positive; FP = false positive; TN = true negative; FN = false negative. |

Disease

|  | | ⊕ | ⊖ |
|---|---|---|---|
| Test | ⊕ | TP | FP |
|  | ⊖ | FN | TN |

| Sensitivity | Proportion of all people with disease who test positive, or the ability of a test to detect a disease when it is present. Value approaching 1 is desirable for ruling **out** disease and indicates a low false-negative rate. Used for screening in diseases with low prevalence. | $= \text{TP} / (\text{TP} + \text{FN})$ <br> = 1 – false-negative rate <br> **SNOUT = SeNsitivity rules OUT.** <br> If 100% sensitivity, $\text{TP} / (\text{TP} + \text{FN}) = 1$, $\text{FN} = 0$, and all negatives must be TNs. |

| Specificity | Proportion of all people without disease who test negative, or the ability of a test to indicate non-disease when disease is not present. Value approaching 1 is desirable for ruling **in** disease and indicates a low false-positive rate. Used as a confirmatory test after a positive screening test. Example: HIV testing. Screen with ELISA (sensitive, high false-positive rate, low threshold); confirm with Western blot (specific, high false-negative rate, high threshold). | $= \text{TN} / (\text{TN} + \text{FP})$ <br> = 1 – false-positive rate <br> **SPIN = SPecificity rules IN.** <br> If 100% specificity, $\text{TN} / (\text{TN} + \text{FP}) = 1$, $\text{FP} = 0$, and all positives must be TPs. |

| Positive predictive value (PPV) | Proportion of positive test results that are true positive. Probability that person actually has the disease given a positive test result. (Note: If the prevalence of a disease in a population is low, even tests with high specificity or high sensitivity will have low positive predictive values!) | $= \text{TP} / (\text{TP} + \text{FP})$ |

| Negative predictive value (NPV) | Proportion of negative test results that are true negative. Probability that person actually is disease free given a negative test result. | $= \text{TN} / (\text{FN} + \text{TN})$ |

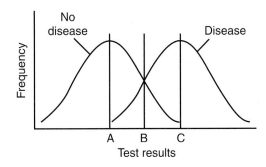

(Adapted, with permission, from McPhee SJ et al. *Current Medical Diagnosis & Treatment,* 47th ed. New York: McGraw-Hill, 2007: Fig. 43-3.)

**Prevalence vs. incidence**

$$\text{Point prevalence} = \frac{\text{total cases in population at a given time}}{\text{total population at risk at a given time}}$$

$$\text{Incidence} = \frac{\text{new cases in population over a given time period}}{\text{total population at risk during that time}}$$

Prevalence $\cong$ incidence $\times$ disease duration.

Prevalence > incidence for chronic diseases (e.g., diabetes).

Prevalence = incidence for acute disease (e.g., common cold).

**Incidence** is new **incidents.**

When calculating incidence, don't forget that people currently with the disease, or those previously positive for it, are not considered at risk.

---

**Odds ratio vs. relative risk**

Odds ratio (OR) for case-control studies
Odds of having disease in exposed group divided by odds of having disease in unexposed group.
Approximates relative risk if prevalence of disease is not too high.

Relative risk (RR) for cohort studies
Relative probability of getting a disease in the exposed group compared to the unexposed group.
Calculated as percent with disease in exposed group divided by percent with disease in unexposed group.

Attributable risk
The difference in risk between exposed and unexposed groups, or the proportion of disease occurrences that are attributable to the exposure (e.g., smoking causes one-third of cases of pneumonia).

Absolute risk reduction
The reduction in risk associated with a treatment as compared to a placebo.

Number needed to treat
1/absolute risk reduction.

Number needed to harm
1/attributable risk.

$$\text{Odds ratio} = \frac{a/b}{c/d} = \frac{ad}{bc}$$

$$\text{Relative risk} = \frac{a/(a+b)}{c/(c+d)}$$

$$\text{Attributable risk} = \frac{a}{a+b} - \frac{c}{c+d}$$

Disease

|  | $\oplus$ | $\ominus$ |
|---|---|---|
| Risk factor $\oplus$ | a | b |
| $\ominus$ | c | d |

---

**Precision vs. accuracy**

Precision is:
1. The consistency and reproducibility of a test (reliability)
2. The absence of random variation in a test

Accuracy is the trueness of test measurements (validity).

Random error—reduced precision in a test.

Systematic error—reduced accuracy in a test.

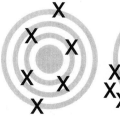 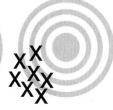 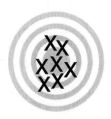 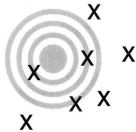

| Accuracy | Precision | Accuracy and precision | No accuracy, no precision |

| **Bias** | Occurs when 1 outcome is systematically favored over another. Systematic errors. | Ways to reduce bias: |
|---|---|---|

Occurs when 1 outcome is systematically favored over another. Systematic errors.

1. **Selection bias**—nonrandom assignment to study group (e.g., Berkson's bias)
2. **Recall bias**—knowledge of presence of disorder alters recall by subjects
3. **Sampling bias**—subjects are not representative relative to general population; therefore, results are not generalizable
4. **Late-look bias**—information gathered at an inappropriate time—e.g., using a survey to study a fatal disease (only those patients still alive will be able to answer survey)
5. **Procedure bias**—subjects in different groups are not treated the same—e.g., more attention is paid to treatment group, stimulating greater compliance
6. **Confounding bias**—occurs with 2 closely associated factors; the effect of 1 factor distorts or confuses the effect of the other
7. **Lead-time bias**—early detection confused with ↑ survival; seen with improved screening (natural history of disease is not changed, but early detection makes it seem as though survival ↑)
8. **Pygmalion effect**—occurs when a researcher's belief in the efficacy of a treatment changes the outcome of that treatment
9. **Hawthorne effect**—occurs when the group being studied changes its behavior owing to the knowledge of being studied

Ways to reduce bias:
1. Blind studies (double blind is better)
2. Placebo responses
3. Crossover studies (each subject acts as own control)
4. Randomization

---

**Statistical distribution**

Terms that describe statistical distributions:

Normal ≈ Gaussian ≈ bell-shaped (mean = median = mode).

Bimodal is simply 2 humps (2 modal peaks).

Positive skew—mean > median > mode. Asymmetry with tail on right.

Negative skew—mean < median < mode. Asymmetry with tail on left.

Mode is least affected by outliers in the sample.

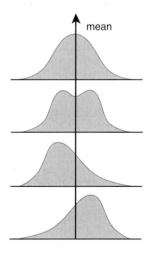

---

**Statistical hypotheses**

| | | Reality | |
|---|---|---|---|
| | | $H_1$ | $H_0$ |
| Study results | $H_1$ | Power $(1 - \beta)$ | $\alpha$ |
| | $H_0$ | $\beta$ | |

Null ($H_0$) — Hypothesis of no difference (e.g., there is no association between the disease and the risk factor in the population).

Alternative ($H_1$) — Hypothesis that there is some difference (e.g., there is some association between the disease and the risk factor in the population).

**Error types**

Type I error ($\alpha$) — Stating that there **is** an effect or difference when none exists (to mistakenly accept the experimental hypothesis and reject the null hypothesis). $p$ = probability of making a type I error. $p$ is judged against $\alpha$, a preset level of significance (usually < .05). "False-positive error."

If $p < .05$, then there is less than a 5% chance that the data will show something that is not really there.

$\alpha$ = you "saw" a difference that did not exist—for example, convicting an innocent man.

Type II error ($\beta$) — Stating that there **is not** an effect or difference when one exists (to fail to reject the null hypothesis when in fact $H_0$ is false). $\beta$ is the probability of making a type II error. "False-negative error."

$\beta$ = you did not "see" a difference that does exist— for example, setting a guilty man free.

**Power (1 – β)** — Probability of rejecting null hypothesis when it is in fact false, or the likelihood of finding a difference if one in fact exists. It depends on:
1. Total number of end points experienced by population
2. Difference in compliance between treatment groups (differences in the mean values between groups)
3. Size of expected effect

If you ↑ sample size, you ↑ power. There is power in numbers.

Power = 1 – $\beta$.

**Standard deviation vs. standard error**

n = sample size.
$\sigma$ = standard deviation.
SEM = standard error of the mean.
SEM = $\sigma/\sqrt{n}$.
Therefore, SEM < $\sigma$ and SEM decreases as n increases.

Normal (Gaussian) distribution:

68%
95%
99.7%

| | | |
|---|---|---|
| **Confidence interval** | Range of values in which a specified probability of the means of repeated samples would be expected to fall.<br>CI = confidence interval.<br>CI = range from [mean − Z(SEM)] to [mean + Z(SEM)].<br>The 95% CI (corresponding to $p = .05$) is often used. For the 95% CI, Z = 1.96. | If the 95% CI for a mean difference between 2 variables includes 0, then there is no significant difference and $H_0$ is not rejected. If the 95% CI for odds ratio or relative risk includes 1, $H_0$ is not rejected.<br>If the CI between 2 groups overlaps, then these groups are not significantly different. |
| **$t$-test vs. ANOVA vs. $\chi^2$** | $t$-test checks difference between the **means** of 2 groups.<br>ANOVA checks difference between the means of 3 or more groups.<br>$\chi^2$ checks difference between 2 or more percentages or proportions of categorical outcomes (not mean values). | Mr. **T** is **mean**.<br><br>**ANOVA** = **AN**alysis **O**f **VA**riance of 3 or more variables.<br>$\chi^2$ = compare percentages (%) or proportions. |
| **Correlation coefficient (r)** | r is always between −1 and +1. The closer the absolute value of r is to 1, the stronger the correlation between the 2 variables.<br>Coefficient of determination = $r^2$ (value that is usually reported). | |
| **Disease prevention** | 1°—prevent disease occurrence (e.g., HPV vaccination).<br>2°—early detection of disease (e.g., Pap smear).<br>3°—reduce disability from disease (e.g., chemotherapy). | **PDR:**<br>**P**revent<br>**D**etect<br>**R**educe disability |

**Important prevention measures**

| Risk factor | Services |
|---|---|
| Diabetes | Eye, foot exams; urine tests |
| Drug use | Hepatitis immunizations; HIV, TB tests |
| Alcoholism | Influenza, pneumococcal immunizations; TB test |
| Overweight | Blood sugar tests for diabetes |
| Homeless, recent immigrant, inmate | TB test |
| High-risk sexual behavior | HIV, hepatitis B, syphilis, gonorrhea, chlamydia tests |

| Reportable diseases | Only some infectious diseases are reportable in all states, including AIDS, chickenpox, gonorrhea, hepatitis A and B, measles, mumps, rubella, salmonella, shigella, syphilis, and TB.<br>Other diseases (including HIV) vary by state. | Hep, Hep, Hep, Hooray, the **SSSMMART Chick** is **Gone**!<br>**Hep** A<br>**Hep** B<br>**Hep** C<br>**H**IV<br>**S**almonella<br>**S**higella<br>**S**yphilis<br>**M**easles<br>**M**umps<br>**A**IDS<br>**R**ubella<br>**T**uberculosis<br>**Chick**enpox<br>**Gon**orrhea |

**Leading causes of death in the United States by age**

| Infants | Congenital anomalies, short gestation/low birth weight, sudden infant death syndrome, maternal complications of pregnancy, respiratory distress syndrome. |
| Age 1–14 | Injuries, cancer, congenital anomalies, homicide, heart disease. |
| Age 15–24 | Injuries, homicide, suicide, cancer, heart disease. |
| Age 25–64 | Cancer, heart disease, injuries, suicide, stroke. |
| Age 65+ | Heart disease, cancer, stroke, COPD, pneumonia, influenza. |

| Health care payment | Physicians' payments—fee-for-service (payment for each procedure), capitation basis (fixed payment for time period, regardless of number of procedures), salary based (hospitals, HMOs, universities pay fixed salary). | |
| | Medicare and Medicaid—federal programs that originated from amendments to the Social Security Act. | MedicarE is for Elderly.<br>MedicaiD is for Destitute. |
| | Medicare Part A = hospital; Part B = doctor bills. | |
| | Medicaid is federal and state assistance for very low income people. | |
| | CHIP (Children's Health Insurance Program)—matching state and federal government funding for child health care coverage. | |
| | Third-party payers—insurance companies collect money from large population to pay all or a portion of the medical bills of current patients. | |

## Core ethical principles

| | |
|---|---|
| Autonomy | Obligation to respect patients as individuals and to honor their preferences in medical care. |
| Beneficence | Physicians have a special ethical (fiduciary) duty to act in the patient's best interest. May conflict with autonomy. If the patient can make an informed decision, ultimately the patient has the right to decide. |
| Nonmaleficence | "Do no harm." However, if the benefits of an intervention outweigh the risks, a patient may make an informed decision to proceed (most surgeries fall into this category). |
| Justice | To treat persons fairly. |

## Informed consent

Legally requires:
1. Discussion of pertinent information
2. Patient's agreement to the plan of care
3. Freedom from coercion

Patients must understand the risks, benefits, and alternatives, which include no intervention.

## Exceptions to informed consent

1. Patient lacks decision-making capacity or is legally incompetent
2. Implied consent in an emergency
3. Therapeutic privilege—withholding information when disclosure would severely harm the patient or undermine informed decision-making capacity
4. Waiver—patient waives the right of informed consent

## Consent for minors

Parental consent must be obtained unless minor is emancipated (e.g., is married, is self-supporting, has children, or is in military).

## Decision-making capacity

1. Patient makes and communicates a choice
2. Patient is informed
3. Decision remains stable over time
4. Decision is consistent with patient's values and goals
5. Decision is not a result of delusions or hallucinations

The patient's family cannot require that a doctor withhold information from the patient.

## Oral advance directive

Incapacitated patient's prior oral statements commonly used as guide. Problems arise from variance in interpretation. If patient was informed, directive is specific, patient made a choice, and decision was repeated over time, the oral directive is more valid.

## Written advance directive

Living will—describes treatments the patient wishes to receive or not receive if he/she becomes incapacitated and cannot communicate about treatment decisions. Usually, patient directs physician to withhold or withdraw life-sustaining treatment if he/she develops a terminal disease or enters a persistent vegetative state.

Durable power of attorney—patient designates a surrogate to make medical decisions in the event that he/she loses decision-making capacity. Patient may also specify decisions in clinical situations. Surrogate retains power unless revoked by patient. More flexible than a living will.

| | |
|---|---|
| **Confidentiality** | Confidentiality respects patient privacy and autonomy. Disclosing information to family and friends should be guided by what the patient would want. The patient may waive the right to confidentiality (e.g., insurance companies). |

| | |
|---|---|
| **Exceptions to confidentiality** | 1. Potential harm to others is serious<br>2. Likelihood of harm to self is great<br>3. No alternative means exist to warn or to protect those at risk<br>4. Physicians can take steps to prevent harm<br>   Examples include:<br>     1. Infectious diseases—physicians may have a duty to warn public officials and identifiable people at risk<br>     2. The Tarasoff decision—law requiring physician to directly inform and protect potential victim from harm; may involve breach of confidentiality<br>     3. Child and/or elder abuse<br>     4. Impaired automobile drivers<br>     5. Suicidal/homicidal patients—physicians may hold patients involuntarily for a period of time |

| | | |
|---|---|---|
| **Malpractice** | Civil suit under negligence requires:<br>  1. Physician had a duty to the patient (**D**uty)<br>  2. Physician breached that duty (**D**ereliction)<br>  3. Patient suffers harm (**D**amage)<br>  4. The breach of the duty was what caused the harm (**D**irect)<br>The most common factor leading to litigation is poor communication between physician and patient. | The **4 D's.**<br>Unlike a criminal suit, in which the burden of proof is "beyond a reasonable doubt," the burden of proof in a malpractice suit is "more likely than not." |

| | |
|---|---|
| **Good Samaritan law** | Relieves health care workers, as well as laypersons in some instances, from liability in certain emergency situations with the objective of encouraging health care workers to offer assistance without expectation of compensation. |

## Ethical situations

| Situation | Appropriate response |
|---|---|
| Patient is noncompliant. | Work to improve the physician-patient relationship. |
| Patient has difficulty taking medications. | Provide written instructions; attempt to simplify treatment regimens. |
| Family members ask for information about patient's prognosis. | Avoid discussing issues with relatives without the permission of the patient. |
| A 17-year-old girl is pregnant and requests an abortion. | Many states require parental notification or consent for minors for an abortion. Parental consent is **not** required for emergency situations, treatment of STDs, medical care during pregnancy, and management of drug addiction. |
| A terminally ill patient requests physician assistance in ending his life. | In the overwhelming majority of states, refuse involvement in any form of physician-assisted suicide. Physicians may, however, prescribe medically appropriate analgesics that coincidentally shorten the patient's life. |
| Patient states that he finds you attractive. | Ask direct, closed-ended questions and use a chaperone if necessary. Romantic relationships with patients are **never** appropriate. Never say, "There can be no relationship while you are a patient," because it implies that a relationship may be possible if the individual is no longer a patient. |
| Patient refuses a necessary procedure or desires an unnecessary one. | Attempt to understand why the patient wants/does not want the procedure. Address the underlying concerns. Avoid performing unnecessary procedures. |
| Patient is angry about the amount of time he spent in the waiting room. | Apologize to the patient for any inconvenience. Stay away from efforts to explain the delay. |
| Patient is upset with the way he was treated by another doctor. | Suggest that the patient speak directly to that physician regarding his/her concerns. If the problem is with a member of the office staff, tell the patient you will speak to that individual. |
| A child wishes to know more about his illness. | Ask what the parents have told the child about his illness. Parents of a child decide what information can be relayed about the illness. |
| Patient continues to smoke, believing that cigarettes are good for him. | Ask how the patient feels about his/her smoking. Offer advice on cessation if the patient seems willing to make an effort to quit. |
| Minor (under age 18) requests condoms. | Physicians can provide counsel and contraceptives to minors without a parent's knowledge or consent. |
| A drug company offers a "referral fee" for every patient a physician enrolls in a study. | Eligible patients who may benefit from the study may be enrolled, but it is never acceptable for a physician to receive compensation from a drug company. |

## ▶ BEHAVIORAL SCIENCE–DEVELOPMENT

**Apgar score** — A 10-point scale evaluated at 1 minute and 5 minutes.

| | 0 points | 1 point | 2 points |
|---|---|---|---|
| Appearance | Blue | Trunk pink | All pink |
| Pulse | None | < 100/min | > 100/min |
| Grimace | None | Grimace | Grimace + cough |
| Activity | Limp | Some | Active |
| Respiration | None | Irregular | Regular |

| | |
|---|---|
| **Low birth weight** | Defined as < 2500 g. Associated with greater incidence of physical and emotional problems. Caused by prematurity or intrauterine growth retardation. Complications include infections, respiratory distress syndrome, necrotizing enterocolitis, intraventricular hemorrhage, and persistent fetal circulation. |

**Early developmental milestones**

| Approximate age | Motor milestone | Cognitive/social milestone |
|---|---|---|
| **Infant** | | |
| Birth–3 mo | Rooting reflex | Orients to voice |
| 3 mo | Holds head up, Moro reflex disappears | Social smile |
| 7–9 mo | Sits alone, crawls | Stranger anxiety |
| 15 mo | Walks, Babinski disappears | Few words, separation anxiety |
| **Toddler** | | |
| 12–24 mo | Climbs stairs; stacks 3 blocks at 1 year, 6 blocks at 2 years (number of blocks stacked = age in years × 3) | Object permanence; 200 words and 2-word sentences at age 2 |
| 24–36 mo | | Core gender identity, parallel play |
| **Preschool** | | |
| 30–36 mo | Stacks 9 blocks | Toilet training ("**pee** at age **3**") |
| 3 yrs | Rides tricycle (rides **3**-cycle at age **3**); copies line or circle drawing | 900 words and complete sentences |
| 4 yrs | Simple drawings (stick figure), hops on 1 foot | Cooperative play, imaginary friends, grooms self, brushes teeth, buttons and zips |

| | |
|---|---|
| **Piaget's stages of cognitive development** | **Sensorimotor stage** (birth to age 2)—egocentric exploration of the world with the 5 senses. Novel use of objects to obtain a goal (e.g., use of stick to reach something). Understanding of **object** permanence is achieved.<br>**Preoperational stage** (ages 2–7)—acquisition of motor skills. Magical thinking predominates, with no "logical" thinking.<br>**Concrete operational stage** (ages 7–12)—start of logical thinking, but confined to concrete concepts. No longer egocentric.<br>**Formal operational stage** (age 12+)—development of abstract reasoning. |
| **Tanner stages of sexual development** | 1. Childhood<br>2. Pubic hair appears (adrenarche); breasts enlarge<br>3. Pubic hair darkens and becomes curly; penis size/length ↑<br>4. Penis width ↑, darker scrotal skin, development of glans, raised areolae<br>5. Adult; areolae are no longer raised |

| | | |
|---|---|---|
| **Changes in the elderly** | 1. Sexual changes:<br>   Men—slower erection/ejaculation, longer refractory period<br>   Women—vaginal shortening, thinning, and dryness<br>2. Sleep patterns—↓ REM, slow-wave sleep; ↑ latency and awakenings<br>3. Common medical conditions—arthritis, hypertension, heart disease, osteoporosis<br>4. ↓ incidence of psychiatric disorders<br>5. ↑ suicide rate (males 65–74 years of age have the highest suicide rate in the United States)<br>6. ↓ vision, hearing, immune response, bladder control<br>7. ↓ renal, pulmonary, GI function<br>8. ↓ muscle mass, ↑ fat | Sexual interest does not ↓.<br>Intelligence does not ↓. |
| **Grief** | Normal bereavement characterized by shock, denial, guilt, and somatic symptoms. Typically lasts 6 months to 1 year. May experience illusions.<br>Pathologic grief includes excessively intense or prolonged grief or grief that is delayed, inhibited, or denied. May experience depressive symptoms, delusions, and hallucinations. | |
| **Kübler-Ross grief stages** | Denial, Anger, Bargaining, Grieving (depression), Acceptance.<br>Stages do not necessarily occur in this order, and > 1 stage can be present at once. | Death Arrives Bringing Grave Adjustments. |

## ▶ BEHAVIORAL SCIENCE–PHYSIOLOGY

| | | |
|---|---|---|
| **Stress effects** | Stress induces production of free fatty acids, 17-OH corticosteroids (immunosuppression), lipids, cholesterol, catecholamines; affects water absorption, muscular tonicity, gastrocolic reflex, and mucosal circulation. | |
| **Sexual dysfunction** | Differential diagnosis includes:<br>1. Drugs (e.g., antihypertensives, neuroleptics, SSRIs, ethanol)<br>2. Diseases (e.g., depression, diabetes)<br>3. Psychological (e.g., performance anxiety) | |
| **Body-mass index (BMI)** | BMI is a measure of weight adjusted for height.<br><br>$$BMI = \frac{\text{weight in kg}}{(\text{height in meters})^2}$$ | < 18.5 underweight;<br>**18.5–24.9 normal;**<br>25.0–29.9 overweight;<br>> 30.0 obese; > 40.0 morbidly obese. |

**Sleep stages**

| Stage (% of total sleep time in young adults) | Description | EEG waveform |
|---|---|---|
| | Awake (eyes open), alert, active mental concentration | Beta (highest frequency, lowest amplitude) |
| | Awake (eyes closed) | Alpha |
| 1 (5%) | Light sleep | Theta |
| 2 (45%) | Deeper sleep; bruxism | Sleep spindles and K complexes |
| 3–4 (25%) | Deepest, non-REM sleep; sleepwalking; night terrors; bedwetting (slow-wave sleep) | Delta (lowest frequency, highest amplitude) |
| REM (25%) | Dreaming, loss of motor tone, possibly a memory processing function, erections, ↑ brain $O_2$ use | Beta<br>At night, **BATS** **D**rink **B**lood. |

1. Serotonergic predominance of raphe nucleus key to initiating sleep
2. NE reduces REM sleep
3. Extraocular movements during REM due to activity of PPRF (paramedian pontine reticular formation/conjugate gaze center)
4. REM sleep having the same EEG pattern as while awake and alert has spawned the terms "paradoxical sleep" and "desynchronized sleep"
5. Benzodiazepines shorten stage 4 sleep; thus useful for night terrors and sleepwalking
6. Imipramine is used to treat enuresis because it ↓ stage 4 sleep

| | | |
|---|---|---|
| **REM sleep** | ↑ and variable pulse, REM, ↑ and variable blood pressure, penile/clitoral tumescence. Occurs every 90 minutes; duration ↑ through the night. ACh is the principal neurotransmitter involved in REM sleep. REM sleep ↓ with age. | REM sleep is like sex:<br> ↑ pulse, penile/<br> clitoral tumescence,<br> ↓ with age. |
| **Narcolepsy** | Disordered regulation of sleep-wake cycles. May include hypnagogic (just before sleep) or hypnopompic (just before awakening) hallucinations. The patient's nocturnal and narcoleptic sleep episodes start off with REM sleep. **Cataplexy** (loss of all muscle tone following a strong emotional stimulus) in some patients. Strong genetic component. Treat with stimulants (e.g., amphetamines, modafinil). | |
| **Circadian rhythm** | Driven by suprachiasmatic nucleus (SCN) of hypothalamus; controls ACTH, prolactin, melatonin, nocturnal NE release. SCN → NE release → pineal gland → melatonin. SCN is regulated by environment (i.e., light). | |

# Biochemistry

*"Biochemistry is the study of carbon compounds that crawl."*
—Mike Adams

*"World, world, O world!*
*But that thy strange mutations make us hate thee,*
*Life would not yield to age."*
—William Shakespeare, *King Lear*, Act IV, Scene I

- Molecular
- Cellular
- Laboratory Techniques
- Genetics
- Nutrition
- Metabolism

This high-yield material includes molecular biology, genetics, cell biology, and principles of metabolism (especially vitamins, cofactors, minerals, and single-enzyme-deficiency diseases). When studying metabolic pathways, emphasize important regulatory steps and enzyme deficiencies that result in disease, as well as reactions targeted by pharmacologic interventions. For example, understanding the defect in Lesch-Nyhan syndrome and its clinical consequences is higher yield than memorizing every intermediate in the purine salvage pathway. Do not spend time on hard-core organic chemistry, mechanisms, and physical chemistry. Detailed chemical structures are infrequently tested; however, many structures have been included here to help students learn reactions and the important enzymes involved. Familiarity with the latest biochemical techniques that have medical relevance—such as enzyme-linked immunosorbent assay (ELISA), immunoelectrophoresis, Southern blotting, and PCR—is useful. Beware if you placed out of your medical school's biochemistry class, for the emphasis of the test differs from that of many undergraduate courses. Review the related biochemistry when studying pharmacology or genetic diseases as a way to reinforce and integrate the material.

| | | |
|---|---|---|
| **Chromatin structure** | DNA exists in the condensed, chromatin form in order to fit into the nucleus. Negatively charged DNA loops twice around positively charged histone octamer (2 sets of H2A, H2B, H3, and H4) to form nucleosome "bead." Octamer subunits consist primarily of lysine and arginine amino acids (postively charged). H1 ties nucleosome beads together in a string. In mitosis, DNA condenses to form mitotic chromosomes. | Think of "**beads on a string.**"  H1 is the only histone that is not in the nucleosome core. |
| Heterochromatin | Condensed, transcriptionally inactive, sterically inaccessible. | HeteroChromatin = Highly Condensed. |
| Euchromatin | Less condensed, transcriptionally active, sterically accessible. | Eu = true, "truly transcribed." |

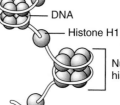

DNA
Histone H1
Nucleosome core histones H2A, H2B, H3, H4

**Nucleotides**

Purines (**A, G**) — 2 rings.
Pyrimidines (**C, T, U**) — 1 ring.
Guanine has a ketone. Thymine has a methyl.
Deamination of cytosine makes uracil.

PURe As Gold: PURines.
CUT the PY (pie):
PYrimidines.

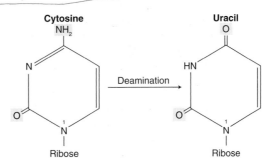

Uracil found in RNA; thymine in DNA.
G-C bond (3 H-bonds) stronger than A-T bond
(2 H-bonds). ↑ G-C content → ↑ melting
temperature.

THYmine has a meTHYl.

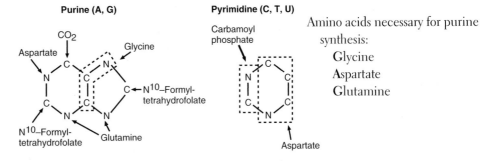

Amino acids necessary for purine
synthesis:
Glycine
Aspartate
Glutamine

Nucleoside = base + ribose.
Nucleotides = base + ribose + phosphate; linked by
3′-5′ phosphodiester bond.

**De novo pyrimidine and purine synthesis**

Purines are made from IMP precursor.

Pyrimidines are made from orotate precursor, with PRPP added later.

Ribonucleotides are synthesized first and are converted to deoxyribonucleotides by ribonucleotide reductase.

Carbamoyl phosphate is involved in 2 metabolic pathways: de novo pyrimidine synthesis and the urea cycle. Ornithine transcarbamoylase deficiency (urea cycle) leads to an accumulation of carbamoyl phosphate, which is then converted to orotic acid.

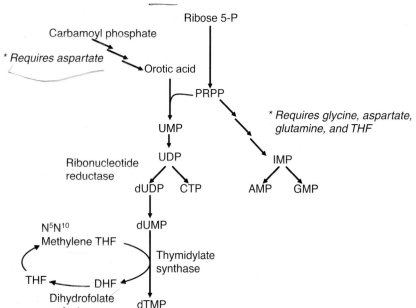

Various antineoplastic and antibiotic drugs function by interfering with nucleotide synthesis.

**Hydroxyurea** inhibits ribonucleotide reductase.

**6-mercaptopurine** (6-MP) blocks de novo purine synthesis.

**5-fluorouracil** (5-FU) inhibits thymidylate synthase ($\downarrow$ dTMP).

**Methotrexate** (MTX) inhibits dihydrofolate reductase ($\downarrow$ dTMP).

**Trimethoprim** inhibits bacterial dihydrofolate reductase ($\downarrow$ dTMP).

**Orotic aciduria**

Inability to convert orotic acid to UMP (de novo pyrimidine synthesis pathway) due to defect in either orotic acid phosphoribosyltransferase or orotidine 5′-phosphate decarboxylase. Autosomal recessive.

Findings: $\uparrow$ orotic acid in urine, megaloblastic anemia (does not improve with administration of vitamin $B_{12}$ or folic acid), failure to thrive. No hyperammonemia (vs. OTC deficiency — $\uparrow$ orotic acid with hyperammonemia).

Treatment: oral uridine administration.

## Purine salvage deficiencies

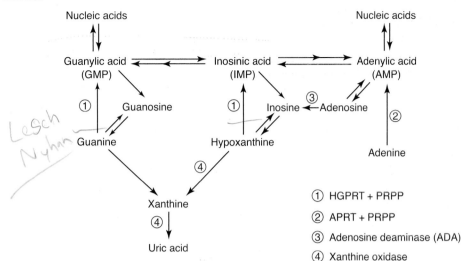

1. HGPRT + PRPP
2. APRT + PRPP
3. Adenosine deaminase (ADA)
4. Xanthine oxidase

| | | |
|---|---|---|
| Adenosine deaminase deficiency | Excess ATP and dATP imbalances nucleotide pool via feedback inhibition of ribonucleotide reductase → prevents DNA synthesis and thus ↓ lymphocyte count. One of the major causes of SCID. | SCID—severe combined immunodeficiency disease. SCID happens to kids (e.g., "bubble boy"). 1st disease to be treated by experimental human gene therapy. |
| Lesch-Nyhan syndrome | Defective purine salvage owing to absence of HGPRT, which converts hypoxanthine to IMP and guanine to GMP. Results in excess uric acid production. Findings: retardation, self-mutilation, aggression, hyperuricemia, gout, choreoathetosis. | X-linked recessive. He's Got Purine Recovery Trouble. |

## Transition vs. transversion

| | | |
|---|---|---|
| Transition | Substituting purine for purine or pyrimidine for pyrimidine. | TransItion = Identical type. |
| Transversion | Substituting purine for pyrimidine or vice versa. | TransVersion = conVersion between types. |

## Genetic code features

| | | |
|---|---|---|
| Unambiguous | Each codon specifies only 1 amino acid. | |
| Degenerate/ redundant | More than 1 codon may code for the same amino acid. | Methionine encoded by only 1 codon (AUG). |
| Commaless, nonoverlapping | Read from a fixed starting point as a continuous sequence of bases. | Some viruses are an exception. |
| Universal | Genetic code is conserved throughout evolution. | Exceptions include mitochondria, archaebacteria, Mycoplasma, and some yeasts. |

## Mutations in DNA

| | | |
|---|---|---|
| Silent | Same aa, often base change in 3rd position of codon (tRNA wobble). | Severity of damage: nonsense > missense > silent. |
| Missense | Changed aa (conservative—new aa is similar in chemical structure). | |
| **Nonsense** | Change resulting in early **stop** codon. | **Stop** the **nonsense!** |
| Frame shift | Change resulting in misreading of all nucleotides downstream, usually resulting in a truncated, nonfunctional protein. | |

## DNA replication

Eukaryotic DNA replication is more complex than the prokaryotic process but uses many enzymes analogous to those listed below. In both cases, DNA replication is semiconservative and involves both continuous and discontinuous (Okazaki fragment) synthesis. For eukaryotes, replication begins at a consensus sequence of base pairs.

| | | |
|---|---|---|
| Origin of replication | Particular sequence in genome where DNA replication begins. May be single (prokaryotes) or multiple (eukaryotes). | |
| Replication fork | Y-shaped region along DNA template where leading and lagging strands are synthesized. | |
| Helicase | Unwinds DNA template at replication fork. | |
| Single-stranded binding proteins | Prevent strands from reannealing. | |
| DNA topoisomerases | Create a nick in the helix to relieve supercoils created during replication. | **Fluoroquinolones**—inhibit DNA gyrase (specific prokaryotic topoisomerase). |
| Primase | Makes an RNA primer on which DNA polymerase III can initiate replication. | |
| DNA polymerase III | Prokaryotic only. Elongates leading strand by adding deoxynucleotides to the 3′ end. Elongates lagging strand until it reaches primer of preceding fragment. 3′ → 5′ exonuclease activity "proofreads" each added nucleotide. | DNA polymerase III has 5′ → 3′ synthesis and proofreads with 3′ → 5′ exonuclease. |
| DNA polymerase I | Prokaryotic only. Degrades RNA primer and fills in the gap with DNA. | DNA polymerase I excises RNA primer with 5′ → 3′ exonuclease. |
| DNA ligase | Seals. | |

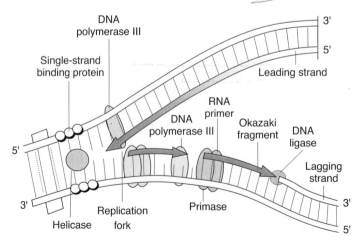

## DNA repair

### Single strand

| | | |
|---|---|---|
| Nucleotide excision repair | Specific endonucleases release the oligonucleotide-containing damaged bases; DNA polymerase and ligase fill and reseal the gap, respectively. | Mutated in **xeroderma pigmentosum** (dry skin with melanoma and other cancers, "children of the night"), which prevents repair of thymidine dimers. |
| Base excision repair | Specific glycosylases recognize and remove damaged bases, AP endonuclease cuts DNA at apyrimidinic site, empty sugar is removed, and the gap is filled and resealed. | |
| Mismatch repair | Unmethylated, newly synthesized string is recognized, mismatched nucleotides are removed, and the gap is filled and resealed. | Mutated in **hereditary nonpolyposis colorectal cancer (HNPCC)**. |

### Double strand

| | | |
|---|---|---|
| Nonhomologous end joining | Brings together 2 ends of DNA fragments. No requirement for homology. | |

| | | |
|---|---|---|
| **DNA/RNA/protein synthesis direction** | DNA and RNA are both synthesized $5' \rightarrow 3'$. Remember that the 5' of the incoming nucleotide bears the triphosphate (energy source for bond). The 3' hydroxyl of the nascent chain is the target. | mRNA is read 5' to 3'. Protein synthesis is N to C. |

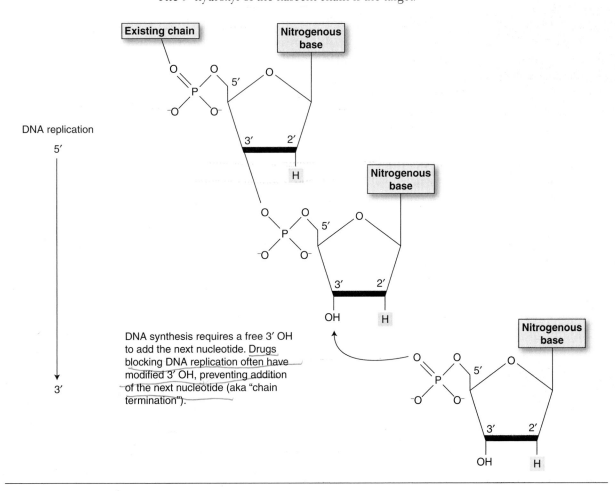

DNA synthesis requires a free 3' OH to add the next nucleotide. Drugs blocking DNA replication often have modified 3' OH, preventing addition of the next nucleotide (aka "chain termination").

| **Types of RNA** | Of the following: | Rampant, Massive, Tiny. |
|---|---|---|
| | rRNA is the most abundant type. | |
| | mRNA is the longest type. | |
| | tRNA is the smallest type. | |

**Start and stop codons**

| mRNA start codons | AUG (or rarely GUG). | AUG inAUGurates protein synthesis. |
|---|---|---|
| Eukaryotes | Codes for methionine, which may be removed before translation is completed. | |
| Prokaryotes | Codes for formyl-methionine (f-Met). | |
| mRNA stop codons | UGA, UAA, UAG. | UGA = U Go Away. |
| | | UAA = U Are Away. |
| | | UAG = U Are Gone. |

**Functional organization of the gene**

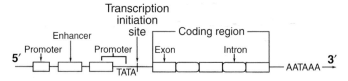

**Regulation of gene expression**

| Promoter | Site where RNA polymerase and multiple other transcription factors bind to DNA upstream from gene locus (AT-rich upstream sequence with TATA and CAAT boxes). | Promoter mutation commonly results in dramatic ↓ in amount of gene transcribed. |
|---|---|---|
| Enhancer | Stretch of DNA that alters gene expression by binding transcription factors. | Enhancers and silencers may be located close to, far from, or even within (in an intron) the gene whose expression it regulates. |
| Silencer | Site where negative regulators (repressors) bind. | |

**RNA polymerases**

| Eukaryotes | RNA polymerase I makes rRNA. | I, II, and III are numbered as their products are used in protein synthesis. |
|---|---|---|
| | RNA polymerase II makes mRNA. | |
| | RNA polymerase III makes tRNA. | |
| | No proofreading function, but can initiate chains. RNA polymerase II opens DNA at promoter site. | α-amanitin (found in death cap mushrooms) inhibits RNA polymerase II. Causes liver failure if ingested. |
| Prokaryotes | 1 RNA polymerase (multisubunit complex) makes all 3 kinds of RNA. | |

**RNA processing (eukaryotes)**

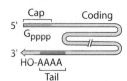

Occurs in nucleus. After transcription:
1. Capping on 5′ end (7-methylguanosine)
2. Polyadenylation on 3′ end (≈ 200 A's)
3. Splicing out of introns

Initial transcript is called heterogeneous nuclear RNA (hnRNA).

Capped and tailed transcript is called mRNA.

Only processed RNA is transported out of the nucleus.

AAUAAA = polyadenylation signal.

Poly-A polymerase does not require a template.

## Splicing of pre-mRNA

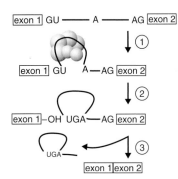

Pre-mRNA splicing occurs in eukaryotes.

1 — Primary transcript combines with snRNPs and other proteins to form spliceosome.

2 — Lariat-shaped (looped) intermediate is generated.

3 — Lariat is released to remove intron precisely and join 2 exons.

Patients with lupus make antibodies to spliceosomal snRNPs.

## Introns vs. exons

Exons contain the actual genetic information coding for protein.

Introns are intervening noncoding segments of DNA.

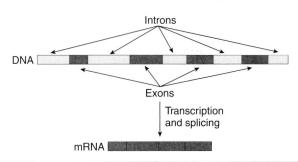

**IN**trons are **IN**tervening sequences and stay **IN** the nucleus, whereas **EX**ons **EX**it and are **EX**pressed.

Different exons can be combined by **alternative splicing** to make unique proteins in different tissues (e.g., β-thalassemia mutations).

## tRNA

| | |
|---|---|
| Structure | 75–90 nucleotides, 2° structure, cloverleaf form, anticodon end is opposite 3′ aminoacyl end. All tRNAs, both eukaryotic and prokaryotic, have CCA at 3′ end along with a high percentage of chemically modified bases. The amino acid is covalently bound to the 3′ end of the tRNA. | |
| Charging | Aminoacyl-tRNA synthetase (1 per aa, "matchmaker," uses ATP) scrutinizes aa before and after it binds to tRNA. If incorrect, bond is hydrolyzed. The aa-tRNA bond has energy for formation of peptide bond. A mischarged tRNA reads usual codon but inserts wrong amino acid. | Aminoacyl-tRNA synthetase and binding of charged tRNA to the codon are responsible for accuracy of amino acid selection. **Tetracyclines** bind 30S subunit, preventing attachment of aminoacyl-tRNA. |

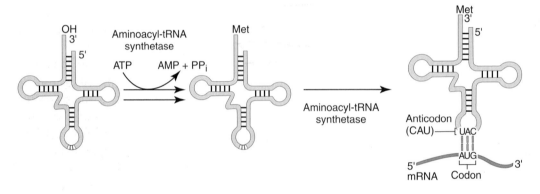

| | |
|---|---|
| **tRNA wobble** | Accurate base pairing is required only in the first 2 nucleotide positions of an mRNA codon, so codons differing in the 3rd "wobble" position may code for the same tRNA/amino acid (due to degeneracy of genetic code). |

## Protein synthesis

| | | |
|---|---|---|
| Initiation | Activated by GTP hydrolysis, initiation factors (eIFs) help assemble the 40S ribosomal subunit with the initiator tRNA and are released when the mRNA and the ribosomal subunit assemble with the complex. | Eukaryotes: 40S + 60S → 80S (Even). PrOkaryotes: 30S + 50S → 70S (Odd). ATP—tRNA Activation (charging). GTP—tRNA Gripping and Going places (translocation). |
| Elongation | 1. Aminoacyl-tRNA binds to A site (except for initiator methionine) <br> 2. Ribosomal rRNA (aka "ribozyme") catalyzes peptide bond formation, transfers growing polypeptide to amino acid in A site <br> 3. Ribosome advances 3 nucleotides toward 3′ end of RNA, moving peptidyl RNA to P site (translocation) | Think of "going APE": <br> A site = incoming Aminoacyl tRNA. <br> P site = accommodates growing Peptide. <br> E site = holds Empty tRNA as it Exits. |
| Termination | Completed protein is released from ribosome through simple hydrolysis and dissociates. | Many antibiotics act as protein synthesis inhibitors. <br> **Aminoglycosides** inhibit formation of the initiation complex and cause misreading of mRNA. <br> **Chloramphenicol** inhibits 50S peptidyltransferase. <br> **Macrolides** bind 50S, blocking translocation. <br> **Clindamycin** binds 50S, blocking translocation. |

Ribosome

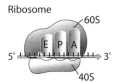

## Energy requirements of translation

| | |
|---|---|
| tRNA aminoacylation | ATP → AMP (2 phosphoanhydride bonds) |
| Loading tRNA onto ribosome | GTP → GDP |
| Translocation | GTP → GDP |
| Total energy expenditure | 4 high-energy phosphoanhydride bonds |

## Posttranslational modifications

| | |
|---|---|
| Trimming | Removal of N- or C-terminal propeptides from zymogens to generate mature proteins. |
| Covalent alterations | Phosphorylation, glycosylation, and hydroxylation. |
| Proteasomal degradation | Attachment of ubiquitin to defective proteins to tag them for breakdown. |

**Cell cycle phases**    Checkpoints control transitions between phases of cell cycle. This process is regulated by cyclins, CDKs, and tumor suppressors. Mitosis (shortest phase): prophase-metaphase-anaphase-telophase. $G_1$ and $G_0$ are of variable duration.

### Regulation of cell cycle

| | | |
|---|---|---|
| CDKs | Cyclin-dependent kinases; constitutive and inactive. | **G** = **G**ap or **G**rowth. |
| Cyclins | Regulatory proteins that control cell cycle events; phase specific; activate CDKs. | **S** = **S**ynthesis. |
| Cyclin-CDK complexes | Must be both activated and inactivated for cell cycle to progress. | |
| Tumor suppressors | Rb and p53 normally inhibit $G_1$-to-S progression; mutations in these genes result in unrestrained growth. | |

### Cell types

| | | |
|---|---|---|
| Permanent | Remain in $G_0$, regenerate from stem cells. | Neurons, skeletal and cardiac muscle, RBCs. |
| Stable (quiescent) | Enter $G_1$ from $G_0$ when stimulated. | Hepatocytes, lymphocytes. |
| Labile | Never go to $G_0$, divide rapidly with a short $G_1$. | Bone marrow, gut epithelium, skin, hair follicles. |

| | | |
|---|---|---|
| **Rough endoplasmic reticulum (RER)** | Site of synthesis of secretory (exported) proteins and of N-linked oligosaccharide addition to many proteins.<br>Nissl bodies (RER in neurons)—synthesize enzymes (e.g., ChAT) and peptide neurotransmitters.<br>Free ribosomes—unattached to any membrane; site of synthesis of cytosolic and organellar proteins. | Mucus-secreting goblet cells of the small intestine and antibody-secreting plasma cells are rich in RER. |
| **Smooth endoplasmic reticulum (SER)** | Site of steroid synthesis and detoxification of drugs and poisons. | Liver hepatocytes and steroid hormone–producing cells of the adrenal cortex are rich in SER. |

**Golgi apparatus**

1. Distribution center of proteins and lipids from ER to the plasma membrane, lysosomes, and secretory vesicles
2. Modifies N-oligosaccharides on asparagine
3. Adds O-oligosaccharides to serine and threonine residues
4. Addition of mannose-6-phosphate to specific lysosomal proteins → targets the protein to the lysosome
5. Proteoglycan assembly from core proteins
6. Sulfation of sugars in proteoglycans and of selected tyrosine on proteins

**Vesicular trafficking proteins:**
COPI: retrograde, Golgi → ER.
COPII: anterograde, RER → cis-Golgi.
Clathrin: trans-Golgi → lysosomes, plasma membrane → endosomes (receptor-mediated endocytosis).

**I-cell disease** (inclusion cell disease)—inherited lysosomal storage disorder; failure of addition of mannose-6-phosphate to lysosome proteins (enzymes are secreted outside the cell instead of being targeted to the lysosome). Results in coarse facial features, clouded corneas, restricted joint movement, and high plasma levels of lysosomal enzymes. Often fatal in childhood.

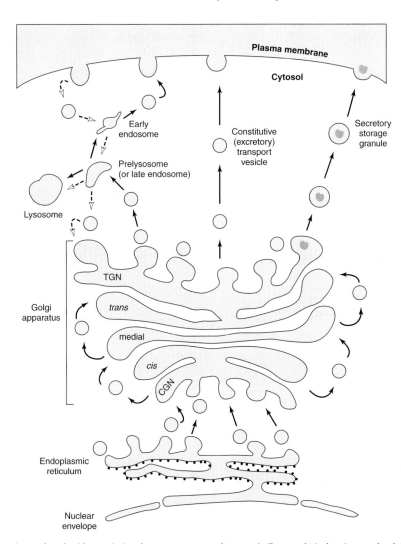

(Reproduced, with permission, from Murray RK et al. *Harper's Illustrated Biochemistry,* 27th ed. New York: McGraw-Hill, 2005: Fig. 45-2.)

**Microtubule**

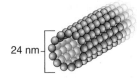

24 nm

Cylindrical structure composed of a helical array of polymerized dimers of α- and β-tubulin. Each dimer has 2 GTP bound. Incorporated into flagella, cilia, mitotic spindles. Grows slowly, collapses quickly. Also involved in slow axoplasmic transport in neurons.

**Molecular motor proteins**—transport cellular cargo toward opposite ends of microtubule tracks.
Dynein = retrograde to microtubule (+ → –).
Kinesin = anterograde to microtubule (– → +).

**Drugs that act on microtubules:**
1. Mebendazole/thiabendazole (antihelminthic)
2. Griseofulvin (antifungal)
3. Vincristine/vinblastine (anti-cancer)
4. Paclitaxel (anti–breast cancer)
5. Colchicine (anti-gout)

**Chédiak-Higashi syndrome**—microtubule polymerization defect resulting in ↓ phagocytosis. Results in recurrent pyogenic infections, partial albinism, and peripheral neuropathy.

**Cilia structure**

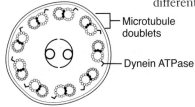

Microtubule doublets

Dynein ATPase

9 + 2 arrangement of microtubules.
Axonemal dynein—ATPase that links peripheral 9 doublets and causes bending of cilium by differential sliding of doublets.

**Kartagener's syndrome**—immotile cilia due to a dynein arm defect. Results in male and female infertility (sperm immotile), bronchiectasis, and recurrent sinusitis (bacteria and particles not pushed out); associated with situs inversus.

**Cytoskeletal elements**

| | |
|---|---|
| Actin and myosin | Microvilli, muscle contraction, cytokinesis, adherens junctions. |
| Microtubule | Cilia, flagella, mitotic spindle, neurons, centrioles. |
| Intermediate filaments | Vimentin, desmin, cytokeratin, glial fibrillary acid proteins (GFAP), neurofilaments. |

**Plasma membrane composition**

Asymmetric fluid bilayer.
Contains cholesterol (~50%), phospholipids (~50%), sphingolipids, glycolipids, and proteins.
High cholesterol or long saturated fatty acid content → ↑ melting temperature, ↓ fluidity.

**Immunohistochemical stains**

| Stain | Cell type |
|---|---|
| Vimentin | Connective tissue |
| Desmin | Muscle |
| Cytokeratin | Epithelial cells |
| GFAP | Neuroglia |
| Neurofilaments | Neurons |

| **Sodium pump** | Na⁺-K⁺ ATPase is located in the plasma membrane with ATP site on cytoplasmic side. For each ATP consumed, 3 Na⁺ go out and 2 K⁺ come in. During cycle, pump is phosphorylated. | **Ouabain** inhibits by binding to K⁺ site.<br>**Cardiac glycosides** (digoxin and digitoxin) directly inhibit the Na⁺-K⁺ ATPase, which leads to indirect inhibition of Na⁺/Ca²⁺ exchange. ↑ [Ca²⁺]ᵢ → ↑ cardiac contractility. |

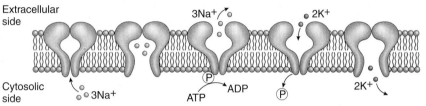

| **Collagen** | Most abundant protein in the human body. Extensively modified.<br>Organizes and strengthens extracellular matrix.<br>Type I (90%)—**B**one, **S**kin, **T**endon, dentin, fascia, cornea, late wound repair.<br>Type II—**C**artilage (including hyaline), vitreous body, nucleus pulposus.<br>Type III (**R**eticulin)—skin, blood vessels, uterus, fetal tissue, granulation tissue.<br>Type IV—**B**asement membrane or basal lamina. | **B**e (**S**o **T**otally) **C**ool, **R**ead **B**ooks.<br><br>Type I: **BONE.**<br><br>Type II: car**TWO**lage.<br><br><br><br>Type IV: Under the **floor** (basement membrane). |

## Collagen synthesis and structure

### Inside fibroblasts

1. Synthesis (RER) — Translation of collagen α chains (**preprocollagen**)—usually Gly-X-Y polypeptide (X and Y are proline, hydroxyproline, or hydroxylysine).

2. Hydroxylation (ER) — Hydroxylation of specific proline and lysine residues (requires **vitamin C**).

3. Glycosylation (ER) — Glycosylation of pro-α-chain lysine residues and formation of **procollagen** (triple helix of 3 collagen α chains).

4. Exocytosis — Exocytosis of procollagen into extracellular space.

### Outside fibroblasts

5. Proteolytic processing — Cleavage of terminal regions of procollagen transforms it into insoluble **tropocollagen.**

6. Cross-linking — Reinforcement of many staggered tropocollagen molecules by covalent lysine-hydroxylysine cross-linkage (by lysyl oxidase) to make **collagen fibrils.**

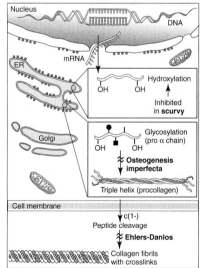

| | | |
|---|---|---|
| **Ehlers-Danlos syndrome** | Faulty collagen synthesis causing:<br>1. Hyperextensible skin<br>2. Tendency to bleed (easy bruising)<br>3. Hypermobile joints<br>6 types. Inheritance and severity vary. Can be autosomal dominant or recessive. May be associated with joint dislocation, berry aneurysms, organ rupture. | **Type III** collagen is most frequently affected. |
| **Osteogenesis imperfecta** | Genetic bone disorder (brittle bone disease) caused by a variety of gene defects.<br>Most common form is autosomal dominant with abnormal type I collagen, causing:<br>1. **Multiple fractures** with minimal trauma; may occur during the birth process<br>2. **Blue sclerae** due to the translucency of the connective tissue over the choroid<br>3. Hearing loss (abnormal middle ear bones)<br>4. Dental imperfections due to lack of dentin | May be confused with child abuse.<br>Type II is fatal in utero or in the neonatal period.<br>Incidence is 1:10,000 (see Image 90). |
| **Alport's syndrome** | Due to a variety of gene defects resulting in abnormal type IV collagen. Most common form is X-linked recessive.<br>Characterized by progressive hereditary nephritis and deafness. May be associated with ocular disturbances. | Type IV collagen is an important structural component of the basement membrane of the kidney, ears, and eyes. |
| **Elastin** | Stretchy protein within lungs, large arteries, elastic ligaments, vocal cords, ligamenta flava (connect vertebrae → relaxed and stretched conformations).<br>Rich in proline and glycine, nonglycosylated forms.<br>Tropoelastin with fibrillin scaffolding.<br>Broken down by elastase, which is normally inhibited by $\alpha_1$-antitrypsin. | **Marfan's syndrome**—caused by a defect in fibrillin.<br>**Emphysema**—can be caused by $\alpha_1$-antitrypsin deficiency, resulting in excess elastase activity. |

| | |
|---|---|
| **Polymerase chain reaction (PCR)** | Molecular biology laboratory procedure used to amplify a desired fragment of DNA. Steps:<br>1. Denaturation—DNA is denatured by heating to generate 2 separate strands<br>2. Annealing—during cooling, excess premade DNA primers anneal to a specific sequence on each strand to be amplified<br>3. Elongation—heat-stable DNA polymerase replicates the DNA sequence following each primer<br>These steps are repeated multiple times for DNA sequence amplification.<br>Agarose gel electrophoresis—used for size separation of PCR products (smaller molecules travel further); compared against DNA ladder. |

**Blotting procedures**

| | | |
|---|---|---|
| Southern blot | A **DNA** sample is electrophoresed on a gel and then transferred to a filter. The filter is then soaked in a denaturant and subsequently exposed to a labeled DNA probe that recognizes and anneals to its complementary strand. The resulting double-stranded labeled piece of DNA is visualized when the filter is exposed to film. | SNoW DRoP:<br>Southern = **DNA**<br>Northern = **RNA**<br>Western = **Protein** |
| Northern blot | Similar technique, except that Northern blotting involves radioactive DNA probe binding to sample **RNA.** | |
| Western blot | Sample protein is separated via gel electrophoresis and transferred to a filter. Labeled antibody is used to bind to relevant **protein.** | |

| | |
|---|---|
| **Microarrays** | Thousands of nucleic acid sequences are arranged in grids on glass or silicon. DNA or RNA probes are hybridized to the chip, and a scanner detects the relative amounts of complementary binding.<br>Used to profile gene expression levels or to detect single nucleotide polymorphisms (SNPs). |

| | | |
|---|---|---|
| **Enzyme-linked immunosorbent assay (ELISA)**<br><br>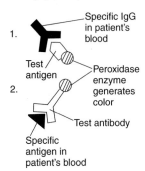 | A rapid immunologic technique testing for **antigen-antibody** reactivity.<br>Patient's blood sample is probed with either<br>1. Test antigen (coupled to color-generating enzyme)—to see if immune system recognizes it; or<br>2. Test antibody (coupled to color-generating enzyme)—to see if a certain antigen is present<br>If the target substance is present in the sample, the test solution will have an intense color reaction, indicating a positive test result. | Used in many laboratories to determine whether a particular antibody (e.g., anti-HIV) is present in a patient's blood sample. Both the sensitivity and the specificity of ELISA approach 100%, but both false-positive and false-negative results do occur. |

| | |
|---|---|
| **Fluorescence in situ hybridization (FISH)** | Fluorescent DNA or RNA probe binds to specific gene site of interest. Used for specific localization of genes and direct visualization of anomalies (e.g., microdeletions) at molecular level (when deletion is too small to be visualized by karyotype). Fluorescence = gene is present; no fluorescence = gene has been deleted. |
| **Cloning methods** | Cloning is the production of a recombinant DNA molecule that is self-perpetuating.<br>1. DNA fragments are inserted into bacterial plasmids that contain antibiotic resistance genes. These plasmids can be selected for by using media containing the antibiotic, and amplified.<br>2. Restriction enzymes cleave DNA at 4- to 6-bp palindromic sequences, allowing for insertion of a fragment into a plasmid.<br>3. Tissue mRNA is isolated and exposed to reverse transcriptase, forming a cDNA (lacks introns) library. |
| **Sanger DNA sequencing** | Dideoxynucleotides halt DNA polymerization at each base, generating sequences of various lengths that encompass the entire original sequence. Terminated fragments are electrophoresed and the original sequence can be deduced. |
| **Model systems** | Transgenic strategies in mice involve:<br>1. Random insertion of gene into mouse genome (constitutive)<br>2. Targeted insertion or deletion of gene through homologous recombination with mouse gene (conditional)<br>Gene can be manipulated at specific developmental points using an inducible Cre-lox system with an antibiotic-controlled promoter (e.g., to study a gene whose deletion causes an embryonic lethal).<br>RNAi—dsRNA is synthesized that is complementary to the mRNA sequence of interest. When transfected into human cells, dsRNA separates and promotes degradation of target mRNA, knocking down gene expression. | Knock-out = removing a gene.<br>Knock-in = inserting a gene. |
| **Karyotyping** | A process in which metaphase chromosomes are stained, ordered, and numbered according to morphology, size, arm-length ratio, and banding pattern. Can be performed on a sample of blood, bone marrow, amniotic fluid, or placental tissue. Used to diagnose chromosomal imbalances (e.g., autosomal trisomies, microdeletions, sex chromosome disorders). |

**Genetic terms**

| Term | Definition | Example |
|---|---|---|
| Codominance | Neither of 2 alleles is dominant. | Blood groups (A, B, AB). |
| Variable expression | Nature and severity of phenotype vary from 1 individual to another. | 2 patients with neurofibromatosis may have varying disease severity. |
| Incomplete penetrance | Not all individuals with a mutant genotype show the mutant phenotype. | – |
| Pleiotropy | 1 gene has > 1 effect on an individual's phenotype. | PKU causes many seemingly unrelated symptoms ranging from mental retardation to hair/skin changes. |
| Imprinting | Differences in phenotype depend on whether the mutation is of maternal or paternal origin. | Prader-Willi and Angelman's syndromes. |
| Anticipation | Severity of disease worsens or age of onset of disease is earlier in succeeding generations. | Huntington's disease. |
| Loss of heterozygosity | If a patient inherits or develops a mutation in a tumor suppressor gene, the complementary allele must be deleted/mutated before cancer develops. This is not true of oncogenes. | Retinoblastoma. |
| Dominant negative mutation | Exerts a **dominant effect**. A heterozygote produces a nonfunctional altered protein that also prevents the normal gene product from functioning. | Mutation of Tx factor in its allosteric site. Nonfunctioning mutant can still bind DNA, preventing wild-type Tx factor from binding. |
| Linkage disequilibrium | Tendency for certain alleles at 2 linked loci to occur together more often than expected by chance. Measured in a population, not in a family, and often varies in different populations. | – |
| Mosaicism | Occurs when cells in the body have different genetic makeup. Can be a germ-line mosaic, which may produce disease that is not carried by parent's somatic cells. | Lyonization—random X inactivation in females. |
| Locus heterogeneity | Mutations at different loci can produce the same phenotype. | Marfan's syndrome, MEN 2B, and homocystinuria; all cause marfanoid habitus. Albinism. |
| Heteroplasmy | Presence of both normal and mutated **mtDNA**, resulting in variable expression in **mitochondrial** inherited disease. | – |
| Uniparental disomy | Offspring receives 2 copies of a chromosome from 1 parent and no copies from the other parent. | – |

| | | |
|---|---|---|
| **Hardy-Weinberg population genetics** | If a population is in Hardy-Weinberg equilibrium and p and q are separate alleles, then:<br>Disease prevalence: $p^2 + 2pq + q^2 = 1$<br>Allele prevalence: $p + q = 1$<br>$2pq$ = heterozygote prevalence.<br>The prevalence of an X-linked recessive disease in males = q and in females = $q^2$. | Hardy-Weinberg law assumes:<br>1. No mutation occurring at the locus<br>2. No selection for any of the genotypes at the locus<br>3. Completely random mating<br>4. No migration |
| **Imprinting** | At a single locus, only 1 allele is active; the other is inactive (imprinted/inactivated by methylation). Deletion of the active allele → disease. | Both syndromes due to inactivation or deletion of genes on chromosome 15.<br>Can also occur as a result of uniparental disomy. |
| Prader-Willi syndrome | Deletion of normally active **P**aternal allele. | Mental retardation, hyperphagia, obesity, hypogonadism, hypotonia. |
| Angel**M**an's syndrome | Deletion of normally active **M**aternal allele. | Mental retardation, seizures, ataxia, inappropriate laughter ("happy puppet"). |

## Modes of inheritance

### Autosomal dominant

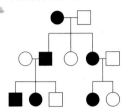

Often due to defects in structural genes. Many generations, both male and female, affected.

Often pleiotropic and, in many cases, present clinically after puberty. Family history crucial to diagnosis.

### Autosomal recessive

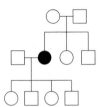

25% of offspring from 2 carrier parents are affected. Often due to enzyme deficiencies. Usually seen in only 1 generation.

Commonly more severe than dominant disorders; patients often present in childhood.

### X-linked recessive

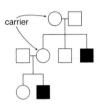

Sons of heterozygous mothers have a 50% chance of being affected. No male-to-male transmission.

Commonly more severe in males. Heterozygous females may be affected.

### X-linked dominant

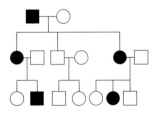

Transmitted through both parents. Either male or female offspring of the affected mother may be affected, while **all** female offspring of the affected father are diseased.

**Hypophosphatemic rickets**—formerly known as vitamin D–resistant rickets. Inherited disorder resulting in ↑ phosphate wasting at proximal tubule. Results in rickets-like presentation.

### Mitochondrial inheritance

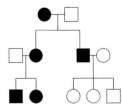

Transmitted only through mother. All offspring of affected females may show signs of disease.

Variable expression in population due to heteroplasmy.

**Mitochondrial myopathies, Leber's hereditary optic neuropathy**—degeneration of retinal ganglion cells and axons. Leads to acute loss of central vision.

## Autosomal-dominant diseases

| | |
|---|---|
| Achondroplasia | Cell-signaling defect of fibroblast growth factor (FGF) receptor 3. Results in dwarfism; short limbs, but head and trunk are normal size. Associated with advanced paternal age. |
| Autosomal-dominant polycystic kidney disease (ADPKD) | Formerly known as adult polycystic kidney disease. **Always bilateral,** massive enlargement of kidneys due to multiple large cysts. Patients present with flank pain, hematuria, hypertension, progressive renal failure. 90% of cases are due to mutation in *APKD1* (chromosome 16; 16 letters in "polycystic kidney"). Associated with polycystic liver disease, **berry aneurysms,** mitral valve prolapse. Infantile form is recessive. |
| Familial adenomatous polyposis | Colon becomes covered with adenomatous polyps after puberty. Progresses to colon cancer unless resected. Deletion on chromosome 5 (*APC gene*); 5 letters in "polyp." |
| Familial hypercholesterolemia (hyperlipidemia type IIA) | Elevated LDL due to defective or absent LDL receptor. Heterozygotes (1:500) have cholesterol ≈ 300 mg/dL. Homozygotes (very rare) have cholesterol ≈ 700+ mg/dL, severe atherosclerotic disease early in life, and tendon xanthomas (classically in the Achilles tendon); MI may develop before age 20. |
| Hereditary hemorrhagic telangiectasia (Osler-Weber-Rendu syndrome) | Inherited disorder of blood vessels. Findings: telangiectasia, recurrent epistaxis, skin discolorations, arteriovenous malformations (AVMs). |
| Hereditary spherocytosis | Spheroid erythrocytes due to spectrin or ankyrin defect; hemolytic anemia; ↑ MCHC. Splenectomy is curative. |
| Huntington's disease | Findings: depression, progressive dementia, choreiform movements, caudate atrophy, and ↓ levels of GABA and ACh in the brain. Symptoms manifest in affected individuals between the ages of 20 and 50. Gene located on chromosome 4; trinucleotide repeat disorder: $(CAG)_n$. "Hunting 4 food." |
| Marfan's syndrome | Fibrillin gene mutation → connective tissue disorder affecting skeleton, heart, and eyes. Findings: tall with long extremities, pectus excavatum, hyperextensive joints, and long, tapering fingers and toes (arachnodactyly; see Image 99); cystic medial necrosis of aorta → aortic incompetence and dissecting aortic aneurysms; floppy mitral valve. Subluxation of lenses. |
| Multiple endocrine neoplasias (MEN) | Several distinct syndromes (1, 2A, 2B) characterized by familial tumors of endocrine glands, including those of the pancreas, parathyroid, pituitary, thyroid, and adrenal medulla. MEN 2A and 2B are associated with *ret* gene. |
| Neurofibromatosis type 1 (von Recklinghausen's disease) | Findings: café-au-lait spots, neural tumors, Lisch nodules (pigmented iris hamartomas). Also marked by skeletal disorders (e.g., scoliosis), optic pathway gliomas, pheochromocytoma, and ↑ tumor susceptibility. On long arm of chromosome 17; 17 letters in von Recklinghausen. |
| Neurofibromatosis type 2 | Bilateral acoustic neuroma, juvenile cataracts. *NF2* gene on chromosome 22; type 2 = 22. |
| Tuberous sclerosis | Findings: facial lesions (adenoma sebaceum), hypopigmented "ash leaf spots" on skin, cortical and retinal hamartomas, seizures, mental retardation, renal cysts and renal angiomyolipomas, cardiac rhabdomyomas, ↑ incidence of astrocytomas. Incomplete penetrance, variable presentation. |
| von Hippel–Lindau disease | Findings: hemangioblastomas of retina/cerebellum/medulla; about half of affected individuals develop multiple bilateral renal cell carcinomas and other tumors. Associated with deletion of *VHL* gene (tumor suppressor) on chromosome 3 (3p). Results in constitutive expression of HIF (transcription factor) and activation of angiogenic growth factors. Von Hippel–Lindau = 3 words for chromosome 3. |

| | | |
|---|---|---|
| **Autosomal-recessive diseases** | Albinism, ARPKD (formerly known as infantile polycystic kidney disease), cystic fibrosis, glycogen storage diseases, hemochromatosis, mucopolysaccharidoses (except Hunter's), phenylketonuria, sickle cell anemias, sphingolipidoses (except Fabry's), thalassemias. | |
| **Cystic fibrosis** | Autosomal-recessive defect in **CFTR gene** on chromosome 7, commonly deletion of Phe 508. CFTR channel actively secretes $Cl^-$ in lungs and GI tract and actively reabsorbs $Cl^-$ from sweat. Defective $Cl^-$ channel → secretion of abnormally thick mucus that plugs lungs, pancreas, and liver → recurrent pulmonary infections (*Pseudomonas* species and *S. aureus*), chronic bronchitis, bronchiectasis, pancreatic insufficiency (malabsorption and steatorrhea), meconium ileus in newborns. Mutation causes abnormal protein folding, resulting in degradation of channel before reaching cell surface. | Infertility in males due to bilateral absence of vas deferens. Fat-soluble vitamin deficiencies (A, D, E, K). Can present as failure to thrive in infancy. Most common lethal genetic disease of Caucasians. ↑ concentration of $Cl^-$ ions in sweat test is diagnostic. Treatment: N-acetylcysteine to loosen mucous plugs (cleaves disulfide bonds within mucous glycoproteins). |
| **X-linked recessive disorders** | Bruton's agammaglobulinemia, Wiskott-Aldrich syndrome, Fabry's disease, G6PD deficiency, Ocular albinism, Lesch-Nyhan syndrome, Duchenne's (and Becker's) muscular dystrophy, Hunter's Syndrome, Hemophilia A and B. Female carriers are rarely affected due to random inactivation of an X chromosome in each cell. | Be Wise, Fool's **GOLD** Heeds Silly Hope. |
| **Muscular dystrophies** | | |
| Duchenne's | X-linked frame-shift mutation → deletion of dystrophin gene → accelerated muscle breakdown. Weakness begins in pelvic girdle muscles and progresses superiorly. Pseudohypertrophy of calf muscles due to fibrofatty replacement of muscle; cardiac myopathy. Use of Gowers' maneuver, requiring assistance of the upper extremities to stand up, is characteristic. Onset before 5 years of age. | Duchenne's = Deleted Dystrophin. Dystrophin gene (**DMD**) is the longest known human gene → ↑ rate of spontaneous mutation. Dystrophin helps anchor muscle fibers, primarily in skeletal and cardiac muscle. Diagnose muscular dystrophies by ↑ CPK and muscle biopsy. |
| Becker's | X-linked mutated dystrophin gene. Less severe than Duchenne's. Onset in adolescence or early adulthood. | |
| **Fragile X syndrome** | X-linked defect affecting the methylation and expression of the **FMR1 gene**. Associated with chromosomal breakage. The 2nd most common cause of genetic mental retardation (after Down syndrome). Findings: macro-orchidism (enlarged testes), long face with a large jaw, large everted ears, autism, mitral valve prolapse. | Trinucleotide repeat disorder $(CGG)_n$. Fragile **X** = eXtra-large testes, jaw, ears. |

| | | |
|---|---|---|
| **Trinucleotide repeat expansion diseases** | Huntington's disease, myotonic dystrophy, Friedreich's ataxia, fragile **X** syndrome.<br><br>Huntington's disease = $(CAG)_n$.<br>MyoTonic dystrophy = $(CTG)_n$.<br>FraGile X syndrome = $(CGG)_n$.<br>Friedreich's ataxia = $(GAA)_n$. | Try (trinucleotide) **hunting** for **my fried** eggs (**X**).<br>May show genetic anticipation (disease severity ↑ and age of onset ↓ in successive generations; germline expansion in females). |

**Autosomal trisomies**

| | | |
|---|---|---|
| Down syndrome (trisomy 21), 1:700 | Findings: mental retardation, **flat facies**, prominent **epicanthal folds, simian crease** (see Image 100), gap between 1st 2 toes, duodenal atresia, congenital heart disease (most commonly septum primum–type ASD). Associated with ↑ risk of ALL and Alzheimer's disease (> 35 years of age).<br>95% of cases due to meiotic nondisjunction of homologous chromosomes (associated with advanced maternal age; from 1:1500 in women < 20 to 1:25 in women > 45).<br>4% of cases due to robertsonian translocation.<br>1% of cases due to Down mosaicism (no maternal association). | Drinking age (21).<br>Most common chromosomal disorder and most common cause of congenital mental retardation.<br>Results of pregnancy quad screen: ↓ α-fetoprotein, ↑ β-hCG, ↓ estriol, ↑ inhibin A.<br>Ultrasound shows ↑ nuchal translucency. |
| Edwards' syndrome (trisomy 18), 1:8000 | Findings: severe mental retardation, rocker-bottom feet, **micrognathia** (small jaw), low-set ears, **clenched hands,** prominent occiput, congenital heart disease. Death usually occurs within 1 year of birth. | Election age (18).<br>Most common trisomy resulting in live birth after Down syndrome. |
| Patau's syndrome (trisomy 13), 1:15,000 | Findings: severe mental retardation, rocker-bottom feet, microphthalmia, microcephaly, **cleft lip/ Palate, holoProsencephaly, Polydactyly,** congenital heart disease. Death usually occurs within 1 year of birth. | Puberty (13). |

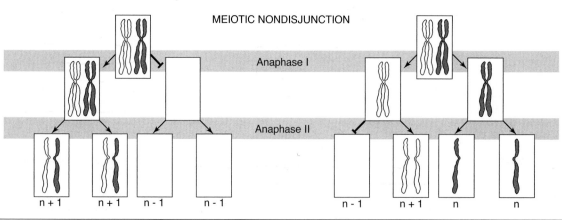

MEIOTIC NONDISJUNCTION

Anaphase I

Anaphase II

n + 1    n + 1    n − 1    n − 1          n − 1    n + 1    n    n

| | | |
|---|---|---|
| **Robertsonian translocation** | Nonreciprocal chromosomal translocation that commonly involves chromosome pairs 13, 14, 15, 21, and 22. One of the most common types of translocation. Occurs when the long arms of 2 acrocentric chromosomes (chromosomes with centromeres near their ends) fuse at the centromere and the 2 short arms are lost. Balanced translocations normally do not cause any abnormal phenotype. Unbalanced translocations can result in miscarriage, stillbirth, and chromosomal imbalance (e.g., Down syndrome, Patau's syndrome). | |
| **Chromosomal inversions** | Chromosome rearrangement in which a segment of a chromosome is reversed end to end. May result in ↓ fertility. | |
|    Pericentric | Involves centromere; proceeds through meiosis. | |
|    Paracentric | Does not involve centromere; does not proceed through meiosis. | |
| **Cri-du-chat syndrome** | Congenital microdeletion of short arm of chromosome 5 (46,XX or XY, 5p–). Findings: microcephaly, moderate to severe mental retardation, high-pitched crying/mewing, epicanthal folds, cardiac abnormalities. | *Cri du chat* = cry of the cat. |
| **Williams syndrome** | Congenital microdeletion of long arm of chromosome 7 (deleted region includes elastin gene). Findings: distinctive "elfin" facies, mental retardation, hypercalcemia (↑ sensitivity to vitamin D), well-developed verbal skills, extreme friendliness with strangers, cardiovascular problems. | |
| **22q11 deletion syndromes** | Variable presentation, including Cleft palate, Abnormal facies, Thymic aplasia → T-cell deficiency, Cardiac defects, Hypocalcemia 2° to parathyroid aplasia, due to microdeletion at chromosome 22q11. DiGeorge syndrome—thymic, parathyroid, and cardiac defects. Velocardiofacial syndrome—palate, facial, and cardiac defects. | CATCH-22. Due to aberrant development of 3rd and 4th branchial pouches. |

## Vitamins

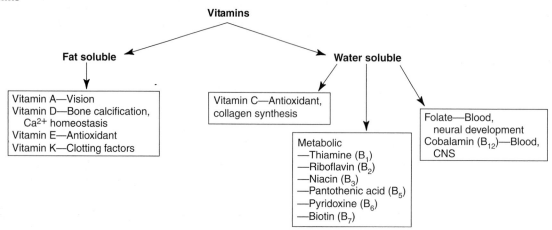

| Vitamins: fat soluble | A, D, E, K. Absorption dependent on gut (ileum) and pancreas. Toxicity more common than for water-soluble vitamins, because these accumulate in fat. | Malabsorption syndromes (steatorrhea), such as cystic fibrosis and sprue, or mineral oil intake can cause fat-soluble vitamin deficiencies. |
|---|---|---|
| Vitamins: water soluble | $B_1$ (thiamine: TPP)<br>$B_2$ (riboflavin: FAD, FMN)<br>$B_3$ (niacin: $NAD^+$)<br>$B_5$ (pantothenic acid: CoA)<br>$B_6$ (pyridoxine: PLP)<br>$B_{12}$ (cobalamin)<br>C (ascorbic acid)<br>Biotin<br>Folate | All wash out easily from body except $B_{12}$ and folate (stored in liver).<br>B-complex deficiencies often result in dermatitis, glossitis, and diarrhea. |

### Vitamin A (retinol)

| Function | Antioxidant; constituent of visual pigments (retinal); essential for normal differentiation of epithelial cells into specialized tissue (pancreatic cells, mucus-secreting cells). | **Retinol** is vitamin **A**, so think **Retin-A** (used topically for wrinkles and acne). |
|---|---|---|
| Deficiency | Night blindness, dry skin. | Found in liver and leafy vegetables. |
| Excess | Arthralgias, fatigue, headaches, skin changes, sore throat, alopecia. Teratogenic (cleft palate, cardiac abnormalities), so a pregnancy test must be done before isotretinoin is prescribed for severe acne. | |

## Vitamin B$_1$ (thiamine)

| | | |
|---|---|---|
| Function | In thiamine pyrophosphate (TPP), a cofactor for several enzymes:<br>1. Pyruvate dehydrogenase (glycolysis)<br>2. α-ketoglutarate dehydrogenase (TCA cycle)<br>3. Transketolase (HMP shunt)<br>4. Branched-chain AA dehydrogenase | Spell beriberi as **Ber1Ber1.**<br>Wernicke-Korsakoff—confusion, ophthalmoplegia, ataxia + memory loss, confabulation, personality change. |
| Deficiency | Impaired glucose breakdown → ATP depletion; highly aerobic tissues (brain and heart) are affected first. Wernicke-Korsakoff syndrome and beriberi. Seen in malnutrition as well as alcoholism (2° to malnutrition and malabsorption). | Dry beriberi—polyneuritis, symmetrical muscle wasting.<br>Wet beriberi—high-output cardiac failure (dilated cardiomyopathy), edema. |

## Vitamin B$_2$ (riboflavin)

| | | |
|---|---|---|
| Function | Cofactor in oxidation and reduction (e.g., FADH$_2$). | FAD and FMN are derived from riboFlavin (B$_2$ = 2 ATP). |
| Deficiency | Cheilosis (inflammation of lips, scaling and fissures at the corners of the mouth), Corneal vascularization. | The **2 C's.** |

## Vitamin B$_3$ (niacin)

| | | |
|---|---|---|
| Function | Constituent of NAD$^+$, NADP$^+$ (used in redox reactions). Derived from tryptophan. Synthesis requires vitamin B$_6$. | **NAD** derived from **N**iacin (B$_3$ = 3 ATP). |
| Deficiency | Glossitis. Severe deficiency leads to pellagra, which can be caused by Hartnup disease (↓ tryptophan absorption), malignant carcinoid syndrome (↑ tryptophan metabolism), and INH (↓ vitamin B$_6$). | The **3 D's:** of pellagra: **D**iarrhea, **D**ermatitis, **D**ementia. |
| Excess | Facial flushing (due to pharmacologic doses for treatment of hyperlipidemia). | Vitamin B$_3$ in corn not absorbable unless treated. Excess untreated corn in diet can lead to pellagra. |

## Vitamin B$_5$ (pantothenate)

| | | |
|---|---|---|
| Function | Essential component of CoA (a cofactor for acyl transfers) and fatty acid synthase. | Pantothen-**A** is in Co-**A.** |
| Deficiency | Dermatitis, enteritis, alopecia, adrenal insufficiency. | |

## Vitamin B$_6$ (pyridoxine)

| | |
|---|---|
| Function | Converted to pyridoxal phosphate, a cofactor used in transamination (e.g., ALT and AST), decarboxylation reactions, glycogen phosphorylase, cystathionine synthesis, and heme synthesis. Required for the synthesis of niacin from tryptophan. |
| Deficiency | Convulsions, hyperirritability, peripheral neuropathy (deficiency inducible by INH and oral contraceptives), sideroblastic anemias. |

## Vitamin B$_{12}$ (cobalamin)

| | | |
|---|---|---|
| Function | Cofactor for homocysteine methyltransferase (transfers CH$_3$ groups as methylcobalamin) and methylmalonyl-CoA mutase. | Found in animal products. Synthesized only by microorganisms. Very large reserve pool (several years) stored primarily in the liver. Deficiency is usually caused by malabsorption (sprue, enteritis, *Diphyllobothrium latum*), lack of intrinsic factor (pernicious anemia, gastric bypass surgery), or absence of terminal ileum (Crohn's disease). Use Schilling test to detect the etiology of the deficiency. |
| Deficiency | Macrocytic, megaloblastic anemia, hypersegmented PMNs, neurologic symptoms (paresthesias, subacute combined degeneration) due to abnormal myelin. Prolonged deficiency leads to irreversible nervous system damage. | |

$$\text{Homocysteine} + \text{N-methyl THF} \xrightarrow{\text{B}_{12}} \text{Methionine} + \text{THF}$$

$$\text{Methylmalonyl-CoA} \xrightarrow{\text{B}_{12}} \text{Succinyl-CoA}$$

## Folic acid

| | | |
|---|---|---|
| Function | Converted to tetrahydrofolate (THF), a coenzyme for 1-carbon transfer/methylation reactions. Important for the synthesis of nitrogenous bases in DNA and RNA. | **FOL**ate from **FOL**iage. Small reserve pool stored primarily in the liver. Eat green leaves. |
| Deficiency | Macrocytic, megaloblastic anemia; no neurologic symptoms (as opposed to vitamin B$_{12}$ deficiency). Most common vitamin deficiency in the United States. Seen in alcoholism and pregnancy. | Deficiency can be caused by several drugs (e.g., phenytoin, sulfonamides, MTX). Supplemental folic acid in early pregnancy reduces neural tube defects. |

## *S*-adenosyl-methionine

| | | |
|---|---|---|
| | ATP + methionine → **SAM**. SAM transfers methyl units. Regeneration of methionine (and thus SAM) is dependent on vitamin B$_{12}$ and folate. | **SAM** the methyl donor man. Required for the conversion of NE to epinephrine. |

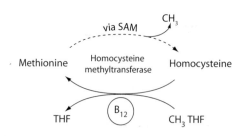

## Biotin

| | | |
|---|---|---|
| Function | Cofactor for carboxylation enzymes (which add a 1-carbon group):<br>1. Pyruvate carboxylase: Pyruvate (3C) $\rightarrow$ oxaloacetate (4C)<br>2. Acetyl-CoA carboxylase: Acetyl-CoA (3C) $\rightarrow$ malonyl-CoA (4C)<br>3. Propionyl-CoA carboxylase: Propionyl-CoA (3C) $\rightarrow$ methylmalonyl-CoA (4C) | "**AVID**in in egg whites **AVID**ly binds biotin." |
| Deficiency | Relatively rare. Dermatitis, alopecia, enteritis. Caused by antibiotic use or excessive ingestion of raw eggs. | |

## Vitamin C (ascorbic acid)

| | | |
|---|---|---|
| Function | Antioxidant. Also:<br>1. Facilitates iron absorption by keeping iron in $Fe^{2+}$ reduced state (more absorbable)<br>2. Necessary for hydroxylation of proline and lysine in collagen synthesis<br>3. Necessary for dopamine β-hydroxylase, which converts dopamine to NE | Found in fruits and vegetables. British sailors carried limes to prevent scurvy (origin of the word "limey"). |
| Deficiency | Scurvy—swollen gums, bruising, anemia, poor wound healing. | |

## Vitamin D

| | | |
|---|---|---|
| | $D_2$ = ergocalciferol—ingested from plants, used as pharmacologic agent.<br>$D_3$ = cholecalciferol—consumed in milk, formed in sun-exposed skin.<br>25-OH $D_3$ = storage form.<br>1,25-$(OH)_2$ $D_3$ (calcitriol) = active form. | Drinking milk (fortified with vitamin D) is good for bones. |
| Function | ↑ intestinal absorption of calcium and phosphate, ↑ bone resorption. | |
| Deficiency | Rickets in children (bending bones), osteomalacia in adults (soft bones), hypocalcemic tetany. | |
| Excess | Hypercalcemia, hypercalciuria, loss of appetite, stupor. Seen in sarcoidosis (↑ activation of vitamin D by epithelioid macrophages). | |

## Vitamin E

| | | |
|---|---|---|
| Function | Antioxidant (protects erythrocytes and membranes from free-radical damage). | E is for Erythrocytes. |
| Deficiency | ↑ fragility of erythrocytes (hemolytic anemia), muscle weakness, neurodysfunction. | |

**Vitamin K**

Function  Catalyzes γ-carboxylation of glutamic acid residues on various proteins concerned with blood clotting. Synthesized by intestinal flora.

**K** for **K**oagulation. Necessary for the synthesis of clotting factors II, VII, IX, X, and protein C and S. Warfarin—vitamin K antagonist.

Deficiency  Neonatal hemorrhage with ↑ PT and ↑ aPTT but normal bleeding time (neonates have sterile intestines and are unable to synthesize vitamin K). Can also occur after prolonged use of broad-spectrum antibiotics.

Neonates are given vitamin K injection at birth to prevent hemorrhage.

**Zinc**

Function  Essential for the activity of 100+ enzymes. Important in the formation of zinc fingers (transcription factor motif).

Deficiency  Delayed wound healing, hypogonadism, ↓ adult hair (axillary, facial, pubic), dysgeusia, anosmia. May predispose to alcoholic cirrhosis.

**Ethanol metabolism**

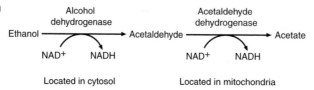

NAD⁺ is the limiting reagent.
Alcohol dehydrogenase operates via zero-order kinetics.

Fomepizole—inhibits alcohol dehydrogenase.
Disulfiram (Antabuse)—inhibits acetaldehyde dehydrogenase (acetaldehyde accumulates, contributing to hangover symptoms).

**Ethanol hypoglycemia**

Ethanol metabolism ↑ NADH/NAD⁺ ratio in liver, causing diversion of pyruvate to lactate and OAA to malate, thereby inhibiting gluconeogenesis and stimulating fatty acid synthesis. Leads to hypoglycemia and hepatic fatty change (hepatocellular steatosis) seen in chronic alcoholics.

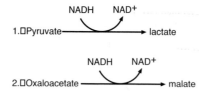

**Kwashiorkor vs. marasmus**

Kwashiorkor—protein malnutrition resulting in skin lesions, edema, liver malfunction (fatty change due to ↓ apolipoprotein synthesis). Clinical picture is small child with swollen belly.

Marasmus—energy malnutrition resulting in tissue and muscle wasting, loss of subcutaneous fat, and variable edema.

Kwashiorkor results from a protein-deficient **MEAL**:
Malnutrition
Edema
Anemia
Liver (fatty)
Marasmus results in
Muscle wasting.

## Metabolism sites

| | |
|---|---|
| Mitochondria | Fatty acid oxidation (β-oxidation), acetyl-CoA production, TCA cycle, oxidative phosphorylation. |
| Cytoplasm | Glycolysis, fatty acid synthesis, HMP shunt, protein synthesis (RER), steroid synthesis (SER). |
| Both | Heme synthesis, Urea cycle, Gluconeogenesis. **HUGs take two.** |

## Enzyme terminology

An enzyme's name often describes its function. For example, glucokinase is an enzyme that catalyzes the phosphorylation of glucose using a molecule of ATP. The following are commonly used enzyme descriptors:

1. Kinase—uses ATP to add high-energy phosphate group onto substrate (e.g., phosphofructokinase)
2. Phosphorylase—adds inorganic phosphate onto substrate without using ATP (e.g., glycogen phosphorylase)
3. Phosphatase—removes phosphate group from substrate (e.g., fructose-1,6-bisphosphatase)
4. Dehydrogenase—oxidizes substrate (e.g., pyruvate dehydrogenase)
5. Carboxylase—adds 1 carbon with the help of biotin (e.g., pyruvate carboxylase)

## Rate-determining enzymes of metabolic processes

| Process | Enzyme |
|---|---|
| Glycolysis | Phosphofructokinase-1 (PFK-1) |
| Gluconeogenesis | Fructose-1,6-bisphosphatase |
| TCA cycle | Isocitrate dehydrogenase |
| Glycogen synthesis | Glycogen synthase |
| Glycogenolysis | Glycogen phosphorylase |
| HMP shunt | Glucose-6-phosphate dehydrogenase (G6PD) |
| De novo pyrimidine synthesis | Carbamoyl phosphate synthetase II |
| De novo purine synthesis | Glutamine-PRPP amidotransferase |
| Urea cycle | Carbamoyl phosphate synthetase I |
| Fatty acid synthesis | Acetyl-CoA carboxylase (ACC) |
| Fatty acid oxidation | Carnitine acyltransferase I |
| Ketogenesis | HMG-CoA synthase |
| Cholesterol synthesis | HMG-CoA reductase |

## Summary of pathways

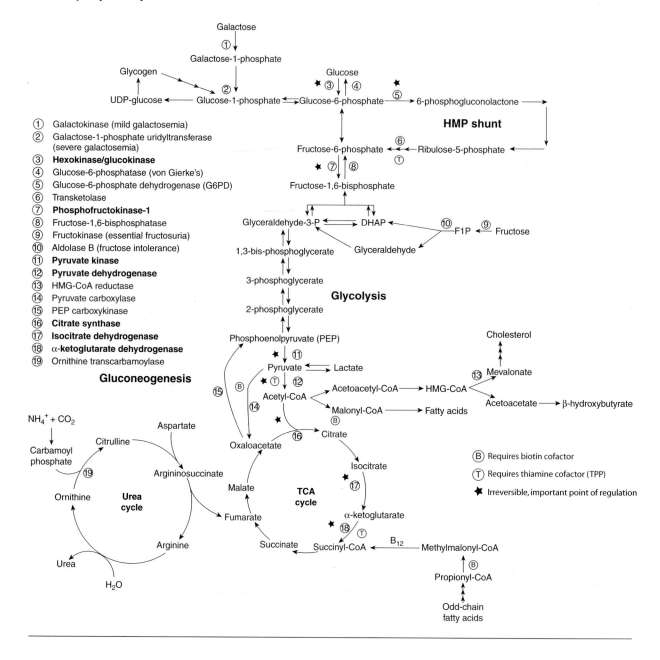

① Galactokinase (mild galactosemia)
② Galactose-1-phosphate uridyltransferase (severe galactosemia)
③ **Hexokinase/glucokinase**
④ Glucose-6-phosphatase (von Gierke's)
⑤ Glucose-6-phosphate dehydrogenase (G6PD)
⑥ Transketolase
⑦ **Phosphofructokinase-1**
⑧ Fructose-1,6-bisphosphatase
⑨ Fructokinase (essential fructosuria)
⑩ Aldolase B (fructose intolerance)
⑪ **Pyruvate kinase**
⑫ **Pyruvate dehydrogenase**
⑬ HMG-CoA reductase
⑭ Pyruvate carboxylase
⑮ PEP carboxykinase
⑯ **Citrate synthase**
⑰ **Isocitrate dehydrogenase**
⑱ **α-ketoglutarate dehydrogenase**
⑲ Ornithine transcarbamoylase

Ⓑ Requires biotin cofactor
Ⓣ Requires thiamine cofactor (TPP)
★ Irreversible, important point of regulation

| | |
|---|---|
| **Glycolysis/ATP production** | Aerobic metabolism of glucose produces 32 ATP via malate-aspartate shuttle (heart and liver), 30 ATP via glycerol-3-phosphate shuttle (muscle).<br>Anaerobic glycolysis produces only 2 net ATP per glucose molecule.<br>ATP hydrolysis can be coupled to energetically unfavorable reactions. |

(Reproduced, with permission, from Murray RK et al. *Harper's Illustrated Biochemistry*, 27th ed. New York: McGraw-Hill, 2005: Fig. 11-4.)

| | | |
|---|---|---|
| **Activated carriers** | Phosphoryl (ATP).<br>Electrons (NADH, NADPH, FADH$_2$).<br>Acyl (coenzyme A, lipoamide).<br>CO$_2$ (biotin).<br>1-carbon units (tetrahydrofolates).<br>CH$_3$ groups (SAM).<br>Aldehydes (TPP). | |
| **Universal electron acceptors** | Nicotinamides (**NAD$^+$**, **NADP$^+$**) and flavin nucleotides (**FAD$^+$**).<br>**NAD$^+$** is generally used in **catabolic** processes to carry reducing equivalents away as NADH.<br>**NADPH** is used in **anabolic** processes (steroid and fatty acid synthesis) as a supply of reducing equivalents. | NADPH is a product of the HMP shunt.<br><br>NADPH is used in:<br>1. Anabolic processes<br>2. Respiratory burst<br>3. P-450<br>4. Glutathione reductase |
| **Hexokinase vs. glucokinase** | Phosphorylation of glucose to yield glucose-6-phosphate serves as the 1st step of glycolysis (also serves as the first step of glycogen synthesis in the liver). Reaction is catalyzed by either hexokinase or glucokinase, depending on the location. | |
| Hexokinase | Ubiquitous. High affinity (low K$_m$), low capacity (low V$_{max}$), uninduced by insulin. | Feedback inhibited by glucose-6-phosphate. |
| Glucokinase | Liver and β cells of pancreas. Low affinity (high K$_m$), high capacity (high V$_{max}$), induced by insulin. (**GLU**cokinase is a **GLU**tton. It has a high V$_{max}$ because it cannot be satisfied.) | No direct feedback inhibition. Phosphorylates excess glucose (e.g., after a meal) to sequester it in the liver. Allows liver to serve as a blood glucose "buffer." |

**Glycolysis regulation, key enzymes**

Net glycolysis (cytoplasm):
Glucose + 2 $P_i$ + 2 ADP + 2 $NAD^+$ → 2 pyruvate + 2 ATP + 2 NADH + $2H^+$ + $2H_2O$.

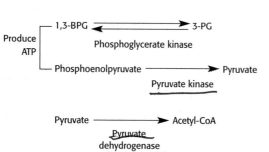

Glucose ⟶ Glucose-6-phosphate
Hexokinase/glucokinase*

Require ATP

Fructose-6-P ⟶ Fructose-1,6-BP
Phosphofructokinase-1
(rate-limiting step)

Glucose-6-P ⊖.

ATP ⊖, AMP ⊕, citrate ⊖, fructose-2,6-BP ⊕.

Produce ATP

1,3-BPG ⟶ 3-PG
Phosphoglycerate kinase

Phosphoenolpyruvate ⟶ Pyruvate
Pyruvate kinase

ATP ⊖, alanine ⊖, fructose-1,6-BP ⊕.

Pyruvate ⟶ Acetyl-CoA
Pyruvate dehydrogenase

ATP ⊖, NADH ⊖, acetyl-CoA ⊖.

* Glucokinase in liver; hexokinase in all other tissues.

---

**Regulation by F2,6BP**

Gluconeogenesis ← Fructose-6-phosphate ⇄ F1,6BP ⟶ Glycolysis
FBPase-1
PFK-1

Fructose bisphosphatase 2 (active in fasting state) | Phosphofructokinase 2 (active in fed state) | (+)

Fructose-2,6-bisphosphate

FBPase-2 and PFK-2 are part of the same complex but respond in opposite manners to phosphorylation by protein kinase A.
Fasting state: ↑ glucagon → ↑ cAMP → ↑ protein kinase A → ↑ FBPase-2, ↓ PFK-2.
Fed state: ↑ insulin → ↓ cAMP → ↓ protein kinase A → ↓ FBPase-2, ↑ PFK-2.

---

**Glycolytic enzyme deficiency**

Associated with **hemolytic anemia**. Inability to maintain activity of $Na^+$-$K^+$ ATPase leads to RBC swelling and lysis.
Due to deficiencies in pyruvate kinase (95%), phosphoglucose isomerase (4%), and other glycolytic enzymes.

RBCs metabolize glucose anaerobically (no mitochondria) and thus depend solely on glycolysis.

| | | |
|---|---|---|
| **Pyruvate dehydrogenase complex** | Reaction: pyruvate + $NAD^+$ + CoA → acetyl-CoA + $CO_2$ + NADH.<br>The complex contains 3 enzymes that require 5 cofactors:<br>    1. Pyrophosphate ($B_1$, thiamine; TPP)<br>    2. FAD ($B_2$, riboflavin)<br>    3. NAD ($B_3$, niacin)<br>    4. CoA ($B_5$, pantothenate)<br>    5. Lipoic acid<br>Activated by exercise:<br>  ↑ $NAD^+$/NADH ratio<br>  ↑ ADP<br>  ↑ $Ca^{2+}$ | The complex is similar to the α-ketoglutarate dehydrogenase complex (same cofactors, similar substrate and action), which converts α-ketoglutarate → succinyl-CoA (TCA cycle).<br>**Arsenic** inhibits lipoic acid.<br>  Findings: vomiting, rice water stools, garlic breath. |
| **Pyruvate dehydrogenase deficiency** | Causes backup of substrate (pyruvate and alanine), resulting in lactic acidosis. Can be congenital or acquired (as in alcoholics due to $B_1$ deficiency).<br>Findings: neurologic defects.<br>Treatment: ↑ intake of ketogenic nutrients (e.g., high fat content or ↑ lysine and leucine). | **Lysine** and **Leucine**—the only purely ketogenic amino acids. |

**Pyruvate metabolism**

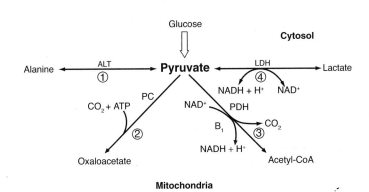

Functions of different pyruvate metabolic pathways:
1. Alanine carries amino groups to the liver from muscle
2. Oxaloacetate can replenish TCA cycle or be used in gluconeogenesis
3. Transition from glycolysis to the TCA cycle
4. End of anaerobic glycolysis (major pathway in RBCs, leukocytes, kidney medulla, lens, testes, and cornea)

**Cori cycle**

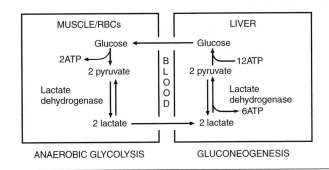

The Cori cycle allows lactate generated during anaerobic metabolism to undergo hepatic gluconeogenesis and become a source of glucose for muscle/RBCs. This comes at the cost of a net loss of 4 ATP/cycle.
Shifts metabolic burden to the liver.

**TCA cycle (Krebs cycle)**

Pyruvate → acetyl-CoA produces 1 NADH, 1 $CO_2$.

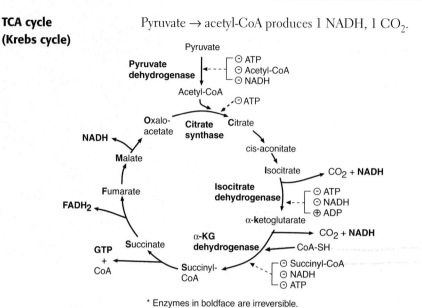

* Enzymes in boldface are irreversible.

The TCA cycle produces 3 NADH, 1 $FADH_2$, 2 $CO_2$, 1 GTP per acetyl-CoA = 12 ATP/acetyl-CoA (2× everything per glucose). TCA cycle reactions occur in the mitochondria.

α-ketoglutarate dehydrogenase complex requires the same cofactors as the pyruvate dehydrogenase complex ($B_1$, $B_2$, $B_3$, $B_5$, lipoic acid).

Citrate Is Krebs' Starting Substrate For Making Oxaloacetate.

---

**Electron transport chain and oxidative phosphorylation**

NADH electrons from glycolysis and the TCA cycle enter mitochondria via the malate-aspartate or glycerol-3-phosphate shuttle. $FADH_2$ electrons are transferred to complex II (at a lower energy level than NADH). The passage of electrons results in the formation of a proton gradient that, coupled to oxidative phosphorylation, drives the production of ATP.

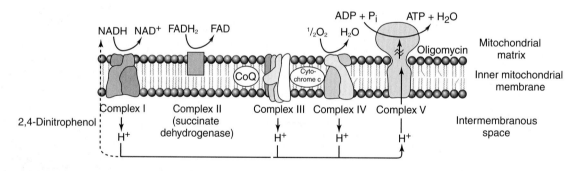

ATP produced via ATP synthase: 1 NADH → 3 ATP; 1 $FADH_2$ → 2 ATP.

**Oxidative phosphorylation poisons**

| | | |
|---|---|---|
| Electron transport inhibitors | Directly inhibit electron transport, causing a ↓ proton gradient and block of ATP synthesis. | Rotenone, $CN^-$, antimycin A, CO. |
| ATPase inhibitors | Directly inhibit mitochondrial ATPase, causing an ↑ proton gradient. No ATP is produced because electron transport stops. | Oligomycin. |
| Uncoupling agents | ↑ permeability of membrane, causing a ↓ proton gradient and ↑ $O_2$ consumption. ATP synthesis stops, but electron transport continues. Produces heat. | 2,4-DNP, aspirin (fevers often occur after aspirin overdose), thermogenin in brown fat. |

## Gluconeogenesis, irreversible enzymes

| | | |
|---|---|---|
| Pyruvate carboxylase | In mitochondria. Pyruvate $\rightarrow$ oxaloacetate. | Requires biotin, ATP. Activated by acetyl-CoA. |
| PEP carboxykinase | In cytosol. Oxaloacetate $\rightarrow$ phosphoenolpyruvate. | Requires GTP. |
| Fructose-1,6-bisphosphatase | In cytosol. Fructose-1,6-bisphosphate $\rightarrow$ fructose-6-P. | |
| Glucose-6-phosphatase | In ER. Glucose-6-P $\rightarrow$ glucose. | **Pathway Produces Fresh Glucose.** |

Occurs primarily in liver. Enzymes also found in kidney, intestinal epithelium. Deficiency of the key gluconeogenic enzymes causes hypoglycemia. (Muscle cannot participate in gluconeogenesis because it lacks glucose-6-phosphatase.)

Odd-chain fatty acids yield 1 propionyl-CoA during metabolism, which can enter the TCA cycle (as succinyl-CoA), undergo gluconeogenesis, and serve as a glucose source. Even-chain fatty acids cannot produce new glucose, since they yield only acetyl-CoA equivalents.

## HMP shunt (pentose phosphate pathway)

Purpose is to provide a source of NADPH from an abundantly available glucose-6-phosphate (NADPH is required for reductive reactions, e.g., glutathione reduction inside RBCs). Additionally, this pathway yields ribose for nucleotide synthesis and glycolytic intermediates. 2 distinct phases (oxidative and nonoxidative), both of which occur in the cytoplasm. No ATP is used or produced.

Sites: lactating mammary glands, liver, adrenal cortex (sites of fatty acid or steroid synthesis), RBCs.

| Reactions | Key enzymes | Products |
|---|---|---|
| Oxidative (irreversible) | Glucose-6-P$_i$ ⟶ **Glucose-6-P dehydrogenase** ⟶ Rate-limiting step | $CO_2$ 2 NADPH Ribulose-5-P$_i$ |
| Nonoxidative (reversible) | Ribulose-5-P$_i$ ⟶ **Transketolases** ⟶ Requires B$_1$ | Ribulose-6-P$_i$ G3P F6P |

**Respiratory burst (oxidative burst)**

Involves the activation of membrane-bound NADPH oxidase (e.g., in neutrophils, macrophages). Plays an important role in the immune response → results in the rapid release of reactive oxygen intermediates (ROIs).

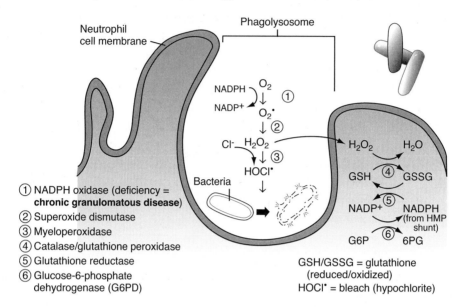

① NADPH oxidase (deficiency = **chronic granulomatous disease**)
② Superoxide dismutase
③ Myeloperoxidase
④ Catalase/glutathione peroxidase
⑤ Glutathione reductase
⑥ Glucose-6-phosphate dehydrogenase (G6PD)

GSH/GSSG = glutathione (reduced/oxidized)
HOCl• = bleach (hypochlorite)

WBCs of patients with CGD can utilize $H_2O_2$ generated by invading organisms and convert it to ROIs. Patients are at ↑ risk for infection by catalase-positive species (e.g., *S. aureus*, *Aspergillus*) because they neutralize their own $H_2O_2$, leaving WBCs without ROIs for fighting infections.

---

**Glucose-6-phosphate dehydrogenase deficiency**

NADPH is necessary to keep glutathione reduced, which in turn detoxifies free radicals and peroxides. ↓ NADPH in RBCs leads to **hemolytic anemia** due to poor RBC defense against oxidizing agents (e.g., fava beans, sulfonamides, primaquine, antituberculosis drugs). Infection can also precipitate hemolysis (free radicals generated via inflammatory response can diffuse into RBCs and cause oxidative damage).

**X-linked recessive** disorder; most common human enzyme deficiency; more prevalent among blacks. ↑ malarial resistance.

**Heinz bodies**—oxidized Hemoglobin precipitated within RBCs.

**Bite cells**—result from the phagocytic removal of Heinz bodies by macrophages.

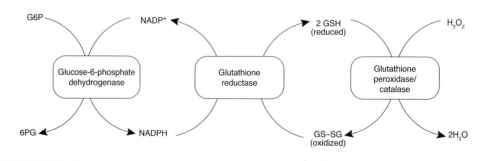

---

## Disorders of fructose metabolism

| | |
|---|---|
| Fructose intolerance | Hereditary deficiency of **aldolase B.** Autosomal recessive. Fructose-1-phosphate accumulates, causing a ↓ in available phosphate, which results in inhibition of glycogenolysis and gluconeogenesis. |
| | Symptoms: hypoglycemia, jaundice, cirrhosis, vomiting. |
| | Treatment: ↓ intake of both fructose and sucrose (glucose + fructose). |
| Essential fructosuria | Involves a defect in **fructokinase.** Autosomal recessive. A benign, asymptomatic condition, since fructose does not enter cells. |
| | Symptoms: fructose appears in blood and urine. |
| | Disorders of fructose metabolism cause milder symptoms than analogous disorders of galactose metabolism. |

**FRUCTOSE METABOLISM (LIVER)**

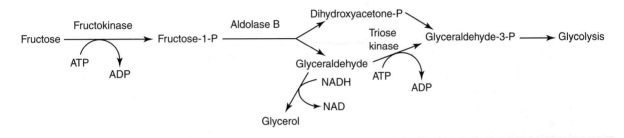

## Disorders of galactose metabolism

| | |
|---|---|
| Classic galactosemia | Absence of **galactose-1-phosphate uridyltransferase.** Autosomal recessive. Damage is caused by accumulation of toxic substances (including galactitol, which accumulates in the lens of the eye). |
| | Symptoms: failure to thrive, jaundice, hepatomegaly, infantile cataracts, mental retardation. |
| | Treatment: exclude galactose and lactose (galactose + glucose) from diet. |
| Galactokinase deficiency | Hereditary deficiency of **galactokinase.** Galactitol accumulates if galactose is present in diet. Relatively mild condition. Autosomal recessive. |
| | Symptoms: galactose appears in blood and urine, infantile cataracts. May initially present as failure to track objects or to develop a social smile. |

**GALACTOSE METABOLISM**

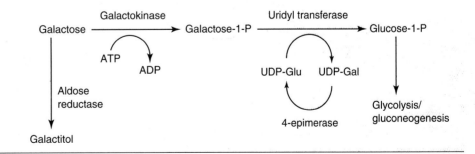

**Sorbitol**

An alternative method of trapping glucose in the cell is to convert it to its alcohol counterpart, called sorbitol, via **aldose reductase.** Some tissues then convert sorbitol to fructose using **sorbitol dehydrogenase;** tissues lacking this enzyme are at risk for sorbitol accumulation.

Liver, ovaries, and seminal vesicles have both enzymes.

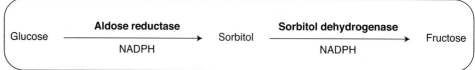

Schwann cells, lens, retina, and kidneys have only aldose reductase.

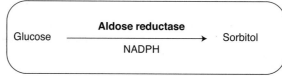

Sorbitol is osmotically active because it cannot freely cross the membrane like glucose. Prolonged hyperglycemic states (e.g., diabetes) lead to sorbitol accumulation, which creates an osmotic pressure that causes water to enter the cell and produce osmotic damage. Examples include cataracts, retinopathy, and peripheral neuropathy, all of which are seen in chronic diabetes.

High blood levels of fructose and galactose also result in conversion to their respective alcohol forms via aldose reductase, and these are also osmotically active.

**Lactase deficiency**

Age-dependent and/or hereditary lactose intolerance (African Americans, Asians) due to loss of brush-border enzyme. May also follow gastroenteritis.

Symptoms: bloating, cramps, osmotic diarrhea.

Treatment: avoid dairy products or add lactase pills to diet.

**Amino acids**

Only L-form amino acids are found in proteins.

Essential

Glucogenic: Met, Val, Arg, His.
Glucogenic/ketogenic: Ile, Phe, Thr, Trp.
Ketogenic: Leu, Lys.

All essential AA need to be supplied in the diet. Glucogenic AA can be converted into glucose via gluconeogenesis. Ketogenic AA form ketone bodies.

Acidic

Asp and Glu (negatively charged at body pH).

Basic

Arg, Lys, and His.

Arg is most basic.
His has no charge at body pH.

Arg and His are required during periods of growth. Arg and Lys are ↑ in histones, which bind negatively charged DNA.

| **Urea cycle** | Amino acid catabolism results in the formation of common metabolites (e.g., pyruvate, acetyl-CoA), which serve as metabolic fuels. Excess nitrogen ($NH_4^+$) generated by this process is converted to urea and excreted by the kidneys. | **O**rdinarily, **C**areless **C**rappers **A**re **A**lso **F**rivolous **A**bout **U**rination. |

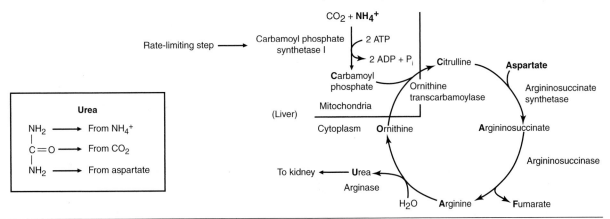

**Transport of ammonium by alanine and glutamine**

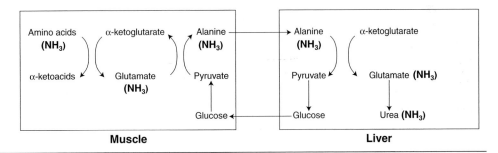

| **Hyperammonemia** | Can be acquired (e.g., liver disease) or hereditary (e.g., urea cycle enzyme deficiencies). Results in excess $NH_4^+$, which depletes α-ketoglutarate, leading to inhibition of TCA cycle. Treatment: limit protein in diet. Benzoate or phenylbutyrate (both of which bind amino acid and lead to excretion) may be given to ↓ ammonia levels. | **Ammonia intoxication**—tremor, slurring of speech, somnolence, vomiting, cerebral edema, blurring of vision. |

| **Ornithine transcarbamoylase (OTC) deficiency** | Most common urea cycle disorder. X-linked recessive (vs. other urea cycle enzyme deficiencies, which are autosomal recessive). Interferes with the body's ability to eliminate ammonia. Often evident in the first few days of life, but may present with late onset. Excess carbamoyl phosphate is converted to orotic acid (part of the pyrimidine synthesis pathway). Findings: orotic acid in blood and urine, ↓ BUN, symptoms of hyperammonemia. | |

**Amino acid derivatives**

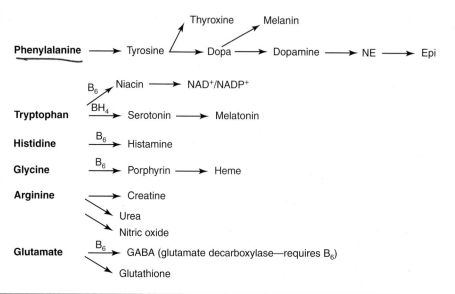

## Catecholamine synthesis

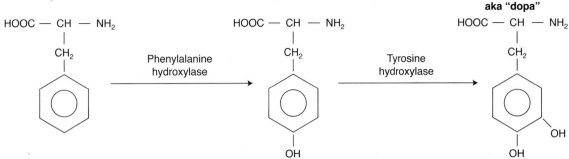

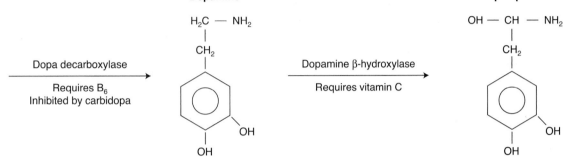

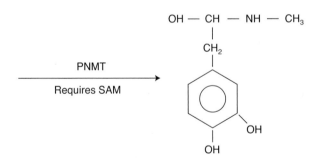

**Breakdown products via MAO and COMT:**
Dopamine → HVA
Norepinephrine → VMA
Epinephrine → Metanephrine

**Enzyme legend:**
• Hydroxylase adds OH
• Decarboxylase removes COOH
• SAM adds CH₃

| | |
|---|---|
| **Phenylketonuria** 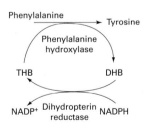 | Due to ↓ phenylalanine hydroxylase or ↓ tetrahydrobiopterin cofactor. Tyrosine becomes essential. ↑ phenylalanine leads to excess phenylketones in urine. |

**Phenylketonuria**

Due to ↓ phenylalanine hydroxylase or ↓ tetrahydrobiopterin cofactor. Tyrosine becomes essential. ↑ phenylalanine leads to excess phenylketones in urine.

Findings: mental retardation, growth retardation, seizures, fair skin, eczema, musty body odor.

Treatment: ↓ **phenylalanine** (contained in aspartame, e.g., NutraSweet) and ↑ **tyrosine** in diet.

**Maternal PKU**—lack of proper dietary therapy during pregnancy. Findings in infant: microcephaly, mental retardation, growth retardation, congenital heart defects.

Screened for 2–3 days after birth (normal at birth because of maternal enzyme during fetal life).

Phenylketones—phenylacetate, phenyllactate, and phenylpyruvate.

Autosomal recessive.

Incidence ≈ 1:10,000.

Disorder of **aromatic** amino acid metabolism → musty body **odor**.

HIGH-YIELD PRINCIPLES

BIOCHEMISTRY

**Alkaptonuria (ochronosis)**

Congenital deficiency of **homogentisic acid oxidase** in the degradative pathway of tyrosine. Autosomal recessive. Benign disease.

Findings: dark connective tissue, pigmented sclera, urine turns black on standing. May have debilitating arthralgias.

**Albinism**

Congenital deficiency of either of the following:
1. Tyrosinase (inability to synthesize melanin from tyrosine)—autosomal recessive
2. Defective tyrosine transporters ($\downarrow$ amounts of tyrosine and thus melanin)

Can result from a lack of migration of neural crest cells.

Lack of melanin results in an $\uparrow$ risk of skin cancer.

Variable inheritance due to locus heterogeneity (vs. ocular albinism—X-linked recessive).

**Homocystinuria**

3 forms (all autosomal recessive):
1. Cystathionine synthase deficiency (treatment: $\downarrow$ Met and $\uparrow$ Cys, and $\uparrow$ $B_{12}$ and folate in diet)
2. $\downarrow$ affinity of cystathionine synthase for pyridoxal phosphate (treatment: $\uparrow\uparrow$ vitamin $B_6$ in diet)
3. Homocysteine methyltransferase deficiency

All forms result in excess homocysteine. Cysteine becomes essential.

Findings: $\uparrow\uparrow$ homocysteine in urine, mental retardation, osteoporosis, tall stature, kyphosis, lens subluxation (downward and inward), and atherosclerosis (stroke and MI).

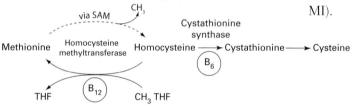

**Cystinuria**

Hereditary defect of renal tubular amino acid transporter for cysteine, ornithine, lysine, and arginine in the PCT of the kidneys.

Excess cystine in urine can lead to the precipitation of **cystine kidney stones** (cystine staghorn calculi).

Autosomal recessive. Common (1:7000). Treatment: acetazolamide to alkalinize the urine.

Cystine is made of 2 cysteines connected by a disulfide bond.

**Maple syrup urine disease**

Blocked degradation of **branched** amino acids (Ile, Leu, Val) due to $\downarrow$ $\alpha$-ketoacid dehydrogenase. Causes $\uparrow$ $\alpha$-ketoacids in the blood, especially Leu.

Causes severe CNS defects, mental retardation, and death.

Urine smells like maple syrup.

**I L**ove **V**ermont maple syrup from maple trees (with **branches**).

**Hartnup disease**

An autosomal-recessive disorder characterized by defective neutral amino acid transporter on renal and intestinal epithelial cells.

Causes tryptophan excretion in urine and absorption from the gut. **Leads to pellagra.**

## Glycogen regulation by insulin and glucagon/epinephrine

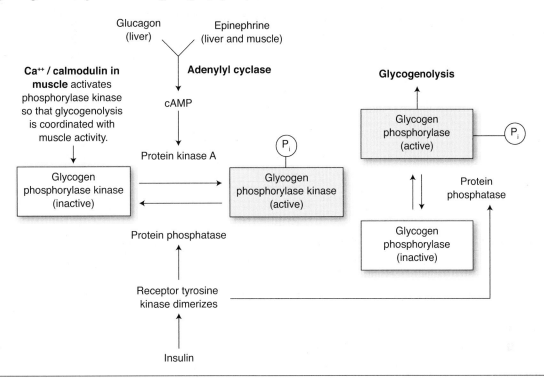

| **Glycogen** | Branches have α (1,6) bonds; linkages have α (1,4) bonds. |
|---|---|
| Skeletal muscle | Glycogen undergoes glycogenolysis to form glucose, which is rapidly metabolized during exercise. |
| Hepatocytes | Glycogen is stored and undergoes glycogenolysis to maintain blood sugar at appropriate levels. |

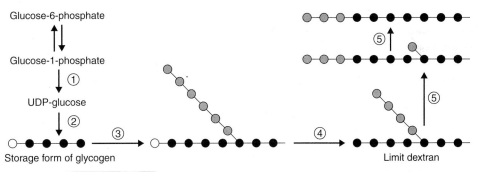

① UDP-glucose pyrophosphorylase
② Glycogen synthase
③ Branching enzyme
④ Glycogen phosphorylase
⑤ Debranching enzyme

Note: A small amount of glycogen is degraded in lysosomes by α-1,4-glucosidase.

## Glycogenolysis/glycogen synthesis

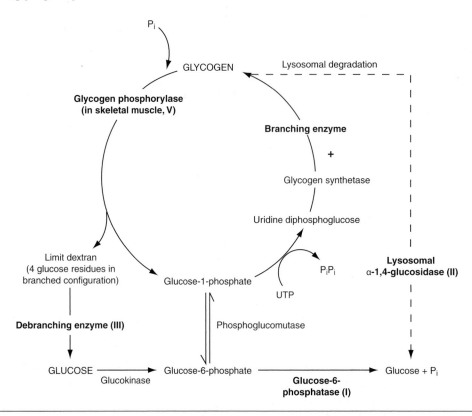

| Glycogen storage diseases | 12 types, all resulting in abnormal glycogen metabolism and an accumulation of glycogen within cells. | Very Poor Carbohydrate Metabolism. |
|---|---|---|

| Disease | Findings | Deficient enzyme | Comments |
|---|---|---|---|
| Von Gierke's disease (type I) | Severe fasting hypoglycemia, ↑↑ glycogen in liver, ↑ blood lactate, hepatomegaly | Glucose-6-phosphatase | |
| Pompe's disease (type II) | Cardiomegaly and systemic findings leading to early death | Lysosomal α-1,4-glucosidase (acid maltase) | Pompe's trashes the Pump (heart, liver, and muscle). |
| Cori's disease (type III) | Milder form of type I with normal blood lactate levels | Debranching enzyme (α-1,6-glucosidase) | Gluconeogenesis is intact. |
| McArdle's disease (type V) | ↑ glycogen in muscle, but cannot break it down, leading to painful muscle cramps, myoglobinuria with strenuous exercise | Skeletal muscle glycogen phosphorylase | McArdle's = Muscle. |

| **Lysosomal storage diseases** | Each is caused by a deficiency in one of the many lysosomal enzymes. Results in an accumulation of abnormal metabolic products. | | | |
|---|---|---|---|---|
| Disease | Findings | Deficient enzyme | Accumulated substrate | Inheritance |
| **Sphingolipidoses** | | | | |
| Fabry's disease | Peripheral neuropathy of hands/feet, angiokeratomas, cardiovascular/renal disease | α-galactosidase A | Ceramide trihexoside | **XR** |
| Gaucher's disease (most common) | Hepatosplenomegaly, aseptic necrosis of femur, bone crises, Gaucher's cells (macrophages that look like crumpled tissue paper) | β-glucocerebrosidase | Glucocerebroside | AR |
| Niemann-Pick disease | Progressive neurodegeneration, hepatosplenomegaly, cherry-red spot on macula, foam cells | Sphingomyelinase | Sphingomyelin | AR |
| Tay-Sachs disease | Progressive neurodegeneration, developmental delay, cherry-red spot on macula, lysosomes with onion skin, no hepatosplenomegaly (vs. Niemann-Pick) | Hexosaminidase A | $GM_2$ ganglioside | AR |
| Krabbe's disease | Peripheral neuropathy, developmental delay, optic atrophy, globoid cells | Galactocerebrosidase | Galactocerebroside | AR |
| Metachromatic leukodystrophy | Central and peripheral demyelination with ataxia, dementia | Arylsulfatase A | Cerebroside sulfate | AR |
| **Mucopolysaccharidoses** | | | | |
| Hurler's syndrome | Developmental delay, gargoylism, airway obstruction, corneal clouding, hepatosplenomegaly | α-L-iduronidase | Heparan sulfate, dermatan sulfate | AR |
| Hunter's syndrome | Mild Hurler's + aggressive behavior, no corneal clouding | Iduronate sulfatase | Heparan sulfate, dermatan sulfate | **XR** |

**No man picks (Niemann-Pick)** his nose with his **sphinger** (**sphing**omyelinase).

Tay-Sa**X** (**Tay-Sachs**) lacks he**X**osaminidase.

**Hunters** see clearly (no corneal clouding) and aim for the **X** (**X**-linked recessive).

↑ incidence of Tay-Sachs, Niemann-Pick, and some forms of Gaucher's disease in Ashkenazi Jews.

## Fatty acid metabolism

SYtrate = SYnthesis.
CARnitine = CARnage of fatty acids.

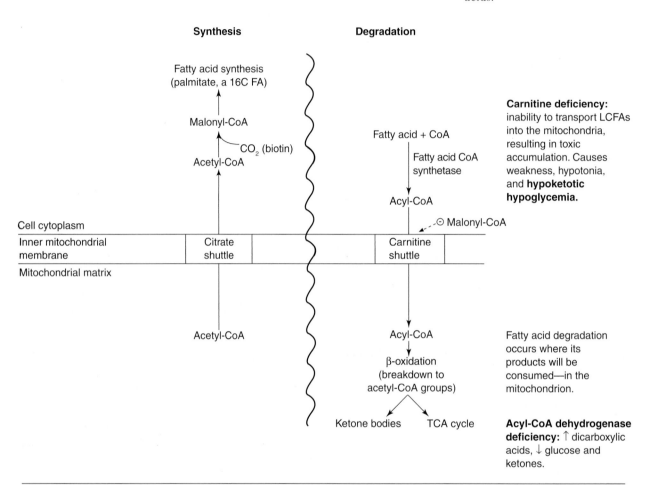

**Carnitine deficiency:** inability to transport LCFAs into the mitochondria, resulting in toxic accumulation. Causes weakness, hypotonia, and **hypoketotic hypoglycemia.**

Fatty acid degradation occurs where its products will be consumed—in the mitochondrion.

**Acyl-CoA dehydrogenase deficiency:** ↑ dicarboxylic acids, ↓ glucose and ketones.

| | |
|---|---|
| **Ketone bodies** | In the liver, fatty acids and amino acids are metabolized to **acetoacetate** and **β-hydroxybutyrate** (to be used in muscle and brain). In prolonged starvation and diabetic ketoacidosis, oxaloacetate is depleted for gluconeogenesis. In alcoholism, excess NADH shunts oxaloacetate to malate. Both processes stall the TCA cycle, which shunts glucose and FFA toward the production of ketone bodies. Made from HMG-CoA. Metabolized by the brain to 2 molecules of acetyl-CoA. Excreted in urine. |

Breath smells like acetone (fruity odor).
Urine test for ketones does not detect β-hydroxybutyrate (favored by high redox state).

## Metabolic fuel use

| | | |
|---|---|---|
| **Exercise** | As distances ↑, ATP is obtained from additional sources. | 1 g protein or carbohydrate = 4 kcal. |
| 100-meter sprint (seconds) | Stored ATP, creatine phosphate, anaerobic glycolysis. | 1 g fat = 9 kcal. |
| 1000-meter run (minutes) | Above + oxidative phosphorylation. | |
| Marathon (hours) | Glycogen and FFA oxidation; glucose conserved for final sprinting. | |
| **Fasting and starvation** | Priorities are to supply sufficient glucose to brain and RBCs and to preserve protein. | |
| Days 1–3 | Blood glucose level maintained by: | |

1. Hepatic glycogenolysis and glucose release
2. Adipose release of FFA
3. Muscle and liver shifting fuel use from glucose to FFA
4. Hepatic gluconeogenesis from peripheral tissue lactate and alanine, and from adipose tissue glycerol and propionyl-CoA from odd-chain FFA metabolism (the only triacylglycerol components that can contribute to gluconeogenesis)

| | |
|---|---|
| After day 3 | Muscle protein loss is maintained by hepatic formation of ketone bodies, supplying the brain and heart. |
| After several weeks | Ketone bodies become main source of energy for brain, so less muscle protein is degraded than during days 1–3. Survival time is determined by amount of fat stores. After this is depleted, vital protein degradation accelerates, leading to organ failure and death. |

| | | |
|---|---|---|
| **Cholesterol synthesis** | Rate-limiting step is catalyzed by **HMG-CoA reductase**, which converts HMG-CoA to mevalonate. ⅔ of plasma cholesterol is esterified by lecithin-cholesterol acyltransferase (LCAT). | Statins (e.g., lovastatin) inhibit HMG-CoA reductase. |
| **Essential fatty acids** | Linoleic and linolenic acids. Arachidonic acid, if linoleic acid is absent. | Eicosanoids are dependent on essential fatty acids. |

### Lipid transport, key enzymes

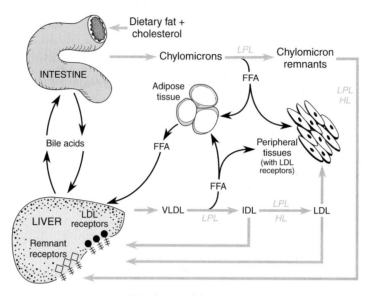

(Reproduced, with permission, from Brunton LL et al. *Goodman & Gilman's The Pharmacological Basis of Therapeutics,* 11th ed. New York: McGraw-Hill, 2005: Fig. 35-1.)

Pancreatic lipase—degradation of dietary TG in small intestine.
Lipoprotein lipase (LPL)—degradation of TG circulating in chylomicrons and VLDLs.
Hepatic TG lipase (HL)—degradation of TG remaining in IDL.
Hormone-sensitive lipase—degradation of TG stored in adipocytes.

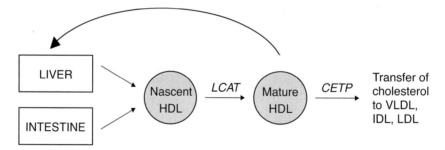

Lecithin-cholesterol acyltransferase (LCAT)—catalyzes esterification of cholesterol.
Cholesterol ester transfer protein (CETP)—mediates transfer of cholesterol esters to other lipoprotein particles.

| Major apolipoproteins | A-I—Activates LCAT.<br>B-100—Binds to LDL receptor, mediates VLDL secretion.<br>C-II—Cofactor for lipoprotein lipase.<br>B-48—Mediates chylomicron secretion.<br>E—Mediates Extra (remnant) uptake. |
|---|---|

**Lipoprotein functions**    Lipoproteins are composed of varying proportions of cholesterol, triglycerides (TGs), and phospholipids. LDL and HDL carry most cholesterol.

|  |  |
|---|---|
| LDL transports cholesterol from liver to tissues. | LDL is Lousy. |
| HDL transports it from periphery to liver. | HDL is Healthy. |

| | **Function and route** | **Apolipoproteins** |
|---|---|---|
| Chylomicron | Delivers dietary TGs to peripheral tissue. Delivers cholesterol to liver in the form of chylomicron remnants, which are mostly depleted of their triacylglycerols. Secreted by intestinal epithelial cells. | B-48, A-IV, C-II, and E |
| VLDL | Delivers hepatic TGs to peripheral tissue. Secreted by liver. | B-100, C-II, and E |
| IDL | Formed in the degradation of VLDL. Delivers triglycerides and cholesterol to liver, where they are degraded to LDL. | B-100 and E |
| LDL | Delivers hepatic cholesterol to peripheral tissues. Formed by lipoprotein lipase modification of VLDL in the peripheral tissue. Taken up by target cells via receptor-mediated endocytosis. | B-100 |
| HDL | Mediates reverse cholesterol transport from periphery to liver. Acts as a repository for apoC and apoE (which are needed for chylomicron and VLDL metabolism). Secreted from both liver and intestine. | |

### Familial dyslipidemias

| Type | Increased | Elevated blood levels | Pathophysiology |
|---|---|---|---|
| I—hyperchylomicronemia | Chylomicrons | TG, cholesterol | Lipoprotein lipase deficiency or altered apolipoprotein C-II. Causes pancreatitis, hepatosplenomegaly, and eruptive/pruritic xanthomas (no ↑ risk for atherosclerosis). |
| IIa—familial hypercholesterolemia | LDL | Cholesterol | Autosomal dominant; absent or ↓ LDL receptors. Causes accelerated atherosclerosis, tendon (Achilles) xanthomas, and corneal arcus. |
| IV—hypertriglyceridemia | VLDL | TG | Hepatic overproduction of VLDL. Causes pancreatitis. |

**Abeta-lipoproteinemia**    Hereditary inability to synthesize lipoproteins due to deficiencies in apoB-100 and apoB-48. Autosomal recessive. Symptoms appear in the first few months of life. Intestinal biopsy shows accumulation within enterocytes due to inability to export absorbed lipid as chylomicrons.

Findings: failure to thrive, steatorrhea, acanthocytosis, ataxia, night blindness.

# Embryology

*"Zygote. This cell, formed by the union of an ovum and a sperm, represents the beginning of a human being."*

—Keith Moore and Vid Persaud,
*Before We Are Born*

*Generally, I've got to say that all sounds, musics, noises since conception are bound to have influenced me.*

—Hugh Hopper

*Is life worth living? This is a question for an embryo, not for a man.*
—Samuel Butler

Embryology is traditionally one of the higher-yield areas within anatomy. This topic can be crammed closer to the exam date. Many questions focus on underlying mechanisms of congenital malformations (e.g., failure of fusion of the maxillary and medial nasal processes leading to cleft lip).

## Important genes of embryogenesis

| | |
|---|---|
| Sonic hedgehog gene | Produced at base of limbs in zone of polarizing activity. Involved in patterning along anterior-posterior axis. |
| *Wnt-7* gene | Produced at apical ectodermal ridge (thickened ectoderm at distal end of each developing limb). Necessary for proper organization along dorsal-ventral axis. |
| *FGF* gene | Produced at apical ectodermal ridge. Stimulates mitosis of underlying mesoderm, providing for lengthening of limbs. |
| Homeobox gene | Involved in segmental organization. |

## Fetal landmarks

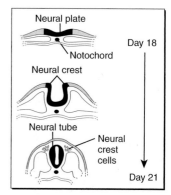

| | |
|---|---|
| Day 0 | Fertilization by sperm forming zygote, initiating embryogenesis. |
| Within week 1 | hCG secretion begins after implantation of blastocyst. |
| Within week 2 | Bilaminar disk (epiblast, hypoblast). |
| Within week 3 | Gastrulation. Primitive streak, notochord, and neural plate begin to form. |
| Weeks 3–8 (embryonic period) | Neural tube formed by neuroectoderm and closes by week 4. Organogenesis. Extremely susceptible to teratogens. |
| Week 4 | Heart begins to beat. Upper and lower limb buds begin to form. |
| Week 8 (fetal period) | Fetal movement, fetus looks like a baby. |
| Week 10 | Genitalia have male/female characteristics. |

| | | |
|---|---|---|
| Alar plate (dorsal) | Sensory | Same orientation as spinal cord. |
| Basal plate (ventral) | Motor | |

## Rules of early development

| | | |
|---|---|---|
| Rule of 2's for 2nd week | 2 germ layers (bilaminar disk): epiblast, hypoblast. 2 cavities: amniotic cavity, yolk sac. 2 components to placenta: cytotrophoblast, syncytiotrophoblast. | The epiblast (precursor to ectoderm) invaginates to form primitive streak. Cells from the primitive streak give rise to both intraembryonic mesoderm and endoderm. |
| Rule of 3's for 3rd week | 3 germ layers (gastrula): ectoderm, mesoderm, endoderm. | |
| Rule of 4's for 4th week | 4 heart chambers. 4 limb buds grow. | |

## Embryologic derivatives

### Ectoderm

| | | |
|---|---|---|
| Surface ectoderm | Adenohypophysis (from Rathke's pouch); lens of eye; epithelial linings of oral cavity, sensory organs of ear, retina, and olfactory epithelium; epidermis; salivary, sweat, and mammary glands. | Craniopharyngioma—benign Rathke's pouch tumor with cholesterol crystals, calcifications. |
| Neuroectoderm | Brain (neurohypophysis, CNS neurons, oligodendrocytes, astrocytes, ependymal cells, pineal gland), retina, spinal cord. | Neuroectoderm—think CNS and brain. |
| Neural crest | ANS, dorsal root ganglia, cranial nerves, celiac ganglion, melanocytes, chromaffin cells of adrenal medulla, enterochromaffin cells, parafollicular (C) cells of thyroid, Schwann cells, pia and arachnoid, bones of the skull, odontoblasts, laryngeal cartilage, aorticopulmonary septum. | Neural crest—think PNS and non-neural structures nearby. Odonto = teeth. Think **Crest** toothpaste. |

### Endoderm

| | | |
|---|---|---|
| **Endoderm** | Gut tube epithelium and derivatives (e.g., lungs, liver, pancreas, thymus, parathyroid, thyroid follicular cells). | |
| **Mesoderm** | Muscle, bone, connective tissue, serous linings of body cavities (e.g., peritoneum), spleen (derived from foregut mesentery), cardiovascular structures, lymphatics, blood, urogenital structures, kidneys, adrenal cortex. | Mesodermal defects = **VACTERL:** **V**ertebral defects, **A**nal atresia, **C**ardiac defects, **T**racheo-**E**sophageal fistula, **R**enal defects, **L**imb defects (bone and muscle). |
| | Notochord induces ectoderm to form neuroectoderm (neural plate). Its postnatal derivative is the nucleus pulposus of the intervertebral disk. | |

**Teratogens**    Most susceptible in 3rd–8th weeks (embryonic period—organogenesis) of pregnancy. Before week 3: all-or-none effects. After week 8: growth and function affected.

| Examples | Effects on fetus |
|---|---|
| ACE inhibitors | Renal damage |
| Alcohol | Leading cause of birth defects and mental retardation; fetal alcohol syndrome |
| Alkylating agents | Absence of digits, multiple anomalies |
| Aminoglycosides | CN VIII toxicity |
| Cocaine | Abnormal fetal development and fetal addiction; placental abruption |
| Diethylstilbestrol (DES) | Vaginal clear cell adenocarcinoma |
| Folate antagonists | Neural tube defects |
| Iodide (lack or excess) | Congenital goiter or hypothyroidism |
| Lithium | Ebstein's anomaly (atrialized right ventricle) |
| Maternal diabetes | Caudal regression syndrome (anal atresia to sirenomelia) |
| Smoking (nicotine, CO) | Preterm labor, placental problems, IUGR, ADHD |
| Tetracyclines | Discolored teeth |
| Thalidomide | Limb defects ("flipper" limbs) |
| Valproate | Inhibition of intestinal folate absorption |
| Vitamin A (excess) | Extremely high risk for spontaneous abortions and birth defects (cleft palate, cardiac abnormalities) |
| Warfarin | Bone deformities, fetal hemorrhage, abortion |
| X-rays, anticonvulsants | Multiple anomalies |

Fetal infections and certain antibiotics can also cause congenital malformations (see the Microbiology chapter).

**Fetal alcohol syndrome**    Leading cause of congenital malformations in the United States. Newborns of mothers who consumed significant amounts of alcohol during pregnancy have an ↑ incidence of congenital abnormalities, including pre- and postnatal developmental retardation, microcephaly, holoprosencephaly, facial abnormalities, limb dislocation, and heart and lung fistulas. Mechanism may include inhibition of cell migration.

## Twinning

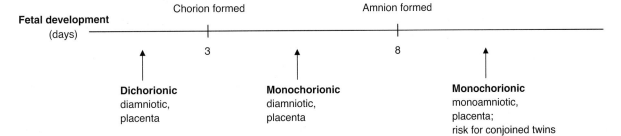

**Fetal development**
(days)

Chorion formed

Amnion formed

3

8

**Dichorionic**
diamniotic,
placenta

**Monochorionic**
diamniotic,
placenta

**Monochorionic**
monoamniotic,
placenta;
risk for conjoined twins

**Monozygotic**

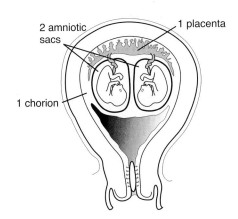

2 amniotic sacs

1 placenta

1 chorion

1 zygote splits evenly to develop 2 amniotic
sacs with a single common chorion and placenta.

Conjoined twins have 1 chorion, 1 amniotic sac.

**Dizygotic (fraternal) or monozygotic**

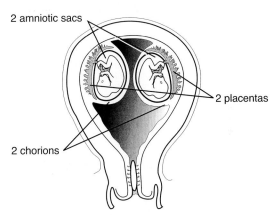

2 amniotic sacs

2 placentas

2 chorions

Monozygotes that split early develop 2 placentas
(separate/fused), chorions, and amniotic sacs.

Dizygotes develop individual placentas, chorions,
and amniotic sacs.

| | |
|---|---|
| **Placental development** | 1° site of nutrient and gas exchange between mother and fetus. |
| Fetal component | Cytotrophoblast—inner layer of chorionic villi. **Cyto** makes **Cells**. |
| | Syncytiotrophoblast—outer layer of chorionic villi; secretes hCG (structurally similar to LH; stimulates corpus luteum to secrete progesterone during first trimester). |
| Maternal component | Decidua basalis—derived from the endometrium. Maternal blood in lacunae. |

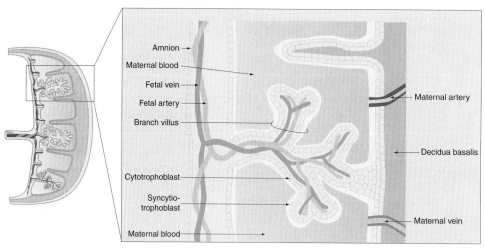

| | | |
|---|---|---|
| **Umbilical cord** | Umbilical arteries (2)—return deoxygenated blood from fetal internal iliac arteries to placenta. Umbilical vein (1)—supplies oxygenated blood from placenta to fetus. | Single umbilical artery is associated with congenital and chromosomal anomalies. Umbilical arteries and veins are derived from allantois. |

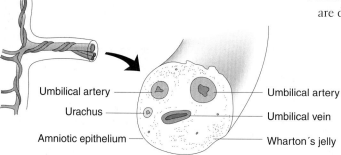

**Urachal duct abnormalities:**

3rd week—yolk sac forms allantois, which extends into urogenital sinus. Allantois becomes urachus, a duct between bladder and yolk sac.

Failure of urachus to obliterate:
1. Patent urachus—urine discharge from umbilicus
2. Vesicourachal diverticulum—outpouching of bladder

**Vitelline duct abnormalities:**

7th week—obliteration of vitelline duct (omphalomesenteric duct), which connects yolk sac to midgut lumen.

Vitelline fistula—failure of duct to close → meconium discharge from umbilicus. Examples: Meckel's diverticulum—partial closure, with patent portion attached to ileum. May have ectopic gastric mucosa → melena and RUQ pain.

**Heart embryology**

| Embryonic structure | Gives rise to |
|---|---|
| Truncus arteriosus (TA) | Ascending aorta and pulmonary trunk |
| Bulbus cordis | Right ventricle and smooth parts (outflow tract) of left and right ventricle |
| Primitive ventricle | Portion of the left ventricle |
| Primitive atria | Trabeculated left and right atrium |
| Left horn of sinus venosus (SV) | Coronary sinus |
| Right horn of SV | Smooth part of right atrium |
| Right common cardinal vein and right anterior cardinal vein | SVC |

**Truncus arteriosus**

Neural crest migration → divide trunk into 2 arteries via fusion and twisting of truncal and bulbar ridges → **ascending aorta and pulmonary trunk.**

Pathology—transposition of great vessels + tetralogy of Fallot.

### Interventricular septum development

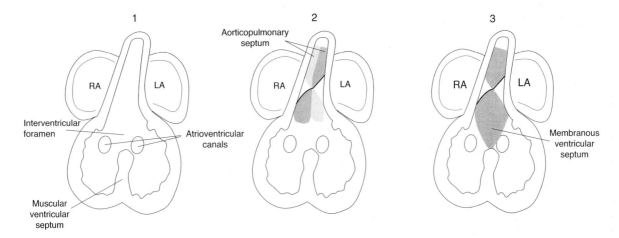

1. Muscular ventricular septum forms. Opening is called interventricular foramen.
2. Aorticopulmonary septum divides TA into aortic and pulmonary trunks.
3. Aorticopulmonary septum meets and fuses with muscular ventricular septum to form membranous interventricular septum, closing interventricular foramen.

## Interatrial septum development

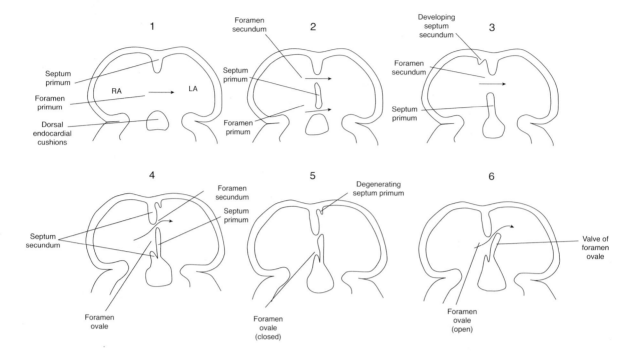

1. Foramen primum narrows as septum primum grows toward endocardial cushions.
2. Perforations in septum primum form foramen secundum (foramen primum disappears).
3. Foramen secundum maintains right-to-left shunt as septum secundum begins to grow.
4. Septum secundum contains a permanent opening (foramen ovale).
5. Foramen secundum enlarges and upper part of septum primum degenerates.
6. Remaining portion of septum primum forms valve of foramen ovale.

| **Fetal erythropoiesis** | Fetal erythropoiesis occurs in: | **Y**oung **L**iver **S**ynthesizes **B**lood. |
|---|---|---|
| | 1. **Y**olk sac (3–8 wk) | |
| | 2. **L**iver (6–30 wk) | Fetal hemoglobin = $\alpha_2\gamma_2$. |
| | 3. **S**pleen (9–28 wk) | Adult hemoglobin = $\alpha_2\beta_2$. |
| | 4. **B**one marrow (28 wk onward) | |

## Fetal circulation

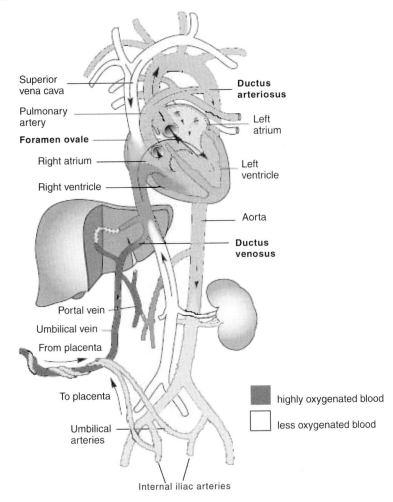

Superior vena cava
Pulmonary artery
**Foramen ovale**
Right atrium
Right ventricle

**Ductus arteriosus**
Left atrium
Left ventricle
Aorta
**Ductus venosus**

Portal vein
Umbilical vein
From placenta

To placenta
Umbilical arteries

Internal iliac arteries

☐ highly oxygenated blood
☐ less oxygenated blood

(Adapted, with permission, from Ganong WF. *Review of Medical Physiology,* 19th ed. Stamford, CT: Appleton & Lange, 1999: 600.)

Blood in umbilical vein is ≈ 80% saturated with $O_2$. Umbilical arteries have low $O_2$ saturation.

3 important shunts:

1. Blood entering the fetus through the umbilical vein is conducted via the **ductus venosus** into the IVC to bypass the hepatic circulation
2. Most oxygenated blood reaching the heart via the IVC is diverted through the **foramen ovale** and pumped out the aorta to the head and body
3. Deoxygenated blood from the SVC is expelled into the pulmonary artery and **ductus arteriosus** to the lower body of the fetus

At birth, infant takes a breath; ↓ resistance in pulmonary vasculature causes ↑ left atrial pressure vs. right atrial pressure; foramen ovale closes (now called fossa ovalis); ↑ in $O_2$ leads to ↓ in prostaglandins, causing closure of ductus arteriosus. Indomethacin helps close PDA. Prostaglandins keep PDA open.

## Fetal-postnatal derivatives

1. Umbilical vein—ligamentum teres hepatis
2. UmbiLical arteries—**mediaL** umbilical ligaments
3. Ductus arteriosus—ligamentum arteriosum
4. Ductus venosus—ligamentum venosum
5. Foramen ovale—fossa ovalis
6. AllaNtois—urachus—**mediaN** umbilical ligament
7. Notochord—nucleus pulposus of intervertebral disk

Contained in falciform ligament.
The urachus is the part of the allantoic duct between the bladder and the umbilicus.
Urachal cyst or sinus is a remnant.

## Aortic arch derivatives

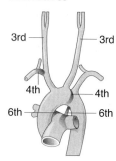

3rd — 3rd
4th — 4th
6th — 6th

1st—part of **MAX**illary artery (branch of external carotid).
2nd—Stapedial artery and hyoid artery.
3rd—common Carotid artery and proximal part of internal carotid artery.
4th—on left, aortic arch; on right, proximal part of right subclavian artery.
6th—proximal part of pulmonary arteries and (on left only) ductus arteriosus.

1st arch is **MAX**imal.

Second = Stapedial.
C is 3rd letter of alphabet.

4th arch (4 limbs) = systemic.

6th arch = pulmonary and the pulmonary-to-systemic shunt (ductus arteriosus).

## Regional specification of developing brain

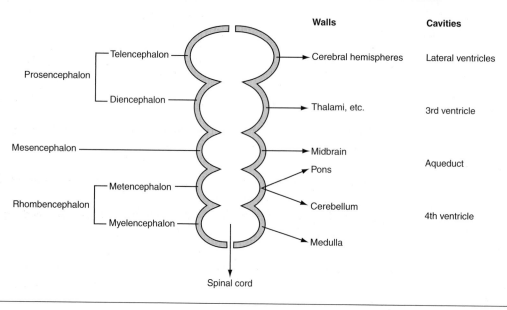

Adult derivatives

| | Walls | Cavities |
|---|---|---|
| Prosencephalon — Telencephalon | Cerebral hemispheres | Lateral ventricles |
| Prosencephalon — Diencephalon | Thalami, etc. | 3rd ventricle |
| Mesencephalon | Midbrain | Aqueduct |
| Rhombencephalon — Metencephalon | Pons / Cerebellum | |
| Rhombencephalon — Myelencephalon | Medulla | 4th ventricle |

Spinal cord

| **Neural tube defects** | Neuropores fail to fuse (4th week) → persistent connection between amniotic cavity and spinal canal. Associated with low folic acid intake during pregnancy. Elevated α-fetoprotein (AFP) in amniotic fluid and maternal serum. ↑ AFP + acetylcholinesterase in CSF. |
|---|---|

Spina bifida occulta—failure of bony spinal canal to close, but no structural herniation. Usually seen at lower vertebral levels. Dura is intact.

Meningocele—meninges herniate through spinal canal defect.

Myelomeningocele—meninges and spinal cord herniate through spinal canal defect (see Image 93).

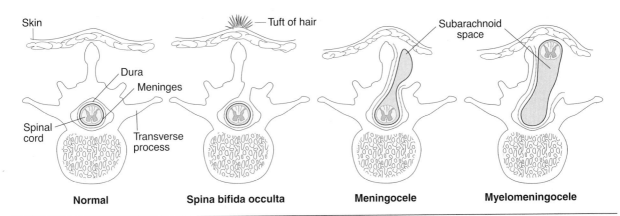

| **Forebrain anomalies** | |
|---|---|
| Anencephaly | Malformation of anterior end of neural tube; no brain/calvarium, elevated AFP, polyhydramnios (no swallowing center in brain). |
| Holoprosencephaly | ↓ separation of hemispheres across midline; results in cyclopia; associated with Patau's syndrome, severe fetal alcohol syndrome, and cleft lip/palate. |

| **Posterior fossa malformations** | Arnold-Chiari type II—cerebellar tonsillar herniation through foramen magnum with aqueductal stenosis and hydrocephaly. Often presents with syringomyelia, thoraco-lumbar myelomeningocele. |
|---|---|
| | Dandy-Walker—large posterior fossa; absent cerebellar vermis with cystic enlargement of 4th ventricle. Can lead to hydrocephalus and spina bifida. |

| **Syringomyelia** | Enlargement of the central canal of spinal cord. Crossing fibers of spinothalamic tract are typically damaged first. "Cape-like," bilateral loss of pain and temperature sensation in upper extremities with preservation of touch sensation. | *Syrinx* (Greek) = tube, as in syringe. Often presents in patients with Arnold-Chiari II malformation. Most common at C8–T1. |
|---|---|---|

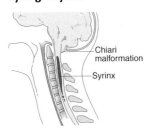

| | | |
|---|---|---|
| **Branchial apparatus** 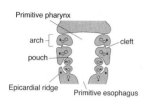 | Also called pharyngeal apparatus. Composed of branchial clefts, arches, and pouches.<br>Branchial clefts—derived from ectoderm. Also called branchial grooves.<br>Branchial arches—derived from mesoderm (muscles, arteries) and neural crests (bones, cartilage).<br>Branchial pouches—derived from endoderm. | **CAP** covers outside from inside:<br>**C**lefts = ectoderm<br>**A**rches = mesoderm<br>**P**ouches = endoderm |
| **Branchial arch innervation** | Arch 1 derivatives supplied by CN $V_2$ and $V_3$.<br>Arch 2 derivatives supplied by CN VII.<br>Arch 3 derivatives supplied by CN IX.<br>Arch 4 and 6 derivatives supplied by CN X.<br>These CNs are the only ones with both sensory and motor components (except $V_2$, which is sensory only).<br>Think of arches in terms of actions—chewing (1), facial expression (2), stylopharyngeus (3), swallowing (4), speaking (6). | 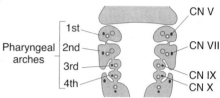<br>One man sat chewing,<br>Two hands on his face.<br>The third with his pharynx<br>Swallowed the fourth plate.<br>"Speak up, speak up!"<br>Said the sixth in return.<br>"Your cricothyroid<br>Makes me want to burn!" |

## Branchial arch derivatives

| Derivative | Cartilage | Muscles | Nerves | Arteries | Abnormalities/ Comments |
|---|---|---|---|---|---|
| 1 | Meckel's cartilage: Mandible, Malleus, incus, spheno-Mandibular ligament | Muscles of **Mastication** (temporalis, **Masseter**, lateral and **Medial** pterygoids), **Mylohyoid**, anterior belly of digastric, tensor tympani, tensor veli palatini, anterior ⅔ of tongue | CN $V_2$ and $V_3$ | Maxillary artery (branch of external carotid) | Treacher Collins syndrome: 1st-arch neural crest fails to migrate → mandibular hypoplasia, facial abnormalities |
| 2 | Reichert's cartilage: **Stapes**, **Styloid** process, lesser horn of hyoid, **Stylohyoid** ligament | Muscles of facial expression, **Stapedius**, **Stylohyoid**, posterior belly of digastric | CN VII | Stapedial artery, hyoid artery | |
| 3 | Cartilage: greater horn of hyoid | Stylopharyngeus (think of stylo-**pharyngeus** innervated by glosso**pharyngeal** nerve) | CN IX | | Congenital pharyngo-cutaneous fistula: persistence of cleft and pouch → fistula between tonsillar area, cleft in lateral neck |
| 4–6 | Cartilages: thyroid, cricoid, arytenoids, corniculate, cuneiform | 4th arch: most pharyngeal constrictors; **cricothyroid**, levator veli palatini 6th arch: all intrinsic muscles of larynx **except cricothyroid** | 4th arch: CN X (superior laryngeal branch—**swallowing**) 6th arch: CN X (recurrent laryngeal branch—**speaking**) | | Arches 3 and 4 form posterior ⅓ of tongue; arch 5 makes no major developmental contributions |

| **Branchial cleft derivatives** | 1st cleft develops into external auditory meatus.<br>2nd through 4th clefts form temporary cervical sinuses, which are obliterated by proliferation of 2nd arch mesenchyme.<br>Persistent cervical sinus → branchial cleft cyst within lateral neck. | |
|---|---|---|
| **Branchial pouch derivatives** | 1st pouch develops into middle ear cavity, eustachian tube, mastoid air cells.<br>2nd pouch develops into epithelial lining of palatine tonsil.<br>3rd pouch (dorsal wings) develops into **inferior** parathyroids.<br>3rd pouch (ventral wings) develops into thymus.<br>4th pouch (dorsal wings) develops into **superior** parathyroids. | 1st pouch contributes to endoderm-lined structures of ear.<br>3rd pouch contributes to 3 structures (thymus, left and right inferior parathyroids).<br>3rd-pouch structures end up **below** 4th-pouch structures.<br>Aberrant development of 3rd and 4th pouches → **DiGeorge syndrome** → leads to T-cell deficiency (thymic aplasia) and hypocalcemia (failure of parathyroid development). |
| | MEN 2A: mutation of germline *RET* (neural crest cells).<br>—Adrenal medulla (pheochromocytoma).<br>—Parathyroid (tumor): 3rd/4th pharyngeal pouch.<br>—Parafollicular cells (medullary thyroid cancer): 4th/5th pharyngeal pouch. | |

**Ear development**

| Origin | Bones | Muscles (innervation) | Miscellaneous |
|---|---|---|---|
| 1st arch | Malleus/incus | Tensor tyMpani ($V_3$) | |
| 2nd arch | Stapes | Stapedius (VII) | |
| 1st cleft | | | External auditory meatus |
| 1st branchial membrane | | | Tympanic membrane |
| 1st pouch | | | Eustachian tube, middle ear cavity, mastoid air cells |

| **Tongue development** | 1st branchial arch forms anterior ⅔ (thus sensation via CN $V_3$, taste via CN VII).<br>3rd and 4th arches form posterior ⅓ (thus sensation and taste mainly via CN IX, extreme posterior via CN X).<br>Motor innervation is via CN XII.<br>Muscles of the tongue are derived from occipital myotomes. | Taste—CN VII, IX, X (solitary nucleus).<br>Pain—CN $V_3$, IX, X.<br>Motor—CN XII. |
|---|---|---|

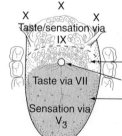

**Thyroid development**

Thyroid diverticulum arises from floor of primitive pharynx, descends into neck. Connected to tongue by thyroglossal duct, which normally disappears but may persist as pyramidal lobe of thyroid. Foramen cecum is normal remnant of thyroglossal duct. Most common ectopic thyroid tissue site is the tongue.

Thyroglossal duct cyst in midline neck and will move with swallowing (vs. persistent cervical sinus leading to branchial cleft cyst in lateral neck).

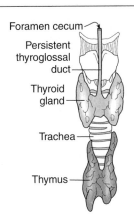

Foramen cecum
Persistent thyroglossal duct
Thyroid gland
Trachea
Thymus

**Cleft lip and cleft palate**

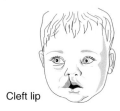

Cleft lip

Cleft lip—failure of fusion of the maxillary and medial nasal processes (formation of 1° palate).

Cleft palate—failure of fusion of the lateral palatine processes, the nasal septum, and/or the median palatine process (formation of 2° palate).

Roof of mouth
Nasal cavity
Palatine shelves (2° palate)
Uvula
Cleft palate (partial)

**Diaphragm embryology**

Diaphragm is derived from:
1. **S**eptum transversum → central tendon
2. **P**leuroperitoneal folds
3. **B**ody wall
4. **D**orsal mesentery of esophagus → crura

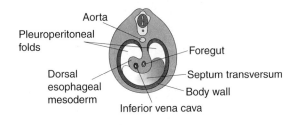

Aorta
Pleuroperitoneal folds
Dorsal esophageal mesoderm
Inferior vena cava
Foregut
Septum transversum
Body wall

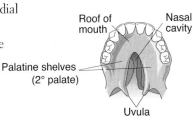

Several **P**arts **B**uild **D**iaphragm.

Diaphragm descends during development but maintains innervation from above. "C3, 4, 5 keeps the diaphragm alive."

Abdominal contents may herniate into the thorax because of incomplete development (diaphragmatic hernia) → hypoplasia of thoracic organs due to space compression, scaphoid abdomen, cyanosis.

| GI embryology | 1. Foregut—pharynx to duodenum<br>2. Midgut—duodenum to transverse colon<br>3. Hindgut—distal transverse colon to rectum<br>Developmental defects of anterior abdominal wall due to failure of:<br>  —Rostral fold closure: sternal defects<br>  —Lateral fold closure: omphalocele, gastroschisis<br>  —Caudal fold closure: bladder exstrophy<br>Duodenal atresia—failure to recanalize (trisomy 21).<br>Jejunal, ileal, colonic atresia—due to vascular accident (apple peel atresia).<br>6th week—midgut herniates through umbilical ring → rapid growth.<br>10th week—return to abdominal cavity + rotate around SMA.<br>Pathology—intestinal obstruction, twisting around SMA (volvulus). | **Gastroschisis**—failure of lateral body folds to fuse → extrusion of abdominal contents through abdominal folds.<br>**Omphalocele**—persistence of herniation of abdominal contents into umbilical cord, covered by peritoneum (see Image 94). |
|---|---|---|

| Tracheoesophageal fistula | Abnormal connection between esophagus and trachea.<br>Most common subtype is blind upper esophagus with lower esophagus connected to trachea. Results in cyanosis, choking and vomiting with feeding, air bubble on CXR, and polyhydramnios. |
|---|---|

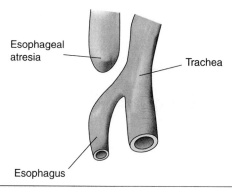

Esophageal atresia

Trachea

Esophagus

| Congenital pyloric stenosis | Hypertrophy of the pylorus causes obstruction. Palpable "olive" mass in epigastric region and nonbilious projectile vomiting at ≈ 2 weeks of age. Treatment is surgical incision. Occurs in 1/600 live births, often in 1st-born males. |
|---|---|

**Pancreas and spleen embryology**

Pancreas—derived from foregut. Ventral pancreatic bud becomes pancreatic head, uncinate process (lower half of head), and main pancreatic duct. Dorsal pancreatic bud becomes everything else (body, tail, isthmus, and accessory pancreatic duct).

Annular pancreas—ventral pancreatic bud abnormally encircles 2nd part of duodenum; forms a ring of pancreatic tissue that may cause duodenal narrowing.

Pancreas divisum—ventral and dorsal parts fail to fuse at 8 weeks.

Spleen—arises from dorsal mesentery (hence is mesodermal) but is supplied by artery of foregut (celiac artery).

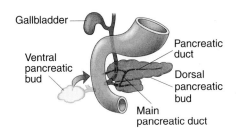

**Kidney embryology**

1. Pronephros—week 4; then degenerates
2. Mesonephros—functions as interim kidney for 1st trimester; later contributes to male genital system
3. Metanephros—permanent; beginnings first appear during 5th week of gestation; nephrogenesis continues through 32–36 weeks of gestation
   —Ureteric bud—derived from caudal end of mesonephros; gives rise to ureter, pelvises, and, through branching, calyces and collecting ducts; fully canalized by 10th week
   —Metanephric mesenchyme—ureteric bud interacts with this tissue; interaction induces differentiation and formation of glomerulus and renal tubules to distal convoluted tubule
   —Aberrant interaction between these 2 tissues may result in several congenital malformations of the kidney
   —Aberrant development of ureteric bud may result in a number of congenital malformations of the lower urinary tract

Uteropelvic junction with kidney—last to canalize → most common site of obstruction (hydronephrosis) in fetus.

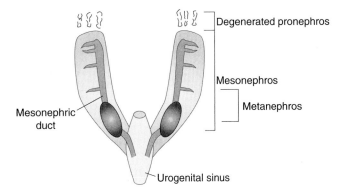

**Potter's syndrome**

Bilateral renal agenesis → oligohydramnios → limb deformities, facial deformities, pulmonary hypoplasia. Caused by malformation of ureteric bud.

Babies who can't "**P**ee" in utero develop **P**otter's.

| | | |
|---|---|---|
| **Horseshoe kidney** | Inferior poles of both kidneys fuse. As they ascend from pelvis during fetal development, horseshoe kidneys get trapped under inferior mesenteric artery and remain low in the abdomen. Kidney functions normally. Note: horseshoe kidney (partial fusion) vs. cake kidney (complete fusion). | 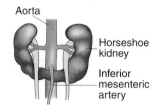 |

**Genital embryology**

| | | |
|---|---|---|
| Female | Default development. Mesonephric duct degenerates and paramesonephric duct develops. | Mesonephric duct must be induced to remain; default program for embryo development is for paramesonephric duct to develop into female. |
| Male | *SRY* gene on Y chromosome codes for testis-determining factor. Müllerian inhibiting substance secreted by testes (Sertoli cells) suppresses development of paramesonephric ducts. ↑ androgens (Leydig cells) → development of mesonephric ducts. | |
| Mesonephric (wolffian) duct | Develops into male internal structures (except prostate)—**S**eminal vesicles, **E**pididymis, **E**jaculatory duct, and **D**uctus deferens. | **SEED.** 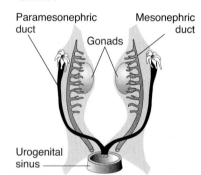 |
| Paramesonephric (müllerian) duct | Develops into fallopian tube, uterus, and upper ⅓ of vagina (lower ⅔ from urogenital sinus). | |

| | | |
|---|---|---|
| **Bicornuate uterus** | Results from incomplete fusion of the paramesonephric ducts. Associated with urinary tract abnormalities and infertility. | 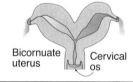 |

## Male/female genital homologues

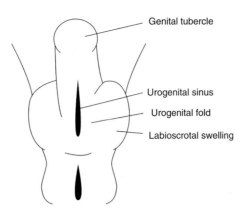

Genital tubercle

Urogenital sinus

Urogenital fold

Labioscrotal swelling

| Male | Dihydrotestosterone | | Estrogen | Female |
|------|---------------------|---|----------|--------|
| Glans penis | ← | Genital tubercle | → | Glans clitoris |
| Corpus cavernosum and spongiosum | ← | Genital tubercle | → | Vestibular bulbs |
| Bulbourethral glands (of Cowper) | ← | Urogenital sinus | → | Greater vestibular glands (of Bartholin) |
| Prostate gland | ← | Urogenital sinus | → | Urethral and paraurethral glands (of Skene) |
| Ventral shaft of penis (penile urethra) | ← | Urogenital folds | → | Labia minora |
| Scrotum | ← | Labioscrotal swelling | → | Labia majora |

## Congenital penile abnormalities

Hypospadias

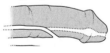

Epispadias

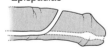

Hypospadias—abnormal opening of penile urethra on inferior (ventral) side of penis due to failure of urethral folds to close.

Epispadias—abnormal opening of penile urethra on superior (dorsal) side of penis due to faulty positioning of genital tubercle.

Hypospadias is more common than epispadias. Fix hypospadias to prevent UTIs.
**Hypo** is **below**.
Exstrophy of the bladder is associated with Epispadias.
When you have Epispadias, you hit your Eye when you pEE.

# Microbiology

*"Support bacteria. They're the only culture some people have."*
— Anonymous

*"What lies behind us and what lies ahead of us are tiny matters compared to what lies within us."*
— Oliver Wendell Holmes

This high-yield material covers the basic concepts of microbiology. The emphasis in previous examinations has been approximately 40% bacteriology (20% basic, 20% quasi-clinical), 25% immunology, 25% virology (10% basic, 15% quasi-clinical), 5% parasitology, and 5% mycology.

Microbiology questions on the Step 1 exam often require two steps: Given a certain clinical presentation, you will first need to identify the most likely causative organism, and you will then need to provide an answer regarding some feature of that organism. For example, a description of a child with fever and a petechial rash will be followed by a question that reads, "From what site does the responsible organism usually enter the blood?"

This section therefore presents organisms in two major ways: in individual microbial "profiles" and in the context of the systems they infect and the clinical presentations they produce. You should become familiar with both formats. When reviewing the systems approach, remind yourself of the features of each microbe by returning to the individual profiles. Also be sure to memorize the laboratory characteristics that allow you to identify microbes.

Additional tables that organize infectious diseases and syndromes according to the most commonly affected hosts and the most likely microbes are available on the First Aid team blog at www.firstaidteam.com.

## Bacterial structures

| Structure | Function | Chemical composition |
| --- | --- | --- |
| Peptidoglycan | Gives rigid support, protects against osmotic pressure. | Sugar backbone with cross-linked peptide side chains. |
| Cell wall/cell membrane (gram positives) | Major surface antigen. | Peptidoglycan for support. Teichoic acid induces TNF and IL-1. |
| Outer membrane (gram negatives) | Site of endotoxin (lipopolysaccharide); major surface antigen. | Lipid A induces TNF and IL-1; polysaccharide is the antigen. |
| Plasma membrane | Site of oxidative and transport enzymes. | Lipoprotein bilayer. |
| Ribosome | Protein synthesis. | 50S and 30S subunits. |
| Periplasm | Space between the cytoplasmic membrane and outer membrane in gram-negative bacteria. | Contains many hydrolytic enzymes, including β-lactamases. |
| Capsule | Protects against phagocytosis. | Polysaccharide (except *Bacillus anthracis*, which contains D-glutamate). |
| Pilus/fimbria | Mediate adherence of bacteria to cell surface; sex pilus forms attachment between 2 bacteria during conjugation. | Glycoprotein. |
| Flagellum | Motility. | Protein. |
| Spore | Provides resistance to dehydration, heat, and chemicals. | Keratin-like coat; dipicolinic acid. |
| Plasmid | Contains a variety of genes for antibiotic resistance, enzymes, and toxins. | DNA. |
| Glycocalyx | Mediates adherence to surfaces, especially foreign surfaces (e.g., indwelling catheters). | Polysaccharide. |

## Cell walls

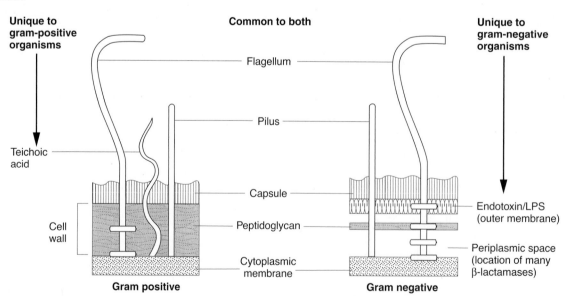

(Adapted, with permission, from Levinson W, Jawetz E. *Medical Microbiology and Immunology: Examination and Board Review,* 9th ed. New York: McGraw-Hill, 2006: 7.)

## Bacterial taxonomy

| Morphology | Gram Positive | Gram Negative |
|---|---|---|
| Circular (coccus) | *Staphylococcus*<br>*Streptococcus* | *Neisseria* |
| Rod (bacillus) | *Clostridium*<br>*Corynebacterium*<br>*Bacillus*<br>*Listeria*<br>*Mycobacterium* (acid fast) | Enterics:<br>  ■ *E. coli*<br>  ■ *Shigella*<br>  ■ *Salmonella*<br>  ■ *Yersinia*<br>  ■ *Klebsiella*<br>  ■ *Proteus*<br>  ■ *Enterobacter*<br>  ■ *Serratia*<br>  ■ *Vibrio*<br>  ■ *Campylobacter*<br>  ■ *Helicobacter*<br>  ■ *Pseudomonas*<br>  ■ *Bacteroides*<br>*Haemophilus*<br>*Legionella* (silver)<br>*Bordetella*<br>*Yersinia*<br>*Francisella*<br>*Brucella*<br>*Pasteurella*<br>*Bartonella*<br>*Gardnerella* (gram variable) |
| Branching filamentous | *Actinomyces*<br>*Nocardia* (weakly acid fast) | |
| Pleomorphic | | Rickettsiae<br>Chlamydiae (Giemsa) |
| Spiral | | Spirochetes:<br>  ■ *Leptospira*<br>  ■ *Borrelia* (Giemsa)<br>  ■ *Treponema* |
| No cell wall | *Mycoplasma* ||

## Bacteria with unusual cell membranes/walls

| | |
|---|---|
| Mycoplasma | Contain sterols and have no cell wall. |
| Mycobacteria | Contain mycolic acid. High lipid content. |

**Gram stain limitations**

These bugs do not Gram stain well:

*Treponema* (too thin to be visualized).
*Rickettsia* (intracellular parasite).
Mycobacteria (high-lipid-content cell wall requires acid-fast stain).
*Mycoplasma* (no cell wall).
*Legionella pneumophila* (primarily intracellular).
*Chlamydia* (intracellular parasite; lacks muramic acid in cell wall).

These **R**ascals **M**ay **M**icroscopically **L**ack **C**olor.
Treponemes—darkfield microscopy and fluorescent antibody staining.

*Legionella*—silver stain.

**Stains**

| | | |
|---|---|---|
| Giemsa | *Borrelia, Plasmodium,* trypanosomes, *Chlamydia.* | |
| PAS (periodic acid-Schiff) | Stains glycogen, mucopolysaccharides; used to diagnose Whipple's disease (*Tropheryma whippelii*). | **PAS**s the sugar. |
| Ziehl-Neelsen | Acid-fast organisms. | |
| India ink | *Cryptococcus neoformans* (mucicarmine can also be used to stain thick polysaccharide capsule red). | |
| Silver stain | Fungi (e.g., *Pneumocystis*), *Legionella.* | |

**Special culture requirements**

| Bug | Media used for isolation |
|---|---|
| *H. influenzae* | Chocolate agar with factors V (NAD$^+$) and X (hematin) |
| *N. gonorrhoeae* | Thayer-Martin (or **VPN**) media—**V**ancomycin (inhibits gram-positive organisms), **P**olymyxin (inhibits gram-negative organisms), and **N**ystatin (inhibits fungi); "to connect to *Neisseria*, please use your **VPN** client" |
| *B. pertussis* | Bordet-Gengou (potato) agar (**Bordet** for *Bordetella*) |
| *C. diphtheriae* | Tellurite plate, Löffler's media |
| *M. tuberculosis* | Löwenstein-Jensen agar |
| *M. pneumoniae* | Eaton's agar |
| Lactose-fermenting enterics | Pink colonies on MacConkey's agar (fermentation produces acid, turning plate pink); *E. coli* is also grown on eosin–methylene blue (EMB) agar as blue-black colonies with metallic sheen |
| *Legionella* | Charcoal yeast extract agar buffered with cysteine |
| Fungi | Sabouraud's agar |

**Obligate aerobes**

Use an $O_2$-dependent system to generate ATP.
Examples include *Nocardia,* **P**seudomonas *aeruginosa,* *Mycobacterium tuberculosis,* and *Bacillus.*
Reactivation of *M. tuberculosis* (e.g., after immune compromise or TNF-α use) has a predilection for the apices of the lung, which have the highest $P_{O_2}$.

**N**agging **P**ests **M**ust **B**reathe.
*P.* **AER**uginosa is an **AER**obe seen in burn wounds, nosocomial pneumonia, and pneumonias in cystic fibrosis patients.

| | | |
|---|---|---|
| **Obligate anaerobes** | Examples include *Clostridium*, *Bacteroides*, and *Actinomyces*. They lack catalase and/or superoxide dismutase and are thus susceptible to oxidative damage. Generally foul smelling (short-chain fatty acids), are difficult to culture, and produce gas in tissue ($CO_2$ and $H_2$). | Anaerobes Can't Breathe Air. Anaerobes are normal flora in GI tract, pathogenic elsewhere. AminO$_2$glycosides are ineffective against anaerobes because these antibiotics require $O_2$ to enter into bacterial cell. |
| **Intracellular bugs** | | |
| Obligate intracellular | *Rickettsia*, *Chlamydia*. Can't make own ATP. | Stay inside (cells) when it is **R**eally **C**old. |
| Facultative intracellular | *Salmonella*, *Neisseria*, *Brucella*, *Mycobacterium*, *Listeria*, *Francisella*, *Legionella*. | **S**ome **N**asty **B**ugs **M**ay **L**ive **F**acultative**L**y. |
| **Encapsulated bacteria** | Positive **quellung** reaction—if encapsulated bug is present, capsule **swells** when specific anticapsular antisera are added.<br>Examples are *Klebsiella pneumoniae*, *Salmonella*, *Streptococcus pneumoniae*, *Haemophilus influenzae* type B (B polysaccharide), and *Neisseria meningitidis*. Their capsules serve as an antiphagocytic virulence factor. **SHiN** can produce IgA protease, cause meningitis, and take up DNA from environment ("transformation"). | **Q**uellung = capsular "swelling." Kapsules Shield **SHiN**. Capsule serves as antigen in vaccines (Pneumovax, *H. influenzae* type B, meningococcal vaccines). Conjugation of polysaccharide with protein ↑ T-cell response and immunity. |
| **Urease-positive bugs** | *Proteus*, *Klebsiella*, *H. pylori*, *Ureaplasma*. | **P**articular **K**inds **H**ave **U**rease. |
| **Pigment-producing bateria** | *Actinomyces israelii*—yellow "sulfur" granules.<br>*S. aureus*—yellow pigment.<br>*Pseudomonas aeruginosa*—blue-**green** pigment.<br>*Serratia marcescens*—red pigment. | **Israel** has **yellow** sand.<br><br>*Aureus* (Latin) = gold.<br>**AERUG**ula is **green**.<br>*Serratia marcescens*—think red maraschino cherries! |
| **Bacterial virulence factors** | These promote evasion of host immune response. | |
| Protein A (*S. aureus*) | Binds Fc region of Ig. Prevents opsonization and phagocytosis. | |
| IgA protease | Enzyme that cleaves IgA. Secreted by *S. pneumoniae*, *H. influenzae* type B, and *Neisseria* (**SHiN**) in order to colonize respiratory mucosa. | |
| M protein (group A streptococcus) | Helps prevent phagocytosis. | |

### Main features of exotoxins and endotoxins

| Property | Exotoxin | Endotoxin |
| --- | --- | --- |
| Source | Certain species of some gram-positive and gram-negative bacteria | Outer cell membrane of most gram-negative bacteria and *Listeria* |
| Secreted from cell | Yes | No |
| Chemistry | Polypeptide | Lipopolysaccharide (structural part of bacteria; released when lysed) |
| Location of genes | Plasmid or bacteriophage | Bacterial chromosome |
| Toxicity | High (fatal dose on the order of 1 μg) | Low (fatal dose on the order of hundreds of micrograms) |
| Clinical effects | Various effects (see text) | Fever, shock |
| Mode of action | Various modes (see text) | Includes TNF and IL-1 |
| Antigenicity | Induces high-titer antibodies called antitoxins | Poorly antigenic |
| Vaccines | Toxoids used as vaccines | No toxoids formed and no vaccine available |
| Heat stability | Destroyed rapidly at 60°C (except staphylococcal enterotoxin) | Stable at 100°C for 1 hour |
| Typical diseases | Tetanus, botulism, diphtheria | Meningococcemia, sepsis by gram-negative rods |

(Adapted, with permission, from Levinson W. *Medical Microbiology and Immunology: Examination and Board Review,* 8th ed. New York: McGraw-Hill, 2004: 39.)

## Bugs with exotoxins

**Superantigens** — Bind directly to MHC II and T-cell receptor simultaneously, activating large numbers of T cells to stimulate release of IFN-$\gamma$ and IL-2.

*S. aureus* — TSST-1 superantigen causes toxic shock syndrome (fever, rash, shock). Other *S. aureus* toxins include enterotoxins that cause food poisoning as well as exfoliatin, which causes staphylococcal scalded skin syndrome.

*S. pyogenes* — Scarlet fever–erythrogenic toxin causes toxic shock–like syndrome.

**ADP ribosylating A-B toxins** — Interfere with host cell function. B (binding) component binds to a receptor on surface of host cell, enabling endocytosis. A (active) component then attaches an ADP-ribosyl to a host cell protein (ADP ribosylation), altering protein function.

*Corynebacterium diphtheriae* — Inactivates elongation factor (EF-2) (similar to *Pseudomonas* exotoxin A); causes pharyngitis and "pseudomembrane" in throat.

*Vibrio cholerae* — ADP ribosylation of G protein stimulates adenylyl cyclase; $\uparrow$ pumping of $Cl^-$ into gut and $\downarrow$ $Na^+$ absorption. $H_2O$ moves into gut lumen; causes voluminous rice-water diarrhea.

*E. coli* — Heat-labile toxin stimulates **A**denylate cyclase. Heat-stable toxin stimulates **G**uanylate cyclase. Both cause watery diarrhea. "Labile like the **A**ir, stable like the **G**round."

*Bordetella pertussis* — Increases cAMP by inhibiting $G\alpha_i$; causes whooping cough; inhibits chemokine receptor, causing lymphocytosis.

### Other toxins

*Clostridium perfringens* — $\alpha$ toxin causes gas gangrene; get double zone of hemolysis on blood agar.

*C. tetani* — Blocks the release of inhibitory neurotransmitters GABA and glycine; causes "lockjaw."

*C. botulinum* — Blocks the release of acetylcholine; causes anticholinergic symptoms, CNS paralysis, especially cranial nerves; spores found in canned food, honey (causes floppy baby).

*Bacillus anthracis* — Edema factor, part of the toxin complex, is an adenylate cyclase.

*Shigella* — Shiga toxin (also produced by *E. coli* O157:H7) cleaves host cell rRNA (inactivates 60S ribosome); also enhances cytokine release, causing HUS.

*S. pyogenes* — Streptolysin O is a hemolysin; antigen for ASO antibody, which is used in the diagnosis of rheumatic fever.

**cAMP inducers**

1. *Vibrio cholerae* toxin permanently activates $G_s$, causing rice-water diarrhea.
2. Pertussis toxin permanently disables $G_i$, causing whooping cough.
3. *E. coli* (ETEC)—heat-labile toxin.
4. *Bacillus anthracis* toxin includes edema factor, a bacterial adenylate cyclase ($\uparrow$ cAMP).

Cholera, pertussis, and *E. coli* toxins act via ADP ribosylation to permanently activate endogenous adenylate cyclase ($\uparrow$ cAMP), while the anthrax edema factor is itself an adenylate cyclase.

Cholera turns the "on" on. Pertussis turns the "off" off. Pertussis toxin also promotes lymphocytosis by inhibiting chemokine receptors.

**Endotoxin**

A lipopolysaccharide found in cell wall of gram-negative bacteria (and *Listeria monocytogenes*, the only gram-positive bacterium with endotoxin).

N-dotoxin is an integral part of gram-Negative outer membrane. Endotoxin is heat stable.

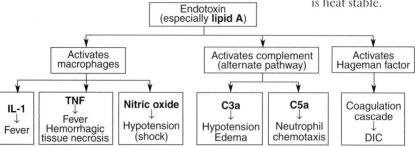

(Adapted, with permission, from Levinson W, Jawetz E. *Medical Microbiology and Immunology: Examination and Board Review*, 6th ed. New York: McGraw-Hill, 2000: 39.)

**Bacterial growth curve**

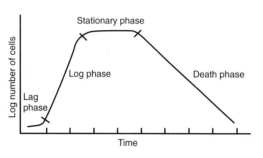

(Adapted, with permission, from Levinson W. *Medical Microbiology and Immunology: Examination and Board Review*, 9th ed. New York: McGraw-Hill, 2006: 15.)

Lag—metabolic activity without division.

Log—rapid cell division.

Stationary—nutrient depletion slows growth. Spore formation in some bacteria.

Death—prolonged nutrient depletion and buildup of waste products lead to death.

## Bacterial genetics

**Transformation**

Ability to take up DNA from environment (also known as "competence"). A feature of many bacteria, especially **S.** *pneumoniae*, **H.** *influenzae* type B, and **N**eisseria (**SHiN**). Any DNA can be used.

**Conjugation**

$F^+ \times F^-$

$F^+$ plasmid contains genes required for conjugation process. Bacteria without this plasmid are termed $F^-$. Plasmid is replicated and transferred through pilus from $F^+$ cell. Plasmid DNA only; no transfer of chromosomal genes.

$Hfr \times F^-$

$F^+$ plasmid can become incorporated into bacterial chromosomal DNA, termed Hfr cell. Replication of incorporated plasmid DNA may include some flanking chromosomal DNA. Transfer of plasmid and chromosomal genes.

**Transduction**

Generalized

A "packaging" event. Lytic phage infects bacterium, leading to cleavage of bacterial DNA and synthesis of viral proteins. Parts of bacterial chromosomal DNA may become packaged in viral capsid. Phage infects another bacterium, transferring these genes.

Specialized

An "excision" event. Lysogenic phage infects bacterium; viral DNA incorporated into bacterial chromosome. When phage DNA is excised, flanking bacterial genes may be excised with it. DNA is packaged into phage viral capsid and can infect another bacterium.

**Transposition**

Segment of DNA that can "jump" (excision and reincorporation) from one location to another, can transfer genes from plasmid to chromosome and vice versa. When excision occurs, may include some flanking chromosomal DNA, which can be incorporated into a plasmid and transferred to another bacterium.

---

**Lysogeny**

Genes for the following 5 bacterial toxins encoded in a lysogenic phage:

ShigA-like toxin

Botulinum toxin (certain strains)

Cholera toxin

Diphtheria toxin

Erythrogenic toxin of *Streptococcus pyogenes*

**ABCDE.**

---

## Gram-positive lab algorithm

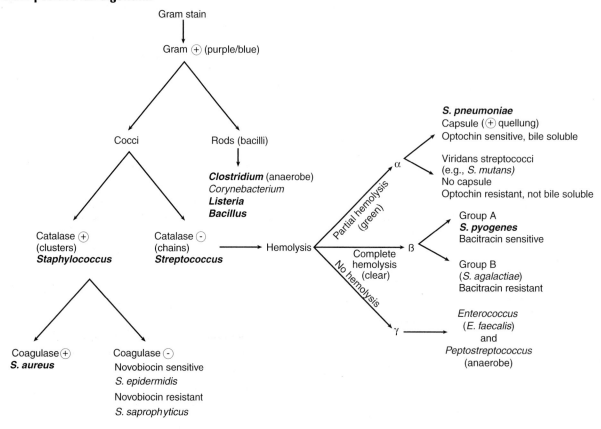

Important pathogens are in **bold type.**
Note: *Enterococcus* is either α- or γ-hemolytic.

---

### Identification of gram-positive cocci

| | | |
|---|---|---|
| Staphylococci | NOvobiocin—*Saprophyticus* is Resistant; *Epidermidis* is Sensitive. | On the office's **staph** retreat, there was **NO StRES.** |
| Streptococci | Optochin—*Viridans* is Resistant; *Pneumoniae* is Sensitive. | OVRPS (overpass). |
| | Bacitracin—group **B** strep are Resistant; group **A** strep are Sensitive. | **B-BRAS.** |

---

**α-hemolytic bacteria**

Form green ring around colonies on blood agar. Include the following organisms:
1. *Streptococcus pneumoniae* (catalase negative and optochin sensitive) (see Image 1)
2. Viridans streptococci (catalase negative and optochin resistant)

---

**β-hemolytic bacteria**

Form clear area of hemolysis on blood agar. Include the following organisms:
1. *Staphylococcus aureus* (catalase and coagulase positive)
2. *Streptococcus pyogenes*—group A strep (catalase negative and bacitracin sensitive)
3. *Streptococcus agalactiae*—group B strep (catalase negative and bacitracin resistant)
4. *Listeria monocytogenes* (tumbling motility, meningitis in newborns, unpasteurized milk)

| **Catalase/coagulase (gram-positive cocci)** | Catalase degrades $H_2O_2$ before it can be converted to microbicidal products by the enzyme myeloperoxidase.<br>Staphylococci make catalase, whereas streptococci do not.<br>*S. aureus* makes coagulase, whereas *S. epidermidis* and *S. saprophyticus* do not. | **Staph** make catalase because they have more "**staff**." Bad staph (*aureus*, because *epidermidis* is skin flora) make coagulase and toxins.<br>Catalase-producing microbes easily degrade what little $H_2O_2$ is present in people with chronic granulomatous disease (NADPH oxidase deficiency), thereby causing recurrent infections. |
|---|---|---|
| ***Staphylococcus aureus***<br> | Protein A (virulence factor) binds Fc-IgG, inhibiting complement fixation and phagocytosis.<br>Causes:<br>1. Inflammatory disease—skin infections, organ abscesses, pneumonia<br>2. Toxin-mediated disease—toxic shock syndrome (TSST-1 toxin), scalded skin syndrome (exfoliative toxin), rapid-onset food poisoning (enterotoxins) (see Image 3)<br>3. MRSA (methicillin-resistant *S. aureus*) infection—important cause of serious nosocomial and community-acquired infections. Resistant to β-lactams due to altered penicillin-binding protein. | TSST is a superantigen that binds to MHC II and T-cell receptor, resulting in polyclonal T-cell activation.<br>*S. aureus* food poisoning is due to ingestion of preformed toxin.<br>Causes acute bacterial endocarditis, osteomyelitis. |
| ***Staphylococcus epidermidis*** | Infects prosthetic devices and intravenous catheters by producing adherent biofilms.<br>Component of normal skin flora; contaminates blood cultures. | |
| ***Streptococcus pneumoniae*** | Most common cause of:<br>**M**eningitis<br>**O**titis media (in children)<br>**P**neumonia<br>**S**inusitis<br>Encapsulated. IgA protease. | *S. pneumoniae* **MOPS** are Most **OP**tochin **S**ensitive.<br>Pneumococcus is associated with "rusty" sputum, sepsis in sickle cell anemia and splenectomy. |
| **Viridans group streptococci** | Viridans streptococci are α-hemolytic. They are normal flora of the oropharynx and cause dental caries (*Streptococcus mutans*) and subacute bacterial endocarditis (*S. sanguis*). Resistant to optochin, differentiating them from *S. pneumoniae*, which is α-hemolytic but is optochin sensitive. | *Sanguis* (Latin) = blood.<br>There is lots of blood in the heart (endocarditis).<br>Viridans group strep live in the mouth because they are not afraid **of-the-chin** (**op-to-chin** resistant). |

| | | |
|---|---|---|
| ***Streptococcus pyogenes* (group A streptococci)** | Causes:<br>1. Pyogenic—pharyngitis, cellulitis, impetigo<br>2. Toxigenic—scarlet fever, toxic shock syndrome<br>3. Immunologic—rheumatic fever, acute glomerulonephritis<br>Bacitracin sensitive. Antibodies to **M protein** enhance host defenses against *S. pyogenes* but can give rise to rheumatic fever.<br>ASO titer detects recent *S. pyogenes* infection. | **PH**aryngitis can result in rheumatic "**PH**ever" and glomerulone**PH**ritis.<br>No "**rheum**" for **SPECC**ulation: Subcutaneous plaques, Polyarthritis, Erythema marginatum, Chorea, Carditis. |
| ***Streptococcus agalactiae* (group B streptococci)** | Bacitracin resistant, β-hemolytic; causes pneumonia, meningitis, and sepsis, mainly in babies. | **B** for **B**abies! |
| **Enterococci (group D streptococci)**<br>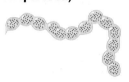 | Enterococci (*Enterococcus faecalis* and *E. faecium*) are normal colonic flora that are penicillin G resistant and cause UTI and subacute endocarditis. Lancefield group D includes the enterococci and the nonenterococcal group D streptococci. Lancefield grouping is based on differences in the C carbohydrate on the bacterial cell wall. Variable hemolysis.<br>VRE (vancomycin-resistant enterococci) are an important cause of nosocomial infection. | Enterococci, hardier than nonenterococcal group D, can thus grow in 6.5% NaCl (lab test).<br>*Entero* = intestine, *faecalis* = feces, *strepto* = twisted (chains), *coccus* = berry. |
| ***Streptococcus bovis* (group D streptococci)** | Colonizes the gut. Can cause bacteremia and subacute endocarditis in colon cancer patients. | |
| **Diphtheria (and exotoxin)** | Caused by *Corynebacterium diphtheriae* via exotoxin encoded by β-prophage. Potent exotoxin inhibits protein synthesis via ADP ribosylation of EF-2.<br>Symptoms include pseudomembranous pharyngitis (grayish-white membrane) with lymphadenopathy.<br>Lab diagnosis based on gram-positive rods with metachromatic (blue and red) granules.<br>Toxoid vaccine prevents diphtheria. | *Coryne* = club shaped.<br>Grows on tellurite agar.<br>**ABCDEFG:**<br>ADP ribosylation<br>Beta-prophage<br>*Corynebacterium*<br>*Diphtheriae*<br>Elongation Factor 2<br>Granules |
| **Spores: bacterial** | Only certain gram-positive rods form spores when nutrients are limited (at end of stationary phase).<br>Spores are highly resistant to destruction by heat and chemicals. Have dipicolinic acid in their core. Have no metabolic activity. Must autoclave to kill spores (as is done to surgical equipment). | Spore-forming gram-positive bacteria found in soil: *Bacillus anthracis*, *Clostridium perfringens*, *C. tetani*. Other spore formers include *B. cereus*, *C. botulinum*. |

| | | |
|---|---|---|
| **Clostridia (with exotoxins)** | Gram-positive, spore-forming, obligate anaerobic bacilli.<br>*Clostridium tetani* produces tetanospasmin, an exotoxin causing tetanus. | **TET**anus is **TET**anic paralysis (blocks glycine release [inhibitory neurotransmitter]) from Renshaw cells in spinal cord. Causes spastic paralysis, trismus (lockjaw), and risus sardonicus. |
| | *C. botulinum* produces a preformed, heat-labile toxin that inhibits ACh release at the neuromuscular junction, causing botulism. In adults, disease is caused by ingestion of preformed toxin. In babies, ingestion of bacterial spores in honey causes disease (floppy baby syndrome). | **BOT**ulinum is from bad **BOT**tles of food and honey (causes a flaccid paralysis). |
| | *C. perfringens* produces α toxin ("lecithinase," a phospholipase) that can cause myonecrosis (gas gangrene) and hemolysis. | *PERF*ringens **PERF**orates a gangrenous leg. |
| | *C. difficile* produces a cytotoxin, an exotoxin that kills enterocytes, causing pseudomembranous colitis. Often 2° to antibiotic use, especially clindamycin or ampicillin. | **DI**fficile causes **DI**arrhea. Treatment: metronidazole. |
| **Anthrax** | Caused by *Bacillus anthracis*, a gram-positive, spore-forming rod that produces anthrax toxin. The only bacterium with a polypeptide capsule (contains D-glutamate).<br>Cutaneous anthrax—contact → black eschar (painless ulcer); can progress to bacteremia and death. | Black skin lesions—black eschar (necrosis) surrounded by edematous ring. Caused by lethal factor and edema factor. |
| | Pulmonary anthrax—inhalation of spores → flulike symptoms that rapidly progress to fever, pulmonary hemorrhage, mediastinitis, and shock. | Woolsorters' disease—inhalation of spores from contaminated wool. |
| **Listeria monocytogenes** | Facultative intracellular microbe; acquired by ingestion of unpasteurized milk/cheese and deli meats or by vaginal transmission during birth. Form "actin rockets" by which they move from cell to cell. The only gram-positive bacteria with endotoxin. Characteristic tumbling motility.<br>Can cause amnionitis, septicemia, and spontaneous abortion in pregnant women; granulomatosis infantiseptica; neonatal meningitis; meningitis in immunocompromised patients; mild gastroenteritis in healthy individuals. | |
| **Actinomyces vs. Nocardia**<br>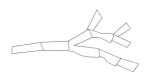 | Both are gram-positive rods forming long branching filaments resembling fungi.<br>*Actinomyces israelii*, a gram-positive anaerobe, causes oral/facial abscesses that may drain through sinus tracts in skin. Normal oral flora.<br>*Nocardia asteroides*, a gram-positive and also a weakly acid-fast aerobe in soil, causes pulmonary infection in immunocompromised patients. | *A. israelii* forms yellow "sulfur granules" in sinus tracts.<br>**SNAP:**<br>Sulfa for *Nocardia*;<br>*Actinomyces* use Penicillin |

### 1° and 2° tuberculosis

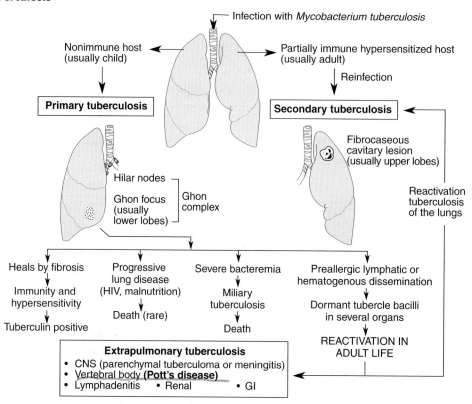

(Adapted, with permission, from Chandrasoma P, Taylor CR. *Concise Pathology,* 3rd ed. Stamford, CT: Appleton & Lange, 1998: 523.)

PPD+ if current infection, past exposure, or BCG vaccinated.
PPD– if no infection or anergic (steroids, malnutrition, immunocompromise, sarcoidosis).

| **Ghon complex** | TB granulomas (Ghon focus) with lobar and perihilar lymph node involvement. Reflects 1° infection or exposure. | |
|---|---|---|
| **Mycobacteria** | *Mycobacterium tuberculosis* (TB, often resistant to multiple drugs).<br>*M. kansasii* (pulmonary TB-like symptoms).<br>*M. avium–intracellulare* (often resistant to multiple drugs; causes disseminated disease in AIDS).<br>All mycobacteria are gram-positive, acid-fast organisms. | TB symptoms include fever, night sweats, weight loss, and hemoptysis (see Image 2). |

**Leprosy (Hansen's disease)**

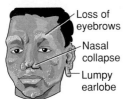

"Leonine facies" of lepromatous leprosy

- Loss of eyebrows
- Nasal collapse
- Lumpy earlobe

Caused by *Mycobacterium leprae*, an acid-fast bacillus that likes cool temperatures (infects skin and superficial nerves) and cannot be grown in vitro. Reservoir in United States: armadillos.

Treatment: long-term oral dapsone; toxicity is hemolysis and methemoglobinemia.

Alternate treatments include rifampin and combination of clofazimine and dapsone.

Hansen's disease has 2 forms: lepromatous (see Image 14) and tuberculoid; lepromatous presents diffusely over skin and is communicable (failed cell-mediated immunity); tuberculoid is limited to a few hypoesthetic nodules. **LE**promatous can be **LE**thal.

**Gram-negative lab algorithm**

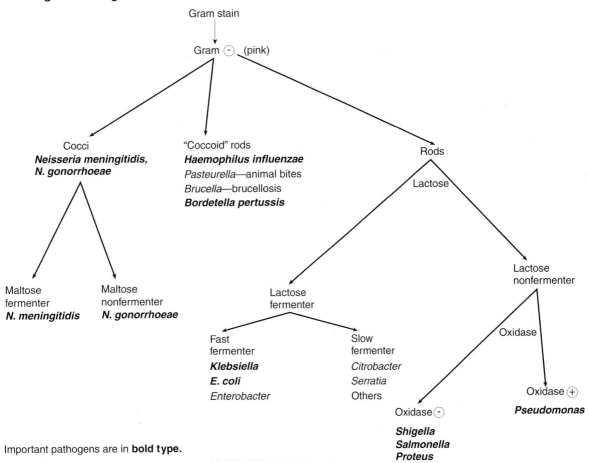

Important pathogens are in **bold type.**

| **Lactose-fermenting enteric bacteria** | These bacteria grow pink colonies on MacConkey's agar. Examples include *Citrobacter*, *Klebsiella*, *E. coli*, *Enterobacter*, and *Serratia*. | Lactose is **KEE**. Test with MacCon**KEE'S** agar. |
|---|---|---|

**Penicillin and gram-negative bugs**

Gram-negative bacilli are resistant to benzylpenicillin G but may be susceptible to penicillin derivatives such as ampicillin. The gram-negative outer membrane layer inhibits entry of penicillin G and vancomycin.

**Neisseria**

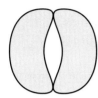

Gram-negative cocci (see Image 4). Both ferment glucose and produce IgA proteases. MeninGococci ferment Maltose and Glucose. Gonococci ferment Glucose.

| Gonococci | Meningococci |
|---|---|
| No polysaccharide capsule | Polysaccharide capsule |
| No maltose fermentation | Maltose fermentation |
| No vaccine (due to rapid antigenic variation) | Vaccine |
| Sexually transmitted | Respiratory and oral secretions |
| Causes gonorrhea, septic arthritis, neonatal conjunctivitis, PID, and Fitz-Hugh–Curtis syndrome | Causes meningococcemia and meningitis, Waterhouse-Friderichsen syndrome |

**Haemophilus influenzae**

HaEMOPhilus causes Epiglottitis ("cherry red" in children), Meningitis, Otitis media, and Pneumonia. Small gram-negative (coccobacillary) rod. Aerosol transmission. Most invasive disease caused by capsular type B. Produces IgA protease. Culture on **chocolate agar** requires factors **V** (NAD$^+$) and **X** (hematin) for growth. Treat meningitis with ceftriaxone. Rifampin prophylaxis in close contacts. Does not cause the flu (influenza virus does).

When a child has "flu," mom goes to five (**V**) and dime (**X**) store to buy some **chocolate.** Vaccine contains type B capsular polysaccharide conjugated to diphtheria toxoid or other protein to improve immune system recognition of polysaccharide and promote class switching. Given between 2 and 18 months of age.

**Legionella pneumophila**

Legionnaires' disease = severe pneumonia and fever. Pontiac fever = mild flulike syndrome.
Gram-negative rod. Gram stains poorly—use silver stain. Grow on charcoal yeast extract culture with iron and cysteine. Detected clinically by presence of antigen in urine. Aerosol transmission from environmental water source habitat. No person-to-person transmission. Treatment: erythromycin.

Think of a French legionnaire (soldier) with his silver helmet, sitting around a campfire (charcoal) with his iron dagger—he is no **sissy** (**cysteine**).

**Pseudomonas aeruginosa**

PSEUDOmonas is associated with wound and burn infections, Pneumonia (especially in cystic fibrosis), Sepsis (black lesions on skin), External otitis (swimmer's ear), UTI, Drug use and Diabetic Osteomyelitis, and hot tub folliculitis. Malignant otitis externa in diabetics. Aerobic gram-negative rod. Non–lactose fermenting, oxidase positive. Produces pyocyanin (blue-green) pigment; has a grapelike odor. Water source. Produces endotoxin (fever, shock) and exotoxin A (inactivates EF-2). Treatment: aminoglycoside plus extended-spectrum penicillin (e.g., piperacillin, ticarcillin).

AERuginosa—AERobic. Think water connection and blue-green pigment. Think *Pseudomonas* in burn victims.

| **Enterobacteriaceae** | Diverse family including *E. coli, Salmonella, Shigella, Klebsiella, Enterobacter, Serratia, Proteus.* All species have somatic (O) antigen (which is the polysaccharide of endotoxin). The capsular (K) antigen is related to the virulence of the bug. The flagellar (H) antigen is found in motile species. All ferment glucose and are oxidase negative. | Think **COFFEe:** <br> **C**apsular <br> **O** antigen <br> **F**lagellar antigen <br> **F**erment glucose <br> **E**nterobacteriaceae |
|---|---|---|

**E. coli**  In addition to the diseases below, ***E. coli*** is a cause of cystitis and pyelonephritis, pneumonia, neonatal meningitis, and septic shock.

| Category[a] | Toxin | Associated Disorders |
|---|---|---|
| **Invade intestinal mucosa** <br> EIEC | Shiga-like toxin | Dysentery (microbe invades **and** toxin causes necrosis and inflammation) |
| **Do not invade intestinal mucosa** <br> EHEC | Shiga-like toxin | Dysentery (toxin alone causes necrosis and inflammation)[b] |
| ETEC | Labile toxin/stable toxin | Traveler's diarrhea |
| EPEC | No toxin produced; adheres to apical surface, flattens villi, prevents absorption | Diarrhea (usually in children) |

[a] EIEC = enteroinvasive *E. coli*; EHEC = enterohemorrhagic *E. coli*; ETEC = enterotoxigenic *E. coli*; EPEC = enteropathogenic *E. coli*.

[b] Some EHEC strains can also cause **H**emolytic-uremic syndrome (triad of anemia, thrombocytopenia, and acute renal failure). The endothelium swells (possibly due to toxins) and narrows the lumen, leading to mechanical hemolysis and reduced renal blood flow; damaged endothelium consumes platelets.

| **Klebsiella** | An intestinal flora that causes pneumonia in alcoholics and diabetics when aspirated. Red currant jelly sputum. Also cause of nosocomial UTIs. | **4 A's:** <br> **A**spiration pneumonia <br> **A**bscess in lungs <br> **A**lcoholics <br> di-**A**-betics |
|---|---|---|
| **Salmonella vs. Shigella** | Both are non–lactose fermenters; both invade intestinal mucosa and can cause bloody diarrhea. *Salmonella* have flagella and can disseminate hematogenously. Only *Salmonella* produce $H_2S$. Symptoms of salmonellosis may be prolonged with antibiotic treatments, and there is typically a monocytic response. *Shigella* is more virulent ($10^1$ organisms) than *Salmonella* ($10^5$ organisms). *Salmonella typhi* causes typhoid fever—fever, diarrhea, headache, rose spots on abdomen. Can remain in gallbladder chronically. | **Salmon swim** (motile and disseminate). *Salmonella* have an animal reservoir (except *S. typhi*, which is found only in humans); *Shigella* do not have flagella but can propel themselves while within a cell by actin polymerization. Transmission is via "Food, Fingers, Feces, and Flies." |

**Yersinia enterocolitica**
Usually transmitted from pet feces (e.g., puppies), contaminated milk, or pork. Outbreaks are common in day-care centers. Can mimic Crohn's or appendicitis, especially in adolescents.

**Helicobacter pylori**
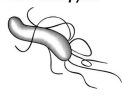
Causes gastritis and up to 90% of duodenal ulcers. Risk factor for peptic ulcer, gastric adenocarcinoma, and lymphoma. Gram-negative rod. Urease positive (e.g., urease breath test). Creates alkaline environment. Treat with triple therapy: (1) metronidazole, bismuth (Pepto-Bismol), and either tetracycline or amoxicillin; or (2) (more costly) metronidazole, omeprazole, and clarithromycin.

**Spirochetes**
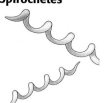
The spirochetes are spiral-shaped bacteria with axial filaments and include *Borrelia* (big size), *Leptospira*, and *Treponema*. Only *Borrelia* can be visualized using aniline dyes (Wright's or Giemsa stain) in light microscopy. *Treponema* is visualized by dark-field microscopy.

**BLT. B** is **B**ig.

**Leptospira interrogans**
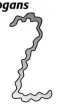
Question mark–shaped bacteria found in water contaminated with animal urine. Leptospirosis includes flulike symptoms, fever, headache, abdominal pain, jaundice, and photophobia with conjunctivitis. Most prevalent in the tropics. Weil's disease (icterohemorrhagic leptospirosis)—severe form with jaundice and azotemia from liver and kidney dysfunction; fever, hemorrhage, and anemia.

**Lyme disease**
Caused by *Borrelia burgdorferi*, which is transmitted by the tick *Ixodes* (also vector for *Babesia*). Presents with erythema chronicum migrans, an expanding "bull's eye" red rash with central clearing. Also affects joints, CNS, and heart. Mice are important reservoirs. Deer required for tick life cycle. Treatment: doxycycline, ceftriaxone. Named after Lyme, Connecticut; disease is common in northeastern United States.

3 stages of Lyme disease:
Stage 1—erythema chronicum migrans, flulike symptoms.
Stage 2—neurologic (Bell's palsy) and cardiac (AV nodal block) manifestations.
Stage 3—chronic monoarthritis, and migratory polyarthritis.
**BAKE** a Key **Lyme** pie: **B**ell's palsy, **A**rthritis, **K**ardiac block, **E**rythema migrans.

**Treponemal disease**
Treponemes are spirochetes.
*Treponema pallidum* causes syphilis.
*T. pertenue* causes yaws; infection of skin, bone, and joints → healing with keloids → severe limb deformities. Disease of the tropics. Not an STD, but VDRL positive.

**Syphilis**
  1° syphilis
  2° syphilis

  3° syphilis

  Congenital
    syphilis

Caused by spirochete *Treponema pallidum*.
Presents with painless chancre (localized disease).
Disseminated disease with constitutional symptoms,
  maculopapular rash (palms and soles),
  condylomata lata. Many treponemes are present
  in chancres of 1° and condylomata lata of 2°
  syphilis.
Gummas (chronic granulomas), aortitis (vasa
  vasorum destruction), neurosyphilis (tabes
  dorsalis), Argyll Robertson pupil (see Image
  12).
Saber shins, saddle nose, CN VIII deafness,
  Hutchinson's teeth, mulberry molars.

Treatment: penicillin G.

Secondary syphilis = Systemic.

Signs: broad-based ataxia,
  positive Romberg, Charcot
  joints, stroke without
  hypertension.

---

**Argyll Robertson pupil**

Argyll Robertson pupil constricts with accommodation
  but is not reactive to light. Associated with 3°
  syphilis.

"Prostitute's pupil"—
  accommodates but does not
  react.

---

**VDRL vs. FTA-ABS**

FTA-ABS is specific for treponemes, turns positive
  earliest in disease, and remains positive longest.

| VDRL | FTA | Interpretation |
|------|-----|----------------|
| + | + | Active infection |
| + | − | Probably false positive |
| − | + | Successfully treated |

**FTA-ABS** = Find **T**he
**A**ntibody-**ABS**olutely:
1. Most specific
2. Earliest positive
3. Remains positive the
   longest

---

**VDRL false positives**

VDRL detects nonspecific antibody that reacts with
  beef cardiolipin. Used for diagnosis of syphilis, but
  many biologic false positives, including viral
  infection (mononucleosis, hepatitis), some drugs,
  rheumatic fever, SLE, and leprosy.

**VDRL:**
  **V**iruses (mono, hepatitis)
  **D**rugs
  **R**heumatic fever
  **L**upus and leprosy

---

**Zoonotic bacteria**

| Species | Disease | Transmission and source | |
|---------|---------|-------------------------|---|
| *Bartonella* spp. | Cat scratch fever | Cat scratch; can cause bacillary angiomatosis in immunocompromised patients (often confused with Kaposi's sarcoma) | **B**ig **B**ad **B**ugs **F**rom **Y**our **P**et named **E**lla. |
| *Borrelia burgdorferi* | Lyme disease | Tick bite; *Ixodes* ticks that live on deer and mice | |
| *Brucella* spp. | Brucellosis/ undulant fever | Dairy products, contact with animals | **U**npasteurized dairy products give you **U**ndulant fever. |
| *Francisella tularensis* | Tularemia | Tick bite; rabbits, deer | |
| *Yersinia pestis* | Plague | Flea bite; rodents, especially prairie dogs | |
| *Pasteurella multocida* | Cellulitis | Animal bite; cats, dogs | |

| | | |
|---|---|---|
| ***Gardnerella vaginalis*** | A pleomorphic, gram-variable rod that causes vaginosis presenting as a gray vaginal discharge with a **fishy** smell; nonpainful. *Mobiluncus*, an anaerobe, is also involved. Associated with sexual activity, but not an STD. Bacterial vaginosis is characterized by overgrowth of certain bacteria in vagina. Treatment: metronidazole. **Clue** cells, or vaginal epithelial cells covered with bacteria, are visible under the microscope (see Image 13). | I don't have a **clue** why I smell **fish** in the **vagina garden!** |
| **Rickettsiae** | Rickettsiae are obligate intracellular organisms that need CoA and $NAD^+$. All except *Coxiella* are transmitted by an arthropod vector and cause headache, fever, and rash; *Coxiella* is an atypical rickettsia because it is transmitted by an aerosol and causes pneumonia.<br>Treatment: tetracycline. | Classic triad—headache, fever, rash (vasculitis). |
| **Rickettsial diseases and vectors** | Rocky Mountain spotted fever (tick)—*Rickettsia rickettsii.*<br>Endemic typhus (fleas)—*R. typhi.*<br>Epidemic typhus (human body louse)—*R. prowazekii.*<br>Ehrlichiosis (tick)—*Ehrlichia.*<br>Q fever (inhaled aerosols)—*Coxiella burnetii.*<br>Treatment for all: tetracycline. | Rickettsial rash starts on hands and feet; typhus rash starts centrally and spreads outward without involving palms or soles: "**R**ickettsia on the w**R**ists, **T**yphus on the **T**runk." **Q** fever is **Q**ueer because it has no rash, has no vector, and has negative Weil-Felix, and its causative organism can survive outside for a long time and does not have *Rickettsia* as its genus name. |
| **Rocky Mountain spotted fever** | Caused by *Rickettsia rickettsii.*<br>Symptoms: rash on palms and soles (migrating to wrists, ankles, then trunk), headache, fever.<br>Endemic to East Coast (in spite of name). | **Palm** and **sole** rash is seen in **C**oxsackievirus **A** infection (hand, foot, and mouth disease), **R**ocky Mountain spotted fever, and **S**yphilis (you drive **CARS** using your **palms** and **soles**). |
| **Weil-Felix reaction** | Patients with rickettsial infection have antibodies against *Rickettsia.* When patient serum is mixed with *Proteus* antigens, antirickettsial antibodies cross-react and agglutinate (Weil-Felix is negative in *Coxiella* infection). | |

**Chlamydiae**

Chlamydiae cannot make their own ATP. They are obligate intracellular organisms that cause mucosal infections. 2 forms:

1. **E**lementary body (small, dense) is **E**nfectious and **E**nters cell via endocytosis
2. **R**eticulate body **R**eplicates in cell by fission

*Chlamydia trachomatis* causes reactive arthritis, conjunctivitis, nongonococcal urethritis, and pelvic inflammatory disease (PID).

*C. pneumoniae* and *C. psittaci* cause atypical pneumonia; transmitted by aerosol.

Treatment: erythromycin or tetracycline.

*Chlamys* = cloak (intracellular).
*Chlamydia psittaci*—notable for an avian reservoir.
The chlamydial cell wall is unusual in that it lacks muramic acid.
Lab diagnosis: cytoplasmic inclusions seen on Giemsa or fluorescent antibody–stained smear.

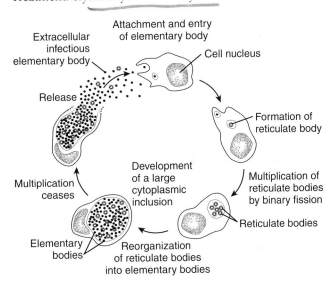

Attachment and entry of elementary body
Cell nucleus
Extracellular infectious elementary body
Release
Formation of reticulate body
Development of a large cytoplasmic inclusion
Multiplication ceases
Multiplication of reticulate bodies by binary fission
Reticulate bodies
Elementary bodies
Reorganization of reticulate bodies into elementary bodies

---

**Chlamydia trachomatis serotypes**

Types A, B, and C—chronic infection, cause blindness in Africa.
Types D–K—urethritis/PID, ectopic pregnancy, neonatal pneumonia, or neonatal conjunctivitis.
Types L1, L2, and L3—lymphogranuloma venereum (acute lymphadenitis—positive Frei test). Do not confuse with granuloma inguinale (donovanosis), which is caused by *Calymmatobacterium granulomatis*.

**ABC** = **A**frica/**B**lindness/**C**hronic infection.
L1–3 = **L**ymphogranuloma venereum.
D–K = everything else.
Neonatal disease can be acquired during passage through infected birth canal.
Treatment: oral erythromycin.

---

**Mycoplasma pneumoniae**

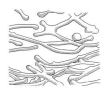

Classic cause of atypical "walking" pneumonia (insidious onset, headache, nonproductive cough, diffuse interstitial infiltrate). X-ray looks worse than patient. High titer of cold agglutinins (IgM), which can agglutinate or lyse RBCs. Grown on Eaton's agar.
Treatment: tetracycline or erythromycin (bugs are penicillin resistant because they have no cell wall).

No cell wall. Not seen on gram stain.
Only bacterial membrane containing cholesterol.
Mycoplasmal pneumonia is more common in patients < 30 years of age.
Frequent outbreaks in military recruits and prisons.

HIGH-YIELD PRINCIPLES

MICROBIOLOGY

| | | |
|---|---|---|
| **Spores: fungal** | Most fungal spores are asexual. Both coccidioidomycosis and histoplasmosis are transmitted by inhalation of asexual spores. | Conidia—asexual fungal spores (e.g., blastoconidia, arthroconidia). |

**Systemic mycoses**

| Disease | Endemic location and pathologic features | Notes |
|---|---|---|
| Histoplasmosis  3–5 μm ↕ Macrophage filled with *Histoplasma* (smaller than RBC) | Mississippi and Ohio river valleys. Causes pneumonia. | Histo Hides (within macrophages). Bird or bat droppings. |
| Blastomycosis 5–15 μm ↕ Broad-base budding (same size as RBC) | States east of Mississippi River and Central America. Causes inflammatory lung disease and can disseminate to skin and bone. Forms granulomatous nodules. *Broad based buds* | Blasto Buds (Broadly). |
| Coccidioidomycosis 20–60 μm ↕ Spherule filled with endospores (much larger than RBC) | Southwestern United States, California. Causes pneumonia and meningitis; can disseminate to bone and skin. Case rate ↑ after earthquakes (spherules are thrown up in the air). | Coccidio Crowds. San Joaquin Valley or desert (desert bumps) "valley fever" (see Image 7). |
| Paracoccidioidomy-cosis 40–50 μm ↕ Budding yeast with "captain's wheel" formation (much larger than RBC) | Latin America. | "Captain's wheel" appearance. Paracoccidio Parasails with the captain's wheel all the way to Latin America. |

All of the above are caused by **dimorphic** fungi, which are mold in soil (at lower temperature) and yeast in tissue (at higher/body temperature: 37°C). **Cold = mold; heat = yeast.** The only exception is coccidioidomycosis, which is a spherule (not yeast) in tissue. All can cause pneumonia and can disseminate. Treatment: fluconazole or ketoconazole for local infection; amphotericin B for systemic infection. Systemic mycoses can mimic TB (granuloma formation).

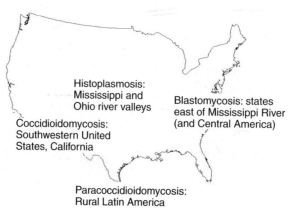

Histoplasmosis: Mississippi and Ohio river valleys

Blastomycosis: states east of Mississippi River (and Central America)

Coccidioidomycosis: Southwestern United States, California

Paracoccidioidomycosis: Rural Latin America

## Cutaneous mycoses

Tinea versicolor

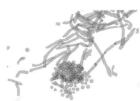

Caused by *Malassezia furfur*. Degradation of lipids produces acids that damage melanocytes and cause hypopigmented patches. Occurs in hot, humid weather. Treatment: topical miconazole, selenium sulfide (Selsun). "Spaghetti and meatball" appearance on KOH prep.

Tinea pedis, cruris, corporis, capitis

Pruritic lesions with central clearing resembling a ring, caused by dermatophytes (*Microsporum*, *Trichophyton*, and *Epidermophyton*). See mold hyphae in KOH prep, not dimorphic. Pets are a reservoir for *Microsporum* and can be treated with topical azoles.

## Opportunistic fungal infections

*Candida albicans*
(*alba* = white)

Systemic or superficial fungal infection. Yeast with pseudohyphae in culture at 20°C; germ tube formation at 37°C (diagnostic). Oral and esophageal thrush in immunocompromised (neonates, steroids, diabetes, AIDS), vulvovaginitis (high pH, diabetes, use of antibiotics), diaper rash, endocarditis in IV drug users, disseminated candidiasis (to any organ), chronic mucocutaneous candidiasis (see Image 9).

Treatment: nystatin for superficial infection; amphotericin B for serious systemic infection.

*Aspergillus fumigatus*

Allergic bronchopulmonary aspergillosis, lung cavity aspergilloma ("fungus ball"), invasive aspergillosis, especially in immunocompromised individuals and those with chronic granulomatous disease. **Mold** with septate hyphae that branch at acute angles (≤ 45°). Think "**A**" for **A**cute **A**ngles in **A**spergillus. Not dimorphic.

*Cryptococcus neoformans*

Cryptococcal meningitis, cryptococcosis. Heavily encapsulated **yeast**. Not dimorphic. Found in soil, pigeon droppings. Culture on Sabouraud's agar. Stains with India ink. Latex agglutination test detects polysaccharide capsular antigen (see Image 8). "Soap bubble" lesions in brain.

*Mucor* and *Rhizopus* spp.

Mucormycosis. **Mold** with irregular nonseptate hyphae branching at wide angles (≥ 90°). Disease mostly in ketoacidotic diabetic and leukemic patients. Fungi also proliferate in the walls of blood vessels and cause infarction and necrosis of distal tissue. Rhinocerebral, frontal lobe abscesses.

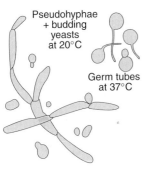

Pseudohyphae + budding yeasts at 20°C

Germ tubes at 37°C

**Candida**

45° angle branching septate hyphae

Rare fruiting bodies

**Aspergillus**

5–10-µm yeasts with wide capsular halo

Narrow-based unequal budding

**Cryptococcus**

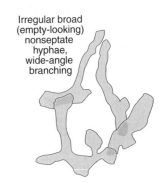

Irregular broad (empty-looking) nonseptate hyphae, wide-angle branching

**Mucor**

***Pneumocystis jiroveci* (formerly *carinii*)**

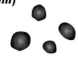

Causes diffuse interstitial pneumonia. Yeast (originally classified as protozoan). Inhaled. Most infections are asymptomatic. Immunosuppression (e.g., AIDS) predisposes to disease. Diffuse, bilateral CXR appearance. Diagnosed by lung biopsy or lavage. Identified by methenamine silver stain of lung tissue. Treatment: TMP-SMX, pentamidine, dapsone. Start prophylaxis when CD4 drops < 200 cells/mL in HIV patients (see Image 19).

***Sporothrix schenckii***

Yeast forms, unequal budding

Sporotrichosis. Dimorphic fungus that lives on vegetation. When traumatically introduced into the skin, typically by a thorn (**"rose gardener's"** disease), causes local pustule or ulcer with nodules along draining lymphatics (ascending lymphangitis). Little systemic illness. Cigar-shaped budding yeast visible in pus. Treatment: itraconazole or potassium iodide.

## Medically important protozoa—single-celled organisms

| Organism | Disease | Transmission | Diagnosis | Treatment |
|---|---|---|---|---|
| **GI infections** | | | | |
| *Giardia lamblia* (see Image 5) Trophozoite Cyst | Giardiasis: bloating, flatulence, foul-smelling, fatty diarrhea (often seen in campers/hikers)—think fat-rich **Ghirardelli** chocolates for fatty stools of *Giardia* | Cysts in water | Trophozoites or cysts in stool | Metronidazole |
| *Entamoeba histolytica* RBCs Trophozoite Cyst with 4 nuclei | Amebiasis: bloody diarrhea (dysentery), liver abscess (reddish brown), RUQ pain (histology shows flask-shaped ulcer if submucosal abscess of colon ruptures) | Cysts in water | Serology and/or trophozoites or cysts in stool; RBCs in cytoplasm of entamoeba | Metronidazole and iodoquinol |
| *Cryptosporidium* Acid-fast cysts | Severe diarrhea in AIDS Mild disease (watery diarrhea) in non-immunocompromised | Cysts in water | Cysts on acid-fast stain | Prevention (by filtering city water supplies) |
| **CNS infections** | | | | |
| *Toxoplasma gondii* | Brain abscess in HIV (seen as ring-enhancing brain lesions on CT/MRI); congenital toxoplasmosis = "classic triad" of chorioretinitis, hydrocephalus, and intracranial calcifications | Cysts in meat or cat feces; crosses placenta (pregnant women should avoid cats) | Serology, biopsy | Sulfadiazine + pyrimethamine |
| *Naegleria fowleri* | Rapidly fatal meningoencephalitis | Swimming in freshwater lakes (think **Nalgene** bottle filled with **freshwater** containing *Naegleria*); enter via cribriform plate | Amoebas in spinal fluid | None |

## Medically important protozoa—single-celled organisms *(continued)*

| Organism | Disease | Transmission | Diagnosis | Treatment |
|---|---|---|---|---|
| **CNS infections *(continued)*** | | | | |
| *Trypanosoma* <br> *T. gambiense* <br> *T. rhodesiense* | African sleeping sickness: enlarged lymph nodes, recurring fever (due to antigenic variation), somnolence, coma | Tsetse fly, a painful bite | Blood smear | **SUR**amin for blood-borne disease or **MELA**rsoprol for CNS penetration (it **SUR**e is nice to go to sleep; **MELA**tonin helps with sleep) |
| **Visceral infections** | | | | |
| *Trypanosoma cruzi* <br> RBC <br> Blood smear | Chagas' disease (dilated cardiomyopathy, megacolon, megaesophagus); predominantly in South America | Reduviid bug ("kissing bug"), a painless bite (much like a kiss) | Blood smear | Nifurtimox |
| *Leishmania donovani* | Visceral leishmaniasis (kala-azar): spiking fevers, hepatosplenomegaly, pancytopenia | Sandfly | Macrophages containing "amastigotes" (form that lacks flagella) | Sodium stibogluconate |
| **Hematologic infections** | | | | |
| *Plasmodium* <br> *P. vivax/ovale* <br> *P. falciparum* <br> *P. malariae* <br> Trophozoite ring form in RBC <br> RBC schizont with merozoites | Malaria: cyclic fever, headache, anemia, splenomegaly. *P. vivax/ovale*—cycles occur every other day; dormant form in liver is treated with primaquine. *P. falciparum*—severe; daily cycles; parasitized RBCs occlude capillaries in brain (cerebral malaria), kidneys, lungs | Mosquito (*Anopheles*) | Blood smear | Begin with chloroquine; if resistant, use mefloquine. *Vivax/ovale*—add primaquine for dormant forms in liver |
| *Babesia* <br> RBC <br> Maltese cross and ring forms | Babesiosis: fever and hemolytic anemia; predominantly in northeastern United States | *Ixodes* tick (same as *Borrelia burgdorferi* of Lyme disease; may often coinfect humans) | Blood smear, no RBC pigment, appears as "Maltese cross" | Quinine, clindamycin |
| **STDs** | | | | |
| *Trichomonas vaginalis* (see Image 10) | Vaginitis: foul-smelling, greenish discharge; itching and burning; do not confuse with *Gardnerella vaginalis*, a gram-negative bacterium that causes vaginosis | Sexual (cannot exist outside human because it cannot form cysts) | Trophozoites (motile) on wet mount | Metronidazole |

**Medically important helminths**

Multicellular organisms. Life cycle involves stages in other organisms.

| Organism | Transmission/Disease | Treatment |
|---|---|---|
| **Nematodes (roundworms)** | | |
| *Enterobius vermicularis* (pinworm) | Food contaminated with eggs; intestinal infection; causes anal pruritus (the Scotch tape test). | -bendazoles or pyrantel pamoate |
| *Ascaris lumbricoides* (giant roundworm) | Eggs are visible in feces; intestinal infection. | -bendazoles or pyrantel pamoate |
| *Trichinella spiralis* | Undercooked meat, usually pork; inflammation of muscle (larvae encyst in muscle), periorbital edema. | -bendazoles |
| *Strongyloides stercoralis* | Larvae in soil penetrate the skin; intestinal infection; causes vomiting, diarrhea, and anemia. | -bendazoles or ivermectin |
| *Ancylostoma duodenale, Necator americanus* (hookworms) | Larvae penetrate skin of feet; intestinal infection can cause anemia (sucks blood from intestinal walls). | -bendazoles or pyrantel pamoate (worms are **BEND**y; treat with me**BEND**azole) |
| *Dracunculus medinensis* | In drinking water; skin inflammation and ulceration. | Niridazole |
| *Onchocerca volvulus* | Transmitted by female blackflies; causes hyperpigmented skin and **river** blindness (remember **blackflies, black** skin nodules, "**black** sight"). Can have allergic reaction to microfilaria. | **Iver**mectin (**IVER**mectin for r**IVER** blindness) |
| *Loa loa* | Transmitted by deer fly, horse fly, and mango fly; causes swelling in skin (can see worm crawling in conjunctiva). | Diethylcarbamazine |
| *Wuchereria bancrofti* | Female mosquito; causes blockage of lymphatic vessels (elephantiasis). Takes 9 months to 1 year after bite to get elephantiasis symptoms. | Diethylcarbamazine |
| *Toxocara canis* | Food contaminated with eggs; causes granulomas (if in retina → blindness) and visceral larva migrans. | Diethylcarbamazine |
| **Cestodes (tapeworms)** | | |
| *Taenia solium* | Ingestion of larvae encysted in undercooked pork leads to intestinal tapeworms. Ingestion of eggs causes cysticercosis and neurocysticercosis, mass lesions in brain ("swiss cheese" appearance). | Praziquantel (use -bendazoles for neurocysticercosis) |
| *Diphyllobothrium latum* | Ingestion of larvae in raw freshwater fish. Causes vitamin $B_{12}$ deficiency, resulting in anemia. | Praziquantel |
| *Echinococcus granulosus* | Eggs in dog feces when ingested can cause cysts in liver; causes anaphylaxis if echinococcal antigens are released from cysts (surgeons inject ethanol before removal to neutralize antigens). | -bendazoles |

### Medically important helminths *(continued)*

| Organism | Transmission/Disease | Treatment |
|---|---|---|
| **Trematodes (flukes)** | | |
| *Schistosoma* | Snails are host; cercariae penetrate skin of humans; causes granulomas, fibrosis, and inflammation of the spleen and liver. Chronic infection with *S. haematobium* can lead to squamous cell carcinoma of the bladder. | Praziquantel |
| *Clonorchis sinensis* | Undercooked fish; causes inflammation of the biliary tract → pigmented gallstones. Also associated with cholangiocarcinoma. | Praziquantel |
| *Paragonimus westermani* | Undercooked crab meat; causes inflammation and 2° bacterial infection of the lung, causing hemoptysis. | Praziquantel |

| | | |
|---|---|---|
| **Nematode routes of infection** | Ingested—*Enterobius, Ascaris, Trichinella.* Cutaneous—*Strongyloides, Ancylostoma, Necator.* | You'll get sick if you **EAT** these! These get into your feet from the **SAN**d. |

**Parasite hints**

| Findings | Organism |
|---|---|
| Brain cysts, seizures | *Taenia solium* (cysticercosis) |
| Liver cysts | *Echinococcus granulosus* |
| B$_{12}$ deficiency | *Diphyllobothrium latum* |
| Biliary tract disease, cholangiosarcoma | *Clonorchis sinensis* |
| Hemoptysis | *Paragonimus westermani* |
| Portal hypertension | *Schistosoma mansoni* |
| Hematuria, bladder cancer | *Schistosoma haematobium* |
| Microcytic anemia | *Ancylostoma, Necator* |
| Perianal pruritus | *Enterobius* |

**"Tricky T's"**

| | |
|---|---|
| Typhoid fever | Caused by bacterium *Salmonella typhi.* |
| Typhus | Caused by bacteria *Rickettsia prowazekii* (epidemic), *Rickettsia typhi* (endemic), and *Rickettsia tsutsugamushi* (scrub typhus). |
| *Chlamydia* **trach**omatis | Bacteria, STD. |
| **Tre**ponema | Spirochete; causes syphilis (*T. pallidum*) or yaws (*T. pertenue*). |
| **Trich**omonas vaginalis | Protozoan, STD. |
| **Try**panosoma | Protozoan, causes Chagas' disease (*T. cruzi*) or African sleeping sickness. |
| **To**xoplasma | Protozoan, a TORCH infection. |
| **Trich**inella spiralis | Nematode in undercooked meat. |
| *Taenia solium* | Tapeworm larvae (intestinal infection) or eggs (neurocysticercosis) in pork. |

## Viral structure—general features

**Naked icosahedral**

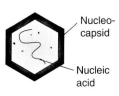

Nucleo-capsid

Nucleic acid

**Enveloped icosahedral**

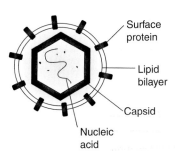

Surface protein

Lipid bilayer

Capsid

Nucleic acid

**Enveloped helical**

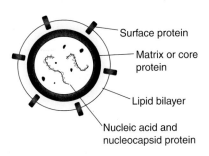

Surface protein

Matrix or core protein

Lipid bilayer

Nucleic acid and nucleocapsid protein

## Viral genetics

| | |
|---|---|
| Recombination | Exchange of genes between 2 chromosomes by crossing over within regions of significant base sequence homology. |
| Reassortment | When viruses with segmented genomes (e.g., influenza virus) exchange segments. High-frequency recombination. Cause of worldwide influenza pandemics. |
| Complementation | When 1 of 2 viruses that infect the cell has a mutation that results in a nonfunctional protein. The nonmutated virus "complements" the mutated one by making a functional protein that serves both viruses. |
| Phenotypic mixing | Occurs with simultaneous infection of a cell with 2 viruses. Genome of virus A can be partially or completely coated (forming pseudovirion) with the surface proteins of virus B. Type B protein coat determines the infectivity of the phenotypically mixed virus. However, the progeny from this infection have a type A coat that is encoded by its type A genetic material. |

## Viral vaccines

Live attenuated vaccines induce humoral and cell-mediated immunity but have reverted to virulence on rare occasions. Killed vaccines induce only humoral immunity but are stable.

**Live** attenuated—**small**pox, **yellow** fever, **chicken**pox (VZV), **Sabin**'s polio virus, **MMR**.

Killed—**R**abies, **I**nfluenza, Salk **P**olio, and HAV vaccines.
Recombinant—HBV (antigen = recombinant HBsAg), HPV (types 6, 11, 16, and 18).

No booster needed for live attenuated vaccines.
Dangerous to give live vaccines to immunocompromised patients or their close contacts.
"**Live!** One night only! See **small yellow chickens** get vaccinated with **Sabin**'s and **MMR!**"
MMR = measles, mumps, rubella (the only live attenuated vaccine that can be given to HIV-positive patients).
Sal**K** = **K**illed.
**RIP** Always.

165

| | | |
|---|---|---|
| **DNA viral genomes** | All DNA viruses except the Parvoviridae are dsDNA. All are linear except papilloma, polyoma, and hepadnaviruses (circular). | All are dsDNA (like our cells), except "**part-of-a-virus**" (**parvovirus**) is ssDNA. *Parvus* = small. |
| **RNA viral genomes** | All RNA viruses except Reoviridae are ssRNA. | All are ssRNA (like our mRNA), except "repeato-virus" (**reo**virus) is dsRNA. |
| **Naked viral genome infectivity** | Purified nucleic acids of most dsDNA (except poxviruses and HBV) and (+) strand ssRNA (≈ mRNA) viruses are infectious. Naked nucleic acids of (−) strand ssRNA and dsRNA viruses are not infectious. They require enzymes contained in the complete virion. | |
| **Virus ploidy** | All viruses are haploid (with 1 copy of DNA or RNA) except retroviruses, which have 2 identical ssRNA molecules (≈ diploid). | |
| **Viral replication** DNA viruses RNA viruses | All replicate in the nucleus (except poxvirus). All replicate in the cytoplasm (except influenza virus and retroviruses). | |
| **Viral envelopes** | **Naked** (nonenveloped) viruses include **C**alicivirus, **P**icornavirus, **R**eovirus, **P**arvovirus, **A**denovirus, **P**apilloma, and **P**olyoma. Generally, enveloped viruses acquire their envelopes from plasma membrane when they exit from cell. Exceptions are herpesviruses, which acquire envelopes from nuclear membrane. | **Naked CPR** and **PAPP** smear. |

**Viral pathogens**

| Structure | Viruses |
|---|---|
| DNA enveloped viruses | Herpesviruses (HSV types 1 and 2, VZV, CMV, EBV), HBV, smallpox virus |
| DNA nucleocapsid viruses | Adenovirus, papillomaviruses, parvovirus |
| RNA enveloped viruses | Influenza virus, parainfluenza virus, RSV, measles virus, mumps virus, rubella virus, rabies virus, HTLV, HIV |
| RNA nucleocapsid viruses | Enteroviruses (poliovirus, coxsackievirus, echovirus, HAV), rhinovirus, reovirus (rotavirus) |

**DNA virus characteristics**

Some general rules—all DNA viruses:

1. Are **HHAPPPP**y viruses

2. Are double stranded
3. Are linear

4. Are icosahedral
5. Replicate in the nucleus

Hepadna, Herpes, Adeno, Pox, Parvo, Papilloma, Polyoma.
EXCEPT parvo (single stranded).
EXCEPT papilloma and polyoma (circular, supercoiled) and hepadna (circular, incomplete).
EXCEPT pox (complex).
EXCEPT pox (carries own DNA-dependent RNA polymerase).

**DNA viruses**

| Viral Family | Envelope | DNA Structure | Medical Importance |
|---|---|---|---|
| Herpesviruses | Yes | DS – linear | HSV-1—oral (and some genital) lesions, keratoconjunctivitis<br>HSV-2—genital (and some oral) lesions<br>VZV (HHV-3)—chickenpox, zoster, shingles<br>EBV (HHV-4)—mononucleosis, Burkitt's lymphoma<br>CMV (HHV-5)—infection in immunosuppressed patients, especially transplant recipients; congenital defects<br>HHV-6—roseola (exanthem subitum)<br>HHV-7—clinically insignificant (included only to complete family)<br>HHV-8—Kaposi's sarcoma–associated herpesvirus (KSHV) |
| Hepadnavirus | Yes | DS – partial circular | HBV<br>Acute or chronic hepatitis<br>Vaccine available—use has increased tremendously<br>Not a retrovirus but has reverse transcriptase |
| Adenovirus | No | DS – linear | Febrile pharyngitis—sore throat<br>Pneumonia<br>Conjunctivitis—"pink eye" (watery) |
| Parvovirus | No | SS – linear (−) (smallest DNA virus) | B19 virus—aplastic crises in sickle cell disease, "slapped cheeks" rash—erythema infectiosum (fifth disease), RBC destruction in fetus leads to hydrops fetalis and death |
| Papillomavirus* | No | DS – circular | HPV—warts, CIN, cervical cancer |
| Polyomavirus* | No | DS – circular | JC—progressive multifocal leukoencephalopathy (PML) in HIV |
| Poxvirus | Yes | DS – linear (largest DNA virus) | Smallpox, although eradicated, could be used in germ warfare<br>Vaccinia—cowpox ("milkmaid's blisters")<br>Molluscum contagiosum |

*Papillomavirus and polyomavirus are two new classifications originally grouped as "papovavirus."

**HIGH-YIELD PRINCIPLES**

**MICROBIOLOGY**

### Herpesviruses

| Virus | Diseases | Route of transmission | |
|---|---|---|---|
| HSV-1 | Gingivostomatitis, keratoconjunctivitis, temporal lobe encephalitis (most common cause of sporadic encephalitis in the United States), herpes labialis | Respiratory secretions, saliva | Get herpes in a **CHEV**rolet: CMV HSV |
| HSV-2 | Herpes genitalis (see Image 11), neonatal herpes | Sexual contact, perinatal | EBV VZV |
| VZV | Varicella-zoster (shingles), encephalitis, pneumonia (see Image 15) | Respiratory secretions | VZV remains dormant in trigeminal and dorsal root ganglia. |
| EBV | Infectious mononucleosis, Burkitt's lymphoma, nasopharyngeal carcinoma | Respiratory secretions, saliva | |
| CMV | Congenital infection, mononucleosis (negative Monospot), pneumonia. Infected cells have characteristic "owl's eye" appearance (see Image 6) | Congenital, transfusion, sexual contact, saliva, urine, transplant | |
| HHV-6 | Roseola: high fevers for several days that can cause seizures, followed by a diffuse macular rash | Not determined | |
| HHV-8 | Kaposi's sarcoma (HIV patients) | Sexual contact | |

| | | |
|---|---|---|
| **HSV identification** | Tzanck test—a smear of an opened skin vesicle to detect multinucleated giant cells. Used to assay for HSV-1, HSV-2, and VZV. Infected cells also have intranuclear Cowdry A inclusions. | **Tzanck** heavens I do not have herpes. |
| **EBV** | A herpesvirus. Can cause mononucleosis. Infects B cells. Characterized by fever, hepatosplenomegaly, pharyngitis, and lymphadenopathy (especially posterior cervical nodes). Peak incidence 15–20 years of age. Abnormal circulating cytotoxic T cells (atypical lymphocytes). Also associated with development of Hodgkin's and endemic Burkitt's lymphomas as well as nasopharyngeal carcinoma. | Most common during peak kissing years ("kissing disease"). Positive Monospot test— heterophil antibodies detected by agglutination of sheep RBCs. |

## RNA viruses

| Viral Family | Envelope | RNA Structure | Capsid Symmetry | Medical Importance |
|---|---|---|---|---|
| Reoviruses | No | DS linear 10–12 segments | Icosahedral (double) | Reovirus—Colorado tick fever<br>Rotavirus—#1 cause of fatal diarrhea in children |
| Picornaviruses | No | SS + linear | Icosahedral | Poliovirus—polio-Salk/Sabin vaccines—IPV/OPV<br>Echovirus—aseptic meningitis<br>Rhinovirus—"common cold"<br>Coxsackievirus—aseptic meningitis<br>  herpangina—febrile pharyngitis<br>  hand, foot, and mouth disease<br>  myocarditis<br>HAV—acute viral hepatitis |
| Hepevirus | No | SS + linear | Icosahedral | HEV |
| Caliciviruses | No | SS + linear | Icosahedral | Norwalk virus—viral gastroenteritis |
| Flaviviruses | Yes | SS + linear | Icosahedral | HCV<br>Yellow fever*<br>Dengue*<br>St. Louis encephalitis*<br>West Nile virus* |
| Togaviruses | Yes | SS + linear | Icosahedral | Rubella (German measles)<br>Eastern equine encephalitis*<br>Western equine encephalitis* |
| Retroviruses | Yes | SS + linear | Icosahedral | Have reverse transcriptase<br>HIV—AIDS<br>HTLV—T-cell leukemia |
| Coronaviruses | Yes | SS + linear | Helical | Coronavirus—"common cold" and SARS |
| Orthomyxoviruses | Yes | SS − linear 8 segments | Helical | Influenza virus |
| Paramyxoviruses | Yes | SS − linear Nonsegmented | Helical | PaRaMyxovirus:<br>  Parainfluenza—croup<br>  RSV—bronchiolitis in babies; Rx—ribavirin<br>  Rubeola (Measles)<br>  Mumps |
| Rhabdoviruses | Yes | SS − linear | Helical | Rabies |
| Filoviruses | Yes | SS − linear | Helical | Ebola/Marburg hemorrhagic fever—often fatal! |
| Arenaviruses | Yes | SS − circular 2 segments | Helical | LCMV—lymphocytic choriomeningitis virus<br>Lassa fever encephalitis—spread by mice |
| Bunyaviruses | Yes | SS − circular 3 segments | Helical | California encephalitis*<br>Sandfly/Rift Valley fevers<br>Crimean-Congo hemorrhagic fever*<br>Hantavirus—hemorrhagic fever, pneumonia |
| Deltavirus | Yes | SS − circular | Helical | HDV |

SS, single-stranded; DS, double-stranded; +, + sense; −, − sense; * = arbovirus

(Adapted, with permission, from Levinson W, Jawetz E. *Medical Microbiology and Immunology: Examination and Board Review*, 6th ed. New York: McGraw-Hill, 2000: 182.)

| | | |
|---|---|---|
| **Negative-stranded viruses** | Must transcribe negative strand to positive. Virion brings its own RNA-dependent RNA polymerase. They include Arenaviruses, Bunyaviruses, Paramyxoviruses, Orthomyxoviruses, Filoviruses, and Rhabdoviruses. | Always Bring Polymerase Or Fail Replication. |
| **Segmented viruses** | All are RNA viruses. They include Bunyaviruses, Orthomyxoviruses (influenza viruses), Arenaviruses, and Reoviruses. Influenza virus consists of 8 segments of negative-stranded RNA. These segments can undergo reassortment, causing antigenic shifts that lead to worldwide pandemics of the flu. | BOAR. |
| **Picornavirus** | Includes Poliovirus, Echovirus, Rhinovirus, Coxsackievirus, HAV. RNA is translated into 1 large polypeptide that is cleaved by proteases into functional viral proteins. Can cause aseptic (viral) meningitis (except rhinovirus and HAV). | PicoRNAvirus = small RNA virus. PERCH on a "peak" (pico). |
| **Rhinovirus** | A picornavirus. Nonenveloped RNA virus. Cause of common cold; > 100 serologic types. | Rhino has a runny nose. |
| **Yellow fever virus** | A flavivirus (also an arbovirus) transmitted by *Aedes* mosquitos. Virus has a monkey or human reservoir. Symptoms: high fever, black vomitus, and jaundice. Councilman bodies (acidophilic inclusions) may be seen in liver. | *Flavi* = yellow. |
| **Rotavirus** | Rotavirus, the most important global cause of infantile gastroenteritis, is a segmented dsRNA virus (a reovirus). Major cause of acute diarrhea in the United States during winter, especially in day-care centers, kindergartens. Villous destruction with atrophy leads to ↓ absorption of $Na^+$ and water. | ROTA = Right Out The Anus. |
| **Influenza viruses** | Orthomyxoviruses. Enveloped, single-stranded RNA viruses with segmented genome. Contain hemagglutinin (promotes viral entry) and neuraminidase (promotes progeny virion release) antigens. Responsible for worldwide influenza epidemics; patients at risk for fatal bacterial superinfection. Rapid genetic changes. | Killed viral vaccine is major mode of protection; reformulated vaccine offered each fall to elderly, health-care workers, etc. |
| Genetic shift (pandemic) Genetic drift (epidemic) | Reassortment of viral genome (such as when human flu A virus recombines with swine flu A virus). Minor (antigenic drift) changes based on random mutation. | Sudden Shift is more deadly than graDual Drift. |

| | | |
|---|---|---|
| **Rubella virus** | A togavirus. Causes German (3-day) measles. Fever, lymphadenopathy, arthralgias, fine truncal rash. Causes mild disease in children but serious congenital disease (a TORCH infection). | |
| **Paramyxoviruses** | Paramyxoviruses cause disease in children. They include those that cause parainfluenza (croup: seal-like barking cough), mumps, and measles as well as RSV, which causes respiratory tract infection (bronchiolitis, pneumonia) in infants. All contain surface F (fusion) protein, which causes respiratory epithelial cells to fuse and form multinucleated cells. Palivizumab is used in RSV to neutralize F protein. | |
| **Rubeola (measles) virus** | A paramyxovirus that causes measles. Koplik spots (red spots with blue-white center on buccal mucosa; see Image 17) are diagnostic. SSPE (years later), encephalitis (1:2000), and giant cell pneumonia (rarely, in immunosuppressed) are possible sequelae. Rash spreads from head to toe (see Image 18). Do not confuse with roseola (caused by HHV-6). | 3 C's of measles:<br>  Cough<br>  Coryza<br>  Conjunctivitis<br>Also look for Koplik spots. |
| **Mumps virus**<br><br>*Parotid*<br>*Paramyxovirus* | A paramyxovirus.<br>Symptoms: **P**arotitis, **O**rchitis (inflammation of testes), and aseptic **M**eningitis. Can cause sterility (especially after puberty). | Mumps makes your parotid glands and testes as big as **POM**-poms. |
| **Rabies virus** | Negri bodies are characteristic cytoplasmic inclusions in neurons infected by rabies virus. Has bullet-shaped capsid. Rabies has long incubation period (weeks to months), which allows for immunization after exposure.<br>Progression of disease: fever, malaise → agitation, photophobia, hydrophobia → paralysis, coma → death.<br>More commonly from bat, raccoon, and skunk bites than from dog bites in the United States. | Travels to the CNS by migrating in a retrograde fashion up nerve axons.<br><br>**Negri bodies**<br>(Reproduced, with permission, from the CDC.) |
| **Arboviruses** | Transmitted by arthropods (mosquitoes, ticks). Classic examples are dengue fever (also known as break-bone fever) and yellow fever. A variant of dengue fever in Southeast Asia is hemorrhagic shock syndrome. | **ARBO**virus—**AR**thropod-**BO**rne virus, including some members of **F**lavivirus, **T**ogavirus, and **B**unyavirus. **F**ever **T**ransmitted by **B**ites. |

**"Lots of spots"**

| | |
|---|---|
| Rubella | Togavirus; German 3-day measles. |
| Rubeola | Paramyxovirus; measles. |
| Roseola | Herpesvirus (HHV-6). High fevers followed by diffuse maculopapular rash. |
| Varicella | Herpesvirus; chickenpox and zoster. |
| Variola | Poxvirus; smallpox (no longer present outside of labs). |

**Hepatitis viruses**

The hepatitis viruses belong to 5 different viral families. Signs and symptoms: episodes of fever, jaundice, elevated ALT and AST.

HAV (RNA picornavirus) is transmitted primarily by fecal-oral route. Short incubation (3 weeks). No carriers.

HBV (DNA hepadnavirus) is transmitted primarily by parenteral, sexual, and maternal-fetal routes. Long incubation (3 months). Carriers. Cellular RNA polymerase transcribes RNA from DNA template. Reverse transcriptase transcribes DNA genome from RNA intermediate. However, the virion enzyme is a DNA-dependent DNA polymerase.

HCV (RNA flavivirus) is transmitted primarily via blood and resembles HBV in its course and severity. Carriers. Common cause of post-transfusion hepatitis and of hepatitis among IV drug users in the United States.

HDV (delta agent) is a defective virus that requires HBsAg as its envelope. HDV can coinfect with HBV or superinfect; the latter has a worse prognosis. Carriers.

HEV (RNA hepevirus) is transmitted enterically and causes water-borne epidemics. Resembles HAV in course, severity, incubation. High mortality rate in pregnant women.

Both HBV and HCV predispose a patient to chronic active hepatitis, cirrhosis, and hepatocellular carcinoma.

Hep **A**: **A**symptomatic (usually), **A**cute, **A**lone (no carriers).

Hep **B**: **B**lood borne.

Hep **C**: **C**hronic, **C**irrhosis, **C**arcinoma, **C**arriers.

Hep **D**: **D**efective, **D**ependent on HBV.

Hep **E**: **E**nteric, **E**xpectant mothers, **E**pidemics.

A and E by fecal-oral route: "The **vowels** hit your **bowels**." (Because naked viruses do not rely on an envelope, they are not destroyed in the gut.)

*[handwritten margin note: Hep E Pregnant women]*

*[handwritten note: A, E naked viruses.]*

## Hepatitis serologic markers

| | |
|---|---|
| IgG HAVAb | Indicates prior infection; protective against reinfection. |
| IgM HAVAb | IgM antibody to HAV; best test to detect active hepatitis A. |
| HBsAg | Antigen found on surface of HBV; continued presence indicates carrier state. |
| HBsAb | Antibody to HBsAg; **provides immunity** to hepatitis B. |
| HBcAg | Antigen associated with core of HBV. |
| HBcAb | Antibody to HBcAg; positive during **window period.** IgM HBcAb is an indicator of recent disease. IgG HBcAb signifies chronic disease. |
| HBeAg | A second, different antigenic determinant in the HBV core. Important indicator of active viral replication and therefore transmissibility. High HBEAg level = high Enfectivity. |
| HBeAb | Antibody to e antigen; indicates low transmissibility. |

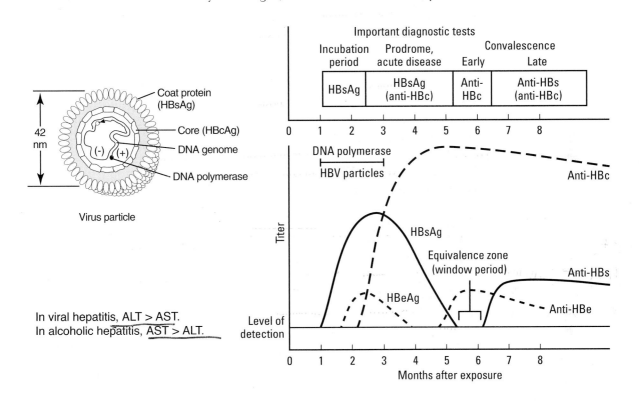

In viral hepatitis, ALT > AST.
In alcoholic hepatitis, AST > ALT.

| Test | Acute Disease | Window Phase | Complete Recovery | Chronic Carrier | Immunized |
|---|---|---|---|---|---|
| HBsAg | + | − | − | + | − |
| HBsAb | − | −[b] | + | − | + |
| HBcAb | +[a] | + | + | + | − |

[a]IgM in acute stage; IgG in chronic or recovered stage.

[b]Patient has surface antibody but available antibody is bound to HBsAg, so not detected in assay.

## HIV

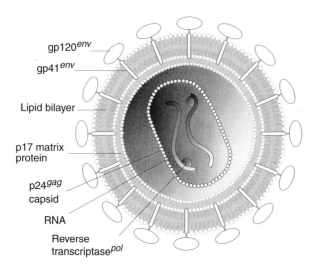

gp120$^{env}$

gp41$^{env}$

Lipid bilayer

p17 matrix protein

p24$^{gag}$ capsid

RNA

Reverse transcriptase$^{pol}$

(Adapted, with permission, from Levinson W. *Medical Microbiology and Immunology: Examination and Board Review,* 8th ed. New York: McGraw-Hill, 2004: 314.)

Diploid genome (2 molecules of RNA).
p24 = capsid protein.
gp41 and gp120 = envelope proteins.

Reverse transcriptase synthesizes dsDNA from RNA; dsDNA integrates into host genome.

Virus binds CXCR4 and CD4 on T cells; binds CCR5 and CD4 on macrophages. Homozygous CCR5 mutation = immunity. Heterozygous CCR5 mutation = slower course.

| **HIV diagnosis** | Presumptive diagnosis made with ELISA (sensitive, high false-positive rate and low threshold, RULE OUT test); positive results are then confirmed with Western blot assay (specific, high false-negative rate and high threshold, RULE IN test). HIV PCR/viral load tests are increasing in popularity: they allow physician to monitor the effect of drug therapy on viral load. AIDS diagnosis ≤ 200 CD4+ (normal: 500–1500). HIV positive with AIDS indicator condition (e.g., *Pneumocystis jiroveci* pneumonia, formerly known as PCP) or CD4/CD8 ratio < 1.5. | ELISA/Western blot tests look for antibodies to viral proteins; these tests are often falsely negative in the first 1–2 months of HIV infection and falsely positive initially in babies born to infected mothers (anti-gp120 crosses placenta). |

HIV test
1. Elisa → sensitive
2. WB → specific

## Time course of HIV infection

4 stages of infection:
1. Flulike (acute)
2. Feeling fine (latent)
3. Falling count
4. Final crisis

During latent phase, virus replicates in lymph nodes.

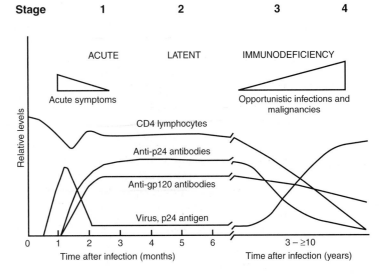

(Adapted, with permission, from Levinson W. *Medical Microbiology and Immunology: Examination and Board Review,* 8th ed. New York: McGraw-Hill, 2004: 318.)

## Opportunistic infections and disease in AIDS

| Organ system | Infection/disease |
|---|---|
| Brain | Cryptococcal meningitis, toxoplasmosis, CMV encephalopathy, AIDS dementia, PML (JC virus) |
| Eyes | CMV retinitis |
| Mouth and throat | Thrush (*Candida albicans*), HSV, CMV, oral hairy leukoplakia (EBV) |
| Lungs | *Pneumocystis jiroveci* pneumonia (formerly known as PCP), TB, histoplasmosis |
| GI | Cryptosporidiosis, *Mycobacterium avium–intracellulare* complex, CMV colitis, non-Hodgkin's lymphoma (EBV), *Isospora belli* |
| Skin | Shingles (VZV), Kaposi's sarcoma (HHV-8) |
| Genitals | Genital herpes, warts, and cervical cancer (HPV) |

## HIV-associated infections and CD4 count

| Risk increases at CD4 level of: | Infection |
|---|---|
| < 400 | Oral thrush, tinea pedis, reactivation VZV, reactivation tuberculosis, other bacterial infections (e.g., *H. influenzae, S. pneumoniae, Salmonella*) |
| < 200 | Reactivation HSV, cryptosporidiosis, *Isospora*, disseminated coccidioidomycosis, *Pneumocystis* pneumonia |
| < 100 | Candidal esophagitis, toxoplasmosis, histoplasmosis |
| < 50 | CMV retinitis and esophagitis, disseminated *M. avium–intracellulare*, cryptococcal meningoencephalitis |

## Neoplasms associated with HIV

Kaposi's sarcoma (HHV-8), invasive cervical carcinoma (HPV), 1° CNS lymphoma, non-Hodgkin's lymphoma.

## HIV encephalitis

Occurs late in the course of HIV infection. Virus gains CNS access via infected macrophages. Microglial nodules with multinucleated giant cells.

**Prions**

PrPc

Prion diseases are caused by the conversion of a normal cellular protein termed *prion protein* (PrPc) to a β-pleated form (PrPsc), which is transmissible. PrPsc resists degradation and facilitates the conversion of still more PrPc to PrPsc. Accumulation of PrPsc results in spongiform encephalopathy and dementia, ataxia, and death. It can be **sporadic** (Creutzfeldt-Jakob disease—rapidly progressive dementia), **inherited** (Gerstmann-Sträussler-Scheinker syndrome), or **acquired** (kuru).

---

**Normal flora: dominant**

Skin—*Staphylococcus epidermidis*.
Nose—*S. epidermidis*; colonized by *S. aureus*.
Oropharynx—viridans group streptococci.
Dental plaque—*Streptococcus mutans*.
Colon—*Bacteroides fragilis* > *E. coli*.
Vagina—*Lactobacillus*, colonized by *E. coli* and group B strep.

Neonates delivered by cesarean section have no flora but are rapidly colonized after birth.

---

**Bugs causing food poisoning**

*Vibrio parahaemolyticus* and *V. vulnificus* in contaminated seafood. *V. vulnificus* can also cause wound infections from contact with contaminated water or shellfish.
*Bacillus cereus* in reheated rice.
*S. aureus* in meats, mayonnaise, custard. Preformed toxin.
*Clostridium perfringens* in reheated meat dishes.
*C. botulinum* in improperly canned foods (bulging cans).
*E. coli* O157:H7 in undercooked meat.
*Salmonella* in poultry, meat, and eggs.

*S. aureus* and *B. cereus* food poisoning starts quickly and ends quickly.
"Food poisoning from reheated rice? **Be serious!**"
(**B. cereus**).

**Bugs causing diarrhea**

| Type | Species | Findings |
|---|---|---|
| Bloody diarrhea | *Campylobacter* | Comma- or S-shaped organisms; growth at 42°C (**Campylobacter** likes the "hot **camp**fire"); oxidase positive |
| | *Salmonella* | Lactose negative; flagellar motility |
| | *Shigella* | Lactose negative; very low $ID_{50}$; produces Shiga toxin |
| | Enterohemorrhagic *E. coli* | O157:H7; can cause HUS; makes Shiga-like toxin |
| | Enteroinvasive *E. coli* | Invades colonic mucosa |
| | *Yersinia enterocolitica* | Day-care outbreaks, pseudoappendicitis |
| | *C. difficile* (can cause both watery and bloody diarrhea) | Pseudomembranous colitis |
| | *Entamoeba histolytica* | Protozoan |
| Watery diarrhea | Enterotoxigenic *E. coli* | Traveler's diarrhea; produces ST and LT toxins |
| | *Vibrio cholerae* | Comma-shaped organisms; rice-water diarrhea |
| | *C. perfringens* | Also causes gas gangrene |
| | Protozoa | *Giardia, Cryptosporidium* (in immunocompromised) |
| | Viruses | Rotavirus, adenovirus, Norwalk virus (norovirus) |

**Common causes of pneumonia**

| Neonates (< 4 wk) | Children (4 wk–18 yr) | Adults (18–40 yr) | Adults (40–65 yr) | Elderly |
|---|---|---|---|---|
| Group B streptococci | Viruses (**R**SV) | *Mycoplasma* | *S. pneumoniae* | S. pneumoniae |
| E. coli | *Mycoplasma* | C. pneumoniae | *H. influenzae* | Viruses |
| | *Chlamydia pneumoniae* | S. pneumoniae | Anaerobes | Anaerobes |
| | *Streptococcus pneumoniae* | | Viruses | *H. influenzae* |
| | **R**unts **M**ay **C**ough **S**putum | | *Mycoplasma* | Gram-negative rods |

Special groups:

| | |
|---|---|
| Nosocomial (hospital acquired) | *Staphylococcus*, enteric gram-negative rods |
| Immunocompromised | *Staphylococcus*, enteric gram-negative rods, fungi, viruses, *Pneumocystis jiroveci*—with HIV |
| Aspiration | Anaerobes , *Bacteroides* |
| Alcoholic/IV drug user | *S. pneumoniae, Klebsiella, Staphylococcus* |
| Cystic fibrosis | *Pseudomonas* |
| Postviral | *Staphylococcus, H. influenzae* |
| Atypical | *Mycoplasma, Legionella, Chlamydia* |

**Common causes of meningitis**

| Newborn (0–6 mos) | Children (6 mos–6 yrs) | 6–60 yrs | 60 yrs + |
|---|---|---|---|
| Group B streptococci | *Streptococcus pneumoniae* | *N. meningitidis* | *S. pneumoniae* |
| *E. coli* | *Neisseria meningitidis* | Enteroviruses | Gram- negative rods |
| *Listeria* | *Haemophilus influenzae* type B | *S. pneumoniae* | *Listeria* |
| | Enteroviruses | HSV | |

Viral causes of meningitis—enteroviruses (esp. coxsackievirus), HSV, HIV, West Nile virus, VZV.

In HIV—*Cryptococcus*, CMV, toxoplasmosis (brain abscess), JC virus (PML).

Note: Incidence of *H. influenzae* meningitis has ↓ greatly with introduction of *H. influenzae* vaccine in last 10–15 years.

**CSF findings in meningitis**

| | Pressure | Cell type | Protein | Sugar |
|---|---|---|---|---|
| Bacterial | ↑ | ↑ PMNs | ↑ | ↓ |
| Fungal/TB | ↑ | ↑ lymphocytes | ↑ | ↓ |
| Viral | Normal/↑ | ↑ lymphocytes | Normal/↑ | Normal |

**Osteomyelitis**

Most people—*S. aureus*.

Sexually active—*Neisseria gonorrhoeae* (rare), septic arthritis more common.

Diabetics and drug addicts—*Pseudomonas aeruginosa*.

Sickle cell—*Salmonella*.

Prosthetic replacement—*S. aureus* and S. *epidermidis*.

Vertebral—*Mycobacterium tuberculosis* (Pott's disease).

Cat and dog bites or scratches—*Pasteurella multocida*.

Assume *S. aureus* if no other information.

Most osteomyelitis occurs in children.

Elevated CRP and ESR classic but nonspecific.

**Urinary tract infections**

Presents with dysuria, frequency, urgency, suprapubic pain, and WBCs (but not WBC casts) in urine. Primarily caused by ascension of microbes from urethra to bladder. Males—infants with congenital defects, vesicoureteral reflux. Elderly—enlarged prostate. Ascension to kidney results in pyelonephritis, which presents with fever, chills, flank pain, CVA tenderness, hematuria, and WBC casts.

Ten times more common in women (shorter urethras colonized by fecal flora). Other predisposing factors include obstruction, kidney surgery, catheterization, GU malformation, diabetes, and pregnancy.

Diagnostic markers:

Positive leukocyte esterase test = bacterial UTI.

Positive nitrite test = gram-negative bacterial UTI.

## UTI bugs

| Species | Features of the organism |
|---|---|
| *Serratia marcescens* | Some strains produce a red pigment; often nosocomial and drug resistant. |
| *Staphylococcus saprophyticus* | 2nd leading cause of community-acquired UTI in sexually active women. |
| *Escherichia coli* | Leading cause of UTI. Colonies show metallic sheen on EMB agar. |
| *Enterobacter cloacae* | Often nosocomial and drug resistant. |
| *Klebsiella pneumoniae* | Large mucoid capsule and viscous colonies. |
| *Proteus mirabilis* | Motility causes "swarming" on agar; produces urease; associated with struvite stones. |
| *Pseudomonas aeruginosa* | Blue-green pigment and fruity odor; usually nosocomial and drug resistant. |

**SSEEK PP.**

Diagnostic markers:
Leukocyte esterase— positive = bacterial.
Nitrite test—positive = gram negative.

## ToRCHeS infections

Microbes that may pass from mother to fetus. Nonspecific signs common to many ToRCHeS infections include hepatosplenomegaly, jaundice, thrombocytopenia, and growth retardation.

Other important infectious agents include *Streptococcus agalactiae* (group B streptococci), *E. coli*, and *Listeria monocytogenes*—all causes of meningitis in neonates.

| Agent | Mode of Transmission | Maternal Manifestations | Neonatal Manifestions |
|---|---|---|---|
| *Toxoplasma gondii* | Aerosolized cat feces or ingestion of undercooked meat | Usually asymptomatic; lymphadenopathy (rarely) | Classic triad: chorioretinitis, hydrocephalus, and intracranial calcifications |
| Rubella | Respiratory droplets | Rash, lymphadenopathy, arthritis | Classic triad: PDA (or pulmonary artery hypoplasia), cataracts, and deafness ± "blueberry muffin" rash |
| CMV | Sexual contact, organ transplants | Usually asymptomatic; mononucleosis-like illness | Hearing loss, seizures |
| HIV | Sexual contact | Variable presentation depending on CD4+ count | Recurrent infections, chronic diarrhea |
| Herpes simplex virus | Skin or mucous membrane contact | Usually asymptomatic; herpetic (vesicular) lesions | Encephalitis, herpetic (vesicular) lesions |
| Syphilis | Sexual contact | Chancre (1°), disseminated rash (2°), or cardiac/neurologic disease (3°) | Often results in stillbirth, hydrops fetalis; if child survives, presents with facial abnormalities (notched teeth, saddle nose, short maxilla), saber shins |

## Red rashes of childhood

| Agent | Associated Syndrome/Disease | Clinical Presentation |
|---|---|---|
| Rubella virus | German measles | Rash begins at head and moves down; postauricular lymphadenopathy. |
| Measles virus | Rubeola, measles | A paramyxovirus; beginning at head and moving down; rash is preceded by cough, coryza, conjunctivitis, and blue-white (Koplik) spots on buccal mucosa. |
| Mumps virus | Mumps | A paramyxovirus; no rash, but can present with parotitis, meningitis (orchitis or oophoritis in young adults). |
| VZV | Chickenpox | Rash begins on trunk; spreads to face and extremities with lesions of different age. |
| HHV-6 | Roseola | A macular rash over body appears after several days of high fever; usually affects infants. |
| Parvovirus B19 | Erythema infectiosum | "Slapped cheek" rash on face later appears over body in reticular, "lace-like" pattern. (Can cause hydrops fetalis in pregnant women.) |
| *Streptococcus pyogenes* | Scarlet fever | Erythematous, sandpaper-like rash with fever and sore throat. |
| Coxsackievirus type A | Hand-foot-mouth disease | Vesicular rash on palms and soles; ulcers in oral mucosa. |

## Sexually transmitted diseases

| Disease | Clinical features | Organism |
|---|---|---|
| Gonorrhea | Urethritis, cervicitis, PID, prostatitis, epididymitis, arthritis, creamy purulent discharge | *Neisseria gonorrhoeae* |
| 1° syphilis | Painless chancre | *Treponema pallidum* |
| 2° syphilis | Fever, lymphadenopathy, skin rashes, condylomata lata | |
| 3° syphilis | Gummas, tabes dorsalis, general paresis, aortitis, Argyll Robertson pupil | |
| Chancroid | Painful genital ulcer, inguinal adenopathy | *Haemophilus* **ducreyi** (it's so painful, you "**do cry**") |
| Genital herpes | Painful penile, vulvar, or cervical ulcers; can cause systemic symptoms such as fever, headache, myalgia. | HSV-2 |
| Chlamydia | Urethritis, cervicitis, conjunctivitis, Reiter's syndrome, PID | *Chlamydia trachomatis* (D–K) |
| Lymphogranuloma venereum | Ulcers, lymphadenopathy, rectal strictures | *C. trachomatis* (L1–L3) |
| Trichomoniasis | Vaginitis, strawberry-colored mucosa | *Trichomonas vaginalis* |
| AIDS | Opportunistic infections, Kaposi's sarcoma, lymphoma | HIV |
| Condylomata acuminata | Genital warts, koilocytes | HPV 6 and 11 |
| Hepatitis B | Jaundice | HBV |
| Bacterial vaginosis | Noninflammatory, malodorous discharge (fishy smell); positive whiff test, clue cells | *Gardnerella vaginalis* |

| **Pelvic inflammatory disease** | Top bugs—*Chlamydia trachomatis* (subacute, often undiagnosed), *Neisseria gonorrhoeae* (acute, high fever). *C. trachomatis*—the most common STD in the United States. Cervical motion tenderness (chandelier sign), purulent cervical discharge. PID may include salpingitis, endometritis, hydrosalpinx, and tubo-ovarian abscess. Can lead to Fitz-Hugh–Curtis syndrome—infection of the liver capsule and "violin string" adhesions of parietal peritoneum to liver. | Salpingitis is a risk factor for ectopic pregnancy, infertility, chronic pelvic pain, and adhesions. Other STDs include *Gardnerella* (clue cells) and *Trichomonas* (corkscrew motility on wet prep). |
|---|---|---|

## Nosocomial infections

| Pathogen | Risk factor | Notes |
|---|---|---|
| CMV, RSV | Newborn nursery | The 2 most common causes of nosocomial infections are *E. coli* (UTI) and S. aureus (wound infection). |
| *E. coli, Proteus mirabilis* | Urinary catheterization | |
| *Pseudomonas aeruginosa* | Respiratory therapy equipment | Presume *Pseudomonas* **AIR**uginosa when **AIR** or burns are involved. |
| HBV | Work in renal dialysis unit | |
| *Candida albicans* | Hyperalimentation | |
| *Legionella* | Water aerosols | *Legionella* when water source is involved. |

## Bugs affecting HIV-positive adults

| Clinical Presentation | Findings/Labs | Pathogen |
|---|---|---|
| **Systemic** | | |
| Low-grade fevers, cough, hepato-splenomegaly | Oval yeast cells within macrophages | *Histoplasma capsulatum* (causes only pulmonary symptoms in immunocompetent hosts) |
| **Dermatologic** | | |
| Fluffy white cottage-cheese lesions | Often on buccal mucosa | *C. albicans* (causes thrush) |
| Superficial vascular proliferation | Biopsy reveals neutrophilic inflammation | *Bartonella henselae* (causes bacillary angiomatosis) |
| Superficial neoplastic proliferation of vasculature | Biopsy reveals lymphocytic inflammation | HHV-8 (causes Kaposi's sarcoma) |
| **Gastrointestinal** | | |
| Chronic, watery diarrhea | Acid-fast cysts seen in stool | *Cryptosporidium* spp. |
| **Neurologic** | | |
| Meningitis | India ink stain reveals narrow-based budding | *Cryptococcus neoformans* (may also cause encephalitis) |
| Encephalopathy | Due to reactivation of a latent virus; results in demyelination | JC virus (cause of PML) |
| Abscesses | Many ring-enhancing lesions on imaging | *Toxoplasma gondii* |
| Retinitis | Cotton-wool spots on funduscopic exam | CMV |
| **Oncologic** | | |
| Hairy leukoplakia | Often on lateral tongue | EBV |
| Non-Hodgkin's lymphoma (large cell type) | Often on oropharynx (Waldeyer's ring) | EBV |
| Squamous cell carcinoma | Often in anus (MSM) or cervix (females) | HPV |
| **Respiratory** | | |
| Interstitial pneumonia | Biopsy reveals cells with intranuclear and cytoplasmic inclusion bodies | CMV |
| Invasive aspergillosis | Pleuritic pain, hemoptysis, infiltrates on imaging | *Aspergillus fumigatus* |
| Pneumonia | Especially with CD4 < 200 cells/mm$^3$ | *Pneumocystis jiroveci* (formerly *carinii*) |
| Tuberculosis-like disease | Especially with CD4 < 50 cells/mm$^3$ | *Mycobacterium avium–intracellulare* |

## Bugs affecting unimmunized children

| Clinical Presentation | Findings/Labs | Pathogen |
|---|---|---|
| **Dermatologic** | | |
| Rash | Beginning at head and moving down with postauricular lymphadenopathy | Rubella virus |
| | Beginning at head and moving down; rash preceded by cough, coryza, conjunctivitis, and blue-white (Koplik) spots on buccal mucosa | Measles virus (paramyxovirus; "rubeola") |
| **Neurologic** | | |
| Meningitis | Microbe colonizes nasopharynx Can also lead to myalgia and paralysis | *H. influenzae* type B Poliovirus |
| **Respiratory** | | |
| Pharyngitis | Grayish oropharyngeal exudate ("pseudomembranes" may obstruct airway); painful throat | *Corynebacterium diphtheriae* (elaborates toxin that causes necrosis in cardiac and CNS tissue) |
| Epiglottitis | Fever with dysphagia, drooling, and difficulty breathing due to edematous "cherry red" epiglottis | *H. influenzae* type B (also capable of causing epiglottitis in fully immunized children) |

## Bug hints (if all else fails)

| | |
|---|---|
| Pus, empyema, abscess | *S. aureus.* |
| Pediatric infection | *Haemophilus influenzae* (including epiglottitis). |
| Pneumonia in cystic fibrosis, burn infection | *Pseudomonas aeruginosa.* |
| Branching rods in oral infection, sulfur granules | *Actinomyces israelii.* |
| Traumatic open wound | *Clostridium perfringens.* |
| Surgical wound | *S. aureus.* |
| Dog or cat bite | *Pasteurella multocida.* |
| Currant jelly sputum | *Klebsiella.* |
| Positive PAS stain | *Tropheryma whippelii* (Whipple's disease). |
| Sepsis/meningitis in newborn | Group B strep. |
| Health care provider | HBV (from needle stick). |
| Fungal infection in diabetic | *Mucor* or *Rhizopus* spp. |
| Asplenic patient | Encapsulated microbes, especially **SHiN** (*S. pneumoniae*, **H.** *influenzae* type B, **N.** *meningitidis*). |
| Chronic granulomatous disease | Catalase-positive microbes—*S. aureus*, *Nocardia* spp., *Serratia marcescens*, *Pseudomonas cepacia*, *Aspergillus* spp. |
| Neutropenic patients | *Candida albicans* (systemic). |
| Bilateral Bell's palsy | *Borrelia burgdorferi* (Lyme disease). |

## Antimicrobial therapy

| Mechanism of action | Drugs |
| --- | --- |
| 1. Block cell wall synthesis by inhibition of peptidoglycan cross-linking | Penicillin, ampicillin, ticarcillin, piperacillin, imipenem, aztreonam, cephalosporins |
| 2. Block peptidoglycan synthesis | Bacitracin, vancomycin |
| 3. Disrupt bacterial cell membranes | Polymyxins |
| 4. Block nucleotide synthesis | Sulfonamides, trimethoprim |
| 5. Block DNA topoisomerases | Fluoroquinolones |
| 6. Block mRNA synthesis | Rifampin |
| 7. Block protein synthesis at 50S ribosomal subunit | Chloramphenicol, macrolides, clindamycin, streptogramins (quinupristin, dalfopristin), linezolid |
| 8. Block protein synthesis at 30S ribosomal subunit | Aminoglycosides, tetracyclines |

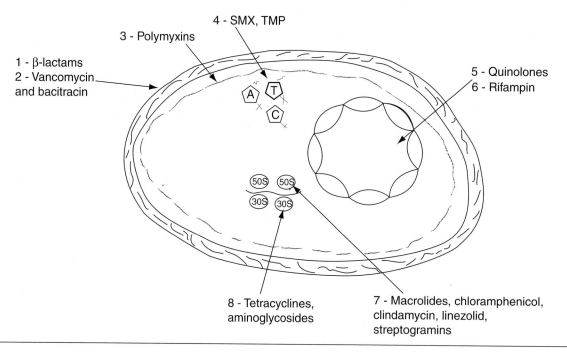

4 - SMX, TMP

3 - Polymyxins

1 - β-lactams
2 - Vancomycin
and bacitracin

5 - Quinolones
6 - Rifampin

8 - Tetracyclines,
aminoglycosides

7 - Macrolides, chloramphenicol,
clindamycin, linezolid,
streptogramins

## Bacteriostatic vs. bactericidal antibiotics

| | | |
| --- | --- | --- |
| Bacteriostatic | Erythromycin, Clindamycin, Sulfamethoxazole, Trimethoprim, Tetracyclines, Chloramphenicol. | "We're ECSTaTiC about bacteriostatics." |
| Bactericidal | Vancomycin, Fluoroquinolones, Penicillin, Aminoglycosides, Cephalosporins, Metronidazole. | "Very Finely Proficient At Cell Murder." |

**Penicillin**

Penicillin G (IV form), penicillin V (oral). Prototype β-lactam antibiotics.

Mechanism
1. Bind penicillin-binding proteins
2. Block transpeptidase cross-linking of cell wall
3. Activate autolytic enzymes

Clinical use
Bactericidal for gram-positive cocci, gram-positive rods, gram-negative cocci, and spirochetes. Not penicillinase resistant.

Toxicity
Hypersensitivity reactions, hemolytic anemia.

---

**Methicillin, nafcillin, dicloxacillin (penicillinase-resistant penicillins)**

Mechanism
Same as penicillin. Narrow spectrum; penicillinase resistant because of bulkier R group.

"Use **naf** (nafcillin) for **staph.**"

Clinical use
*S. aureus* (except MRSA; resistant because of altered penicillin-binding protein target site).

Toxicity
Hypersensitivity reactions; methicillin—interstitial nephritis.

---

**Ampicillin, amoxicillin (aminopenicillins)**

Mechanism
Same as penicillin. Wider spectrum; penicillinase sensitive. Also combine with clavulanic acid (penicillinase inhibitor) to enhance spectrum. AmOxicillin has greater Oral bioavailability than ampicillin.

**AMP**ed up penicillin.

Clinical use
Extended-spectrum penicillin—certain gram-positive bacteria and gram-negative rods (*Haemophilus influenzae*, *E. coli*, *Listeria monocytogenes*, *Proteus mirabilis*, *Salmonella*, enterococci).

Coverage: ampicillin/ amoxicillin **HELPS** kill enterococci.

Toxicity
Hypersensitivity reactions; ampicillin rash; pseudomembranous colitis.

---

**Ticarcillin, carbenicillin, piperacillin (antipseudomonals)**

Mechanism
Same as penicillin. Extended spectrum.

**TCP**: Takes Care of *Pseudomonas*.

Clinical use
*Pseudomonas* spp. and gram-negative rods; susceptible to penicillinase; use with clavulanic acid (β-lactamase inhibitor).

Toxicity
Hypersensitivity reactions.

### Cephalosporins

| | | |
|---|---|---|
| Mechanism | β-lactam drugs that inhibit cell wall synthesis but are less susceptible to penicillinases. Bactericidal. | |
| Clinical use | 1st generation (cefazolin, cephalexin)—gram-positive cocci, *Proteus mirabilis*, *E. coli*, *Klebsiella pneumoniae*. | 1st generation—**PEcK**. |
| | 2nd generation (cefoxitin, cefaclor, cefuroxime)—gram-positive cocci, *Haemophilus influenzae*, *Enterobacter aerogenes*, *Neisseria* spp., *Proteus mirabilis*, *E. coli*, *Klebsiella pneumoniae*, *Serratia marcescens*. | 2nd generation—**HEN PEcKS**. |
| | 3rd generation (ceftriaxone, cefotaxime, ceftazidime)—serious gram-negative infections resistant to other β-lactams; meningitis (most penetrate the blood-brain barrier). Examples: ceftazidime for *Pseudomonas*; ceftriaxone for gonorrhea. | |
| | 4th generation (cefepime)—↑ activity against *Pseudomonas* and gram-positive organisms. | |
| Toxicity | Hypersensitivity reactions. Cross-hypersensitivity with penicillins occurs in 5–10% of patients. ↑ nephrotoxicity of aminoglycosides; disulfiram-like reaction with ethanol (in cephalosporins with a methylthiotetrazole group, e.g., cefamandole). | |

### Aztreonam

| | |
|---|---|
| Mechanism | A monobactam resistant to β-lactamases. Inhibits cell wall synthesis (binds to PBP3). Synergistic with aminoglycosides. No cross-allergenicity with penicillins. |
| Clinical use | Gram-negative rods—*Klebsiella* spp., *Pseudomonas* spp., *Serratia* spp. No activity against gram-positives or anaerobes. For penicillin-allergic patients and those with renal insufficiency who cannot tolerate aminoglycosides. |
| Toxicity | Usually nontoxic; occasional GI upset. No cross-sensitivity with penicillins or cephalosporins. |

### Imipenem/cilastatin, meropenem

| | | |
|---|---|---|
| Mechanism | Imipenem is a broad-spectrum, β-lactamase-resistant carbapenem. Always administered with cilastatin (inhibitor of renal dihydropeptidase I) to ↓ inactivation in renal tubules. | With imipenem, "the kill is **LASTIN'** with ci**LASTATIN**." |
| Clinical use | Gram-positive cocci, gram-negative rods, and anaerobes. Drug of choice for *Enterobacter*. The significant side effects limit use to life-threatening infections, or after other drugs have failed. Meropenem, however, has a reduced risk of seizures and is stable to dihydropeptidase I. | |
| Toxicity | GI distress, skin rash, and CNS toxicity (seizures) at high plasma levels. | |

## Vancomycin

**Mechanism**  Inhibits cell wall mucopeptide formation by binding D-ala D-ala portion of cell wall precursors. Bactericidal. Resistance occurs with amino acid change of D-ala D-ala to D-ala D-lac.

**Clinical use**  Used for serious, gram-positive multidrug-resistant organisms, including S. *aureus* and *Clostridium difficile* (pseudomembranous colitis).

**Toxicity**  Nephrotoxicity, Ototoxicity, Thrombophlebitis, diffuse flushing—"red man syndrome" (can largely prevent by pretreatment with antihistamines and slow infusion rate). Well tolerated in general—does **NOT** have many problems.

---

**Protein synthesis inhibitors**

30S inhibitors:
A = Aminoglycosides (streptomycin, gentamicin, tobramycin, amikacin) [bactericidal]
T = Tetracyclines [bacteriostatic]

50S inhibitors:
C = Chloramphenicol, Clindamycin [bacteriostatic]
E = Erythromycin [bacteriostatic]
L = Lincomycin [bacteriostatic]
L = Linezolid [variable]

"Buy **AT 30, CCELL** (sell) at **50**."

---

**Aminoglycosides**  Gentamicin, Neomycin, Amikacin, Tobramycin, Streptomycin.

**Mechanism**  Bactericidal; inhibit formation of initiation complex and cause misreading of mRNA. Require $O_2$ for uptake; therefore ineffective against anaerobes.

**Clinical use**  Severe gram-negative rod infections. Synergistic with β-lactam antibiotics. Neomycin for bowel surgery.

**Toxicity**  Nephrotoxicity (especially when used with cephalosporins), Ototoxicity (especially when used with loop diuretics). Teratogen.

"**Mean**" GNATS can**NOT** kill anaerobes.

| | | |
|---|---|---|
| **Tetracyclines** | Tetracycline, doxycycline, demeclocycline, minocycline. | Demeclocycline—ADH antagonist; acts as a Diuretic in SIADH. |
| Mechanism | Bacteriostatic; bind to 30S and prevent attachment of aminoacyl-tRNA; limited CNS penetration. Doxycycline is fecally eliminated and can be used in patients with renal failure. Must NOT take with milk, antacids, or iron-containing preparations because divalent cations inhibit its absorption in the gut. | |
| Clinical use | *Vibrio cholerae*, **A**cne, *Chlamydia*, *Ureaplasma Urealyticum*, *Mycoplasma pneumoniae*, **T**ularemia, *H. pylori*, *Borrelia burgdorferi* (Lyme disease), *Rickettsia*. | **VACUUM TH**e **BedR**oom. |
| Toxicity | GI distress, discoloration of teeth and inhibition of bone growth in children, photosensitivity. Contraindicated in pregnancy. | |

| | |
|---|---|
| **Macrolides** | Erythromycin, azithromycin, clarithromycin. |
| Mechanism | Inhibit protein synthesis by blocking translocation; bind to the 23S rRNA of the 50S ribosomal subunit. Bacteriostatic. |
| Clinical use | URIs, pneumonias, STDs—gram-positive cocci (streptococcal infections in patients allergic to penicillin), *Mycoplasma*, *Legionella*, *Chlamydia*, *Neisseria*. |
| Toxicity | Prolonged QT interval (especially erythromycin), GI discomfort (most common cause of noncompliance), acute cholestatic hepatitis, eosinophilia, skin rashes. Increases serum concentration of theophyllines, oral anticoagulants. |

| | |
|---|---|
| **Chloramphenicol** | |
| Mechanism | Inhibits 50S peptidyltransferase activity. Bacteriostatic. |
| Clinical use | Meningitis (*Haemophilus influenzae*, *Neisseria meningitidis*, *Streptococcus pneumoniae*). Conservative use owing to toxicities. |
| Toxicity | Anemia (dose dependent), aplastic anemia (dose independent), gray baby syndrome (in premature infants because they lack liver UDP-glucuronyl transferase). |

| | | |
|---|---|---|
| **Clindamycin** | | |
| Mechanism | Blocks peptide bond formation at 50S ribosomal subunit. Bacteriostatic. | Treats anaerobes above the diaphragm. |
| Clinical use | Treat anaerobic infections (e.g., *Bacteroides fragilis*, *Clostridium perfringens*). | |
| Toxicity | Pseudomembranous colitis (*C. difficile* overgrowth), fever, diarrhea. | |

**Sulfonamides**

Sulfamethoxazole (SMX), sulfisoxazole, sulfadiazine.

Mechanism — PABA antimetabolites inhibit dihydropteroate synthetase. Bacteriostatic.

Clinical use — Gram-positive, gram-negative, *Nocardia*, *Chlamydia*. Triple sulfas or SMX for simple UTI.

Toxicity — Hypersensitivity reactions, hemolysis if G6PD deficient, nephrotoxicity (tubulointerstitial nephritis), photosensitivity, kernicterus in infants, displace other drugs from albumin (e.g., warfarin).

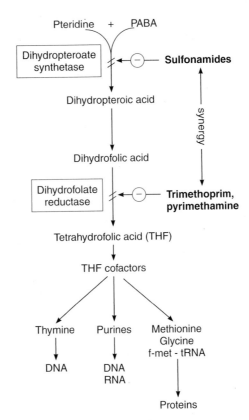

(Adapted, with permission, from Katzung BG. *Basic and Clinical Pharmacology,* 7th ed. Stamford, CT: Appleton & Lange, 1997: 762.)

**Trimethoprim**

Mechanism — Inhibits bacterial dihydrofolate reductase. Bacteriostatic.

Clinical use — Used in combination with sulfonamides (trimethoprim-sulfamethoxazole [TMP-SMX]), causing sequential block of folate synthesis. Combination used for recurrent UTIs, *Shigella*, *Salmonella*, *Pneumocystis jiroveci* pneumonia.

Toxicity — Megaloblastic anemia, leukopenia, granulocytopenia. (May alleviate with supplemental folinic acid.)

Trimethoprim = **TMP:** "Treats **M**arrow **P**oorly."

**Sulfa drug allergies**

Patients who do not tolerate sulfa drugs should not be given sulfonamides or other sulfa drugs, such as sulfasalazine, sulfonylureas, thiazide diuretics, acetazolamide, or furosemide.

| | | |
|---|---|---|
| **Fluoroquinolones** | Ciprofloxacin, norfloxacin, ofloxacin, sparfloxacin, moxifloxacin, gatifloxacin, enoxacin (fluoroquinolones), nalidixic acid (a quinolone). | |
| Mechanism | Inhibit DNA gyrase (topoisomerase II). Bactericidal. Must not be taken with antacids. | FluoroquinoLONES hurt attachments to your BONES. |
| Clinical use | Gram-negative rods of urinary and GI tracts (including *Pseudomonas*), *Neisseria*, some gram-positive organisms. | |
| Toxicity | GI upset, superinfections, skin rashes, headache, dizziness. Contraindicated in pregnant women and in children because animal studies show damage to cartilage. Tendonitis and tendon rupture in adults; leg cramps and myalgias in kids. | |

| | | |
|---|---|---|
| **Metronidazole** | | |
| Mechanism | Forms toxic metabolites in the bacterial cell that damage DNA. Bactericidal, antiprotozoal. | |
| Clinical use | Treats *Giardia*, *Entamoeba*, *Trichomonas*, *Gardnerella vaginalis*, Anaerobes (*Bacteroides*, *Clostridium*). Used with bismuth and amoxicillin (or tetracycline) for "triple therapy" against *H. Pylori*. | **GET GAP** on the **Metro!** Anaerobic infection below the diaphragm. |
| Toxicity | Disulfiram-like reaction with alcohol; headache, metallic taste. | |

| | | |
|---|---|---|
| **Polymyxins** | Polymyxin B, polymyxin E. | **'MYXins MIX up** membranes. |
| Mechanism | Bind to cell membranes of bacteria and disrupt their osmotic properties. Polymyxins are cationic, basic proteins that act like detergents. | |
| Clinical use | Resistant gram-negative infections. | |
| Toxicity | Neurotoxicity, acute renal tubular necrosis. | |

**Antimycobacterial drugs**

| Bacterium | Prophylaxis | Treatment |
|---|---|---|
| *M. tuberculosis* | Isoniazid | Rifampin, Isoniazid, Pyrazinamide, Ethambutol (**RIPE** for **treatment**) |
| *M. avium–intracellulare* | Azithromycin | Azithromycin, rifampin, ethambutol, streptomycin |
| *M. leprae* | N/A | Dapsone, rifampin, clofazimine |

| | | |
|---|---|---|
| **Anti-TB drugs** | Streptomycin, Pyrazinamide, Isoniazid (**INH**), Rifampin, Ethambutol. Cycloserine (2nd-line therapy). Important side effect of ethambutol is optic neuropathy (red-green color blindness). For other drugs, hepatotoxicity. | **INH-SPIRE** (inspire). |

### Isoniazid (INH)

| | | |
|---|---|---|
| Mechanism | ↓ synthesis of mycolic acids. | **INH** Injures **N**eurons and **H**epatocytes. |
| Clinical use | *Mycobacterium tuberculosis*. The only agent used as solo prophylaxis against TB. | Different INH half-lives in fast vs. slow acetylators. |
| Toxicity | Neurotoxicity, hepatotoxicity. Pyridoxine (vitamin B$_6$) can prevent neurotoxicity. | |

### Rifampin

| | | |
|---|---|---|
| Mechanism | Inhibits DNA-dependent RNA polymerase. | Rifampin's **4 R's:** |
| Clinical use | *Mycobacterium tuberculosis*; delays resistance to dapsone when used for leprosy. Used for meningococcal prophylaxis and chemoprophylaxis in contacts of children with *Haemophilus influenzae* type B. | **R**NA polymerase inhibitor<br>**R**evs up microsomal P-450<br>**R**ed/orange body fluids<br>**R**apid resistance if used alone |
| Toxicity | Minor hepatotoxicity and drug interactions (↑ P-450); orange body fluids (nonhazardous side effect). | |

### Resistance mechanisms for various antibiotics

| Drug | Most common mechanism |
|---|---|
| Penicillins/ cephalosporins | β-lactamase cleavage of β-lactam ring, or altered PBP in cases of MRSA or penicillin-resistant S. *pneumoniae* |
| Aminoglycosides | Modification via acetylation, adenylation, or phosphorylation |
| Vancomycin | Terminal D-ala of cell wall component replaced with D-lac; ↓ affinity |
| Chloramphenicol | Modification via acetylation |
| Macrolides | Methylation of rRNA near erythromycin's ribosome-binding site |
| Tetracycline | ↓ uptake or ↑ transport out of cell |
| Sulfonamides | Altered enzyme (bacterial dihydropteroate synthetase), ↓ uptake, or ↑ PABA synthesis |
| Quinolones | Altered gyrase or reduced uptake |

### Nonsurgical antimicrobial prophylaxis

| | |
|---|---|
| Meningococcal infection | Rifampin (drug of choice), minocycline. |
| Gonorrhea | Ceftriaxone. |
| Syphilis | Benzathine penicillin G. |
| History of recurrent UTIs | TMP-SMX. |
| *Pneumocystis jiroveci* pneumonia | TMP-SMX (drug of choice), aerosolized pentamidine. |
| Endocarditis with surgical or dental procedures | Penicillins. |

### Treatment of highly resistant bacteria

MRSA—vancomycin.
VRE—linezolid and streptogramins (quinupristin/dalfopristin).

### Antifungal therapy

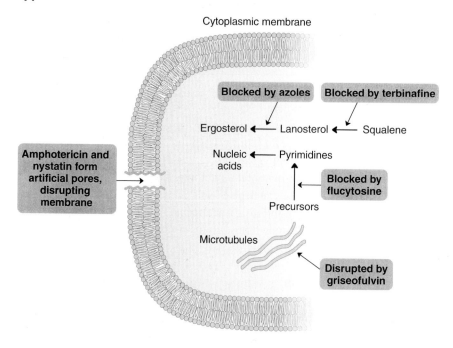

(Adapted, with permission, from Katzung BG, Trevor AJ. *USMLE Road Map: Pharmacology*, 1st ed. New York: McGraw-Hill, 2003: 120.)

### Amphotericin B

| | | |
|---|---|---|
| Mechanism | Binds ergosterol (unique to fungi); forms membrane pores that allow leakage of electrolytes. | Amphotericin "tears" holes in the fungal membrane by forming pores. |
| Clinical use | Used for wide spectrum of systemic mycoses. *Cryptococcus, Blastomyces, Coccidioides, Aspergillus, Histoplasma, Candida, Mucor* (systemic mycoses). Intrathecally for fungal meningitis; does not cross blood-brain barrier. | |
| Toxicity | Fever/chills ("shake and bake"), hypotension, nephrotoxicity, arrhythmias, anemia, IV phlebitis ("amphoterrible"). Hydration reduces nephrotoxicity. Liposomal amphotericin reduces toxicity. | |

### Nystatin

| | |
|---|---|
| Mechanism | Binds to ergosterol, disrupting fungal membranes. Too toxic for systemic use. |
| Clinical use | "Swish and swallow" for oral candidiasis (thrush); topical for diaper rash or vaginal candidiasis. |

### Azoles

| | |
|---|---|
| | Fluconazole, ketoconazole, clotrimazole, miconazole, itraconazole, voriconazole. |
| Mechanism | Inhibit fungal sterol (ergosterol) synthesis. |
| Clinical use | Systemic mycoses. Fluconazole for cryptococcal meningitis in AIDS patients (because it can cross blood-brain barrier) and candidal infections of all types (i.e., yeast infections). Ketoconazole for *Blastomyces, Coccidioides, Histoplasma, Candida albicans*; hypercortisolism. Clotrimazole and miconazole for topical fungal infections. |
| Toxicity | Hormone synthesis inhibition (gynecomastia), liver dysfunction (inhibits cytochrome P-450), fever, chills. |

**Flucytosine**

| | |
|---|---|
| Mechanism | Inhibits DNA synthesis by conversion to 5-fluorouracil. |
| Clinical use | Used in systemic fungal infections (e.g., *Candida*, *Cryptococcus*) in combination with amphotericin B. |
| Toxicity | Nausea, vomiting, diarrhea, bone marrow suppression. |

**Caspofungin**

| | |
|---|---|
| Mechanism | Inhibits cell wall synthesis by inhibiting synthesis of β-glucan. |
| Clinical use | Invasive aspergillosis. |
| Toxicity | GI upset, flushing. |

**Terbinafine**

| | |
|---|---|
| Mechanism | Inhibits the fungal enzyme squalene epoxidase. |
| Clinical use | Used to treat dermatophytoses (especially onychomycosis). |

**Griseofulvin**

| | |
|---|---|
| Mechanism | Interferes with microtubule function; disrupts mitosis. Deposits in keratin-containing tissues (e.g., nails). |
| Clinical use | Oral treatment of superficial infections; inhibits growth of dermatophytes (tinea, ringworm). |
| Toxicity | Teratogenic, carcinogenic, confusion, headaches, ↑ P-450 and warfarin metabolism. |

**Antiviral chemotherapy**

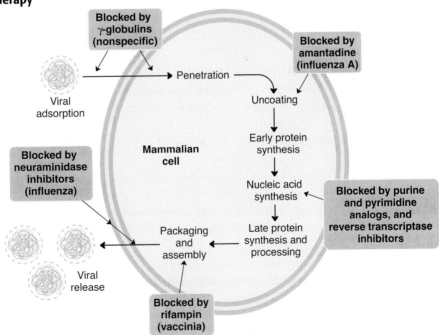

(Adapted, with permission, from Katzung BG, Trevor AJ. *USMLE Road Map: Pharmacology*, 1st ed. New York: McGraw-Hill, 2003: 120.)

### Amantadine

| | |
|---|---|
| Mechanism | Blocks viral penetration/uncoating (M2 protein); may buffer pH of endosome. Also causes the release of dopamine from intact nerve terminals. |
| Clinical use | Prophylaxis and treatment for influenza A; Parkinson's disease. |
| Toxicity | Ataxia, dizziness, slurred speech. |
| Mechanism of resistance | Mutated M2 protein. 90% of all influenza A strains are resistant to amantadine, so not used. |

**"A man to dine"** takes off his **coat.**
Amantadine blocks influenza A and rubellA and causes problems with the cerebellA.
Rimantidine is a derivative with fewer CNS side effects. Does not cross the blood-brain barrier.

### Zanamivir, oseltamivir

| | |
|---|---|
| Mechanism | Inhibit influenza neuraminidase, decreasing the release of progeny virus. |
| Clinical use | Both influenza A and B. |

### Ribavirin

| | |
|---|---|
| Mechanism | Inhibits synthesis of guanine nucleotides by competitively inhibiting IMP dehydrogenase. |
| Clinical use | RSV, chronic hepatitis C. |
| Toxicity | Hemolytic anemia. Severe teratogen. |

### Acyclovir

| | |
|---|---|
| Mechanism | Monophosphorylated by HSV/VZV thymidine kinase. Guanosine analog. Triphosphate formed by cellular enzymes. Preferentially inhibits viral DNA polymerase by chain termination. |
| Clinical use | HSV, VZV, EBV. Used for HSV-induced mucocutaneous and genital lesions as well as for encephalitis. Prophylaxis in immunocompromised patients. For herpes zoster, use a related agent, famciclovir. No effect on latent forms of HSV and VZV. |
| Toxicity | Generally well tolerated. |
| Mechanism of resistance | Lack of thymidine kinase. |

### Ganciclovir

| | |
|---|---|
| Mechanism | 5′-monophosphate formed by a CMV viral kinase or HSV/VZV thymidine kinase. Guanosine analog. Triphosphate formed by cellular kinases. Preferentially inhibits viral DNA polymerase. |
| Clinical use | CMV, especially in immunocompromised patients. |
| Toxicity | Leukopenia, neutropenia, thrombocytopenia, renal toxicity. More toxic to host enzymes than acyclovir. |
| Mechanism of resistance | Mutated CMV DNA polymerase or lack of viral kinase. |

HIGH-YIELD PRINCIPLES

MICROBIOLOGY

## Foscarnet

| | | |
|---|---|---|
| Mechanism | Viral DNA polymerase inhibitor that binds to the pyrophosphate-binding site of the enzyme. Does not require activation by viral kinase. | FOScarnet = pyroFOSphate analog. |
| Clinical use | CMV retinitis in immunocompromised patients when ganciclovir fails; acyclovir-resistant HSV. | |
| Toxicity | Nephrotoxicity. | |
| Mechanism of resistance | Mutated DNA polymerase. | |

## HIV therapy

| | | |
|---|---|---|
| **Protease inhibitors** | Saqui**navir**, rito**navir**, indi**navir**, nelfi**navir**, ampre**navir**. | All protease inhibitors end in *-navir*. |
| Mechanism | Inhibit maturation of new virus by blocking protease in progeny virions. | **NAVIR** (never) **TEASE** a pro**TEASE**. |
| Toxicity | GI intolerance (nausea, diarrhea), hyperglycemia, lipodystrophy, thrombocytopenia (indinavir). | |
| **Reverse transcriptase inhibitors** | | |
| Nucleosides | Zidovudine (ZDV, formerly AZT), didanosine (ddI), zalcitabine (ddC), stavudine (d4T), lamivudine (3TC), abacavir. | Have **you dined (vudine)** with my **nuclear (nucleosides)** family? |
| Non-nucleosides | **N**evirapine, **E**favirenz, **D**elavirdine. | **N**ever **E**ver **D**eliver nucleosides. |
| Mechanism | Preferentially inhibit reverse transcriptase of HIV; prevent incorporation of DNA copy of viral genome into host DNA. | |
| Toxicity | Bone marrow suppression (neutropenia, anemia), peripheral neuropathy, lactic acidosis (nucleosides), rash (non-nucleosides), megaloblastic anemia (ZDV). | GM-CSF and erythropoietin can be used to reduce bone marrow suppression. |
| Clinical use | Highly active antiretroviral therapy (HAART) generally entails combination therapy with protease inhibitors and reverse transcriptase inhibitors. Initiated when patients have low CD4 counts (< 500 cells/mm$^3$) or high viral load. ZDV is used for general prophylaxis and during pregnancy to reduce risk of fetal transmission. | |
| **Fusion inhibitors** | Enfuvirtide. | |
| Mechanism | Bind viral gp41 subunit; inhibit conformational change required for fusion with CD4 cells. Therefore block entry and subsequent replication. | |
| Toxicity | Hypersensitivity reactions, reactions at subcutaneous injection site, ↑ risk of bacterial pneumonia. | |
| Clinical use | In patients with persistent viral replication in spite of antiretroviral therapy. Used in combination with other drugs. | |

**Interferons**

| | |
|---|---|
| Mechanism | Glycoproteins from human leukocytes that block various stages of viral RNA and DNA synthesis. Induce ribonuclease that degrades viral mRNA. |
| Clinical use | IFN-α—chronic hepatitis B and C, Kaposi's sarcoma. IFN-β—MS. IFN-γ—NADPH oxidase deficiency. |
| Toxicity | Neutropenia. |

---

**Antibiotics to avoid in pregnancy**

Sulfonamides—kernicterus.

Aminoglycosides—ototoxicity.

Fluoroquinolones—cartilage damage.

Erythromycin—acute cholestatic hepatitis in mom (and clarithromycin—embryotoxic).

Metronidazole—mutagenesis.

Tetracyclines—discolored teeth, inhibition of bone growth.

Ribavirin (antiviral)—teratogenic.

Griseofulvin (antifungal)—teratogenic.

Chloramphenicol—"gray baby."

**SAFE** Moms **T**ake **R**eally **G**ood **C**are.

# Immunology

*"I hate to disappoint you, but my rubber lips are immune to your charms."*
—*Batman & Robin*

*"No State shall abridge the privileges or immunities of its citizens."*
—The United States Constitution

▶ Lymphoid Structures

▶ Lymphocytes

▶ Immune Responses

▶ Immunosuppressants

Immunology can be confusing and complicated, but luckily the USMLE tests only basic principles and facts in this area. Cell surface markers are important to know because they are clinically useful (i.e., in identifying specific types of immune deficiency or cancer) and are functionally critical to the jobs immune cells carry out. By spending a little extra effort here, it is possible to turn a traditionally difficult subject into one that is high yield.

**Lymph node**     A 2° lymphoid organ that has many afferents, 1 or more efferents. Encapsulated, with trabeculae. Functions are nonspecific filtration by macrophages, storage and activation of B and T cells, antibody production.

Follicle     Site of B-cell localization and proliferation. In outer cortex. 1° follicles are dense and dormant. 2° follicles have pale central germinal centers and are active.

Medulla     Consists of medullary cords (closely packed lymphocytes and plasma cells) and medullary sinuses. Medullary sinuses communicate with efferent lymphatics and contain reticular cells and macrophages.

Paracortex     Houses T cells. Region of cortex between follicles and medulla. Contains high endothelial venules through which T and B cells enter from blood. In an extreme cellular immune response, paracortex becomes greatly enlarged. Not well developed in patients with DiGeorge syndrome.

Paracortex enlarges in an extreme cellular immune response (i.e., viral).

**Lymph drainage**

| Area of body | 1° lymph node drainage site |
| --- | --- |
| 1. Upper limb, lateral breast | 1. Axillary |
| 2. Stomach | 2. Celiac |
| 3. Duodenum, jejunum | 3. Superior mesenteric |
| 4. Sigmoid colon | 4. Colic → inferior mesenteric |
| 5. Rectum (lower part), anal canal above pectinate line | 5. Internal iliac |
| 6. Anal canal below pectinate line | 6. Superficial inguinal |
| 7. Testes | 7. Superficial and deep plexuses → para-aortic |
| 8. Scrotum | 8. Superficial inguinal |
| 9. Thigh (superficial) | 9. Superficial inguinal |
| 10. Lateral side of dorsum of foot | 10. Popliteal |

Right lymphatic duct—drains right arm and right half of head.

Thoracic duct—drains everything else.

**Sinusoids of spleen**
Long, vascular channels in red pulp with fenestrated "barrel hoop" basement membrane. Macrophages found nearby.

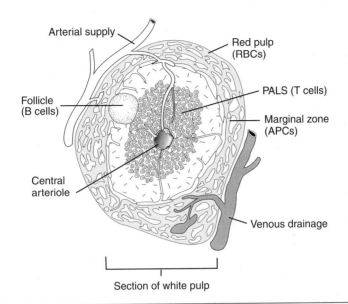

Arterial supply

Red pulp (RBCs)

PALS (T cells)

Follicle (B cells)

Marginal zone (APCs)

Central arteriole

Venous drainage

Section of white pulp

T cells are found in the periarterial lymphatic sheath (PALS) and in the red pulp of the spleen. B cells are found in follicles within the white pulp of the spleen.

Macrophages in the spleen remove encapsulated bacteria.

Splenic dysfunction: ↓ IgM → ↓ complement activation → ↓ C3b opsonization → ↑ susceptibility to encapsulated organisms (*S. pneumoniae, H. influenzae, Salmonella, N. meningitidis*).

Postsplenectomy:
—Howell-Jolly bodies (nuclear remnants)
—Target cells
—Thrombocytosis

**Thymus**
Site of T-cell differentiation and maturation. Encapsulated. From epithelium of 3rd branchial pouches. Lymphocytes of mesenchymal origin. Cortex is dense with immature T cells; medulla is pale with mature T cells and epithelial reticular cells and contains Hassall's corpuscles. Positive (MHC restriction) and negative selection (nonreactive to self) occur at the corticomedullary junction.

**T** cells = **T**hymus.
**B** cells = **B**one marrow.

▶ **IMMUNOLOGY–LYMPHOCYTES**

**Innate vs. adaptive immunity**
Innate—receptors that recognize pathogens are germline encoded. Response to pathogens is fast and nonspecific. No memory. Consists of neutrophils, macrophages, dendritic cells, natural killer cells, and complement.
Adaptive—receptors that recognize pathogens undergo V(D)J recombination during lymphocyte development. Response is slow on first exposure, but memory response is faster and more robust. Consists of T cells, B cells, and circulating antibody.

## Differentiation of T cells

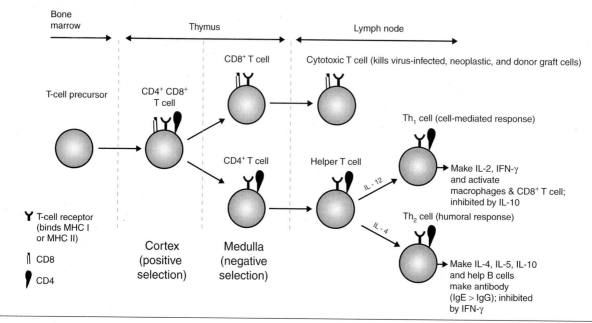

## MHC I and II

MHC = major histocompatibility complex, encoded by **H**uman **L**eukocyte **A**ntigen (HLA) genes; present antigen fragments to T cells and bind TCR.

MHC I = HLA-A, HLA-B, HLA-C.
   Expressed on almost all nucleated cells.
   Antigen is loaded in RER of mostly intracellular peptides.
   Mediates viral immunity.
   Pairs with $\beta_2$-microglobulin (aids in transport to cell surface).

MHC II = HLA-DR, HLA-DP, HLA-DQ.
   Expressed only on antigen-presenting cells (APCs).
   Antigen is loaded following release of invariant chain in an acidified endosome.

MHC I—HLA I letter (A, B, C).
MHC II—HLA II letters (DR, DP, DQ).

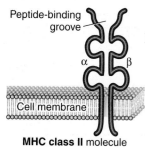

Peptide-binding groove

α       β

Cell membrane

**MHC class II molecule**

Peptide-binding groove

α

$\beta_2$-microglobulin

Cell membrane

**MHC class I molecule**

## HLA subtypes associated with diseases

| | | |
|---|---|---|
| A3 | Hemochromatosis | |
| B27 | **P**soriasis, **A**nkylosing spondylitis, **I**nflammatory bowel disease, **R**eiter's syndrome. | **PAIR.** |
| B8 | Graves' disease. | |
| DR2 | Multiple sclerosis, hay fever, SLE, Goodpasture's. | |
| DR3 | Diabetes mellitus type 1. | |
| DR4 | Rheumatoid arthritis, diabetes mellitus type 1. | |
| DR5 | Pernicious anemia → $B_{12}$ deficiency, Hashimoto's thyroiditis. | |
| DR7 | Steroid-responsive nephrotic syndrome. | |

## Major functions of B and T cells

| B-cell functions | T-cell functions |
|---|---|
| Make antibody | CD4+ T cells help B cells make antibody and produce γ-interferon, which activates macrophages |
| IgG antibodies opsonize bacteria, neutralize viruses | Kill virus-infected cells directly (CD8+ T cells) |
| Allergy (type I hypersensitivity): IgE | Delayed cell-mediated hypersensitivity (type IV) |
| Cytotoxic (type II) and immune complex (type III) hypersensitivity: IgG | |
| Antibodies cause organ rejection (hyperacute) | Organ (allograft) rejection (acute and chronic) |

| | |
|---|---|
| **Natural killer cells** | Use perforin and granzymes to induce apoptosis of virally infected cells and tumor cells. Only lymphocyte member of innate immune system.<br>Activity enhanced by IL-12, IFN-β, and IFN-α.<br>Induced to kill when exposed to a nonspecific activation signal on target cell and/or to an absence of class I MHC on target cell surface. |

**T-cell glycoproteins**

Helper T cells have CD4, which binds to MHC II on APCs. Cytotoxic T cells have CD8, which binds to MHC I on virus-infected cells.

Product of CD and MHC = 8 (CD4 × MHC II = 8 = CD8 × MHC I).

**CD3 complex**—cluster of polypeptides associated with a T-cell receptor. Important in signal transduction.

APCs:
1. Macrophage
2. B cell
3. Dendritic cell

Macrophage-lymphocyte interaction—activated lymphocytes (release IFN-γ) and macrophages (release IL-1, TNF-α) stimulate one another.

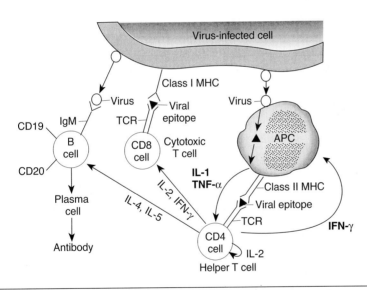

**Effects of bacterial toxins**

Superantigens (*S. pyogenes* and *S. aureus*)—cross-link the β-region of the T-cell receptor to the MHC class II on APCs. Results in the uncoordinated release of IFN-γ from Th$_1$ cells and subsequent release of IL-1, IL-6, and TNF-α from macrophages.

Endotoxins/lipopolysaccharide (gram-negative bacteria)—directly stimulate macrophages by binding to endotoxin receptor CD14; Th cells are not involved.

**T- and B-cell activation**

2 signals are required for T-cell activation and B-cell class switching—signal 1 and signal 2.

Th activation:
1. Foreign body is phagocytosed by APC
2. Foreign antigen is presented on MHC II and recognized by TCR on Th cell (signal 1)
3. "Costimulatory signal" is given by interaction of B7 and CD28 (signal 2)
4. Th cell activated to produce cytokines

Tc activation:
1. Endogenously synthesized (viral or self) proteins are presented on MHC I and recognized by TCR on Tc cell (signal 1)
2. IL-2 from Th cell activates Tc cell to kill virus-infected cell (signal 2)

B-cell class switching:
1. IL-4, IL-5, or IL-6 from Th$_2$ cell (signal 1)
2. CD40 receptor activation by binding CD40 ligand on Th cell (signal 2)

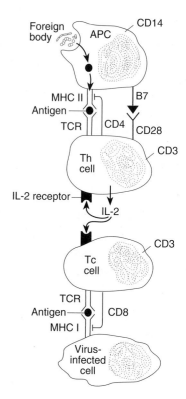

**Antibody structure and function**

Variable part of L and H chains recognizes antigens. Fc portion of IgM and IgG fixes complement. Heavy chain contributes to Fc and Fab fractions. Light chain contributes only to Fab fraction.

Fab:
Antigen-binding fragment
Determines idiotype: unique antigen-binding pocket; only 1 antigenic specificity expressed per B cell

Fc:
Constant
Carboxy terminal
Complement binding at $C_H2$ (IgG + IgM only)
Carbohydrate side chains
Determines isotype (IgM, IgD, etc.)

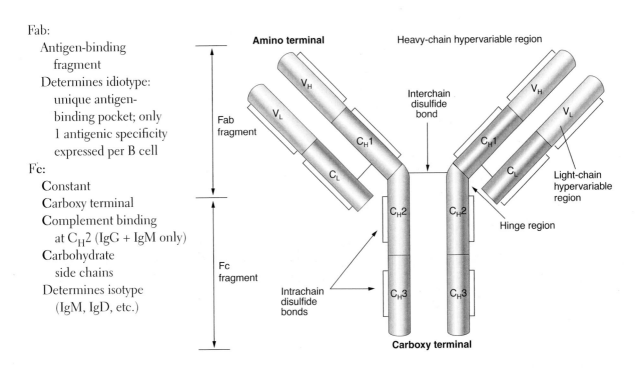

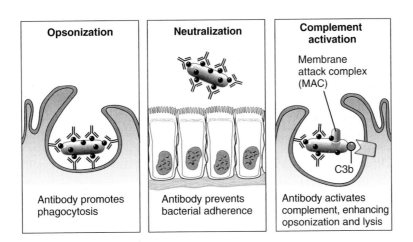

| Opsonization | Neutralization | Complement activation |
|---|---|---|
| Antibody promotes phagocytosis | Antibody prevents bacterial adherence | Antibody activates complement, enhancing opsonization and lysis |

Antibody diversity is generated by:
1. Random "recombination" of VJ (light-chain) or V(D)J (heavy-chain) genes
2. Random combination of heavy chains with light chains
3. Somatic hypermutation (following antigen stimulation)
4. Addition of nucleotides to DNA during "recombination" (see #1) by terminal deoxynucleotidyl transferase

**HIGH-YIELD PRINCIPLES**

**IMMUNOLOGY**

| | |
|---|---|
| **Immunoglobulin isotypes** | Mature B lymphocytes express IgM and IgD on their surfaces. They may differentiate by isotype switching (alternative splicing of mRNA; mediated by cytokines and CD40 ligand) into plasma cells that secrete IgA, IgE, or IgG. |
| IgG | Main antibody in 2° (**delayed**) response to an antigen. Most abundant. Fixes complement, crosses the placenta (provides infants with passive immunity), opsonizes bacteria, neutralizes bacterial toxins and viruses. |
| IgA | Prevents attachment of bacteria and viruses to mucous membranes; does not fix complement. Monomer (in circulation) or dimer (when secreted). Found in secretions (tears, saliva, mucus) and breast milk (known as "colostrum"). Picks up secretory component from epithelial cells before secretion. |
| IgM | Produced in the 1° (**immediate**) response to an antigen. Fixes complement but does not cross the placenta. Antigen receptor on the surface of B cells. Monomer on B cell or pentamer. Shape of pentamer allows it to efficiently trap free antigens out of tissue while humoral response evolves. |
| IgD | Unclear function. Found on the surface of many B cells and in serum. |
| IgE | Binds mast cells and basophils; cross-links when exposed to allergen, mediating immediate (type I) hypersensitivity through release of inflammatory mediators such as histamine. Mediates immunity to worms by activating eosinophils. Lowest concentration in serum. |

| | | |
|---|---|---|
| **Ig epitopes** | Allotype (polymorphism)—Ig epitope that differs among members of same species. Can be on light chain or heavy chain. | **ALL**otypes represent different **ALL**eles. |
| | Isotype (IgG, IgA, etc.)—Ig epitope common to a single class of Ig (5 classes, determined by heavy chain). | Isotype = *iso* (same). Common to same class. |
| | Idiotype (specific for a given antigen)—Ig epitope determined by antigen-binding sites. | Idiotype = *idio* (unique). Hypervariable region is unique. |

| | |
|---|---|
| **Antigen type and memory** | Thymus-independent antigens—antigens lacking a peptide component; cannot be presented by MHC to T cells (e.g., lipopolysaccharide from cell envelope of gram-negative bacteria and polysaccharide capsular antigen). Stimulate release of IgM antibodies only and do not result in immunologic memory. |
| | Thymus-dependent antigens—antigens containing a protein component (e.g., conjugated *H. influenzae* vaccine). Class switching and immunologic memory occur as a result of direct contact of B cells with Th cells (CD40–CD40 ligand interaction) and release of IL-4, IL-5, and IL-6. |

**Important cytokines**

| | | |
|---|---|---|
| IL-1 | Secreted by macrophages. Causes acute inflammation. Induces chemokine production to recruit leukocytes; activates endothelium to express adhesion molecules. An endogenous pyrogen. | "Hot T-Bone stEAk": IL-1: fever (hot). |
| IL-2 | Secreted by Th cells. Stimulates growth of helper and cytotoxic T cells. | IL-2: stimulates T cells. |
| IL-3 | Secreted by activated T cells. Supports the growth and differentiation of bone marrow stem cells. Has a function similar to GM-CSF. | IL-3: stimulates Bone marrow. |
| IL-4 | Secreted by $Th_2$ cells. Promotes growth of B cells. Enhances class switching to IgE and IgG. | IL-4: stimulates IgE production. |
| IL-5 | Secreted by $Th_2$ cells. Promotes differentiation of B cells. Enhances class switching to IgA. Stimulates production and activation of eosinophils. | IL-5: stimulates IgA production. |
| IL-6 | Secreted by Th cells and macrophages. Stimulates production of acute-phase reactants and immunoglobulins. | |
| IL-8 | Secreted by macrophages. Major chemotactic factor for neutrophils. | "Clean up on aisle 8." Neutrophils are recruited by IL-8 to clear infections. |
| IL-10 | Secreted by regulatory T cells. Inhibits actions of activated T cells. Activates $Th_2$, inhibits $Th_1$. | |
| IL-12 | Secreted by B cells and macrophages. Activates NK and $Th_1$ cells. | |
| γ-interferon | Secreted by $Th_1$ cells. Stimulates macrophages. Activates $Th_1$, inhibits $Th_2$. | |
| TNF | Secreted by macrophages. Mediates septic shock. Causes leukocyte recruitment, vascular leak. | |

**Cell surface proteins**

| | |
|---|---|
| Helper T cells | CD4, TCR, CD3, CD28, CD40L. |
| Cytotoxic T cells | CD8, TCR, CD3. |
| B cells | IgM, CD19, CD20, CD21 (receptor for EBV), CD40, MHC II, B7. |
| Macrophages | MHC II, B7, CD40, CD14. Receptors for Fc and C3b. |
| NK cells | Receptors for MHC I, CD16 (binds Fc of IgG), CD56. |
| All cells except mature red cells | MHC I. |

**Complement**

System of proteins that interact to play a role in humoral immunity and inflammation.

Membrane attack complex of complement defends against gram-negative bacteria. Activated by **IgG** or **IgM** in the **classic** pathway, and activated by molecules on the surface of microbes (especially endotoxin) in the **alternative** pathway.

C3b and IgG are the two 1° opsonins in bacterial defense. C3b aids in clearance of immune complexes.

Decay-accelerating factor (DAF) and C1 esterase inhibitor help prevent complement activation on self-cells.

**GM** makes **classic** cars.

C1, C2, C3, C4—viral neutralization.

C3b—opsonization. **B**inds **B**acteria.

C3a, C5a—Anaphylaxis.

C5a—neutrophil chemotaxis.

C5b-9—cytolysis by membrane attack complex (MAC).

Deficiency of C1 esterase inhibitor leads to hereditary angioedema.

Deficiency of C3 leads to severe, recurrent pyogenic sinus and respiratory tract infections; ↑ susceptibility to type III hypersensitivity reactions.

Deficiency of C5–C8 leads to *Neisseria* bacteremia.

Deficiency of DAF (GPI-anchored enzyme) leads to complement-mediated lysis of RBCs and paroxysmal nocturnal hemoglobinuria (PNH).

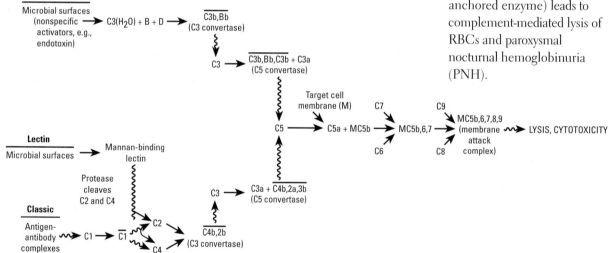

(Adapted, with permission, from Levinson W. *Medical Microbiology and Immunology: Examination and Board Review,* 8th ed. New York: McGraw-Hill, 2004: 432.)

**Interferon mechanism**

Interferons (α, β, γ) are proteins that place uninfected cells in an antiviral state. Interferons induce the production of a ribonuclease that inhibits viral protein synthesis by degrading viral mRNA (but not host mRNA).

**Interfer**es with viruses:

1. α- and β-interferons inhibit viral protein synthesis
2. γ-interferons ↑ MHC I and II expression and antigen presentation in all cells
3. Activates NK cells to kill virus-infected cells

## Passive vs. active immunity

| | | |
|---|---|---|
| Active | Induced after exposure to foreign antigens. Slow onset. Long-lasting protection (memory). | After exposure to **T**etanus toxin, **B**otulinum toxin, **H**BV, or **R**abies virus, patients are given preformed antibodies (passive)—**To Be Healed Rapidly.** |
| Passive | Based on receiving preformed antibodies from another host. Rapid onset. Short life span of antibodies (half-life = 3 weeks). Example: IgA in breast milk. | |

## Antigen variation

Classic examples:
    Bacteria—*Salmonella* (2 flagellar variants), *Borrelia* (relapsing fever), *Neisseria gonorrhoeae* (pilus protein).
    Virus—influenza (major = shift, minor = drift).
    Parasites—trypanosomes (programmed rearrangement).

Some mechanisms for variation include DNA rearrangement and RNA segment reassortment (e.g., influenza major shift).

## Anergy

Self-reactive T cells become nonreactive without costimulatory molecule.
B cells also become anergic, but tolerance is less complete than in T cells.

## Granulomatous diseases

1. Tuberculosis
2. Fungal infections (e.g., histoplasmosis)
3. Syphilis
4. Leprosy
5. Cat scratch fever
6. Sarcoidosis
7. Crohn's disease
8. Berylliosis

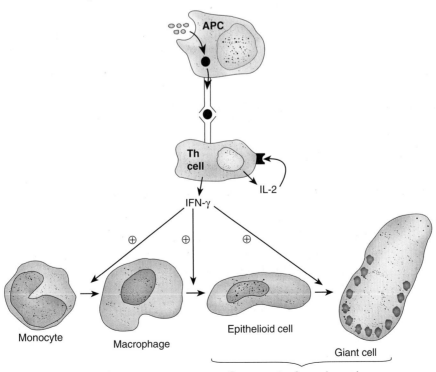

Components of granuloma along with fibroblasts and lymphocytes

**HIGH-YIELD PRINCIPLES**

**IMMUNOLOGY**

## Hypersensitivity

### Type I

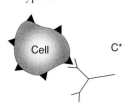

Mast cell or basophil

Fc receptor

IgE

Ag

**Anaphylactic and atopic**—free antigen cross-links IgE on presensitized mast cells and basophils, triggering release of vasoactive amines that act at postcapillary venules (i.e., histamine). Reaction develops rapidly after antigen exposure due to preformed antibody.

First and Fast (anaphylaxis). Types I, II, and III are all antibody mediated.
Test: scratch test and radioimmunosorbent assay.

### Type II

Cell C*

**Antibody mediated**—IgM, IgG bind to fixed antigen on "enemy" cell, leading to lysis (by complement) or phagocytosis.
3 mechanisms:
1. Opsonize cells or activate complement
2. Antibodies recruit neutrophils and macrophages that incite tissue damage
3. Bind to normal cellular receptors and interfere with functioning

Cy-2-toxic.
Antibody and complement lead to membrane attack complex (MAC).
Test: direct and indirect Coombs.

### Type III

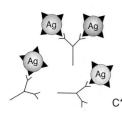

Ag  Ag

Ag  Ag

C*

**Immune complex**—antigen-antibody (IgG) complexes activate complement, which attracts neutrophils; neutrophils release lysosomal enzymes.
**Serum sickness**—an immune complex disease (type III) in which antibodies to the foreign proteins are produced (takes 5 days). Immune complexes form and are deposited in membranes, where they fix complement (leads to tissue damage). More common than Arthus reaction.
**Arthus reaction**—a local subacute antibody-mediated hypersensitivity (type III) reaction. Intradermal injection of antigen induces antibodies, which form antigen-antibody complexes in the skin. Characterized by edema, necrosis, and activation of complement.

Imagine an immune complex as 3 things stuck together: antigen-antibody-complement.
Most serum sickness is now caused by drugs (not serum). Fever, urticaria, arthralgias, proteinuria, lymphadenopathy 5–10 days after antigen exposure.
Antigen-antibody complexes cause the Arthus reaction.
Test: immunofluorescent staining.

### Type IV

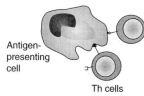

Antigen-presenting cell

Th cells

C* = complement

**Delayed (T-cell-mediated) type**—sensitized T lymphocytes encounter antigen and then release lymphokines (leads to macrophage activation; no antibody involved).

**ACID:**
Anaphylactic and Atopic (type I)
Cytotoxic (antibody mediated) (type II)
Immune complex (type III)
Delayed (cell mediated) (type IV)

4th and last—delayed. Cell mediated; therefore, it is not transferable by serum.
4 T's = T lymphocytes, Transplant rejections, TB skin tests, Touching (contact dermatitis).
Test: patch test (e.g., PPD).

**Hypersensitivity disorders**

| Reaction | Disorder | Presentation |
|---|---|---|
| Type I | Anaphylaxis (e.g., bee sting, some food/drug allergies)<br>Allergic and atopic disorders (e.g., rhinitis, hay fever, eczema, hives, asthma) | Immediate, anaphylactic, atopic |
| Type II | Hemolytic anemia<br>Pernicious anemia<br>Idiopathic thrombocytopenic purpura<br>Erythroblastosis fetalis<br>Acute hemolytic transfusion reactions<br>Rheumatic fever<br>Goodpasture's syndrome<br>Bullous pemphigoid<br>Pemphigus vulgaris<br>Graves' disease<br>Myasthenia gravis | Disease tends to be specific to tissue or site where antigen is found |
| Type III | SLE<br>Rheumatoid arthritis<br>Polyarteritis nodosa<br>Poststreptococcal glomerulonephritis<br>Serum sickness<br>Arthus reaction (e.g., swelling and inflammation following tetanus vaccine)<br>Hypersensitivity pneumonitis (e.g., farmer's lung) | Can be associated with vasculitis and systemic manifestations |
| Type IV | Type 1 DM<br>Multiple sclerosis<br>Guillain-Barré syndrome<br>Hashimoto's thyroiditis<br>Graft-versus-host disease<br>PPD (test for *M. tuberculosis*)<br>Contact dermatitis (e.g., poison ivy, nickel allergy) | Response is delayed and does **not** involve antibodies (vs. types I, II, and III) |

**Autoantibodies**

| Autoantibody | Associated disorder |
|---|---|
| Antinuclear antibodies (ANA) | SLE |
| Anti-dsDNA, anti-Smith | Specific for SLE |
| Antihistone | Drug-induced lupus |
| Anti-IgG (rheumatoid factor) | Rheumatoid arthritis |
| Anticentromere | Scleroderma (CREST) |
| Anti-Scl-70 (anti-DNA topoisomerase I) | Scleroderma (diffuse) |
| Antimitochondrial | 1° biliary cirrhosis |
| Antigliadin, antiendomysial | Celiac disease |
| Anti–basement membrane | Goodpasture's syndrome |
| Anti-desmoglein | Pemphigus vulgaris |
| Antimicrosomal, antithyroglobulin | Hashimoto's thyroiditis |
| Anti-Jo-1 | Polymyositis, dermatomyositis |
| Anti-SS-A (anti-Ro) | Sjögren's syndrome |
| Anti-SS-B (anti-La) | Sjögren's syndrome |
| Anti-U1 RNP (ribonucleoprotein) | Mixed connective tissue disease |
| Anti–smooth muscle | Autoimmune hepatitis |
| Anti–glutamate decarboxylase | Type 1 diabetes mellitus |
| c-ANCA | Wegener's granulomatosis |
| p-ANCA | Other vasculitides |

**Immune deficiencies**

| Disease | Defect | Presentation | Labs |
|---|---|---|---|
| **B-cell disorders** | | | |
| Bruton's agammaglobulinemia | X-linked recessive ($\uparrow$ in **B**oys). Defect in *BTK*, a **tyrosine kinase** gene → blocks B-cell differentiation/ maturation. | Recurrent bacterial infections after 6 months ($\downarrow$ maternal IgG) due to opsonization defect. | Normal pro-B, $\downarrow$ maturation, $\downarrow$ number of B cells, $\downarrow$ immunoglobulins of all classes. |
| Hyper-IgM syndrome | Defective CD40L on helper T cells = inability to class switch. | Severe pyogenic infections early in life. | $\uparrow$ IgM; $\downarrow\downarrow$ IgG, IgA, IgE. |
| Selective Ig deficiency | Defect in isotype switching → deficiency in specific class of immunoglobulins. | Sinus and lung infections, milk allergies and diarrhea, Anaphylaxis on exposure to blood products with Ig**A**. | IgA deficiency most common. Failure to mature into plasma cells. $\downarrow$ secretory IgA. |
| Common variable immunodeficiency (CVID) | Defect in B-cell maturation; many causes. | Can be acquired in 20s–30s; $\uparrow$ risk of autoimmune disease, lymphoma, sinopulmonary infections. | Normal number of B cells; $\downarrow$ plasma cells, immunoglobulin. |
| **T-cell disorders** | | | |
| Thymic aplasia (DiGeorge syndrome) | 22q11 deletion; failure to develop 3rd and 4th pharyngeal pouches. | Tetany (hypocalcemia), recurrent viral/fungal infections (T-cell deficiency), congenital heart and great vessel defects. | Thymus and parathyroids fail to develop → $\downarrow$ T cells, $\downarrow$ PTH, $\downarrow$ Ca$^{2+}$. Absent thymic shadow on CXR. |
| IL-12 receptor deficiency | $\downarrow$ Th$_1$ response. | Disseminated mycobacterial infections. | $\downarrow$ IFN-$\gamma$. |
| Hyper-IgE syndrome (Job's syndrome) | Th cells fail to produce IFN-$\gamma$ → inability of neutrophils to respond to chemotactic stimuli. | **FATED**: coarse **F**acies, cold (noninflamed) staphylococcal **A**bscesses, retained primary **T**eeth, $\uparrow$ Ig**E**, **D**ermatologic problems (eczema). | $\uparrow$ IgE. |
| Chronic mucocutaneous candidiasis | T-cell dysfunction. | *Candida albicans* infections of skin and mucous membranes. | |

**Immune deficiencies** *(continued)*

| Disease | Defect | Presentation | Labs |
|---------|--------|--------------|------|
| **B- and T-cell disorders** | | | |
| Severe combined immunodeficiency (SCID) | Several types: defective IL-2 receptor (most common, X-linked), adenosine deaminase deficiency, failure to synthesize MHC II antigens. | Recurrent viral, bacterial, fungal, and protozoal infections due to both B- and T-cell deficiency. Treatment: bone marrow transplant (no allograft rejection). | ↓ IL-2R = ↓ T-cell activation. ↑ adenine = toxic to B and T cells. (↓ dNTPs, ↓ DNA synthesis.) |
| Ataxia-telangiectasia | Defect in DNA repair enzymes. | Triad: cerebellar defects (ataxia), spider angiomas (telangiectasia), IgA deficiency. | IgA deficiency. |
| Wiskott-Aldrich syndrome | X-linked recessive defect. Progressive deletion of B and T cells. | Triad (**TIE**): Thrombocytopenic purpura, Infections, Eczema. | ↑ IgE, IgA; ↓ **IgM**. |
| **Phagocyte dysfunction** | | | |
| Leukocyte adhesion deficiency (type 1) | Defect in LFA-1 integrin (CD18) protein on phagocytes. | Recurrent bacterial infections, absent pus formation, delayed separation of umbilicus. | Neutrophilia. |
| Chédiak-Higashi syndrome | Autosomal recessive; defect in microtubular function with ↓ phagocytosis. | Recurrent pyogenic infections by staphylococci and streptococci; partial albinism, peripheral neuropathy. | |
| Chronic granulomatous disease | Lack of NADPH oxidase → ↓ reactive oxygen species (e.g., superoxide) and absent respiratory burst in neutrophils. | ↑ susceptibility to catalase-positive organisms (e.g., *S. aureus*, *E. coli*, *Aspergillus*). | Negative Nitroblue tetrazolium dye reduction test. |

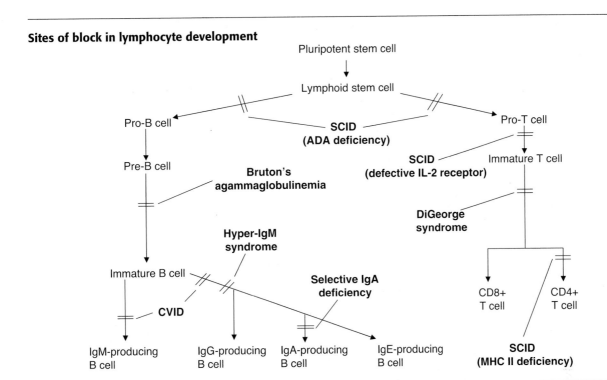

## Sites of block in lymphocyte development

## Grafts

| | |
|---|---|
| Autograft | From self. |
| Syngeneic graft | From identical twin or clone. |
| Allograft | From nonidentical individual of same species. |
| Xenograft | From different species. |

## Transplant rejection

| | |
|---|---|
| Hyperacute rejection | Antibody mediated (type II) due to the presence of preformed antidonor antibodies in the transplant recipient. Occurs within minutes after transplantation. |
| Acute rejection | Cell mediated due to cytotoxic T lymphocytes reacting against foreign MHCs. Occurs weeks after transplantation. Reversible with immunosuppressants such as cyclosporine and OKT3. |
| Chronic rejection | T-cell- and antibody-mediated vascular damage (obliterative vascular fibrosis); occurs months to years after transplantation. Irreversible. Class I-MHC$_{non-self}$ is perceived by CTLs as class I-MHC$_{self}$ presenting a non-self antigen. |
| Graft-versus-host disease | Grafted immunocompetent T cells proliferate in the irradiated immunocompromised host and reject cells with "foreign" proteins, resulting in severe organ dysfunction. Major symptoms include a maculopapular rash, jaundice, hepatosplenomegaly, and diarrhea. |

### ▶ IMMUNOLOGY—IMMUNOSUPPRESSANTS

## Cyclosporine

| | |
|---|---|
| Mechanism | Binds to cyclophilins. Complex blocks the differentiation and activation of T cells by inhibiting calcineurin, thus preventing the production of IL-2 and its receptor. |
| Clinical use | Suppresses organ rejection after transplantation; selected autoimmune disorders. |
| Toxicity | Predisposes patients to viral infections and lymphoma; nephrotoxic (preventable with mannitol diuresis). |

**Tacrolimus (FK506)**

| | |
|---|---|
| Mechanism | Similar to cyclosporine; binds to FK-binding protein, inhibiting secretion of IL-2 and other cytokines. |
| Clinical use | Potent immunosuppressive used in organ transplant recipients. |
| Toxicity | Significant—nephrotoxicity, peripheral neuropathy, hypertension, pleural effusion, hyperglycemia. |

**Azathioprine**

| | |
|---|---|
| Mechanism | Antimetabolite precursor of 6-mercaptopurine that interferes with the metabolism and synthesis of nucleic acids. Toxic to proliferating lymphocytes. |
| Clinical use | Kidney transplantation, autoimmune disorders (including glomerulonephritis and hemolytic anemia). |
| Toxicity | Bone marrow suppression. Active metabolite mercaptopurine is metabolized by xanthine oxidase; thus, toxic effects may be ↑ by allopurinol. |

**Muromonab-CD3 (OKT3)**

| | |
|---|---|
| Mechanism | Monoclonal antibody that binds to CD3 (epsilon chain) on the surface of T cells. Blocks cellular interaction with CD3 protein responsible for T-cell signal transduction. |
| Clinical use | Immunosuppression after kidney transplantation. |
| Toxicity | Cytokine release syndrome, hypersensitivity reaction. |

**Sirolimus (rapamycin)**

| | |
|---|---|
| Mechanism | Binds to mTOR. Inhibits T-cell proliferation in response to IL-2. |
| Clinical use | Immunosuppression after kidney transplantation in combination with cyclosporine and corticosteroids. |
| Toxicity | Hyperlipidemia, thrombocytopenia, leukopenia. |

**Mycophenolate mofetil**

| | |
|---|---|
| Mechanism | Inhibits de novo guanine synthesis and blocks lymphocyte production. |

**Daclizumab**

| | |
|---|---|
| Mechanism | Monoclonal antibody with high affinity for the IL-2 receptor on activated T cells. |

**Recombinant cytokines and clinical uses**

| Agent | Clinical uses |
|---|---|
| Aldesleukin (interleukin-2) | Renal cell carcinoma, metastatic melanoma |
| Erythropoietin (epoetin) | Anemias (especially in renal failure) |
| Filgrastim (granulocyte colony-stimulating factor) | Recovery of bone marrow |
| Sargramostim (granulocyte-macrophage colony-stimulating factor) | Recovery of bone marrow |
| α-interferon | Hepatitis B and C, Kaposi's sarcoma, leukemias, malignant melanoma |
| β-interferon | Multiple sclerosis |
| γ-interferon | Chronic granulomatous disease |
| Oprelvekin (interleukin-11) | Thrombocytopenia |
| Thrombopoietin | Thrombocytopenia |

# Pathology

*"Digressions, objections, delight in mockery, carefree mistrust are signs of health; everything unconditional belongs in pathology."*

—Friedrich Nietzsche

▶ Inflammation

▶ Neoplasia

The fundamental principles of pathology are key to understanding diseases in all organ systems. Major topics such as inflammation and neoplasia appear frequently in questions aimed at many different organ systems, and such topics are definitely high yield. For example, the concepts of cell injury and inflammation are key to understanding the inflammatory response that follows myocardial infarction, a very common subject of boards questions. Similarly, a familiarity with the early cellular changes that culminate in the development of neoplasias—for example, esophageal or colon cancer—is critical. Finally, make sure you recognize the major tumor-associated genes and are comfortable with key cancer concepts such as tumor staging and metastasis.

**Apoptosis**

Programmed cell death; ATP required.

Intrinsic pathway—occurs during embryogenesis, hormone induction (e.g., menstruation), and atrophy (e.g., endometrial lining during menopause) and as a result of injurious stimuli (e.g., radiation, toxins, hypoxia). Changes in the levels of anti- and pro-apoptotic factors lead to ↑ mitochondrial permeability and release of cytochrome c.

Extrinsic pathway—occurs with ligand-receptor interactions (e.g., Fas ligand binding to Fas [CD95]) or immune cell (T$_{killer}$) release of perforin and granzyme B.

Both pathways lead to activation of cytosolic caspases that mediate cellular breakdown.

Characterized by cell shrinkage, nuclear shrinkage and basophilia (pyknosis), membrane blebbing, pyknotic nuclear fragmentation (karyorrhexis), nuclear fading (karyolysis), and formation of apoptotic bodies, which are then phagocytosed. No significant inflammation.

**Necrosis**

Enzymatic degradation of a cell resulting from exogenous injury.

Characterized by enzymatic digestion and protein denaturation, with release of intracellular components.

Inflammatory.

Morphologically occurs as coagulative (heart, liver, kidney), liquefactive (brain), caseous (tuberculosis), fat (pancreas), or fibrinoid (blood vessels). Gangrenous necrosis can be dry (ischemic coagulative) or wet (with bacteria) and is common in limbs and GI tract.

**Cell injury**

| **Reversible** | **Irreversible** |
|---|---|
| Cellular swelling | Nuclear pyknosis, karyolysis, karyorrhexis |
| Nuclear chromatin clumping | |
| ↓ ATP synthesis | $Ca^{2+}$ influx → caspase activation |
| ↓ glycogen | Plasma membrane damage |
| Fatty change | Lysosomal rupture |
| Ribosomal detachment | Mitochondrial permeability |

**Infarcts: red vs. pale**

Red (hemorrhagic) infarcts occur in loose tissues with collaterals, such as liver, lungs, or intestine, or following reperfusion.

Pale infarcts occur in solid tissues with single blood supply, such as heart, kidney, and spleen.

**RE**d = **RE**perfusion.
Reperfusion injury is due to damage by free radicals.

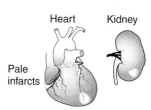

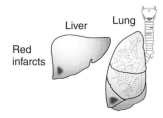

| Inflammation | Characterized by *rubor* (redness), *dolor* (pain), *calor* (heat), *tumor* (swelling), and *functio laesa* (loss of function). | |
|---|---|---|
| Fluid exudation | ↑ vascular permeability, vasodilation, endothelial injury. | |
| Leukocyte activation | Emigration (rolling, tight binding, diapedesis); chemotaxis (bacterial products, complement, chemokines); phagocytosis and killing. | Neutrophils love the feeling of **CILK**: **C**5a, **I**L-8, **L**eukotriene B4, and **K**allikrein recruit neutrophils to sites of injury/inflammation. |
| Fibrosis | Fibroblast emigration and proliferation; deposition of ECM. | |
| Acute | Neutrophil, eosinophil, and antibody mediated. | Acute inflammation is rapid onset (seconds to minutes), lasts minutes to days. |
| Chronic | Mononuclear cell mediated: Characterized by persistent destruction and repair. Associated with blood vessel proliferation, fibrosis. Granuloma—nodular collections of epithelioid macrophages and giant cells. | Granulomatous diseases: TB (caseating), syphilis, *Listeria monocytogenes*, Wegener's granulomatosis, leprosy, *Bartonella*, some fungal pneumonias, sarcoidosis, Crohn's disease. Granuloma formation is IL-2, interferon-γ mediated. |
| Resolution | Restoration of normal structure. Granulation tissue—highly vascularized, fibrotic. Abscess—fibrosis surrounding pus. Fistula—abnormal communication. Scarring—collagen deposition resulting in altered structure and function. | |

| Transudate vs. exudate | **Transudate** | **Exudate** |
|---|---|---|
| | Hypocellular | Cellular |
| | Protein poor | Protein rich |
| | Specific gravity < 1.012 | Specific gravity > 1.020 |
| | Due to: ↑ hydrostatic pressure ↓ oncotic pressure $Na^+$ retention | Due to: Lymphatic obstruction Inflammation |

**Leukocyte extravasation**

Neutrophils exit from blood vessels at sites of tissue injury and inflammation in 4 steps:

| Step | Vasculature/Stroma | Leukocyte |
|---|---|---|
| 1. Rolling | E-selectin <br> P-selectin | Sialyl Lewis$^X$ |
| 2. Tight binding | ICAM-1 | LFA-1 ("integrin") |
| 3. Diapedesis—leukocyte travels between endothelial cells and exits blood vessel | PECAM-1 | PECAM-1 |
| 4. Migration—leukocyte travels through interstitium to site of injury or infection guided by chemotactic signals | Bacterial products <br> **CILK:** <br> C5a <br> IL-8 <br> LTB4 <br> **K**allikrein | Various |

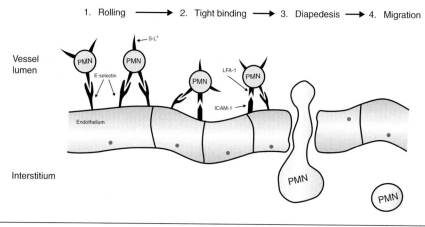

**Free radical injury**

Initiated via radiation exposure, metabolism of drugs (phase I), redox reaction, nitric oxide, transition metals, leukocyte oxidative burst.

Induces cell injury through membrane lipid peroxidation, protein modification, DNA breakage.

Free radical degradation produced through enzymes (catalase, superoxide dismutase, glutathione peroxidase), spontaneous decay, antioxidants (vitamins A, C, E).

Reperfusion after anoxia induces free radical production (e.g., superoxide) and is a major cause of injury after thrombolytic therapy.

**Amyloidosis** β-pleated sheet demonstrable by apple-green birefringence of Congo red stain under polarized light; affected tissue has waxy appearance.

| Types | Protein | Derived from | |
|---|---|---|---|
| Primary | AL | Ig light chains (multiple myeloma) | AL = **L**ight chain. |
| Secondary | AA | Serum amyloid-associated (SAA) protein (chronic inflammatory disease) | AA = **A**cute-phase reactant. |
| Senile cardiac | Transthyretin | AF | AF = old **F**ogies. |
| Diabetes mellitus type 2 | Amylin | AE | AE = **E**ndocrine. |
| Medullary carcinoma of the thyroid | A-CAL | Calcitonin | A-**CAL** = **CAL**citonin. |
| Alzheimer's disease | β-amyloid | Amyloid precursor protein (APP) | |
| Dialysis-associated | $\beta_2$-microglobulin | MHC class I proteins | |

| **Shock** | **Hypovolemic/cardiogenic** | **Septic** |
|---|---|---|
| | **Low**-output failure | **High**-output failure |
| | ↑ TPR | ↓ TPR |
| | Low cardiac output | Dilated arterioles, high mixed venous pressure |
| | Cold, clammy patient | Hot patient |

**Neoplastic progression**     Hallmarks of cancer—evading apoptosis, self-sufficiency in growth signals, insensitivity to anti-growth signals, sustained angiogenesis, limitless replicative potential, tissue invasion, and metastasis.

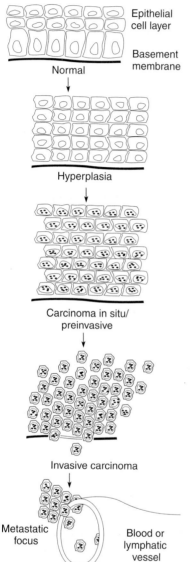

Epithelial cell layer

Basement membrane

Normal

• Normal cells with basal → apical differentiation

Hyperplasia

• Cells have increased in number—**hyperplasia**
• Abnormal proliferation of cells with loss of size, shape, and orientation—**dysplasia**

Carcinoma in situ/ preinvasive

• **In situ carcinoma**
• Neoplastic cells have not invaded basement membrane
• High nuclear/cytoplasmic ratio and clumped chromatin
• Neoplastic cells encompass entire thickness
• Tumor cells are monoclonal

Invasive carcinoma

• Cells have invaded basement membrane using **collagenases** and **hydrolases**
• Can metastasize if they reach a blood or lymphatic vessel

Metastatic focus

Blood or lymphatic vessel

**Metastasis**—spread to distant organ
• Must survive immune attack
• "Seed and soil" theory of metastasis
   • Seed = tumor embolus
   • Soil = target organ—liver, lungs, bone, brain . . .
   • Angiogenesis allows for tumor survival
   • ↓ cadherin, ↑ laminin, integrin receptors

(Adapted, with permission, from McPhee SJ et al. *Pathophysiology of Disease: An Introduction to Clinical Medicine,* 3rd ed. New York: McGraw-Hill, 2000: 84.)

## *-plasia* definitions

Reversible  Hyperplasia—↑ in number of cells.

Metaplasia—1 adult cell type is replaced by another. Often 2° to irritation and/or environmental exposure (e.g., squamous metaplasia in trachea and bronchi of smokers).

Dysplasia—abnormal growth with loss of cellular orientation, shape, and size in comparison to normal tissue maturation; commonly preneoplastic.

Irreversible  Anaplasia—abnormal cells lacking differentiation; like primitive cells of same tissue, often equated with undifferentiated malignant neoplasms. Little or no resemblance to tissue of origin.

Neoplasia—a clonal proliferation of cells that is uncontrolled and excessive.

Desmoplasia—fibrous tissue formation in response to neoplasm.

## Tumor grade vs. stage

Grade  Degree of cellular differentiation based on histologic appearance of tumor. Usually graded I–IV based on degree of differentiation and number of mitoses per high-power field; character of tumor itself.

Stage  Degree of localization/spread based on site and size of 1° lesion, spread to regional lymph nodes, presence of metastases; spread of tumor in a specific patient.

Stage usually has more prognostic value than grade.
Stage = **S**pread.
TNM staging system:
  **T** = size of **T**umor
  **N** = **N**ode involvement
  **M** = **M**etastases

## Tumor nomenclature

| Cell type | Benign | Malignant[a] |
|---|---|---|
| **Epithelium** | Adenoma, papilloma | Adenocarcinoma, papillary carcinoma |
| **Mesenchyme** | | |
| Blood cells | | Leukemia, lymphoma |
| Blood vessels | Hemangioma | Angiosarcoma |
| Smooth muscle | Leiomyoma | Leiomyosarcoma |
| Skeletal muscle | Rhabdomyoma | Rhabdomyosarcoma |
| Bone | Osteoma | Osteosarcoma |
| Fat | Lipoma | Liposarcoma |
| > 1 cell type | Mature teratoma (women) | Immature teratoma and mature teratoma (men) |

[a]The term **carcinoma** implies epithelial origin, whereas **sarcoma** denotes mesenchymal origin. Both terms imply malignancy.

## Tumor differences

Benign  Usually well differentiated, slow growing, well demarcated, no metastasis.

Malignant  May be poorly differentiated, erratic growth, locally invasive/diffuse, may metastasize.

| Disease conditions associated with neoplasms | Condition | Neoplasm |
|---|---|---|
| | 1. **Down** syndrome | 1. **ALL** (we **ALL** fall **Down**), AML |
| | 2. Xeroderma pigmentosum, albinism | 2. Melanoma, basal cell carcinoma, and especially squamous cell carcinomas of skin |
| | 3. Chronic atrophic gastritis, pernicious anemia, postsurgical gastric remnants | 3. Gastric adenocarcinoma |
| | 4. Tuberous sclerosis (facial angiofibroma, seizures, mental retardation) | 4. Astrocytoma, angiomyolipoma, and cardiac rhabdomyoma |
| | 5. Actinic keratosis | 5. Squamous cell carcinoma of skin |
| | 6. Barrett's esophagus (chronic GI reflux) | 6. Esophageal adenocarcinoma |
| | 7. Plummer-Vinson syndrome (atrophic glossitis, esophageal webs, anemia; all due to iron deficiency) | 7. Squamous cell carcinoma of esophagus |
| | 8. Cirrhosis (alcoholic, hepatitis B or C) | 8. Hepatocellular carcinoma |
| | 9. Ulcerative colitis | 9. Colonic adenocarcinoma |
| | 10. Paget's disease of bone | 10. 2° osteosarcoma and fibrosarcoma |
| | 11. Immunodeficiency states | 11. Malignant lymphomas |
| | 12. AIDS | 12. Aggressive malignant lymphomas (non-Hodgkin's) and Kaposi's sarcoma |
| | 13. Autoimmune diseases (e.g., Hashimoto's thyroiditis, myasthenia gravis) | 13. Lymphoma |
| | 14. Acanthosis nigricans (hyperpigmentation and epidermal thickening) | 14. Visceral malignancy (stomach, lung, breast, uterus) |
| | 15. Dysplastic nevus | 15. Malignant melanoma |
| | 16. Radiation exposure | 16. Sarcoma, papillary thyroid cancer |

| Oncogenes | Gain of function → cancer. Need damage to only 1 allele. | |
|---|---|---|
| **Gene** | **Associated tumor** | |
| *abl* | CML | |
| c-*myc* | Burkitt's lymphoma | |
| *bcl*-2 | Follicular and undifferentiated lymphomas (inhibits apoptosis) | |
| *erb*-B2 | Breast, ovarian, and gastric carcinomas | |
| *ras* | Colon carcinoma | |
| **L**-*myc* | Lung tumor | |
| **N**-*myc* | Neuroblastoma | |
| *ret* | Multiple endocrine neoplasia (MEN) types II and III | |
| c-*kit* | Gastrointestinal stromal tumor (GIST) | |

| **Tumor suppressor genes** | Loss of function → cancer; both alleles must be lost for expression of disease. | | |
|---|---|---|---|
| Gene | Chromosome | Associated tumor | |
| *Rb* | 13q | Retinoblastoma, osteosarcoma | |
| *BRCA1* | 17q | Breast and ovarian cancer | |
| *BRCA2* | 13q | Breast cancer | |
| *p53* | 17p | Most human cancers, Li-Fraumeni syndrome | |
| *p16* | 9p | Melanoma | MelaNoma is on Nine. |
| APC | 5q | Colorectal cancer (associated with FAP) | |
| WT1 | 11p | Wilms' tumor | |
| NF1 | 17q | Neurofibromatosis type 1 | |
| NF2 | 22q | Neurofibromatosis type 2 | Type 2 = 22. |
| DPC | 18q | Pancreatic cancer | DPC—Deleted in Pancreatic Cancer. |
| DCC | 18q | Colon cancer | DCC—Deleted in Colon Cancer. |

**Tumor markers**

| | | |
|---|---|---|
| PSA | Prostate-specific antigen. Used to screen for prostate carcinoma. Can also be elevated in BPH and prostatitis. | Tumor markers should not be used as the 1° tool for cancer diagnosis. They may be used to confirm diagnosis, to monitor for tumor recurrence, and to monitor response to therapy. |
| Prostatic acid phosphatase | Prostate carcinoma. | |
| CEA | Carcinoembryonic antigen. Very nonspecific but produced by ~ 70% of colorectal and pancreatic cancers; also produced by gastric and breast carcinomas. | |
| α-fetoprotein | Normally made by fetus. Hepatocellular carcinomas. Nonseminomatous germ cell tumors of the testis (e.g., yolk sac tumor). | |
| β-hCG | Hydatidiform moles, Choriocarcinomas, and Gestational trophoblastic tumors. | |
| CA-125 | Ovarian, malignant epithelial tumors. | |
| S-100 | Melanoma, neural tumors, astrocytomas. | |
| Alkaline phosphatase | Metastases to bone, obstructive biliary disease, Paget's disease of bone. | |
| Bombesin | Neuroblastoma, lung and gastric cancer. | |
| **TRAP** | Tartrate-resistant acid phosphatase. **Hairy** cell leukemia—a B-cell neoplasm. | **TRAP** the **hairy** animal. |
| CA-19-9 | Pancreatic adenocarcinoma. | |

**Oncogenic viruses**

| Virus | Associated cancer |
|---|---|
| HTLV-1 | Adult T-cell leukemia/lymphoma |
| HBV, HCV | Hepatocellular carcinoma |
| EBV | Burkitt's lymphoma, nasopharyngeal carcinoma |
| HPV | Cervical carcinoma (16, 18), penile/anal carcinoma |
| HHV-8 (Kaposi's sarcoma–associated herpesvirus) | Kaposi's sarcoma, body cavity fluid B-cell lymphoma |

**Chemical carcinogens**

| Toxin | Affected organ |
|---|---|
| Aflatoxins (produced by *Aspergillus*) | Liver (hepatocellular carcinoma) |
| Vinyl chloride | Liver (angiosarcoma) |
| $CCl_4$ | Liver (centrilobular necrosis, fatty change) |
| Nitrosamines (e.g., in smoked foods) | Esophagus, stomach |
| Cigarette smoke | Larynx (squamous cell carcinoma), lung (squamous cell and small cell carcinomas), kidney (renal cell carcinoma), bladder (transitional cell carcinoma) |
| Asbestos | Lung (mesothelioma and bronchogenic carcinoma) |
| Arsenic | Skin (squamous cell carcinoma), liver (angiosarcoma) |
| Naphthalene (aniline) dyes | Bladder (transitional cell carcinoma) |
| Alkylating agents | Blood (leukemia) |

**Paraneoplastic effects of tumors**

| Neoplasm | Causes | Effect |
|---|---|---|
| Small cell lung carcinoma | ACTH or ACTH-like peptide | Cushing's syndrome |
| Small cell lung carcinoma and intracranial neoplasms | ADH | SIADH |
| Squamous cell lung carcinoma, renal cell carcinoma, and breast carcinoma | PTH-related peptide, TGF-β, TNF, IL-1 | Hypercalcemia |
| Renal cell carcinoma, hemangioblastoma | Erythropoietin | Polycythemia |
| Thymoma, small cell lung carcinoma | Antibodies against presynaptic $Ca^{2+}$ channels at neuromuscular junction | Lambert-Eaton syndrome (muscle weakness) |
| Leukemias and lymphomas | Hyperuricemia due to excess nucleic acid turnover (i.e., cytotoxic therapy) | Gout, urate nephropathy |

**Psammoma bodies**

Laminated, concentric, calcific spherules seen in:
1. Papillary adenocarcinoma of thyroid
2. Serous papillary cystadenocarcinoma of ovary
3. Meningioma
4. Malignant mesothelioma

**PSaMMoma:**
Papillary (thyroid)
Serous (ovary)
Meningioma
Mesothelioma

HIGH-YIELD PRINCIPLES

PATHOLOGY

| **Erythrocyte sedimentation rate (ESR)** | Products of inflammation (e.g., fibrinogen) coat RBCs and cause aggregation. When aggregated, RBCs fall at a faster rate within the test tube. | |
|---|---|---|
| | ↑ ESR<br>Infections<br>Inflammation (e.g., temporal arteritis)<br>Cancer<br>Pregnancy<br>SLE | ↓ ESR<br>Sickle cell (altered shape)<br>Polycythemia (too many)<br>CHF (unknown) |
| **Metastasis to brain** | 1° tumors that metastasize to brain—Lung, Breast, Skin (melanoma), Kidney (renal cell carcinoma), GI. Overall, approximately 50% of brain tumors are from metastases. | Lots of **B**ad **S**tuff **K**ills **G**lia.<br>Typically multiple well-circumscribed tumors at gray-white border. |
| **Metastasis to liver** | The liver and lung are the most common sites of metastasis after the regional lymph nodes. 1° tumors that metastasize to the liver—Colon > Stomach > Pancreas > Breast > Lung. | Metastases >> 1° liver tumors.<br>**C**ancer **S**ometimes **P**enetrates **B**enign **L**iver. |
| **Metastasis to bone** | These 1° tumors metastasize to bone—Prostate, Thyroid, Testes, Breast, Lung, Kidney.<br>Metastases from breast and prostate are most common.<br>Metastatic bone tumors are far more common than 1° bone tumors. | **P. T. B**arnum **L**oves **K**ids.<br>Lung = **L**ytic.<br>Prostate = blastic.<br>**B**reast = **B**oth lytic and blastic. |

**Cancer epidemiology**

| | Male | Female | |
|---|---|---|---|
| Incidence | Prostate (32%)<br>Lung (16%)<br>Colon and rectum (12%) | Breast (32%)<br>Lung (13%)<br>Colon and rectum (13%) | Deaths from lung cancer have plateaued in males but continue to ↑ in females.<br>Cancer is the 2nd leading cause of death in the United States (heart disease is 1st). |
| Mortality | Lung (33%)<br>Prostate (13%) | Lung (23%)<br>Breast (18%) | |

# Pharmacology

*"Take me, I am the drug; take me, I am hallucinogenic."*
—Salvador Dali

*"I was under medication when I made the decision not to burn the tapes."*
—Richard Nixon

Preparation for questions on pharmacology is straightforward. Memorizing all the key drugs and their characteristics (e.g., mechanisms, clinical use, and important side effects) is high yield. Focus on understanding the prototype drugs in each class. Avoid memorizing obscure derivatives. Learn the "classic" and distinguishing toxicities of the major drugs. Do not bother with drug dosages or trade names. Reviewing associated biochemistry, physiology, and microbiology can be useful while studying pharmacology. There is a strong emphasis on ANS, CNS, antimicrobial, and cardiovascular agents as well as on NSAIDs. Much of the material is clinically relevant. Newer drugs on the market are also fair game.

### Enzyme kinetics

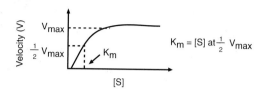

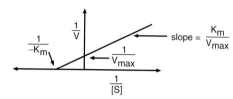

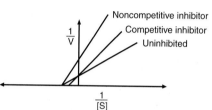

$K_m$ reflects the affinity of the enzyme for its substrate.

$V_{max}$ is directly proportional to the enzyme concentration.

$\downarrow K_m$, $\uparrow$ affinity.

$\uparrow$ y-intercept, $\downarrow V_{max}$. The further to the right the x-intercept, the greater the $K_m$.

HINT: Competitive inhibitors cross each other competitively, while noncompetitive inhibitors do not.

| | Competitive inhibitors | Noncompetitive inhibitors |
|---|---|---|
| Resemble substrate | Yes | No |
| Overcome by $\uparrow$ [S] | Yes | No |
| Bind active site | Yes | No |
| Effect on $V_{max}$ | Unchanged | $\downarrow$ |
| Effect on $K_m$ | $\uparrow$ | Unchanged |
| Pharmacodynamics | $\downarrow$ potency | $\downarrow$ efficacy |

### Pharmacokinetics

| | |
|---|---|
| Volume of distribution ($V_d$) | Relates the amount of drug in the body to the plasma concentration. $V_d$ of plasma protein–bound drugs can be altered by liver and kidney disease.<br><br>$V_d = \dfrac{\text{amount of drug in the body}}{\text{plasma drug concentration}}$<br><br>Drugs with:<br>Low $V_d$ (4–8 L) distribute in blood.<br>Medium $V_d$ distribute in extracellular space or body water.<br>High $V_d$ (> body weight) distribute in tissues. |
| Clearance (CL) | Relates the rate of elimination to the plasma concentration.<br><br>$CL = \dfrac{\text{rate of elimination of drug}}{\text{plasma drug concentration}} = V_d \times K_e$ (elimination constant) |
| Half-life ($t_{1/2}$) | The time required to change the amount of drug in the body by ½ during elimination (or during a constant infusion). A drug infused at a constant rate reaches about 94% of steady state after 4 $t_{1/2}$. Property of first-order elimination.<br><br>$t_{1/2} = \dfrac{0.7 \times V_d}{CL}$ |

| # of half-lives | 1 | 2 | 3 | 4 |
|---|---|---|---|---|
| Concentration | 50% | 75% | 87.5% | 93.75% |

HIGH-YIELD PRINCIPLES

PHARMACOLOGY

| **Dosage calculations** | Loading dose = $C_p \times V_d/F$. <br> Maintenance dose = $C_p \times CL/F$ where $C_p$ = target plasma concentration and $F$ = bioavailability = 1 when drug is given IV. <br> In patients with impaired renal or hepatic function, the loading dose remains unchanged, although the maintenance dose is $\downarrow$. | |

**Elimination of drugs**

| Zero-order elimination | Rate of elimination is constant regardless of C (i.e., constant **amount** of drug eliminated per unit time). <br> $C_p \downarrow$ linearly with time. Examples of drugs—**P**henytoin, **E**thanol, and **A**spirin (at high or toxic concentrations). | **PEA.** (A pea is round, shaped like the "0" in "zero-order.") |
| First-order elimination | Rate of elimination is proportional to the drug concentration (i.e., constant **fraction** of drug eliminated per unit time). <br> $C_p \downarrow$ exponentially with time. | |

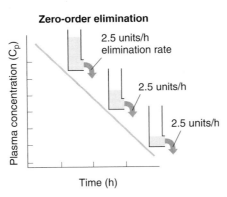 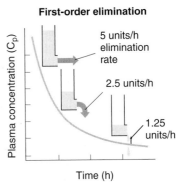

(Adapted, with permission, from Katzung BG, Trevor AJ. *Pharmacology: Examination & Board Review,* 5th ed. Stamford, CT: Appleton & Lange, 1998: 5.)

| **Urine pH and drug elimination** | Ionized species get trapped. | |
| Weak acids | Examples: phenobarbital, methotrexate, TCAs, aspirin. Trapped in basic environments. Treat overdose with bicarbonate. <br><br> $$RCOOH \rightleftharpoons RCOO^- + H^+$$ <br> (lipid soluble)     (trapped) | |
| Weak bases | Example: amphetamines. Trapped in acidic environments. Treat overdose with ammonium chloride. <br><br> $$RNH_3^+ \rightleftharpoons RNH_2 + H^+$$ <br> (trapped)     (lipid soluble) | |

| **Phase I vs. phase II metabolism** | Phase I (reduction, oxidation, hydrolysis) usually yields slightly polar, water-soluble metabolites (often still active). <br> Phase II (acetylation, glucuronidation, sulfation) usually yields very polar, inactive metabolites (renally excreted). | Phase I—cytochrome P-450. <br> Phase II—conjugation. <br> Geriatric patients lose phase I first. |

| **Efficacy vs. potency** | Efficacy—maximal effect a drug can produce. <br> Potency—amount of drug needed for a given effect. | |

**HIGH-YIELD PRINCIPLES**

**PHARMACOLOGY**

## Pharmacodynamics

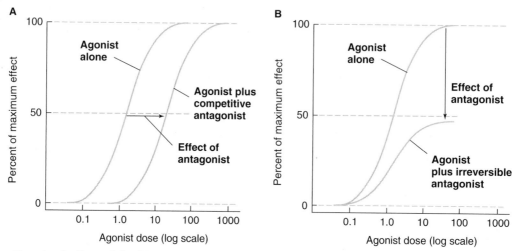

(Reproduced, with permission, from Trevor AJ, Katzung BG, Masters S. *Katzung & Trevor's Pharmacology: Examination & Board Review*, 8th ed. New York: McGraw-Hill, 2008: 14.)

**A.** A competitive antagonist shifts curve to the right, **decreasing potency** and increasing $EC_{50}$ (half maximally Effective Concentration for producing a given effect). **B.** A noncompetitive antagonist shifts the agonist curve downward, **decreasing efficacy.**

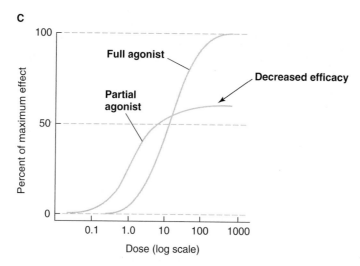

(Adapted, with permission, from Katzung BG. *Basic and Clinical Pharmacology*, 7th ed. Stamford, CT: Appleton & Lange, 1997: 13.)

**C.** Comparison of dose-response curves for a full agonist and a partial agonist. The **partial agonist** acts on the same receptor system as the full agonist but has a **lower maximal efficacy** regardless of the dose. A partial agonist may be more potent (as in the figure), less potent, or equally potent; **potency is an independent factor.**

| Therapeutic index | Measurement of drug safety. |
|---|---|

$$\frac{LD_{50}}{ED_{50}} = \frac{\text{median toxic dose}}{\text{median effective dose}}$$

TILE:
$TI = LD_{50} / ED_{50}$.
Safer drugs have higher TI values.

## Central and peripheral nervous system

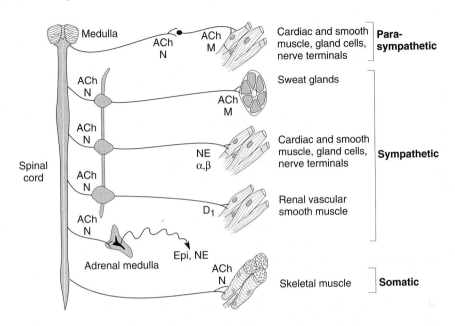

(Adapted, with permission, from Katzung BG. *Basic and Clinical Pharmacology*, 7th ed. Stamford, CT: Appleton & Lange, 1997: 74.)

| | |
|---|---|
| **ACh receptors** | Nicotinic ACh receptors are ligand-gated $Na^+/K^+$ channels; $N_N$ (found in autonomic ganglia) and $N_M$ (found in neuromuscular junction) subtypes.<br>Muscarinic ACh receptors are G-protein-coupled receptors that act through 2nd messengers; 5 subtypes: $M_1$, $M_2$, $M_3$, $M_4$, and $M_5$. |

## G-protein-linked 2nd messengers

| Receptor | G-protein class | Major functions |
|---|---|---|
| $\alpha_1$ | q | ↑ vascular smooth muscle contraction, ↑ pupillary dilator muscle contraction (mydriasis), ↑ intestinal and bladder sphincter muscle contraction |
| $\alpha_2$  — Sympathetic | i | ↓ sympathetic outflow, ↓ insulin release |
| $\beta_1$ | s | ↑ heart rate, ↑ contractility, ↑ renin release, ↑ lipolysis |
| $\beta_2$ | s | Vasodilation, bronchodilation, ↑ heart rate, ↑ contractility, ↑ lipolysis, ↑ insulin release, ↓ uterine tone |
| $M_1$  — Para-sympathetic | q | CNS, enteric nervous system |
| $M_2$ | i | ↓ heart rate and contractility of atria |
| $M_3$ | q | ↑ exocrine gland secretions (e.g., sweat, gastric acid), ↑ gut peristalsis, ↑ bladder contraction, bronchoconstriction, ↑ pupillary sphincter muscle contraction (miosis), ciliary muscle contraction (accommodation) |
| $D_1$  — Dopamine | s | Relaxes renal vascular smooth muscle |
| $D_2$ | i | Modulates transmitter release, especially in brain |
| $H_1$  — Histamine | q | ↑ nasal and bronchial mucus production, contraction of bronchioles, pruritus, and pain |
| $H_2$ | s | ↑ gastric acid secretion |
| $V_1$  — Vasopressin | q | ↑ vascular smooth muscle contraction |
| $V_2$ | s | ↑ $H_2O$ permeability and reabsorption in the collecting tubules of the kidney (V2 is found in the 2 kidneys) |

"**Q**iss (kiss) and **qiq** (kick) till you're **siq** (sick) of **sqs** (sex)."

$H_1$, $\alpha_1$, $V_1$, $M_1$, $M_3$  Receptor $\xrightarrow{G_q}$ Phospholipase **C** $\longrightarrow$ Lipids ↓ $PIP_2$ → $IP_3$ → ↑ $[Ca^{2+}]_{in}$ ; → DAG → Protein kinase **C**  ⠀⠀ **HAV**e 1 M&M.

$\beta_1$, $\beta_2$, $D_1$, $H_2$, $V_2$  Receptor $\xrightarrow{G_s}$ **A**denylyl cyclase $\longrightarrow$ ATP ↓ cAMP → Protein kinase **A**

$M_2$, $\alpha_2$, $D_2$  Receptor $\xrightarrow{G_i}$ **A**denylyl cyclase $\longrightarrow$ cAMP ↓ $\longrightarrow$ Protein kinase **A** ↓ ⠀⠀ MAD 2's.

## Autonomic drugs

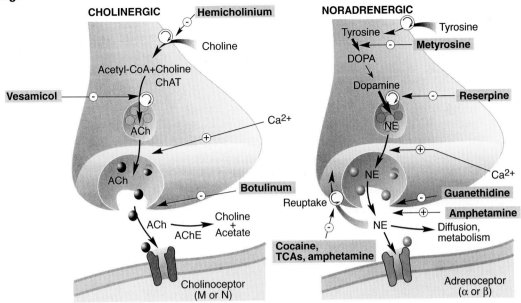

(Adapted, with permission, from Katzung BG, Trevor AJ. *Pharmacology: Examination & Board Review,* 5th ed. Stamford, CT: Appleton & Lange, 1998: 42.)

Circles with rotating arrows represent transporters; ChAT, choline acetyltransferase; ACh, acetylcholine; AChE, acetylcholinesterase; NE, norepinephrine.

**Noradrenergic nerve terminal**

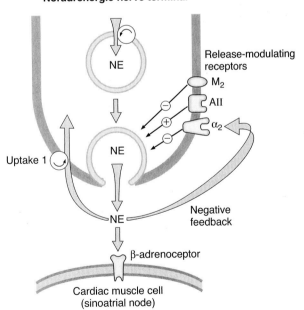

(Adapted, with permission, from Katzung BG, Trevor AJ. *Pharmacology: Examination & Board Review,* 5th ed. Stamford, CT: Appleton & Lange, 1998: 42.)

Release of NE from a sympathetic nerve ending is modulated by NE itself, acting on presynaptic $\alpha_2$ autoreceptors, and by ACh, angiotensin II, and other substances.

## Cholinomimetic agents

| Drug | Clinical applications | Action |
|------|----------------------|--------|
| **1. Direct agonists** | | |
| Bethanechol | Postoperative and neurogenic ileus and urinary retention | Activates **B**owel and **B**ladder smooth muscle; resistant to AChE. **Beth Anne, call (bethanechol)** me if you want to activate your **B**owels and **B**ladder. |
| Carbachol | Glaucoma, pupillary contraction, and release of intraocular pressure | |
| Pilocarpine | Potent stimulator of sweat, tears, saliva | Contracts ciliary muscle of eye (open angle), pupillary sphincter (narrow angle); resistant to AChE. **PILE** on the sweat and tears. |
| Methacholine | Challenge test for diagnosis of asthma | Stimulates muscarinic receptors in airway when inhaled. |
| **2. Indirect agonists (anticholinesterases)** | | |
| Neostigmine | Postoperative and neurogenic ileus and urinary retention, myasthenia gravis, reversal of neuromuscular junction blockade (postoperative) | ↑ endogenous ACh; no CNS penetration. **NEO** CNS = **NO** CNS penetration. |
| Pyridostigmine | Myasthenia gravis (long acting); does not penetrate CNS | ↑ endogenous ACh; ↑ strength. |
| Edrophonium | Diagnosis of myasthenia gravis (extremely short acting) | ↑ endogenous ACh. |
| Physostigmine | Glaucoma (crosses blood-brain barrier → CNS) and atropine overdose | ↑ endogenous ACh. **PHYS** is for **EYES**. |
| Echothiophate | Glaucoma | ↑ endogenous ACh. |

| | | |
|------|----------------------|--------|
| **Cholinesterase inhibitor poisoning** | Symptoms include **D**iarrhea, **U**rination, **M**iosis, **B**ronchospasm, **B**radycardia, **E**xcitation of skeletal muscle and CNS, **L**acrimation, **S**weating, and **S**alivation (also abdominal cramping). Antidote—atropine (muscarinic antagonist) plus pralidoxime (chemical antagonist used to regenerate active cholinesterase). | **DUMBBELSS.** Parathion and other organophosphates. Irreversible inhibitors. |

## Muscarinic antagonists

| Drug | Organ system | Application |
|---|---|---|
| Atropine, homatropine, tropicamide | Eye | Produce mydriasis and cycloplegia |
| **Benz**tropine | CNS | **PARK**inson's disease—**PARK** my **BENZ** |
| Scopolamine | CNS | Motion sickness |
| **Ipra**tropium | Respiratory | Asthma, COPD (**I pray** I can breathe soon!) |
| Oxybutynin, glycopyrrolate | Genitourinary | Reduce urgency in mild cystitis and reduce bladder spasms |
| Methscopolamine, pirenzepine, propantheline | Gastrointestinal | Peptic ulcer treatment |

---

**Atropine** — Muscarinic antagonist.

**Organ system**

| | | |
|---|---|---|
| Eye | ↑ pupil dilation, cycloplegia. | Blocks **DUMBBELSS** (see previous page). |
| Airway | ↓ secretions. | |
| Stomach | ↓ acid secretion. | |
| Gut | ↓ motility. | |
| Bladder | ↓ urgency in cystitis. | |

**Toxicity** — ↑ body temperature; rapid pulse; dry mouth; dry, flushed skin; cycloplegia; constipation; disorientation.

Can cause acute angle-closure glaucoma in elderly, urinary retention in men with prostatic hyperplasia, and hyperthermia in infants.

Side effects:
- Hot as a hare
- Dry as a bone
- Red as a beet
- Blind as a bat
- Mad as a hatter

---

**Hexamethonium** — Nicotinic antagonist.

**Clinical use** — Ganglionic blocker. Used in experimental models to prevent vagal reflex responses to changes in blood pressure—e.g., prevents reflex bradycardia caused by NE.

**Toxicity** — Severe orthostatic hypotension, blurred vision, constipation, sexual dysfunction.

Put a **hex** on smokers (**nicotine**) to help them quit.

### Sympathomimetics

| Drug | Mechanism/selectivity | Applications |
|---|---|---|
| **1. Direct sympatho- mimetics** | | |
| Epinephrine | $\alpha_1, \alpha_2, \beta_1, \beta_2$, **low** doses selective for $\beta_1$ (**Blow**) | Anaphylaxis, glaucoma (open angle), asthma, hypotension |
| NE | $\alpha_1, \alpha_2 > \beta_1$ | Hypotension (but ↓ renal perfusion) |
| **Iso**proterenol | $\beta_1 = \beta_2$ (**iso**lated to $\beta$) | AV block (rare) |
| Dopamine | $D_1 = D_2 > \beta > \alpha$, inotropic and chronotropic | Shock (↑ renal perfusion), heart failure |
| Dobutamine | $\beta_1 > \beta_2$, inotropic but not chronotropic | Shock, heart failure, cardiac stress testing |
| Phenylephrine | $\alpha_1 > \alpha_2$ | Pupillary dilation, vasoconstriction, nasal decongestion |
| **M**etaproterenol, **a**lbuterol, **s**almeterol, **t**erbutaline | Selective $\beta_2$-agonists ($\beta_2 > \beta_1$) | **MAST: M**etaproterenol and **A**lbuterol for acute asthma; **S**almeterol for long-term treatment; **T**erbutaline to reduce premature uterine contractions |
| Ritodrine | $\beta_2$ | Reduces premature uterine contractions |
| **2. Indirect sympatho- mimetics** | | |
| Amphetamine | Indirect general agonist, releases stored catecholamines | Narcolepsy, obesity, attention deficit disorder |
| Ephedrine | Indirect general agonist, releases stored catecholamines | Nasal decongestion, urinary incontinence, hypotension |
| Cocaine | Indirect general agonist, uptake inhibitor | Causes vasoconstriction and local anesthesia |

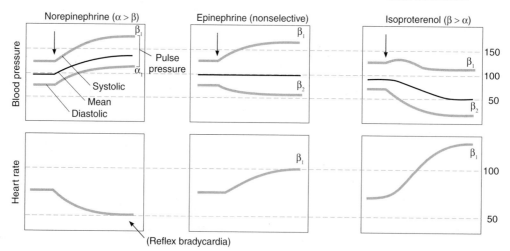

(Adapted, with permission, from Katzung BG, Trevor AJ. *Pharmacology: Examination & Board Review,* 5th ed. Stamford, CT: Appleton & Lange, 1998: 72.)

## Sympathoplegics

| | | |
|---|---|---|
| Clonidine, α-methyldopa | Centrally acting $\alpha_2$-agonists, ↓ central adrenergic outflow | Hypertension, especially with renal disease (no ↓ in blood flow to kidney) |

## α-blockers

| Drug | Application | Toxicity |
|---|---|---|
| **Nonselective** | | |
| Phenoxybenzamine (irreversible) and phentolamine (reversible) | Pheochromocytoma (use phenoxybenzamine before removing tumor, since high levels of released catecholamines will not be able to overcome blockage) | Orthostatic hypotension, reflex tachycardia |
| **$\alpha_1$ selective (-zosin ending)** | | |
| Prazosin, terazosin, doxazosin | Hypertension, urinary retention in BPH | 1st-dose orthostatic hypotension, dizziness, headache |
| **$\alpha_2$ selective** | | |
| Mirtazapine | Depression | Sedation, ↑ serum cholesterol, ↑ appetite |

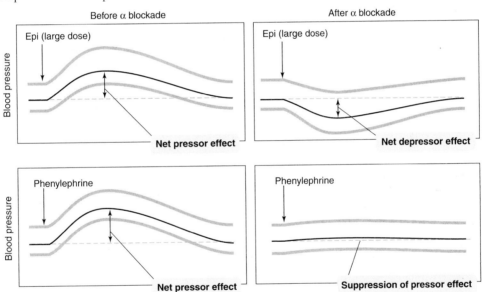

(Adapted, with permission, from Katzung BG, Trevor AJ. *Pharmacology: Examination & Board Review*, 5th ed. Stamford, CT: Appleton & Lange, 1998: 80.)

Shown above are the effects of an α-blocker (e.g., phentolamine) on blood pressure responses to epinephrine and phenylephrine. The epinephrine response exhibits reversal of the mean blood pressure change, from a net increase (the α response) to a net decrease (the $\beta_2$ response). The response to phenylephrine is suppressed but not reversed because phenylephrine is a "pure" α-agonist without β action.

**β-blockers**   Acebutolol, betaxolol, esmolol, atenolol, metoprolol, propranolol, timolol, pindolol, labetalol.

| Application | Effect |
|---|---|
| Hypertension | ↓ cardiac output, ↓ renin secretion (due to β-receptor blockade on JGA cells) |
| Angina pectoris | ↓ heart rate and contractility, resulting in ↓ $O_2$ consumption |
| MI | β-blockers ↓ mortality |
| SVT (propranolol, esmolol) | ↓ AV conduction velocity (class II antiarrhythmic) |
| CHF | Slows progression of chronic failure |
| Glaucoma (timolol) | ↓ secretion of aqueous humor |

**Toxicity**   Impotence, exacerbation of asthma, cardiovascular adverse effects (bradycardia, AV block, CHF), CNS adverse effects (sedation, sleep alterations); use with caution in diabetics

**Selectivity**   Nonselective antagonists ($\beta_1 = \beta_2$) — propranolol, timolol, nadolol, pindolol, and labetalol

$\beta_1$-selective antagonists ($\beta_1 > \beta_2$) — **A**cebutolol (partial agonist), **B**etaxolol, **E**smolol (short acting), **A**tenolol, **M**etoprolol

**A BEAM** of $\beta_1$-blockers.

Nonselective α- and β-antagonists — carvedilol, labetalol

Partial β-Agonists — **P**indolol, **A**cebutolol

| Specific antidotes | Toxin | Antidote/treatment |
|---|---|---|
| | 1. Acetaminophen | 1. N-acetylcysteine |
| | 2. Salicylates | 2. $NaHCO_3$ (alkalinize urine), dialysis |
| | 3. Amphetamines (basic) | 3. $NH_4Cl$ (acidify urine) |
| | 4. Anticholinesterases, organophosphates | 4. Atropine, pralidoxime |
| | 5. Antimuscarinic, anticholinergic agents | 5. Physostigmine salicylate |
| | 6. β-blockers | 6. Glucagon |
| | 7. Digitalis | 7. Stop dig, normalize $K^+$, lidocaine, anti-dig Fab fragments, $Mg^{2+}$ |
| | 8. Iron | 8. Deferoxamine |
| | 9. Lead | 9. CaEDTA, dimercaprol, succimer, penicillamine |
| | 10. Mercury, arsenic, gold | 10. Dimercaprol (BAL), succimer |
| | 11. Copper, arsenic, gold | 11. Penicillamine |
| | 12. Cyanide | 12. Nitrite, hydroxocobalamin, thiosulfate |
| | 13. **Meth**emoglobin | 13. **Meth**ylene blue, vitamin C |
| | 14. Carbon monoxide | 14. 100% $O_2$, hyperbaric $O_2$ |
| | 15. Methanol, ethylene glycol (antifreeze) | 15. Ethanol, dialysis, fomepizole |
| | 16. Opioids | 16. Naloxone/naltrexone |
| | 17. Benzodiazepines | 17. Flumazenil |
| | 18. TCAs | 18. $NaHCO_3$ (serum alkalinization) |
| | 19. Heparin | 19. Protamine |
| | 20. Warfarin | 20. Vitamin K, fresh frozen plasma |
| | 21. tPA, streptokinase | 21. Aminocaproic acid |
| | 22. Theophylline | 22. β-blocker |

| Iron poisoning | One of the leading causes of fatality from toxicologic agents in children. |
|---|---|
| Mechanism | Cell death due to peroxidation of membrane lipids. |
| Symptoms | Acute—gastric bleeding. |
| | Chronic—metabolic acidosis, scarring leading to GI obstruction. |

**Drug reactions**

| Drug reaction by system | Causal agent |
| --- | --- |
| **1. Cardiovascular** | |
| Atropine-like side effects | TCAs |
| Coronary vasospasm | Cocaine, sumatriptan |
| Cutaneous flushing | **VANC: V**ancomycin, **A**denosine, **N**iacin, **C**a$^{2+}$ channel blockers |
| Dilated cardiomyopathy | Doxorubicin (Adriamycin), daunorubicin |
| Torsades de pointes | Class III (sotalol), class IA (quinidine) antiarrhythmics, cisapride |
| **2. Hematologic** | |
| Agranulocytosis | Clozapine, carbamazepine, colchicine, propylthiouracil, methimazole, dapsone |
| Aplastic anemia | Chloramphenicol, benzene, NSAIDs, propylthiouracil, methimazole |
| Direct Coombs-positive hemolytic anemia | Methyldopa |
| Gray baby syndrome | Chloramphenicol |
| Hemolysis in G6PD-deficient patients | **I**soniazid (INH), **S**ulfonamides, **P**rimaquine, **A**spirin, **I**buprofen, **N**itrofurantoin (hemolysis **IS PAIN**) |
| Megaloblastic anemia | **P**henytoin, **M**ethotrexate, **S**ulfa drugs (having a **blast** with **PMS**) |
| Thrombotic complications | OCPs (e.g., estrogens and progestins) |
| **3. Respiratory** | |
| Cough | ACE inhibitors (note: ARBs like losartan—no cough) |
| Pulmonary fibrosis | **BL**eomycin, **A**miodarone, **B**usulfan (it's hard to **BLAB** when you have pulmonary fibrosis) |
| **4. GI** | |
| Acute cholestatic hepatitis | Macrolides |
| Focal to massive hepatic necrosis | Halothane, valproic acid, acetaminophen, *Amanita phalloides* |
| Hepatitis | INH |
| Pseudomembranous colitis | Clindamycin, ampicillin |
| **5. Reproductive/endocrine** | |
| Adrenocortical insufficiency | Glucocorticoid withdrawal (HPA suppression) |
| Gynecomastia | **S**pironolactone, **D**igitalis, **C**imetidine, chronic **A**lcohol use, estrogens, **K**etoconazole (**S**ome **D**rugs **C**reate **A**wesome **K**nockers) |
| Hot flashes | Tamoxifen, clomiphene |
| Hypothyroidism | Lithium, amiodarone |

### Drug reactions *(continued)*

**6. Musculoskeletal/ connective tissue**

| | |
|---|---|
| Gingival hyperplasia | Phenytoin |
| Gout | Furosemide, thiazides |
| Osteoporosis | Corticosteroids, heparin |
| Photosensitivity | Sulfonamides, Amiodarone, Tetracycline (**SAT** for a **photo**) |
| Rash (Stevens-Johnson syndrome) | Ethosuximide, lamotrigine, carbamazepine, phenobarbital, phenytoin, sulfa drugs, penicillin, allopurinol |
| SLE-like syndrome | Hydralazine, INH, Procainamide, Phenytoin (it's not **HIPP** to have lupus) |
| Tendonitis, tendon rupture, and cartilage damage (kids) | Fluoroquinolones |

**7. Renal/GU**

| | |
|---|---|
| Fanconi's syndrome | Expired tetracycline |
| Interstitial nephritis | Methicillin, NSAIDs, furosemide |
| Hemorrhagic cystitis | Cyclophosphamide, ifosfamide (prevent by coadministrating with mesna) |

**8. Neurologic**

| | |
|---|---|
| Cinchonism | Quinidine, quinine |
| Diabetes insipidus | Lithium, demeclocycline |
| Parkinson-like syndrome | Haloperidol, chlorpromazine, reserpine, metoclopramide |
| Seizures | Bupropion, imipenem/cilastatin, isoniazid |
| Tardive dyskinesia | Antipsychotics |

**9. Multiorgan**

| | |
|---|---|
| Disulfiram-like reaction | Metronidazole, certain cephalosporins, procarbazine, 1st-generation sulfonylureas |
| Nephrotoxicity/ neurotoxicity | Polymyxins |
| Nephrotoxicity/ ototoxicity | Aminoglycosides, vancomycin, loop diuretics, cisplatin |

---

**P-450 interactions**

| Inducers (+) | Inhibitors (−) | |
|---|---|---|
| Quinidine* | Sulfonamides | **Inducers:** |
| Barbiturates | Isoniazid | Queen Barb Steals Phen-phen |
| St. John's wort | Cimetidine | and Refuses Greasy Carbs |
| Phenytoin | Ketoconazole | Chronically. |
| Rifampin | Erythromycin | |
| Griseofulvin | Grapefruit juice | **Inhibitors:** |
| Carbamazepine | Acute alcohol use | Inhibit yourself from drinking |
| Chronic alcohol use | | beer from a KEG because it |
| | | makes you Acutely SICk. |

*Quinidine can both induce and inhibit different isoforms of P-450. Induction is the more important effect.

241

**Alcohol toxicity**

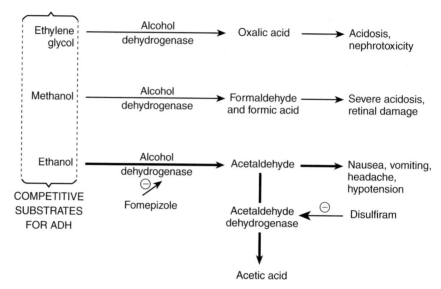

(Adapted, with permission, from Katzung BG, Trevor AJ. *Pharmacology: Examination & Board Review*, 5th ed. Appleton & Lange, 1998: 181.)

| **Sulfa drugs** | Celecoxib, furosemide, probenecid, thiazides, TMP-SMX, sulfasalazine, sulfonylureas, sumatriptan. |
|---|---|
| | Patients with sulfa allergies may develop fever, pruritic rash, Stevens-Johnson syndrome, hemolytic anemia, thrombocytopenia, agranulocytosis, and urticaria (hives). |
| | Symptoms range from mild to life-threatening. |

**Drug name**

| Ending | Category | Example |
|--------|----------|---------|
| -afil | Erectile dysfunction | Sildenafil |
| -ane | Inhalational general anesthetic | Halothane |
| -azepam | Benzodiazepine | Diazepam |
| -azine | Phenothiazine (neuroleptic, antiemetic) | Chlorpromazine |
| -azole | Antifungal | Ketoconazole |
| -barbital | Barbiturate | Phenobarbital |
| -caine | Local anesthetic | Lidocaine |
| -cillin | Penicillin | Methicillin |
| -cycline | Antibiotic, protein synthesis inhibitor | Tetracycline |
| -etine | SSRI | Fluoxetine |
| -ipramine | TCA | Imipramine |
| -navir | Protease inhibitor | Saquinavir |
| -olol | $\beta$ antagonist | Propranolol |
| -operidol | Butyrophenone (neuroleptic) | Haloperidol |
| -oxin | Cardiac glycoside (inotropic agent) | Digoxin |
| -phylline | Methylxanthine | Theophylline |
| -pril | ACE inhibitor | Captopril |
| -terol | $\beta_2$ agonist | Albuterol |
| -tidine | $H_2$ antagonist | Cimetidine |
| -triptan | 5-HT$_{1B/1D}$ agonists (migraine) | Sumatriptan |
| -triptyline | TCA | Amitriptyline |
| -tropin | Pituitary hormone | Somatotropin |
| -zolam | Benzodiazepine | Alprazolam |
| -zosin | $\alpha_1$ antagonist | Prazosin |

# SECTION III

# High-Yield Organ Systems

In this section, we have divided the High-Yield Facts into the major **Organ Systems.** Within each Organ System are several subsections, including **Anatomy, Physiology, Pathology,** and **Pharmacology.** As you progress through each Organ System, refer back to information in the previous subsections to organize these basic science subsections into a "vertical" framework for learning. Below is some general advice for studying the organ systems by these subsections.

## Anatomy

Several topics fall under this heading, including embryology, gross anatomy, histology, and neuroanatomy. Do not memorize all the small details; however, do not ignore anatomy altogether. Review what you have already learned and what you wish you had learned. Many questions require two steps. The first step is to identify a structure on anatomic cross section, electron micrograph, or photomicrograph. The second step may require an understanding of the clinical significance of the structure.

When studying, stress clinically important material. For example, be familiar with gross anatomy related to specific diseases (e.g., Pancoast's tumor, Horner's syndrome), traumatic injuries (e.g., fractures, sensory and motor nerve deficits), procedures (e.g., lumbar puncture), and common surgeries (e.g., cholecystectomy). There are also many questions on the exam involving x-rays, CT scans, and neuro MRI scans. Many students suggest browsing through a general radiology atlas, pathology atlas, and histology atlas. Focus on learning basic anatomy at key levels in the body (e.g., sagittal brain MRI; axial CT of the midthorax, abdomen, and pelvis). Basic neuroanatomy (especially pathways, blood supply, and functional anatomy) also has good yield. Use this as an opportunity to learn associated neuropathology and neurophysiology. Basic embryology (especially congenital malformations) is worth reviewing as well.

## Physiology

The portion of the examination dealing with physiology is broad and concept oriented and thus does not lend itself as well to fact-based review. Diagrams are often the best study aids, especially given the increasing number of questions requiring the interpretation of diagrams. Learn to apply basic physiologic relationships in a variety of ways (e.g., the Fick equation, clearance equations). You are seldom asked to perform complex calculations. Hormones are the focus of many questions, so learn their sites of production and action as well as their regulatory mechanisms.

A large portion of the physiology tested on the USMLE Step 1 is now clinically relevant and involves understanding physiologic changes associated with pathologic processes (e.g., changes in pulmonary function with COPD). Thus, it is worthwhile to review the physiologic changes that are found with common pathologies of the major organ systems (e.g., heart, lungs, kidneys, GI tract) and endocrine glands.

## Pathology

Questions dealing with this discipline are difficult to prepare for because of the sheer volume of material involved. Review the basic principles and hallmark characteristics of the key diseases. Given the increasingly clinical orientation of Step 1, it is no longer sufficient to know only the "trigger word" associations of certain diseases (e.g., café-au-lait macules and neurofibromatosis); you must also know the clinical descriptions of these findings.

Given the clinical slant of the USMLE Step 1, it is also important to review the classic presenting signs and symptoms of diseases as well as their associated laboratory findings. Delve into the signs, symptoms, and pathophysiology of major diseases that have a high prevalence in the United States (e.g., alcoholism, diabetes, hypertension, heart failure, ischemic heart disease, infectious disease). Be prepared to think one step beyond the simple diagnosis to treatment or complications.

The examination includes a number of color photomicrographs and photographs of gross specimens that are presented in the setting of a brief clinical history. However, read the question and the choices carefully before looking at the illustration, because the history will help you identify the pathologic process. Flip through an illustrated pathology textbook, color atlases, and appropriate Web sites in order to look at the pictures in the days before the exam. Pay attention to potential clues such as age, sex, ethnicity, occupation, recent activities and exposures, and specialized lab tests.

## Pharmacology

Preparation for questions on pharmacology is straightforward. Memorizing all the key drugs and their characteristics (e.g., mechanisms, clinical use, and important side effects) is high yield. Focus on understanding the prototype drugs in each class. Avoid memorizing obscure derivatives. Learn the "classic" and distinguishing toxicities of the major drugs. Do not bother with drug dosages or trade names. Reviewing associated biochemistry, physiology, and microbiology can be useful while studying pharmacology. There is a strong emphasis on ANS, CNS, antimicrobial, and cardiovascular agents as well as on NSAIDs. Much of the material is clinically relevant. Newer drugs on the market are also fair game.

# Cardiovascular

*"As for me, except for an occasional heart attack, I feel as young as I ever did."*
— Robert Benchley

*"Hearts will never be practical until they are made unbreakable."*
— The Wizard of Oz

*"As the arteries grow hard, the heart grows soft."*
— H. L. Mencken

*"Nobody has ever measured, not even poets, how much the heart can hold."*
— Zelda Fitzgerald

*"Only from the heart can you touch the sky."*
— Rumi

Starting in 2008, the USMLE Step 1 began to include audio questions, which include heart sounds.

**Carotid sheath**

3 structures inside:
1. Internal jugular **V**ein (lateral)
2. Common carotid **A**rtery (medial)
3. Vagus **N**erve (posterior)

VAN.

**Coronary artery anatomy**

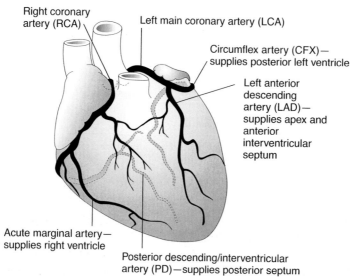

Right coronary artery (RCA)

Left main coronary artery (LCA)

Circumflex artery (CFX)— supplies posterior left ventricle

Left anterior descending artery (LAD)— supplies apex and anterior interventricular septum

Acute marginal artery— supplies right ventricle

Posterior descending/interventricular artery (PD)—supplies posterior septum

(Adapted, with permission, from Ganong WF. *Review of Medical Physiology,* 19th ed. Stamford, CT: Appleton & Lange, 1999: 592.)

In the majority of cases, the SA and AV nodes are supplied by the RCA. 80% of the time, the RCA supplies the inferior portion of the left ventricle via the PD artery (= right dominant). 20% of the time, the PD arises from the CFX.

Coronary artery occlusion most commonly occurs in the LAD, which supplies the anterior interventricular septum.

Coronary arteries fill during diastole.

The most posterior part of the heart is the left atrium; enlargement can cause dysphagia (due to compression of the esophageal nerve) or hoarseness (due to compression of the recurrent laryngeal nerve, a branch of the vagus).

**Cardiac output (CO)**

Cardiac output (CO) = (stroke volume) × (heart rate).
Fick principle:

$$CO = \frac{\text{rate of } O_2 \text{ consumption}}{\text{arterial } O_2 \text{ content} - \text{venous } O_2 \text{ content}}$$

$$\begin{pmatrix}\text{Mean arterial} \\ \text{pressure}\end{pmatrix} = \begin{pmatrix}\text{cardiac} \\ \text{output}\end{pmatrix} \times \begin{pmatrix}\text{total peripheral} \\ \text{resistance}\end{pmatrix}$$

MAP = ⅔ diastolic pressure + ⅓ systolic pressure.
Pulse pressure = systolic pressure – diastolic pressure.
Pulse pressure is proportional to stroke volume.

$$SV = \frac{CO}{HR} = EDV - ESV$$

During exercise, CO ↑ initially as a result of an ↑ in SV. After prolonged exercise, CO ↑ as a result of an ↑ in HR.

If HR is too high, diastolic filling is incomplete and CO ↓ (e.g., ventricular tachycardia).

HIGH-YIELD SYSTEMS

CARDIOVASCULAR

| | | |
|---|---|---|
| **Cardiac output variables** | Stroke Volume affected by Contractility, Afterload, and Preload. ↑ SV when ↑ preload, ↓ afterload, or ↑ contractility.<br><br>Contractility (and SV) ↑ with:<br>1. Catecholamines (↑ activity of $Ca^{2+}$ pump in sarcoplasmic reticulum)<br>2. ↑ intracellular calcium<br>3. ↓ extracellular sodium (↓ activity of $Na^+/Ca^{2+}$ exchanger)<br>4. Digitalis (↑ intracellular $Na^+$, resulting in ↑ $Ca^{2+}$)<br><br>Contractility (and SV) ↓ with:<br>1. $\beta_1$ blockade<br>2. Heart failure<br>3. Acidosis<br>4. Hypoxia/hypercapnea<br>5. Non-dihydropyridine $Ca^{2+}$ channel blockers | **SV CAP.**<br><br>SV ↑ in anxiety, exercise, and pregnancy.<br>A failing heart has ↓ SV.<br>Myocardial $O_2$ demand is ↑ by:<br>1. ↑ afterload ($\propto$ arterial pressure)<br>2. ↑ contractility<br>3. ↑ heart rate<br>4. ↑ heart size (↑ wall tension) |
| **Preload and afterload** | Preload = ventricular EDV.<br>Afterload = mean arterial pressure (proportional to peripheral resistance).<br>Venodilators (e.g., nitroglycerin) ↓ preload.<br>Vasodilators (e.g., hydrAlAzine) ↓ Afterload (Arterial). | Preload ↑ with exercise (slightly), ↑ blood volume (overtransfusion), and excitement (sympathetics).<br>Preload pumps up the heart. |
| **Starling curve** | Force of contraction is proportional to initial length of cardiac muscle fiber (preload).<br><br>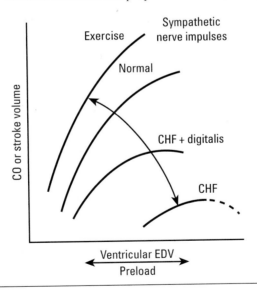 | **CONTRACTILE STATE OF MYOCARDIUM**<br>⊕  ⊖<br><br>Circulating catecholamines   Pharmacologic depressants<br>Digitalis   Loss of myocardium (MI)<br>Sympathetic stimulation |
| **Ejection fraction (EF)** | $$EF = \frac{SV}{EDV} = \frac{EDV - ESV}{EDV}$$<br>EF is an index of ventricular contractility.<br>EF is normally $\geq 55\%$. | |

| | | |
|---|---|---|
| **Resistance, pressure, flow** | $\Delta P = Q \times R$<br>Similar to Ohm's law: $\Delta V = IR$.<br><br>$\text{Resistance} = \dfrac{\text{driving pressure } (\Delta P)}{\text{flow } (Q)} = \dfrac{8\eta \text{ (viscosity)} \times \text{length}}{\pi r^4}$<br><br>Total resistance of vessels in series $= R_1 + R_2 + R_3 \ldots$<br>1/Total resistance of vessels in parallel $= 1/R_1 + 1/R_2$<br>$\qquad + 1/R_3 \ldots$<br>Viscosity depends mostly on hematocrit.<br>Viscosity $\uparrow$ in:<br>1. Polycythemia<br>2. Hyperproteinemic states (e.g., multiple myeloma)<br>3. Hereditary spherocytosis | Pressure gradient drives flow from high pressure to low.<br>Resistance is directly proportional to viscosity and inversely proportional to the radius to the 4th power.<br>Arterioles account for most of total peripheral resistance $\rightarrow$ regulate capillary flow. |

## Cardiac and vascular function curves

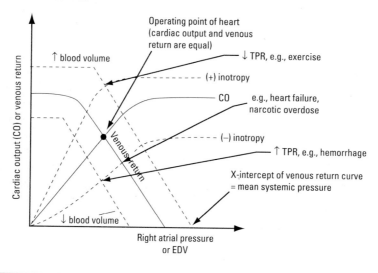

## Cardiac cycle

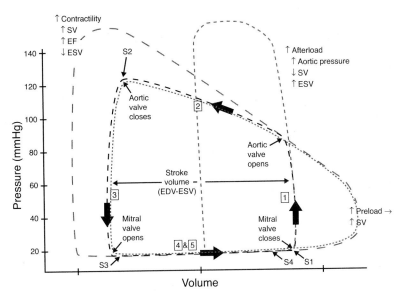

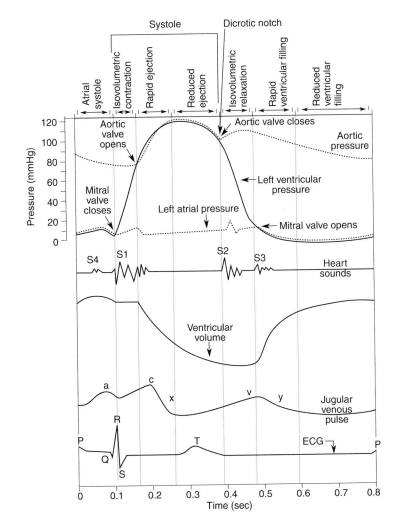

Phases—left ventricle:
1. Isovolumetric contraction—period between mitral valve closure and aortic valve opening; period of highest $O_2$ consumption
2. Systolic ejection—period between aortic valve opening and closing
3. Isovolumetric relaxation—period between aortic valve closing and mitral valve opening
4. Rapid filling—period just after mitral valve opening
5. Reduced filling—period just before mitral valve closure

Sounds:
S1—mitral and tricuspid valve closure. Loudest at mitral area.
S2—aortic and pulmonary valve closure. Loudest at left sternal border.
S3—in early diastole during rapid ventricular filling phase. Associated with ↑ filling pressures and more common in dilated ventricles (but normal in children and pregnant women).
S4 ("atrial kick")—in late diastole. High atrial pressure. Associated with ventricular hypertrophy. Left atrium must push against stiff LV wall.

Jugular venous pulse (JVP):
a wave—atrial contraction.
c wave—RV contraction (tricuspid valve bulging into atrium).
v wave—↑ atrial pressure due to filling against closed tricuspid valve.

S2 splitting: aortic valve closes before pulmonic; inspiration ↑ this difference.

Normal:
| Expiration | | |
| --- | --- | --- |
| | | | | |
| | $S_1$ | $A_2$ $P_2$ |
| Inspiration | | |
| | | | | |

Wide splitting (associated with pulmonic stenosis or right bundle branch block):
| Expiration | | |
| --- | --- | --- |
| | | | | | |
| | $S_1$ | $A_2$ $P_2$ |
| Inspiration | | |
| | | | | | |

Fixed splitting (associated with ASD):
| Expiration | | |
| --- | --- | --- |
| | | | | | |
| | $S_1$ | $A_2$ $P_2$ |
| Inspiration | | |
| | | | | | |

Paradoxical splitting (associated with aortic stenosis or left bundle branch block):
| Expiration | | |
| --- | --- | --- |
| | | | | |
| | $S_1$ | $P_2$ $A_2$ |
| Inspiration | | |
| | | | | | |

**Splitting**

**Normal splitting**—inspiration leads to drop in intrathoracic pressure, which ↑ capacity of pulmonary circulation. Pulmonic valve closes later to accommodate more blood entering lungs; aortic valve closes earlier because of ↓ return to left heart.

**Wide splitting**—seen in conditions that delay RV emptying (pulmonic stenosis, right bundle branch block). Delay in RV emptying causes delayed pulmonic sound (regardless of breath). An exaggeration of normal splitting.

**Fixed splitting**—seen in ASD. ASD leads to left-to-right shunt and therefore ↑ flow through pulmonic valve such that regardless of breath, pulmonic closure is greatly delayed.

**Paradoxical splitting**—seen in conditions that delay LV emptying (aortic stenosis, left bundle branch block). Normal order of valve closure is reversed so that P2 sound occurs before delayed A2 sound. Therefore on inspiration, the later P2 and earlier A2 sounds move closer to one another, "paradoxically" eliminating the split.

## Auscultation of the heart

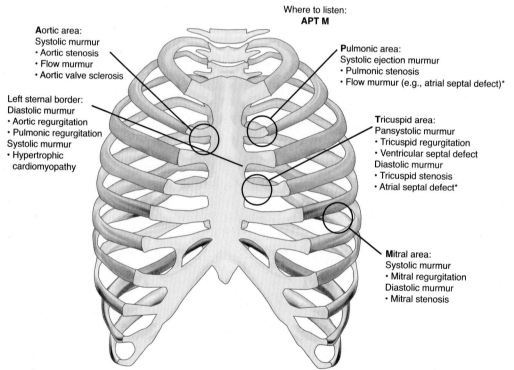

Where to listen:
**APT M**

**A**ortic area:
Systolic murmur
• Aortic stenosis
• Flow murmur
• Aortic valve sclerosis

Left sternal border:
Diastolic murmur
• Aortic regurgitation
• Pulmonic regurgitation
Systolic murmur
• Hypertrophic cardiomyopathy

**P**ulmonic area:
Systolic ejection murmur
• Pulmonic stenosis
• Flow murmur (e.g., atrial septal defect)*

**T**ricuspid area:
Pansystolic murmur
• Tricuspid regurgitation
• Ventricular septal defect
Diastolic murmur
• Tricuspid stenosis
• Atrial septal defect*

**M**itral area:
Systolic murmur
• Mitral regurgitation
Diastolic murmur
• Mitral stenosis

\* ASD commonly presents with a pulmonary flow murmur (↑ flow through pulmonary valve) and a diastolic rumble (↑ flow across tricuspid); blood flow across the actual ASD does not cause a murmur because there is no pressure gradient. The murmur later progresses to a louder diastolic murmur of pulmonic regurgitation from dilatation of the pulmonary artery.

## Heart murmurs

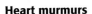

S1           S2

Mitral/tricuspid regurgitation (MR/TR)

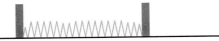

Holosystolic, high-pitched "blowing murmur."

Mitral—loudest at apex and radiates toward axilla. Enhanced by maneuvers that ↑ TPR (e.g., squatting, hand grip) or LA return (e.g., expiration). MR is often due to ischemic heart disease, mitral valve prolapse, or LV dilation.

Tricuspid—loudest at tricuspid area and radiates to right sternal border. Enhanced by maneuvers that ↑ RA return (e.g., inspiration). TR is due to RV dilation or endocarditis. Rheumatic fever can cause both.

Aortic stenosis

EC

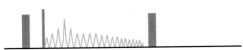

Crescendo-decrescendo systolic ejection murmur following ejection click (EC; due to abrupt halting of valve leaflets). LV >> aortic pressure during systole. Radiates to carotids/apex. "Pulsus parvus et tardus"—pulses weak compared to heart sounds. Can lead to syncope. Often due to age-related calcific aortic stenosis or bicuspid aortic valve (see Image 77).

VSD

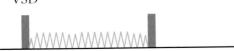

Holosystolic, harsh-sounding murmur. Loudest at tricuspid area.

Mitral prolapse

MC

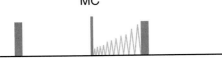

Late systolic crescendo murmur with midsystolic click (MC; due to sudden tensing of chordae tendineae). Most frequent valvular lesion. Loudest at S2. Usually benign. Can predispose to infective endocarditis. Can be caused by myxomatous degeneration, rheumatic fever, or chordae rupture. Enhanced by maneuvers that ↑ TPR (e.g., squatting, hand grip).

Aortic regurgitation

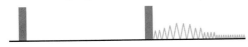

Immediate high-pitched "blowing" diastolic murmur. Wide pulse pressure when chronic; can present with bounding pulses and head bobbing. Often due to aortic root dilation, bicuspid aortic valve, or rheumatic fever.

Mitral stenosis

OS

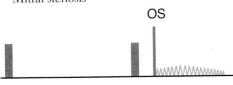

Follows opening snap (OS; due to tensing of chordae tendineae). Delayed rumbling late diastolic murmur. LA >> LV pressure during diastole. Often occurs 2° to rheumatic fever. Chronic MS can result in LA dilation. Enhanced by maneuvers that ↑ LA return (e.g., expiration).

PDA

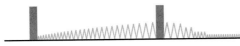

Continuous machine-like murmur. Loudest at S2.

**Cardiac myocyte physiology**

Cardiac muscle contraction is dependent on extracellular calcium, which enters the cells during plateau of action potential and stimulates calcium release from the cardiac muscle sarcoplasmic reticulum (calcium-induced calcium release).

In contrast to skeletal muscle:

1. Cardiac muscle action potential has a plateau, which is due to $Ca^{2+}$ influx
2. Cardiac nodal cells spontaneously depolarize, resulting in automaticity due to $I_f$ channels
3. Cardiac myocytes are electrically coupled to each other by gap junctions

**Ventricular action potential**

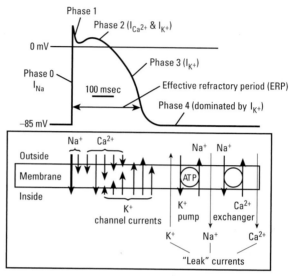

Also occurs in bundle of His and Purkinje fibers.

**Phase 0** = rapid upstroke—voltage-gated $Na^+$ channels open.

**Phase 1** = initial repolarization—inactivation of voltage-gated $Na^+$ channels. Voltage-gated $K^+$ channels begin to open.

**Phase 2** = plateau—$Ca^{2+}$ influx through voltage-gated $Ca^{2+}$ channels balances $K^+$ efflux. $Ca^{2+}$ influx triggers $Ca^{2+}$ release from sarcoplasmic reticulum and myocyte contraction.

**Phase 3** = rapid repolarization—massive $K^+$ efflux due to opening of voltage-gated slow $K^+$ channels and closure of voltage-gated $Ca^{2+}$ channels.

**Phase 4** = resting potential—high $K^+$ permeability through $K^+$ channels.

**Pacemaker action potential**

Occurs in the SA and AV nodes. Key differences from the ventricular action potential include:

**Phase 0** = upstroke—opening of voltage-gated $Ca^{2+}$ channels. These cells lack fast voltage-gated $Na^+$ channels. Results in a slow conduction velocity that is used by the AV node to prolong transmission from the atria to ventricles.

**Phase 2** = plateau is absent.

**Phase 3** = inactivation of the $Ca^{2+}$ channels and ↑ activation of $K^+$ channels → ↑ $K^+$ efflux.

**Phase 4** = slow diastolic depolarization—membrane potential spontaneously depolarizes as $Na^+$ conductance ↑ ($I_f$ different from $I_{Na}$ above). Accounts for automaticity of SA and AV nodes. The slope of phase 4 in the SA node determines heart rate. ACh ↓ the rate of diastolic depolarization and ↓ heart rate, while catecholamines ↑ depolarization and ↑ heart rate. Sympathetic stimulation ↑ the chance that $I_f$ channels are open.

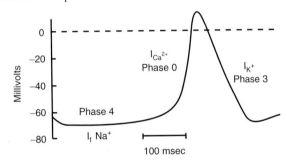

**Electrocardiogram**

P wave—atrial depolarization.

PR interval—conduction delay through AV node (normally < 200 msec).

QRS complex—ventricular depolarization (normally < 120 msec).

QT interval—mechanical contraction of the ventricles.

T wave—ventricular repolarization. T-wave inversion indicates recent MI.

Atrial repolarization is masked by QRS complex.

ST segment—isoelectric, ventricles depolarized.

U wave—caused by hypokalemia, bradycardia.

Speed of conduction— Purkinje > atria > ventricles > AV node.
Pacemakers—SA > AV > bundle of His/Purkinje/ ventricles.

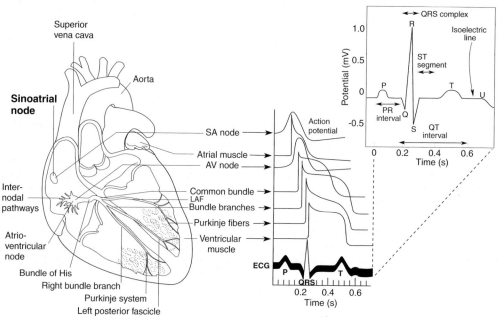

SA node "pacemaker" inherent dominance with slow phase of upstroke
AV node—100-msec delay—atrioventricular delay; allows time for ventricular filling

(Adapted, with permission, from Ganong WF. *Review of Medical Physiology,* 22nd ed. New York: McGraw-Hill, 2005: 548, 550.)

**Torsades de pointes**

Ventricular tachycardia is characterized by shifting sinusoidal waveforms on ECG. Can progress to V-fib. Anything that prolongs the QT interval can predispose to torsades de pointes.

Congenital long QT syndromes are most often due to defects in cardiac sodium or potassium channels. Can present with severe congenital sensorineural deafness (Jervell and Lange-Nielsen syndrome).

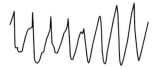

## Wolff-Parkinson-White syndrome

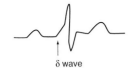

δ wave

Also known as ventricular preexcitation syndrome. Accessory conduction pathway from atria to ventricle (bundle of Kent), bypassing AV node. As a result, ventricles begin to partially depolarize earlier, giving rise to characteristic delta wave on ECG. May result in reentry current leading to supraventricular tachycardia.

## ECG tracings

### Atrial fibrillation

Chaotic and erratic baseline (**irregularly irregular**) with **no discrete P waves** in between irregularly spaced QRS complexes. Can result in atrial stasis and lead to stroke. Treat with β-blocker or calcium channel blocker; prophylaxis against thromboembolism with warfarin (Coumadin).

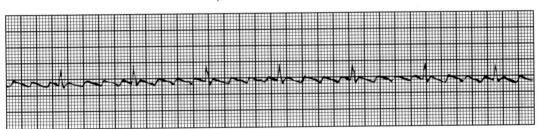

### Atrial flutter

A rapid succession of identical, back-to-back atrial depolarization waves. The identical appearance accounts for the "**sawtooth**" appearance of the flutter waves. Attempt to convert to sinus rhythm. Use class IA, IC, or III antiarrhythmics.

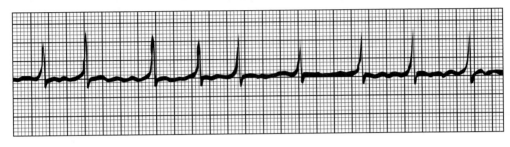

### AV block

#### 1st degree

The PR interval is prolonged (> 200 msec). Asymptomatic.

Prolonged PR interval

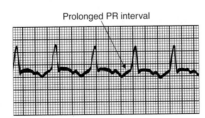

**ECG tracings** *(continued)*

2nd degree

Mobitz type I (Wenckebach)

Progressive lengthening of the PR interval until a beat is "dropped" (a P wave not followed by a QRS complex). Usually asymptomatic.

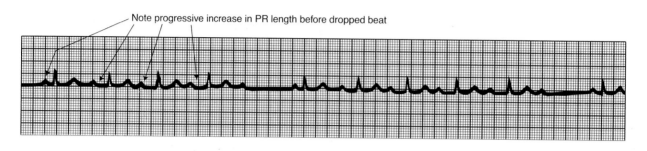

Note progressive increase in PR length before dropped beat

Mobitz type II

Dropped beats that are not preceded by a change in the length of the PR interval (as in type I). These abrupt, nonconducted P waves result in a pathologic condition. It is often found as 2:1 block, where there are 2 P waves to 1 QRS response. May progress to 3rd-degree block.

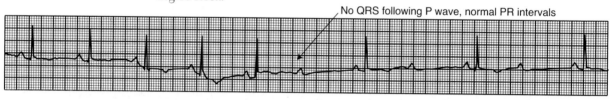

No QRS following P wave, normal PR intervals

3rd degree (complete)

The atria and ventricles beat independently of each other. Both P waves and QRS complexes are present, although the **P waves bear no relation to the QRS complexes.** The atrial rate is faster than the ventricular rate. Usually treated with pacemaker. Lyme disease can result in 3rd-degree heart block.

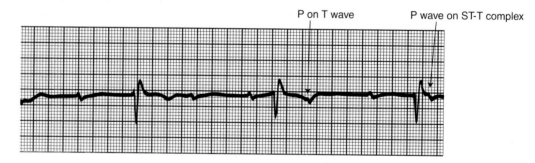

P on T wave          P wave on ST-T complex

Ventricular fibrillation

A completely erratic rhythm with no identifiable waves. Fatal arrhythmia without immediate CPR and defibrillation.

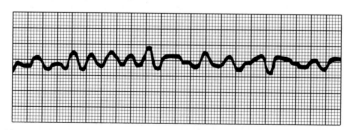

(Adapted, with permission, from Hurst JW. *Introduction to Electrocardiography.* New York: McGraw-Hill, 2001.)

HIGH-YIELD SYSTEMS

CARDIOVASCULAR

## Maintenance of mean arterial pressure

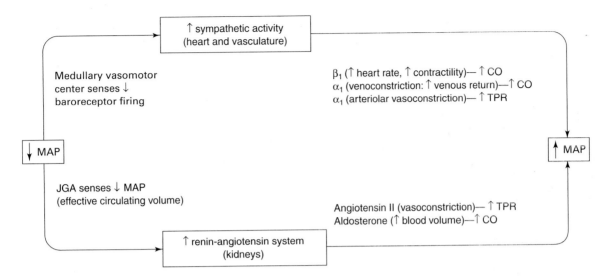

ANP, a diuretic, is released from atria in response to ↑ blood volume and atrial pressure. Causes generalized vascular relaxation. Constricts efferent renal arterioles, dilates afferent arterioles. Involved in "escape from aldosterone" mechanism.

## Baroreceptors and chemoreceptors

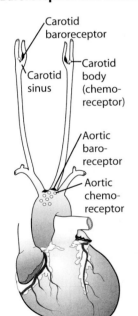

Carotid baroreceptor
Carotid sinus
Carotid body (chemoreceptor)
Aortic baroreceptor
Aortic chemoreceptor

**Receptors:**
1. Aortic arch transmits via vagus nerve to medulla (responds **only** to ↑ BP)
2. Carotid sinus transmits via glossopharyngeal nerve to solitary nucleus of medulla (responds to ↓ and ↑ in BP).

**Baroreceptors:**
1. Hypotension—↓ arterial pressure → ↓ stretch → ↓ afferent baroreceptor firing → ↑ efferent sympathetic firing and ↓ efferent parasympathetic stimulation → vasoconstriction, ↑ HR, ↑ contractility, ↑ BP. Important in the response to severe hemorrhage.
2. Carotid massage—↑ pressure on carotid artery → ↑ stretch → ↑ afferent baroreceptor firing → ↓ HR.

**Chemoreceptors:**
1. Peripheral—carotid and aortic bodies respond to ↓ $P_{O_2}$ (< 60 mmHg), ↑ $P_{CO_2}$, and ↓ pH of blood.
2. Central—respond to changes in pH and $P_{CO_2}$ of brain interstitial fluid, which in turn are influenced by arterial $CO_2$. Do not directly respond to $P_{O_2}$. Responsible for Cushing reaction— ↑ intracranial pressure constricts arterioles → cerebral ischemia → hypertension (sympathetic response) → reflex bradycardia. Note: Cushing triad = hypertension, bradycardia, respiratory depression.

## Circulation through organs

| | |
|---|---|
| Liver | Largest share of systemic cardiac output. |
| Kidney | Highest blood flow per gram of tissue. |
| Heart | Large arteriovenous $O_2$ difference because $O_2$ extraction is always ~ 100%. ↑ $O_2$ demand is met by ↑ coronary blood flow, not by ↑ extraction of $O_2$. |

### Normal pressures

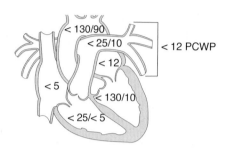

< 130/90
< 25/10
< 12 PCWP
< 12
< 5
< 130/10
< 25/< 5

PCWP—pulmonary capillary wedge pressure (in mmHg) is a good approximation of left atrial pressure. In mitral stenosis, PCWP > LV diastolic pressure.
Measured with Swan-Ganz catheter.

### Autoregulation

How blood flow to an organ remains constant over a wide range of perfusion pressures.

| Organ | Factors determining autoregulation |
|---|---|
| Heart | Local metabolites—$O_2$, adenosine, NO |
| Brain | Local metabolites—$CO_2$ (pH) |
| Kidneys | Myogenic and tubuloglomerular feedback |
| Lungs | Hypoxia causes vasoconstriction |
| Skeletal muscle | Local metabolites—lactate, adenosine, $K^+$ |
| Skin | Sympathetic stimulation most important mechanism—temperature control |

Note: the pulmonary vasculature is unique in that hypoxia causes vasoconstriction so that only well-ventilated areas are perfused. In other organs, hypoxia causes vasodilation.

### Capillary fluid exchange

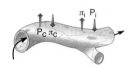

Starling forces determine fluid movement through capillary membranes:
1. $P_c$ = capillary pressure—pushes fluid out of capillary
2. $P_i$ = interstitial fluid pressure—pushes fluid into capillary
3. $\pi_c$ = plasma colloid osmotic pressure—pulls fluid into capillary
4. $\pi_i$ = interstitial fluid colloid osmotic pressure—pulls fluid out of capillary

Thus, net filtration pressure = $P_{net} = [(P_c - P_i) - (\pi_c - \pi_i)]$.
$K_f$ = filtration constant (capillary permeability).
Net fluid flow = $(P_{net}) (K_f)$.
Edema—excess fluid outflow into interstitium commonly caused by:
1. ↑ capillary pressure (↑ $P_c$; heart failure)
2. ↓ plasma proteins (↓ $\pi_c$; nephrotic syndrome, liver failure)
3. ↑ capillary permeability (↑ $K_f$; toxins, infections, burns)
4. ↑ interstitial fluid colloid osmotic pressure (↑ $\pi_i$; lymphatic blockage)

HIGH-YIELD SYSTEMS

CARDIOVASCULAR

**Congenital heart disease**

| Right-to-left shunts (early cyanosis)— "blue babies" | 1. Tetralogy of Fallot (most common cause of early cyanosis)<br>2. Transposition of great vessels<br>3. Truncus arteriosus<br>4. Tricuspid atresia<br>5. Total anomalous pulmonary venous return (TAPVR) | The **5 T**'s:<br>**T**etralogy<br>**T**ransposition<br>**T**runcus<br>**T**ricuspid<br>**TAPVR** |
|---|---|---|
| | Persistent truncus arteriosus—failure of truncus arteriosus to divide into pulmonary trunk and aorta.<br>Tricuspid atresia—characterized by absence of tricuspid valve and hypoplastic right ventricle. Requires both ASD and VSD for viability.<br>TAPVR—pulmonary veins drain into right heart circulation (SVC, coronary sinus, etc.) | |
| Left-to-right shunts (late cyanosis)— "blue kids" | 1. VSD (most common congenital cardiac anomaly)<br>2. ASD (loud S1; wide, fixed split S2)<br>3. PDA (close with indomethacin) | Frequency—VSD > ASD > PDA.<br>↑ pulmonary resistance due to arteriolar thickening.<br>→ progressive pulmonary hypertension; right-to-left shunt (Eisenmenger's). |

| **Eisenmenger's syndrome** | Uncorrected VSD, ASD, or PDA causes compensatory vascular hypertrophy, which results in progressive pulmonary hypertension. As pulmonary resistance ↑, the shunt reverses from L → R to R → L, which causes late cyanosis (clubbing and polycythemia). | 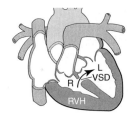 |
|---|---|---|

| **Tetralogy of Fallot** | 1. **P**ulmonary stenosis (most important determinant for prognosis)<br>2. **R**VH<br>3. **O**verriding aorta (overrides the VSD)<br>4. **V**SD<br>Early cyanosis is caused by a right-to-left shunt across the VSD. Right-to-left shunt exists because of the ↑ pressure caused by stenotic pulmonic valve. On x-ray, boot-shaped heart due to RVH. Patients suffer "cyanotic spells."<br>Tetralogy of Fallot is caused by anterosuperior displacement of the infundibular septum. | **PROV**e.<br>Patient learns to squat to improve symptoms: compression of femoral arteries ↑ pressure, thereby ↓ the right-to-left shunt and directing more blood from the RV to the lungs. Compression → resistance → pressure. |
|---|---|---|

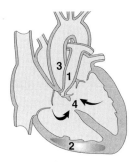

HIGH-YIELD SYSTEMS

CARDIOVASCULAR

**D-transposition of great vessels**

Aorta leaves RV (anterior) and pulmonary trunk leaves LV (posterior) → separation of systemic and pulmonary circulations. Not compatible with life unless a shunt is present to allow adequate mixing of blood (e.g., VSD, PDA, or patent foramen ovale).

Due to failure of the aorticopulmonary septum to spiral.
Without surgical correction, most infants die within the first few months of life.

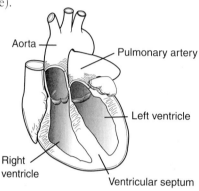

Aorta
Pulmonary artery
Left ventricle
Right ventricle
Ventricular septum

**Coarctation of the aorta**

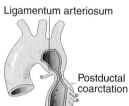

Ligamentum arteriosum
Postductal coarctation
Descending aorta

**Infantile type**—aortic stenosis proximal to insertion of ductus arteriosus (preductal).
**Adult type**—stenosis is distal to ductus arteriosus (postductal). Associated with notching of the ribs (due to collateral circulation), hypertension in upper extremities, weak pulses in lower extremities. Associated with Turner's syndrome.
Can result in aortic regurgitation.

Check femoral pulses on physical exam.
**IN**fantile: **IN** close to the heart.
**AD**ult: Distal to **D**uctus.
Most commonly associated with bicuspid aortic valve.

**Patent ductus arteriosus**

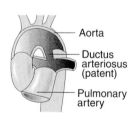

Aorta
Ductus arteriosus (patent)
Pulmonary artery

In fetal period, shunt is right to left (normal). In neonatal period, lung resistance ↓ and shunt becomes left to right with subsequent RVH and failure (abnormal). Associated with a continuous, "machine-like" murmur. Patency is maintained by PGE synthesis and low $O_2$ tension. Uncorrected PDA can eventually result in late cyanosis in the lower extremities.

**END**omethacin (indomethacin) **END**s patency of PDA; **PGEE kEE**ps it open (may be necessary to sustain life in conditions such as transposition of the great vessels).
PDA is normal in utero and normally closes only after birth.

**Congenital cardiac defect associations**

| Disorder | Defect |
| --- | --- |
| 22q11 syndromes | Truncus arteriosus, tetralogy of Fallot |
| Down syndrome | ASD, VSD, AV septal defect (endocardial cushion defect) |
| Congenital rubella | Septal defects, PDA, pulmonary artery stenosis |
| Turner's syndrome | Coarctation of aorta |
| Marfan's syndrome | Aortic insufficiency (late complication) |
| Infant of diabetic mother | Transposition of great vessels |

| | |
|---|---|
| **Hypertension** | Defined as BP ≥ 140/90. |
| Risk factors | ↑ age, obesity, diabetes, smoking, genetics, black > white > Asian. |
| Features | 90% of hypertension is 1° (essential) and related to ↑ CO or ↑ TPR; remaining 10% mostly 2° to renal disease. Malignant hypertension is severe and rapidly progressing. |
| Predisposes to | Atherosclerosis, left ventricular hypertrophy, stroke, CHF, renal failure, retinopathy, and aortic dissection. |

| | |
|---|---|
| **Hyperlipidemia signs** | |
| Atheromas | Plaques in blood vessel walls. |
| Xanthomas | Plaques or nodules composed of lipid-laden histiocytes in the skin, especially the eyelids (xanthelasma). |
| Tendinous xanthoma | Lipid deposit in tendon, especially Achilles. |
| Corneal arcus | Lipid deposit in cornea, nonspecific (arcus senilis). |

| | |
|---|---|
| **Arteriosclerosis** | |
| Mönckeberg | Calcification in the media of the arteries, especially radial or ulnar. Usually benign; "pipestem" arteries. Does not obstruct blood flow; intima not involved. |
| Arteriolosclerosis | Hyaline thickening of small arteries in essential hypertension or diabetes mellitus. Hyperplastic "onion skinning" in malignant hypertension. |
| Atherosclerosis | Fibrous plaques and atheromas form in intima of arteries. |

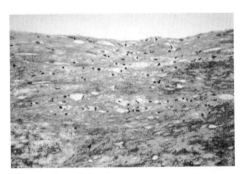

Atherosclerosis

(Reproduced, with permission, from the PEIR Digital Library.)

| | |
|---|---|
| **Aortic dissection** | Longitudinal intraluminal tear forming a false lumen. Associated with hypertension or cystic medial necrosis (component of Marfan's syndrome). Presents with tearing chest pain radiating to the back. CXR shows mediastinal widening. The false lumen occupies most of the descending aorta. Can result in aortic rupture and death. |

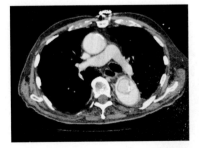

(Reproduced, with permission, from USMLERx.com.)

**Atherosclerosis**  Disease of elastic arteries and large and medium-sized muscular arteries.

Risk factors  Smoking, hypertension, diabetes mellitus, hyperlipidemia, family history.

Progression  Endothelial cell dysfunction → macrophage and LDL accumulation → foam cell formation → fatty streaks → smooth muscle cell migration (involves PDGF and FGF-β) → fibrous plaque → complex atheromas.

Complications  Aneurysms, ischemia, infarcts, peripheral vascular disease, thrombus, emboli.

Location  Abdominal aorta > coronary artery > popliteal artery > carotid artery.

Symptoms  Angina, claudication, but can be asymptomatic.

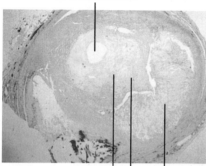

Lumen of vessel
(narrowed to about
5% of original lumen)

Calcification

Fibrous cap

Fatty atherosclerotic
plaque (lipid zone)

**Ischemic heart disease**  Possible manifestations:

1. **Angina** (CAD narrowing > 75%):
   a. Stable—mostly 2° to atherosclerosis; ST depression on ECG (retrosternal chest pain with exertion)
   b. Prinzmetal's variant—occurs at rest 2° to coronary artery spasm; ST elevation on ECG
   c. Unstable/crescendo—thrombosis but no necrosis; ST depression on ECG (worsening chest pain at rest or with minimal exertion)
2. **Myocardial infarction**—most often acute thrombosis due to coronary artery atherosclerosis; results in myocyte necrosis
3. **Sudden cardiac death**—death from cardiac causes within 1 hour of onset of symptoms, most commonly due to a lethal arrhythmia (e.g., V-fib)
4. **Chronic ischemic heart disease**—progressive onset of CHF over many years due to chronic ischemic myocardial damage

HIGH-YIELD SYSTEMS

CARDIOVASCULAR

**Evolution of MI**

Coronary artery occlusion: LAD > RCA > circumflex.

Symptoms: diaphoresis, nausea, vomiting, severe retrosternal pain, pain in left arm and/or jaw, shortness of breath, fatigue, adrenergic symptoms.

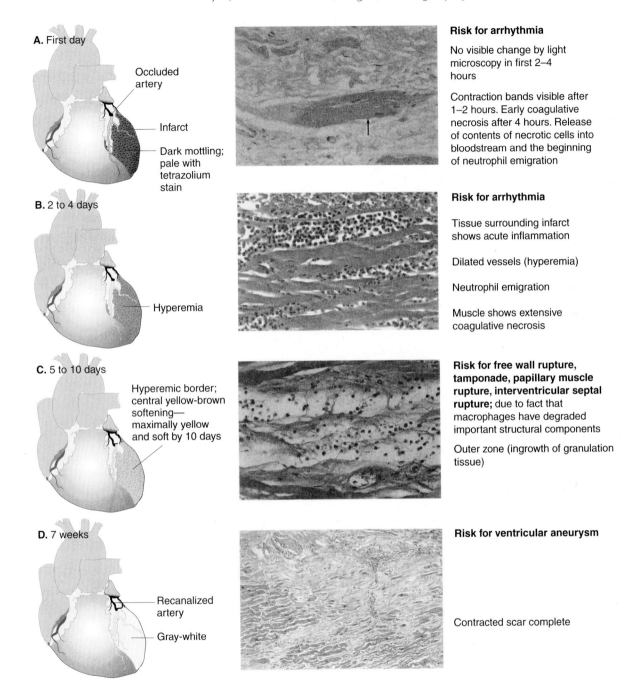

**A. First day**

Occluded artery

Infarct

Dark mottling; pale with tetrazolium stain

**Risk for arrhythmia**

No visible change by light microscopy in first 2–4 hours

Contraction bands visible after 1–2 hours. Early coagulative necrosis after 4 hours. Release of contents of necrotic cells into bloodstream and the beginning of neutrophil emigration

**B. 2 to 4 days**

Hyperemia

**Risk for arrhythmia**

Tissue surrounding infarct shows acute inflammation

Dilated vessels (hyperemia)

Neutrophil emigration

Muscle shows extensive coagulative necrosis

**C. 5 to 10 days**

Hyperemic border; central yellow-brown softening— maximally yellow and soft by 10 days

**Risk for free wall rupture, tamponade, papillary muscle rupture, interventricular septal rupture;** due to fact that macrophages have degraded important structural components

Outer zone (ingrowth of granulation tissue)

**D. 7 weeks**

Recanalized artery

Gray-white

**Risk for ventricular aneurysm**

Contracted scar complete

**Diagnosis of MI**　In the first 6 hours, ECG is the gold standard.

Cardiac troponin I rises after 4 hours and is elevated for 7–10 days; more specific than other protein markers.

CK-MB is predominantly found in myocardium but can also be released from skeletal muscle.

AST is nonspecific and can be found in cardiac, liver, and skeletal muscle cells.

ECG changes can include ST elevation (transmural infarct), ST depression (subendocardial infarct), and pathologic Q waves (transmural infarct).

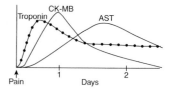

**Types of infarcts**

| Transmural infarcts | Subendocardial infarcts |
|---|---|
| ↑ necrosis | Due to ischemic necrosis of < 50% of ventricle wall |
| Affects entire wall | Subendocardium especially vulnerable to ischemia |
| ST elevation on ECG | Due to fewer collaterals, higher pressure |
| | ST depression on ECG |

**MI complications**
1. Cardiac arrhythmia—important cause of death before reaching hospital; common in first few days
2. LV failure and pulmonary edema
3. Cardiogenic shock (large infarct—high risk of mortality)
4. Ventricular free wall rupture → cardiac tamponade; papillary muscle → severe mitral regurgitation; and interventricular septal rupture → VSD
5. Aneurysm formation—↓ CO, risk of arrhythmia, embolus from mural thrombus
6. Postinfarction fibrinous pericarditis—friction rub (3–5 days post-MI)
7. Dressler's syndrome—autoimmune phenomenon resulting in fibrinous pericarditis (several weeks post-MI)

## Cardiomyopathies

| | | |
|---|---|---|
| Dilated (congestive) cardiomyopathy | Most common cardiomyopathy (90% of cases). Etiologies include chronic **A**lcohol abuse, wet **B**eriberi, **C**oxsackie B virus myocarditis, chronic **C**ocaine use, **C**hagas' disease, **D**oxorubicin toxicity, hemochromatosis, and peripartum cardiomyopathy.<br>Findings: S3, dilated heart on ultrasound, balloon appearance on chest x-ray. | Systolic dysfunction ensues.<br>Eccentric hypertrophy (sarcomeres added in series). |
| Hypertrophic cardiomyopathy | Hypertrophied IV septum is "too close" to mitral valve leaflet, leading to outflow tract obstruction. 50% of cases are familial, autosomal dominant. Associated with Friedreich's ataxia. Disoriented, tangled, hypertrophied myocardial fibers. Cause of sudden death in young athletes.<br>Findings: normal-sized heart, S4, apical impulses, systolic murmur. Treat with β-blocker or non-dihydropyridine calcium channel blocker (e.g., verapamil). | Diastolic dysfunction ensues.<br>Concentric hypertrophy (sarcomeres added in parallel).<br>Proximity of hypertrophied IV septum to mitral leaflet obstructs outflow tract, resulting in systolic murmur and syncopal episodes. |

(Reproduced, with permission, from Fuster V et al. *Hurst's the Heart,* 12th ed. New York: McGraw-Hill, 2008, Fig. 30-3.)

| | | |
|---|---|---|
| Restrictive/obliterative cardiomyopathy | Major causes include sarcoidosis, amyloidosis, postradiation fibrosis, endocardial fibroelastosis (thick fibroelastic tissue in endocardium of young children), Löffler's syndrome (endomyocardial fibrosis with a prominent eosinophilic infiltrate), and hemochromatosis (dilated cardiomyopathy can also occur). | Diastolic dysfunction ensues. |

**CHF**   A clinical syndrome that occurs in patients with an inherited or acquired abnormality of cardiac structure or function, who develop a constellation of clinical symptoms (dyspnea, fatigue) and signs (edema, rales).

| Abnormality | Cause |
|---|---|
| Dyspnea on exertion | Failure of LV output to ↑ during exercise. |
| Cardiac dilation | Greater ventricular end-diastolic volume. |
| Pulmonary edema, paroxysmal nocturnal dyspnea | LV failure → ↑ pulmonary venous pressure → pulmonary venous distention and transudation of fluid. Presence of hemosiderin-laden macrophages ("heart failure" cells) in the lungs due to microhemorrhages from ↑ pulmonary capillary pressure. |
| Orthopnea (shortness of breath when supine) | ↑ venous return in supine position exacerbates pulmonary vascular congestion. |
| Hepatomegaly (nutmeg liver) | ↑ central venous pressure → ↑ resistance to portal flow. Rarely, leads to "cardiac cirrhosis." |
| Ankle, sacral edema | RV failure → ↑ venous pressure → fluid transudation. |
| Jugular venous distention | Right heart failure → ↑ venous pressure. |

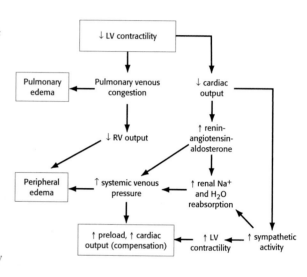

Right heart failure most often results from left heart failure. Isolated right heart failure is usually due to cor pulmonale.

| | | |
|---|---|---|
| **Bacterial endocarditis** | **Fever** (most common symptom), Roth's spots (round white spots on retina surrounded by hemorrhage), Osler's nodes (tender raised lesions on finger or toe pads), new **murmur, Janeway lesions** (small erythematous lesions on palm or sole), anemia, **splinter hemorrhages** on nail bed. Valvular damage may cause new murmur (see damaged aortic valve below). Multiple blood cultures necessary for diagnosis.<br>    1. Acute—*S. aureus* (high virulence). Large vegetations on previously normal valves. Rapid onset.<br>    2. Subacute—viridans streptococci (low virulence). Smaller vegetations on congenitally abnormal or diseased valves. Sequela of dental procedures. More insidious onset.<br>Endocarditis may also be nonbacterial 2° to malignancy or hypercoagulable state (marantic/thrombotic endocarditis). *S. bovis* is present in colon cancer, *S. epidermidis* on prosthetic valves; HACEK organisms cause culture-negative endocarditis. | Mitral valve is most frequently involved.<br>**Tri**cuspid valve endocarditis is associated with IV **drug** abuse (don't **tri drugs**). Associated with *S. aureus, Pseudomonas,* and *Candida.*<br>Complications: chordae rupture, glomerulonephritis, suppurative pericarditis, emboli.<br>Bacteria **FROM JANE:**<br>  **F**ever<br>  **R**oth's spots<br>  **O**sler's nodes<br>  **M**urmur<br>  **J**aneway lesions<br>  **A**nemia<br>  **N**ail-bed hemorrhage<br>  **E**mboli |

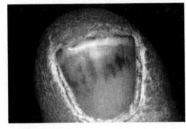

Splinter hemorrhage
(Reproduced, with permission, from USMLERx.)

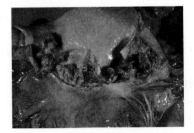

Acute bacterial endocarditis

| | | |
|---|---|---|
| **Libman-Sacks endocarditis** | Verrucous (wartlike), sterile vegetations occur on both sides of the valve. Most often benign; can be associated with mitral regurgitation and, less commonly, mitral stenosis. The most common heart manifestation of SLE. | **SLE** causes **LSE.** |

| | | |
|---|---|---|
| **Rheumatic heart disease** | A consequence of pharyngeal infection with group A β-hemolytic streptococci. Early deaths due to myocarditis. Late sequelae include rheumatic heart disease, which affects heart valves—mitral > aortic >> tricuspid (high-pressure valves affected most). Early lesion is mitral valve prolapse; late lesion is mitral stenosis. Associated with Aschoff bodies (granuloma with giant cells), Anitschkow's cells (activated histiocytes), elevated ASO titers. | **FEVERSS:** |
| | | **F**ever |
| | | **E**rythema marginatum |
| | | **V**alvular damage (vegetation and fibrosis) |
| | | **E**SR ↑ |
| | | **R**ed-hot joints (migratory polyarthritis) |
| | Immune mediated (type II hypersensitivity); not direct effect of bacteria. Antibodies to M protein. | **S**ubcutaneous nodules (Aschoff bodies) |
| | | **S**t. Vitus' dance (chorea) |

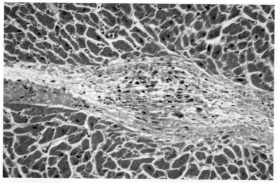

Aschoff body

(Reproduced, with permission, from the PEIR Digital Library.)

| | |
|---|---|
| **Cardiac tamponade** | Compression of heart by fluid (e.g., blood, effusions) in pericardium, leading to ↓ CO. Equilibration of diastolic pressures in all 4 chambers. |
| | Findings: hypotension, ↑ venous pressure (JVD), distant heart sounds, ↑ HR, pulsus paradoxus. |
| | **Pulsus paradoxus** (Kussmaul's pulse)—exaggerated ↓ in amplitude of pulse during inspiration. Seen in severe cardiac tamponade, asthma, obstructive sleep apnea, pericarditis, and croup. |

| | |
|---|---|
| **Pericarditis** | |
| Serous | Caused by SLE, rheumatoid arthritis, viral infection, uremia. |
| Fibrinous | Uremia, MI (Dressler's syndrome), rheumatic fever. |
| Hemorrhagic | TB, malignancy (e.g., melanoma). |
| | Findings: pericardial pain, friction rub, pulsus paradoxus, distant heart sounds. ECG changes with ST-segment elevation in multiple leads. |
| | Can resolve without scarring or lead to chronic adhesive or chronic constrictive pericarditis. |

| | | |
|---|---|---|
| **Syphilitic heart disease** | 3° syphilis disrupts the vasa vasorum of the aorta with consequent dilation of the aorta and valve ring. May see calcification of the aortic root and ascending aortic arch. Leads to "tree bark" appearance of the aorta. | Can result in aneurysm of the ascending aorta or aortic arch and aortic valve incompetence. |

| | | |
|---|---|---|
| **Cardiac tumors** | Myxomas are the most common 1° cardiac tumor in adults (see Image 80). 90% occur in the atria (mostly left atrium). Myxomas are usually described as a "ball-valve" obstruction in the left atrium (associated with multiple syncopal episodes). Rhabdomyomas are the most frequent 1° cardiac tumor in children (associated with tuberous sclerosis). Metastases most common heart tumor (melanoma, lymphoma). Kussmaul's sign: ↑ in jugular venous pressure on inspiration. | |
| **Telangiectasia** | Arteriovenous malformation in small vessels. Dilated vessels on skin and mucous membranes. Hereditary hemorrhagic telangiectasia (Osler-Weber-Rendu syndrome)—autosomal-dominant inheritance. Presents with recurrent epistaxis, skin discolorations, mucosal telangiectasias, and GI bleeds. | Affects small vessels. |

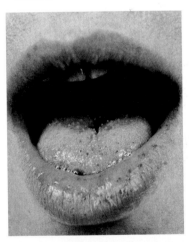

**Hereditary hemorrhagic telangiectasia**
(Reproduced, with permission, from Wolff K et al. *Fitzpatrick's Color Atlas & Synopsis of Clinical Dermatology*, 5th ed. New York: McGraw-Hill, 2005, Fig. 15-31.)

| | | |
|---|---|---|
| **Varicose veins** | Dilated, tortuous superficial veins due to chronically ↑ venous pressure. Predisposes to poor wound healing and varicose ulcers. | Thromboembolism is rare (compare with stasis of deep veins). |
| **Raynaud's disease** | ↓ blood flow to the skin due to arteriolar vasospasm in response to cold temperature or emotional stress. Most often in the fingers and toes (see Image 97). Called Raynaud's phenomenon when 2° to a mixed connective tissue disease, SLE, or CREST syndrome. | Affects small vessels. |

| **Wegener's granulomatosis** | Characterized by triad of focal necrotizing vasculitis, necrotizing granulomas in the **lung and upper airway,** and necrotizing glomerulonephritis. | Affects small vessels. |
|---|---|---|
| Symptoms | Hemoptysis, hematuria, perforation of nasal septum, chronic sinusitis, otitis media, mastoiditis, cough, dyspnea. | |
| Findings | **c-ANCA** is a strong marker of disease; chest x-ray may reveal large nodular densities; hematuria and red cell casts. | |
| Treatment | Cyclophosphamide and corticosteroids. | |

| **Other ANCA-positive vasculitides** | | |
|---|---|---|
| Microscopic polyangiitis | Like Wegener's but lacks granulomas. **p-ANCA.** | All affect small vessels. |
| 1° pauci-immune crescentic glomerulo-nephritis | Vasculitis limited to kidney. **Pauci-**immune = **pauci**ty of antibodies. | |
| Churg-Strauss syndrome | Granulomatous vasculitis with eosinophilia. Most often presents with asthma, sinusitis, skin lesions, and peripheral neuropathy (e.g., wrist/foot drop); can also involve heart, GI, and kidneys. **p-ANCA.** | |

| **Sturge-Weber disease** | Congenital vascular disorder that affects capillary-sized blood vessels. Manifests with port-wine stain (aka nevus flammeus) on face, ipsilateral leptomeningeal angiomatosis (intracerebral AVM), seizures, and early-onset glaucoma. | Affects small vessels. |
|---|---|---|

| **Henoch-Schönlein purpura** | Most common form of childhood systemic vasculitis. Skin rash on buttocks and legs (palpable purpura), arthralgia, intestinal hemorrhage, abdominal pain, and melena. Follows URIs. IgA immune complexes. Association with IgA nephropathy. | Affects small vessels. Common triad: 1. Skin 2. Joints 3. GI Multiple lesions of the same age. |
|---|---|---|

| | | |
|---|---|---|
| **Buerger's disease** | Also known as thromboangiitis obliterans; idiopathic, segmental, thrombosing vasculitis of small and medium peripheral arteries and veins. Seen in **heavy smokers.** | Affects small and medium vessels. Note: Medium-vessel diseases cause thrombosis/infarction of arteries. |
| Symptoms | Intermittent claudication, superficial nodular phlebitis, cold sensitivity (Raynaud's phenomenon), severe pain in affected part. May lead to gangrene and autoamputation of digits. | |
| Treatment | Smoking cessation. | |
| **Kawasaki disease** | Acute, self-limiting necrotizing vasculitis in infants/children. Association with Asian ethnicity. | Affects small and medium vessels. |
| Symptoms | Fever, conjunctivitis, changes in lips/oral mucosa ("strawberry tongue"), lymphadenitis, desquamative skin rash. May develop coronary aneurysms. | |
| Treatment | IV immunoglobulin, aspirin. | |
| **Polyarteritis nodosa** | Immune complex–mediated transmural vasculitis with fibrinoid necrosis. | Affects small and medium arteries. |
| Symptoms | Fever, weight loss, malaise, abdominal pain, melena, headache, myalgia, hypertension, neurologic dysfunction, cutaneous eruptions. | Typically involves renal and visceral vessels, **not** pulmonary arteries. |
| Findings | **Hepatitis B** seropositivity in 30% of patients. Multiple aneurysms and constrictions on arteriogram. | Lesions are of different ages. |
| Treatment | Corticosteroids, cyclophosphamide. | |
| **Takayasu's arteritis** | Known as **"pulseless disease"** — granulomatous thickening of aortic arch and/or proximal great vessels. Associated with an ↑ ESR. Primarily affects Asian females < 40 years of age. | Affects medium and large arteries. |
| Symptoms | Fever, Arthritis, Night sweats, MYalgia, SKIN nodules, Ocular disturbances, Weak pulses in upper extremities. | **FAN MY SKIN On** Wednesday. |
| **Temporal arteritis (giant cell arteritis)** | Most common vasculitis affecting medium and large arteries, usually branches of carotid artery. Focal, granulomatous inflammation. Affects elderly females. | Affects medium and large arteries. TEMporal arteritis has signs near TEMples. |
| Symptoms | Unilateral headache, jaw claudication, impaired vision (occlusion of ophthalmic artery that may lead to irreversible blindness). | |
| Findings | Associated with an ↑ ESR. Half of patients have systemic involvement and polymyalgia rheumatica. | |
| Treatment | High-dose steroids. | |

**Vascular tumors**

| | |
|---|---|
| Strawberry hemangioma | Benign capillary hemangioma of infancy. Initially grows with child; then spontaneously regresses. |
| Cherry hemangioma | Benign capillary hemangioma of the elderly. Does not regress. Frequency ↑ with age. |
| Pyogenic granuloma | Polypoid capillary hemangioma that can ulcerate and bleed. Associated with trauma and pregnancy. |
| Cystic hygroma | Cavernous lymphangioma of the neck. Associated with Turner's syndrome. |
| Glomus tumor | Benign, painful, red-blue tumor under fingernails. Arises from modified smooth muscle cells of glomus body. |
| Bacillary angiomatosis | Benign capillary skin papules found in AIDS patients. Caused by *Bartonella henselae* infections. Frequently mistaken for Kaposi's sarcoma. |
| Angiosarcoma | Highly lethal malignancy of the liver. Associated with vinyl chloride, arsenic, and $ThO_2$ (Thorotrast) exposure. |
| Lymphangiosarcoma | Lymphatic malignancy associated with persistent lymphedema (e.g., post–radical mastectomy). |
| Kaposi's sarcoma | Endothelial malignancy of the skin associated with HHV-8 and HIV. Frequently mistaken for bacillary angiomatosis. |

▶ CARDIOVASCULAR–PHARMACOLOGY

**Antihypertensive therapy**

| | | |
|---|---|---|
| Essential hypertension | Diuretics, ACE inhibitors, angiotensin II receptor blockers (ARBs), calcium channel blockers. | See the Renal chapter for more details about diuretics and ACE inhibitors/ARBs. |
| CHF | Diuretics, ACE inhibitors/ARBs, β-blockers (compensated CHF), $K^+$-sparing diuretics. | β-blockers are contraindicated in decompensated CHF. |
| Diabetes mellitus | ACE inhibitors/ARBs, calcium channel blockers, diuretics, β-blockers, α-blockers. | ACE inhibitors are protective against diabetic nephropathy. See the Pharmacology chapter for more details about α-blockers. |

**Hydralazine**

| | |
|---|---|
| Mechanism | ↑ cGMP → smooth muscle relaxation. Vasodilates arterioles > veins; afterload reduction. |
| Clinical use | Severe hypertension, CHF. First-line therapy for hypertension in pregnancy, with methyldopa. Frequently coadministered with a β-blocker to prevent reflex tachycardia. |
| Toxicity | Compensatory tachycardia (contraindicated in angina/CAD), fluid retention, nausea, headache, angina. Lupus-like syndrome. |

**Minoxidil**

| | |
|---|---|
| Mechanism | $K^+$ channel opener—hyperpolarizes and relaxes vascular smooth muscle. |
| Clinical use | Severe hypertension. |
| Toxicity | Hypertrichosis, pericardial effusion, reflex tachycardia, angina, salt retention. |

| Calcium channel blockers | Nifedipine, verapamil, diltiazem. |
|---|---|
| Mechanism | Block voltage-dependent L-type calcium channels of cardiac and smooth muscle and thereby reduce muscle contractility. Vascular smooth muscle—nifedipine > diltiazem > verapamil (**Verapamil = Ventricle**). Heart—verapamil > diltiazem > nifedipine. |
| Clinical use | Hypertension, angina, arrhythmias (not nifedipine), Prinzmetal's angina, Raynaud's. |
| Toxicity | Cardiac depression, AV block, peripheral edema, flushing, dizziness, and constipation. |

## Nitroglycerin, isosorbide dinitrate

| | |
|---|---|
| Mechanism | Vasodilate by releasing nitric oxide in smooth muscle, causing $\uparrow$ in cGMP and smooth muscle relaxation. Dilate veins >> arteries. $\downarrow$ preload. |
| Clinical use | Angina, pulmonary edema. Also used as an aphrodisiac and erection enhancer. |
| Toxicity | Reflex tachycardia, hypotension, flushing, headache, "Monday disease" in industrial exposure; development of tolerance for the vasodilating action during the work week and loss of tolerance over the weekend, resulting in tachycardia, dizziness, and headache on reexposure. |

## Malignant hypertension treatment

| | |
|---|---|
| Nitroprusside | Short acting; $\uparrow$ cGMP via direct release of NO. Can cause cyanide toxicity (releases CN). |
| Fenoldopam | Dopamine $D_1$ receptor agonist—relaxes renal vascular smooth muscle. |
| Diazoxide | $K^+$ channel opener—hyperpolarizes and relaxes vascular smooth muscle. Can cause hyperglycemia (reduces insulin release). |

## Antianginal therapy

Goal—reduction of myocardial $O_2$ consumption ($MVO_2$) by decreasing 1 or more of the determinants of $MVO_2$: end diastolic volume, blood pressure, heart rate, contractility, ejection time.

| Component | Nitrates (affect preload) | β-blockers (affect afterload) | Nitrates + β-blockers |
|---|---|---|---|
| End diastolic volume | $\downarrow$ | $\uparrow$ | No effect or $\downarrow$ |
| Blood pressure | $\downarrow$ | $\downarrow$ | $\downarrow$ |
| Contractility | $\uparrow$ (reflex response) | $\downarrow$ | Little/no effect |
| Heart rate | $\uparrow$ (reflex response) | $\downarrow$ | $\downarrow$ |
| Ejection time | $\downarrow$ | $\uparrow$ | Little/no effect |
| $MVO_2$ | $\downarrow$ | $\downarrow$ | $\downarrow\downarrow$ |

Calcium channel blockers—**N**ifedipine is similar to **N**itrates in effect; verapamil is similar to β-blockers in effect.

Note: Pindolol and acebutolol are partial β-agonists—contraindicated in angina.

**Lipid-lowering agents**

| Drug | Effect on LDL "Bad Cholesterol" | Effect on HDL "Good Cholesterol" | Effect on Triglycerides | Mechanisms of Action | Side Effects/ Problems |
|---|---|---|---|---|---|
| HMG-CoA reductase inhibitors (lovastatin, pravastatin, simvastatin, atorvastatin, rosuvastatin) | ↓↓↓ | ↑ | ↓ | Inhibit cholesterol precursor, mevalonate | Hepatotoxicity (↑ LFTs), rhabdomyolysis |
| Niacin | ↓↓ | ↑↑ | ↓ | Inhibits lipolysis in adipose tissue; reduces hepatic VLDL secretion into circulation | Red, flushed face, which is ↓ by aspirin or long-term use Hyperglycemia (acanthosis nigricans) Hyperuricemia (exacerbates gout) |
| Bile acid resins (cholestyramine, colestipol, colesevelam) | ↓↓ | Slightly ↑ | Slightly ↑ | Prevent intestinal reabsorption of bile acids; liver must use cholesterol to make more | Patients hate it—tastes bad and causes GI discomfort, ↓ absorption of fat-soluble vitamins Cholesterol gallstones |
| Cholesterol absorption blockers (ezetimibe) | ↓↓ | — | — | Prevent cholesterol reabsorption at small intestine brush border | Rare ↑ LFTs |
| "Fibrates" (gemfibrozil, clofibrate, bezafibrate, fenofibrate) | ↓ | ↑ | ↓↓↓ | Upregulate LPL → ↑ TG clearance | Myositis, hepatotoxicity (↑ LFTs), cholesterol gallstones |

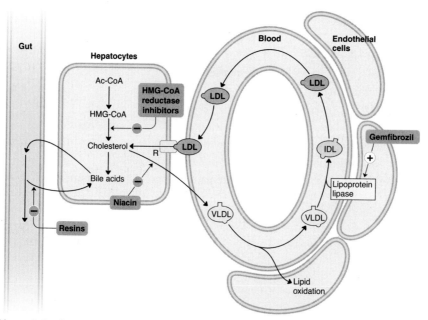

(Adapted, with permission, from Katzung BG, Trevor AJ. *USMLE Road Map: Pharmacology*, 1st ed. New York: McGraw-Hill, 2003: 56.)

## Cardiac drugs: sites of action

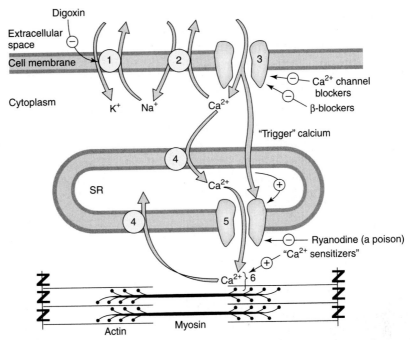

(Adapted, with permission, from Katzung BG. *Basic and Clinical Pharmacology*, 7th ed. Stamford, CT: Appleton & Lange, 1997: 198.)

Cardiac sarcomere is shown above with the cellular components involved in excitation-contraction coupling. Factors involved in excitation-contraction coupling are numbered. (1) $Na^+/K^+$ ATPase; (2) $Na^+$-$Ca^{2+}$ exchanger; (3) voltage-gated (L-type) calcium channel; (4) calcium pump in the wall of the sarcoplasmic reticulum (SR); (5) ryanodine receptors and calcium release channels in the SR, which are closely coupled to L-type calcium channels in the cell membrane; (6) site of calcium interaction with troponin-tropomyosin system.

$\beta_1$ receptors are $G_s$ and activate protein kinase A, which phosphorylates L-type $Ca^{2+}$ channels and phospholamban, both of which $\uparrow$ intracellular $Ca^{2+}$ during contraction.

| | |
|---|---|
| **Cardiac glycosides** | Digoxin—75% bioavailability, 20–40% protein bound, $t_{1/2}$ = 40 hours, urinary excretion. |
| Mechanism | Direct inhibition of $Na^+/K^+$ ATPase leads to indirect inhibition of $Na^+/Ca^{2+}$ exchanger/antiport. $\uparrow [Ca^{2+}]_i \rightarrow$ positive inotropy. Stimulates vagus nerve. |
| Clinical use | CHF ($\uparrow$ contractility); atrial fibrillation ($\downarrow$ conduction at AV node and depression of SA node). |
| Toxicity | Cholinergic—nausea, vomiting, diarrhea, blurry yellow vision (think Van Gogh). ECG—$\uparrow$ PR, $\downarrow$ QT, scooping, T-wave inversion, arrhythmia, hyperkalemia. Worsened by renal failure ($\downarrow$ excretion), hypokalemia (permissive for digoxin binding at $K^+$-binding site on $Na^+/K^+$ ATPase), quinidine ($\downarrow$ digoxin clearance; displaces digoxin from tissue-binding sites). |
| Antidote | Slowly normalize $K^+$, lidocaine, cardiac pacer, anti-dig Fab fragments, $Mg^{2+}$. |

| | | |
|---|---|---|
| **Antiarrhythmics—Na⁺ channel blockers (class I)** | Local anesthetics. Slow or block (↓) conduction (especially in depolarized cells). ↓ slope of phase 4 depolarization and ↑ threshold for firing in abnormal pacemaker cells. Are state dependent (selectively depress tissue that is frequently depolarized, e.g., fast tachycardia). | |
| Class IA | Quinidine, Procainamide, Disopyramide. ↑ AP duration, ↑ effective refractory period (ERP), ↑ QT interval. Affect both atrial and ventricular arrhythmias, especially reentrant and ectopic supraventricular and ventricular tachycardia.<br><br>Toxicity: quinidine (cinchonism—headache, tinnitus; thrombocytopenia; torsades de pointes due to ↑ QT interval); procainamide (reversible SLE-like syndrome). | "The **Q**ueen **P**roclaims **D**iso's **pyramid**." |
| Class **IB** | **Lid**ocaine, **Mexi**letine, **T**ocainide. ↓ AP duration. Preferentially affect ischemic or depolarized Purkinje and ventricular tissue. Useful in acute ventricular arrhythmias (especially post-MI) and in digitalis-induced arrhythmias.<br><br>Toxicity: local anesthetic. CNS stimulation/depression, cardiovascular depression. | "I'd **B**uy **Lid**y's **Mexi**can **T**acos." Phenytoin can also fall into the IB category. |
| Class IC | **F**lecainide, **E**ncainide, **P**ropafenone. No effect on AP duration. Useful in V-tachs that progress to VF and in intractable SVT. Usually used only as last resort in refractory tachyarrhythmias. For patients without structural abnormalities.<br><br>Toxicity: proarrhythmic, especially post-MI (contraindicated). Significantly prolongs refractory period in AV node. | "**C**hipotle's **F**ood has **E**xcellent **P**roduce." IB is **B**est post-MI. IC is **C**ontraindicated post-MI. |

Hyperkalemia causes ↑ toxicity for all class I drugs.

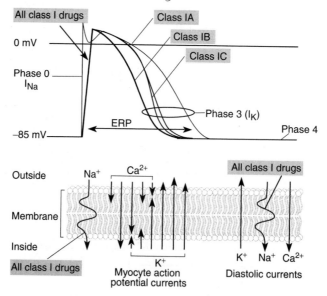

(Adapted, with permission, from Katzung BG, Trevor AJ. *Pharmacology: Examination & Board Review*, 5th ed. Stamford, CT: Appleton & Lange, 1998: 118.)

CARDIOVASCULAR

HIGH-YIELD SYSTEMS

| **Antiarrhythmics—**<br>**β-blockers**<br>**(class II)** | Propranolol, esmolol, metoprolol, atenolol, timolol. |
|---|---|
| Mechanism | ↓ cAMP, ↓ $Ca^{2+}$ currents. Suppress abnormal pacemakers by ↓ slope of phase 4. AV node particularly sensitive—↑ PR interval. Esmolol very short acting. |
| Clinical use | V-tach, SVT, slowing ventricular rate during atrial fibrillation and atrial flutter. |
| Toxicity | Impotence, exacerbation of asthma, cardiovascular effects (bradycardia, AV block, CHF), CNS effects (sedation, sleep alterations). May mask the signs of hypoglycemia. Metoprolol can cause dyslipidemia. Treat overdose with glucagon. |

| **Antiarrhythmics—**<br>**K⁺ channel**<br>**blockers (class III)** | Sotalol, ibutilide, bretylium, dofetilide, amiodarone. | |
|---|---|---|
| Mechanism | ↑ AP duration, ↑ ERP. Used when other antiarrhythmics fail. ↑ QT interval. | |
| Toxicity | Sotalol—torsades de pointes, excessive β block; ibutilide—torsades; bretylium—new arrhythmias, hypotension; amiodarone—**pulmonary fibrosis, hepatotoxicity, hypothyroidism/hyperthyroidism** (amiodarone is 40% iodine by weight), corneal deposits, skin deposits (blue/gray) resulting in photodermatitis, neurologic effects, constipation, cardiovascular effects (bradycardia, heart block, CHF).<br><br>Amiodarone has class I, II, III, and IV effects because it alters the lipid membrane. | Remember to check **PFT**s, **LFT**s, and **TFT**s when using amiodarone. |

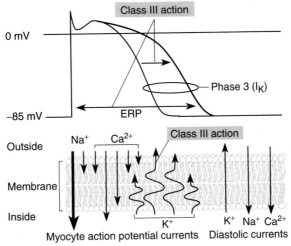

(Adapted, with permission, from Katzung BG, Trevor AJ. *Pharmacology: Examination & Board Review,* 5th ed. Stamford, CT: Appleton & Lange, 1998: 120.)

**Antiarrhythmics—
Ca²⁺ channel
blockers (class IV)**

Verapamil, diltiazem.

   Mechanism

Primarily affect AV nodal cells. ↓ conduction velocity, ↑ ERP, ↑ PR interval. Used in prevention of nodal arrhythmias (e.g., SVT).

   Toxicity

Constipation, flushing, edema, CV effects (CHF, AV block, sinus node depression).

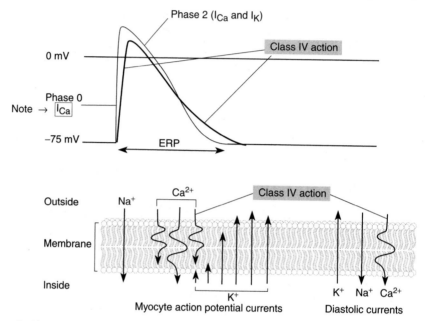

(Adapted, with permission, from Katzung BG, Trevor AJ. *Pharmacology: Examination & Board Review,* 5th ed. Stamford, CT: Appleton & Lange, 1998: 121.)

**Other antiarrhythmics**

   Adenosine

↑ K⁺ out of cells → hyperpolarizing the cell + ↓ $I_{Ca}$. Drug of choice in diagnosing/ abolishing supraventricular tachycardia. Very short acting (∼ 15 sec). Toxicity includes flushing, hypotension, chest pain. Effects blocked by theophylline.

   K⁺

Depresses ectopic pacemakers in hypokalemia (e.g., digoxin toxicity).

   Mg²⁺

Effective in torsades de pointes and digoxin toxicity.

# Endocrine

*"Chocolate causes certain endocrine glands to secrete hormones that affect your feelings and behavior by making you happy."*
— Elaine Sherman, *Book of Divine Indulgences*

▶ Anatomy

▶ Physiology

▶ Pathology

▶ Pharmacology

## Adrenal cortex and medulla

Cortex (from mesoderm)

Medulla (from neural crest)

| Primary regulatory control | Anatomy | Secretory products |
|---|---|---|
| | Capsule | |
| Renin-angiotensin | → Zona **G**lomerulosa | → Aldosterone |
| ACTH, hypothalamic CRH | → Zona **F**asciculata | → Cortisol, sex hormones |
| ACTH, hypothalamic CRH | → Zona **R**eticularis | → Sex hormones (e.g., androgens) |
| Preganglionic sympathetic fibers | → Medulla | → Catecholamines (epi, NE) |

Chromaffin cells ⟶

**GFR** corresponds with **S**alt (Na⁺), **S**ugar (glucocorticoids), and **S**ex (androgens).

"The deeper you go, the sweeter it gets."

**Pheochromocytoma**—most common tumor of the adrenal medulla in adults.

**Neuroblastoma**—most common in children.

Pheochromocytoma causes episodic hypertension; neuroblastoma does not.

| **Adrenal gland drainage** | Left adrenal → left adrenal vein → left renal vein → IVC. <br> Right adrenal → right adrenal vein → IVC. | Same as left and right gonadal vein. |
|---|---|---|
| **Pituitary gland** | Posterior pituitary (neurohypophysis) → vasopressin (ADH) and oxytocin, made in the hypothalamus and shipped to pituitary. Derived from neuroectoderm. <br> Anterior pituitary (adenohypophysis) → FSH, LH, ACTH, TSH, prolactin, GH, melanotropin (MSH). Derived from oral ectoderm. <br> α subunit—common subunit to TSH, LH, FSH, and hCG. <br> β subunit—determines hormone specificity. | **Acidophils**—GH, prolactin. <br> **B-FLAT: B**asophils—FSH, LH, ACTH, TSH. <br> **FLAT PiG:** <br> FSH <br> LH <br> ACTH <br> TSH <br> Prolactin <br> GH |
| **Endocrine pancreas cell types** | Islets of Langerhans are collections of α, β, and δ endocrine cells (most numerous in tail of pancreas). Islets arise from pancreatic buds. <br> α = glucagon (peripheral); β = insulin (central); δ = somatostatin (interspersed). | **INS**ulin (beta cells) **INS**ide. |

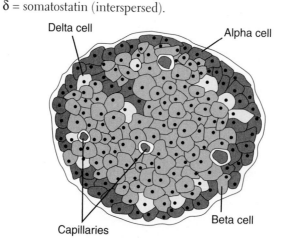

Delta cell

Alpha cell

Capillaries

Beta cell

## Insulin

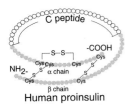

C peptide

-COOH

NH₂-

Cys Cys    Cys    Cys
S—S
S    α chain    S
Cys              Cys
β chain

Human proinsulin

Made in β cells of pancreas in response to ATP from glucose metabolism closing $K^+$ channels and depolarizing cells. Required for adipose and skeletal muscle uptake of glucose.

Inhibits glucagon release by α cells of pancreas.

Serum C-peptide is not present with exogenous insulin intake (proinsulin → insulin + C-peptide).

Anabolic effects of insulin:
1. ↑ glucose transport
2. ↑ glycogen synthesis and storage
3. ↑ triglyceride synthesis and storage
4. ↑ $Na^+$ retention (kidneys)
5. ↑ protein synthesis (muscles)
6. ↑ cellular uptake of $K^+$

Insulin moves glucose **In**to cells.

**BRICK L** (don't need insulin for glucose uptake):
- **B**rain
- **R**BCs
- **I**ntestine
- **C**ornea
- **K**idney
- **L**iver

GLUT-1: RBCs, brain.

GLUT-2 (bidirectional): β islet cells, liver, kidney.

GLUT-4 (insulin responsive): adipose tissue, skeletal muscle.

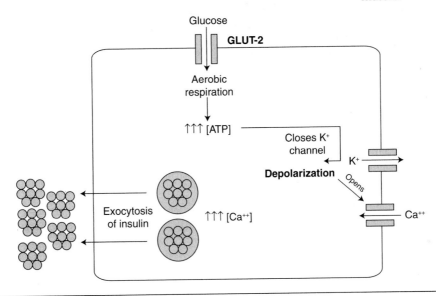

Glucose

**GLUT-2**

Aerobic respiration

↑↑↑ [ATP] — Closes $K^+$ channel

$K^+$

**Depolarization**

Opens

Exocytosis of insulin    ↑↑↑ [Ca⁺⁺]    Ca⁺⁺

## Insulin-dependent organs

Skeletal muscle and adipose tissue depend on insulin for ↑ glucose uptake (GLUT-4). Brain and RBCs take up glucose independent of insulin levels (GLUT-1). Brain depends on glucose for metabolism under normal circumstances and uses ketone bodies in starvation. RBCs always depend on glucose.

| | |
|---|---|
| **Hypothalamic-pituitary hormone regulation** | TRH—$\oplus$→ TSH, prolactin.<br>Dopamine—$\ominus$→ prolactin.<br>CRH—$\oplus$→ ACTH.<br>GHRH—$\oplus$→ GH.<br>Somatostatin—$\ominus$→ GH, TSH.<br>GnRH—$\oplus$→ FSH, LH.<br>Prolactin—$\ominus$→ GnRH. |

---

**Prolactin regulation**

Regulation—prolactin secretion from anterior pituitary is tonically inhibited by dopamine from hypothalamus. Prolactin in turn inhibits its own secretion by increasing dopamine synthesis and secretion from hypothalamus. TRH ↑ prolactin secretion.

Function—stimulates milk production in breast; inhibits ovulation (in females) and spermatogenesis (in males) by inhibiting GnRH synthesis and release.

Dopamine agonists (bromocriptine) inhibit prolactin secretion and can be used in treatment of prolactinoma.

Dopamine antagonists (most antipsychotics) stimulate prolactin secretion.

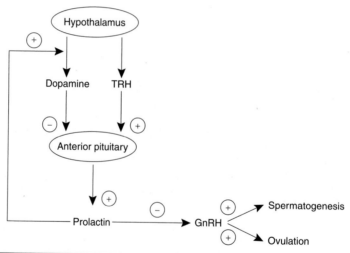

---

## Adrenal steroids

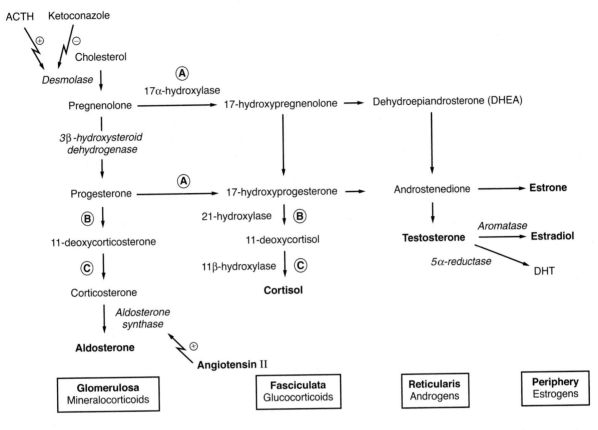

**A = 17α-hydroxylase deficiency.** ↓ sex hormones, ↓ cortisol, ↑ mineralocorticoids. Sx = **HYPER**tension, hypokalemia. XY: ↓ DHT → pseudohermaphroditism (externally phenotypic female, no internal reproductive structures due to MIF). XX: externally phenotypic female with normal internal sex organs, but lacking 2° sexual characteristics ("sexual infantilism").

Congenital bilateral adrenal hyperplasias*

**B = 21-hydroxylase deficiency.** Most common form. ↓ cortisol (increased ACTH), ↓ mineralocorticoids, ↑ sex hormones. Sx = masculinization, female pseudohermaphroditism, **HYPO**tension, hyperkalemia, ↑ plasma renin activity, and volume depletion. Salt wasting can lead to hypovolemic shock in the newborn.

**C = 11ß-hydroxylase deficiency.** ↓ cortisol, ↓ aldosterone and corticosterone, ↑ sex hormones. Sx = masculinization, **HYPER**tension (like aldosterone, 11-deoxycorticosterone is a mineralocorticoid and is secreted in excess).

*All congenital adrenal enzyme deficiencies are characterized by an enlargement of the adrenal glands due to an ↑ in ACTH stimulation because of the ↓ levels of cortisol.

## Cortisol

| | | |
|---|---|---|
| Source | Adrenal zona fasciculata. | Bound to corticosteroid-binding globulin (CBG). |
| Function | Cortisol is **BBIIG**: | Chronic stress induces prolonged secretion. |

    1. Maintains **B**lood pressure (by upregulating $\alpha_1$ receptors on arterioles)
    2. ↓ **B**one formation
    3. Anti-**I**nflammatory
    4. ↓ **I**mmune function
    5. ↑ **G**luconeogenesis, lipolysis, proteolysis

Regulation     CRH (hypothalamus) stimulates ACTH release (pituitary), causing cortisol production in adrenal zona fasciculata.

**PTH**

Source — Chief cells of parathyroid.

Function —
1. ↑ bone resorption of calcium and phosphate
2. ↑ kidney reabsorption of calcium in distal convoluted tubule
3. ↓ kidney reabsorption of phosphate
4. ↑ $1,25\text{-}(OH)_2$ vitamin D (calcitriol) production by stimulating kidney $1\alpha$-hydroxylase

PTH ↑ serum $Ca^{2+}$, ↓ serum $(PO_4)^{3-}$, ↑ urine $(PO_4)^{3-}$.
PTH stimulates both osteoclasts (indirectly) and osteoblasts (directly).

**PTH** = **P**hosphate **T**rashing **H**ormone.

Regulation —
↓ free serum $Ca^{2+}$ ↑ PTH secretion.
↓ free serum $Mg^{2+}$ ↓ PTH secretion.
Common causes of ↓ $Mg^{2+}$ include diarrhea, aminoglycosides, diuretics, and alcohol abuse.

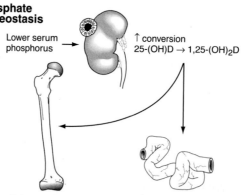

Low ionized calcium

**Calcium homeostasis**

Four parathyroid glands

⊖ Feedback inhibition of PTH secretion

PTH (1-84) released into circulation

Renal tubular cells → Bone

- Stimulates reabsorption of calcium
- Inhibits phosphate reabsorption
- ↑ urinary cAMP
- Stimulates production of $1,25\text{-}(OH)_2D$

- Stimulates calcium release from bone mineral compartment
- **Directly stimulates osteoblastic cells,** indirectly stimulates osteoclastic cells
- Stimulates bone resorption via indirect effect on osteoclasts
- Enhances bone matrix degradation

- Increases intestinal calcium absorption → Increases serum calcium

**Phosphate homeostasis**

Lower serum phosphorus → ↑ conversion $25\text{-}(OH)D \rightarrow 1,25\text{-}(OH)_2D$

- Releases phosphate from matrix
- Increases calcium and phosphate absorption

(Adapted, with permission, from Chandrasoma P et al. *Concise Pathology*, 3rd ed. Stamford, CT: Appleton & Lange, 1998.)

### Vitamin D (cholecalciferol)

Source — Vitamin $D_3$ from sun exposure in skin. $D_2$ ingested from plants. Both converted to 25-OH vitamin D in liver and to 1,25-$(OH)_2$ vitamin D (active form) in kidney.

Function —
1. ↑ absorption of dietary calcium
2. ↑ absorption of dietary phosphate
3. ↑ bone resorption of $Ca^{2+}$ and $(PO_4)^{3-}$

Regulation —
↑ PTH causes ↑ 1,25-$(OH)_2$ vitamin D production.
↓ $[Ca^{2+}]$ causes ↑ 1,25-$(OH)_2$ vitamin D production.
↓ phosphate causes ↑ 1,25-$(OH)_2$ vitamin D production.
1,25-$(OH)_2$ vitamin D feedback inhibits its own production.

If you do not get vitamin D, you get rickets (kids) or osteomalacia (adults).
24,25-$(OH)_2$ vitamin D is an inactive form of vitamin D.
PTH ↑ calcium reabsorption and ↓ phosphate reabsorption, while 1,25-$(OH)_2$ vitamin D ↑ absorption of **both** calcium and phosphate.

### Calcitonin

Source — Parafollicular cells (C cells) of thyroid.
Function — ↓ bone resorption of calcium.
Regulation — ↑ serum $Ca^{2+}$ causes calcitonin secretion.

Calcitonin opposes actions of PTH. Not important in normal calcium homeostasis. CalciTONin TONes down calcium levels.

### Signaling pathways of endocrine hormones

| cAMP | cGMP | $IP_3$ | Steroid receptor | Tyrosine kinase |
|---|---|---|---|---|
| FSH | ANP | GnRH | Glucocorticoid | Insulin |
| LH | NO (EDRF) | GHRH | Estrogen | IGF-1 |
| ACTH | (Think | Oxytocin | Progesterone | FGF |
| TSH | vasodilators) | ADH ($V_1$ | Testosterone | PDGF |
| CRH | | receptor) | Aldosterone | Prolactin |
| hCG | | TRH | Vitamin D | GH |
| ADH ($V_2$ receptor) | | ("GGOAT") | $T_3/T_4$ | |
| MSH | | | | |
| PTH | | | | |
| Calcitonin | | | | |
| Glucagon | | | | |
| ("FLAT CHAMP") | | | | |

### Steroid/thyroid hormone mechanism

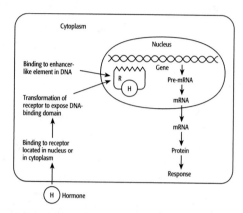

(Adapted, with permission, from Ganong WF. *Review of Medical Physiology,* 22th ed. New York: McGraw-Hill, 2005, Fig. 1-35.)

Steroid/thyroid hormones—
**PET CAT:**
  **P**rogesterone
  **E**strogen
  **T**estosterone
  **C**ortisol
  **A**ldosterone
  **T**hyroxine and $T_3$
In men, ↑ levels of sex hormone–binding globulin (SHBG) lower free testosterone → gynecomastia.
In women, ↓ SHBG raises free testosterone → hirsutism.

Steroid hormones are lipophilic and relatively insoluble in plasma; therefore, they must circulate bound to specific binding globulins, which ↑ solubility and allow for ↑ delivery of steroid to the target organ. The need for gene transcription and protein synthesis delays the onset of action of these hormones.

---

| **Thyroid hormones ($T_3$/$T_4$)** | Iodine-containing hormones that control the body's metabolic rate. | |
|---|---|---|
| Source | Follicles of thyroid. Most $T_3$ formed in blood. | $T_3$ functions—**4 B's:** |
| Function | 1. Bone growth (synergism with GH) | **B**rain maturation |
| | 2. CNS maturation | **B**one growth |
| | 3. ↑ $\beta_1$ receptors in heart = ↑ CO, HR, SV, contractility | **B**eta-adrenergic effects |
| | 4. ↑ basal metabolic rate via ↑ $Na^+/K^+$-ATPase activity = ↑ $O_2$ consumption, RR, body temperature | **B**MR ↑ |
| | 5. ↑ glycogenolysis, gluconeogenesis, lipolysis | Thyroxine-binding globulin (TBG) binds most $T_3$/$T_4$ in blood; only free hormone is active. ↓ TBG in hepatic failure; ↑ TBG in pregnancy or OCP use (estrogen ↑ TBG). |
| Regulation | TRH (hypothalamus) stimulates TSH (pituitary), which stimulates follicular cells. Negative feedback by free $T_3$ to anterior pituitary ↓ sensitivity to TRH. TSI, like TSH, stimulates follicular cells (Graves' disease). | $T_4$ is major product; converted to $T_3$ by peripheral tissue. $T_3$ binds receptors with greater affinity than $T_4$. Peroxidase—enzyme responsible for oxidation and organification of iodide as well as coupling of MIT and DIT. |

Blood   Cell   Lumen

Thyroglobulin → TG
                     } MIT
I⁻ → Oxidation → I₂   DIT ← ⊖
$T_3$/$T_4$ ← Proteolysis ← $T_3$/$T_4$

Antithyroid drugs (propylthiouracil, methimazole)

HIGH-YIELD SYSTEMS

ENDOCRINE

| | | |
|---|---|---|
| **Cushing's syndrome** | ↑ cortisol due to a variety of causes. Exogenous (iatrogenic) steroids—#1 cause; ↓ ACTH. Endogenous causes: <br> 1. **Cushing's disease** (70%)—due to ACTH secretion from pituitary adenoma; ↑ ACTH <br> 2. **Ectopic ACTH** (15%)—from nonpituitary tissue making ACTH (e.g., small cell lung cancer, bronchial carcinoids); ↑ ACTH <br> 3. **Adrenal** (15%)—adenoma (see Image 68), carcinoma, nodular adrenal hyperplasia; ↓ ACTH <br> Findings: hypertension, weight gain, moon facies, truncal obesity, buffalo hump, hyperglycemia (insulin resistance), skin changes (thinning, striae), osteoporosis, amenorrhea, and immune suppression (see Image 70). | Dexamethasone (synthetic glucocorticoid) suppression test: <br> Healthy: ↓ cortisol after low dose. <br> ACTH-producing pituitary tumor: ↑ cortisol after low dose; ↓ cortisol after high dose. <br> Ectopic ACTH-producing tumor (e.g., small cell carcinoma): ↑ cortisol after low dose; ↑ cortisol after high dose. <br> Cortisol-producing tumor: ↑ cortisol after low and high dose. |

**Hyperaldosteronism**

| | | |
|---|---|---|
| Primary (Conn's syndrome) | Caused by an aldosterone-secreting tumor, resulting in hypertension, hypokalemia, metabolic alkalosis, and **low** plasma renin. May be bilateral or unilateral. | Treatment: spironolactone, a K+-sparing diuretic that works by acting as an aldosterone antagonist. |
| Secondary | Kidney perception of low intravascular volume results in an overactive renin-angiotensin system. Due to renal artery stenosis, chronic renal failure, CHF, cirrhosis, or nephrotic syndrome. Associated with **high** plasma renin. | |

| | |
|---|---|
| **Addison's disease** | **Chronic** adrenal insufficiency due to adrenal atrophy or destruction by disease (e.g., autoimmune, TB, metastasis). 1° deficiency of aldosterone and cortisol, causing hypotension (hyponatremic volume contraction) and skin hyperpigmentation (due to MSH, a by-product of ↑ ACTH production from POMC). Characterized by **A**drenal **A**trophy and **A**bsence of hormone production; involves **A**ll 3 cortical divisions. Distinguish from 2° adrenal insufficiency (↓ pituitary ACTH production), which has no skin hyperpigmentation and no hyperkalemia. |
| **Waterhouse-Friderichsen syndrome** | **Acute** adrenocortical insufficiency due to adrenal hemorrhage associated with *Neisseria meningitidis* septicemia, DIC, and endotoxic shock. |

**Pheochromocytoma**

Most common tumor of the adrenal medulla in adults. Derived from chromaffin cells (arise from neural crest; see Image 69).

Most tumors secrete epinephrine, NE, and dopamine and can cause episodic hypertension. Urinary VMA (a breakdown product of norepinephrine) and plasma catecholamines are elevated. Associated with neurofibromatosis, MEN types 2A and 2B. Treatment: α-antagonists, especially **phenoxybenzamine**, a nonselective, **irreversible** α-blocker.

Episodic hyperadrenergic symptoms (**5 P's**):
**P**ressure (elevated blood pressure)
**P**ain (headache)
**P**erspiration
**P**alpitations (tachycardia)
**P**allor

Rule of 10's:
10% malignant
10% bilateral
10% extra-adrenal
10% calcify
10% kids
10% familial
Symptoms occur in "spells"— relapse and remit.

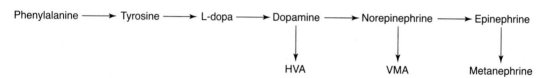

**Neuroblastoma**

The most common tumor of the adrenal medulla in children. Can occur anywhere along the sympathetic chain. HVA (a breakdown product of dopamine) in urine. Less likely to develop hypertension. N-*myc* oncogene.

**Hypothyroidism vs. hyperthyroidism**

|  | Hypothyroidism | Hyperthyroidism |
|---|---|---|
| Signs/symptoms | Cold intolerance (↓ heat production) | Heat intolerance (↑ heat production) |
|  | Weight gain, ↓ appetite | Weight loss, ↑ appetite |
|  | Hypoactivity, lethargy, fatigue, weakness | Hyperactivity |
|  | Constipation | Diarrhea |
|  | ↓ reflexes | ↑ reflexes |
|  | Myxedema (facial/periorbital) | Chest pain, palpitations, arrhythmias |
|  | Dry, cool skin; coarse, brittle hair | Warm, moist skin; fine hair |
| Lab findings | ↑ TSH (sensitive test for 1° hypothyroidism) | ↓ TSH (if 1°) |
|  | ↓ total $T_4$ | ↑ total $T_4$ |
|  | ↓ free $T_4$ | ↑ free $T_4$ |
|  | ↓ $T_3$ uptake | ↑ $T_3$ uptake |

## Hypothyroidism

| | | |
|---|---|---|
| Hashimoto's thyroiditis | The most common cause of hypothyroidism; an autoimmune disorder (can have thyrotoxicosis during follicular rupture). Slow course; moderately enlarged, nontender thyroid. Lymphocytic infiltrate with germinal centers. Antimicrosomal and antithyroglobulin antibodies. Associated with HLA-DR5 and Hürthle cells on histology. | May be hyperthyroid early in course. |
| Cretinism | Due to severe fetal hypothyroidism. Endemic cretinism occurs wherever endemic goiter is prevalent (lack of dietary iodine); sporadic cretinism is caused by defect in $T_4$ formation or developmental failure in thyroid formation. Findings: pot-bellied, pale, puffy-faced child with protruding umbilicus and protuberant tongue. | Cretin means Christlike (French *chrétien*). Those affected were considered so mentally retarded as to be incapable of sinning. Still common in China. |
| Subacute thyroiditis (de Quervain's) | Self-limited hypothyroidism often following a flulike illness. Elevated ESR, jaw pain, early inflammation, and very tender thyroid gland. Histology shows granulomatous inflammation. | May be hyperthyroid early in course. Lymphocytic subacute thyroiditis is painless. |
| Riedel's thyroiditis | Thyroid replaced by fibrous tissue (hypothyroid). Presents with fixed, hard (rock-like), and painless goiter. | |

## Hyperthyroidism

| | | |
|---|---|---|
| Graves' disease | An autoimmune hyperthyroidism with thyroid-stimulating/TSH receptor antibodies. Ophthalmopathy (proptosis, EOM swelling), pretibial myxedema, diffuse goiter (see Image 105). Often presents during stress (e.g., childbirth) (see Image 71). Stress-induced catecholamine surge leading to death by arrhythmia. Seen as a serious complication of Graves' and other hyperthyroid disorders. | Graves' is a type II hypersensitivity. |
| Toxic multinodular goiter | Focal patches of hyperfunctioning follicular cells working independently of TSH due to mutation in TSH receptor. ↑ release of $T_3$ and $T_4$. Nodules are not malignant. Jod-Basedow phenomenon—thyrotoxicosis if a patient with iodine deficiency goiter is made iodine replete. | |

## Thyroid cancer

1. Papillary carcinoma—most common, excellent prognosis, "ground-glass" nuclei (Orphan Annie), psammoma bodies, nuclear grooves. ↑ risk with childhood irradiation.
2. Follicular carcinoma—good prognosis, uniform follicles.
3. Medullary carcinoma—from parafollicular "C cells"; produces calcitonin, sheets of cells in amyloid stroma. Associated with MEN types 2A and 2B.
4. Undifferentiated/anaplastic—older patients; very poor prognosis.
5. Lymphoma—associated with Hashimoto's thyroiditis.

| | | |
|---|---|---|
| **Hypercalcemia** | Caused by Calcium ingestion (milk-alkali syndrome), Hyperparathyroid, Hyperthyroid, Iatrogenic (thiazides), Multiple myeloma, Paget's disease, Addison's disease, Neoplasms, Zollinger-Ellison syndrome, Excess vitamin D, Excess vitamin A, Sarcoidosis. | **CHIMPANZEES.** Patients with Paget's disease are usually normocalcemic but can become hypercalcemic if immobilized. |

**Hyperparathyroidism**

| | | |
|---|---|---|
| Primary | Usually an adenoma. **Hypercalcemia**, hypercalciuria **(renal stones)**, hypophosphatemia, ↑ PTH, ↑ alkaline phosphatase, ↑ cAMP in urine. Often asymptomatic, or may present with weakness and constipation (**"groans"**). | **"Stones, bones, and groans."** **Osteitis fibrosa cystica** (von Recklinghausen's syndrome)—cystic bone spaces filled with brown fibrous tissue (**bone pain**). |
| Secondary | 2° hyperplasia due to ↓ gut $Ca^{2+}$ absorption and ↑ phosphorus, most often in chronic renal disease (causes hypovitaminosis D → ↓ $Ca^{2+}$ absorption). **Hypocalcemia**, hyperphosphatemia, ↑ alkaline phosphatase, ↑ PTH. | **Renal osteodystrophy**—bone lesions due to 2° hyperparathyroidism due in turn to renal disease. |

| | | |
|---|---|---|
| **Hypoparathyroidism** | Due to accidental surgical excision (thyroid surgery), autoimmune destruction, or DiGeorge syndrome. Findings: hypocalcemia, tetany. Chvostek's sign—tapping of facial nerve → contraction of facial muscles. Trousseau's sign—occlusion of brachial artery with BP cuff → carpal spasm. | **Pseudohypoparathyroidism** (Albright's hereditary osteodystrophy)—autosomal-dominant kidney unresponsiveness to PTH. Hypocalcemia, shortened 4th/5th digits, short stature. |

| | |
|---|---|
| **Pituitary adenoma** | Most commonly prolactinoma. Findings: amenorrhea, galactorrhea, low libido, infertility. Bromocriptine or cabergoline (dopamine agonists) causes shrinkage. Can impinge on optic chiasm → bitemporal hemianopia. |

| | | |
|---|---|---|
| **Acromegaly** | Excess GH in adults. Findings: large tongue with deep furrows, deep voice, large hands and feet, coarse facial features, impaired glucose tolerance (insulin resistance). ↑ GH in children → gigantism (↑ linear bone growth). Treatment: pituitary adenoma resection followed by octreotide administration. | ↑ GH is normal in stress, exercise, and hypoglycemia. Diagnosis: ↑ serum IGF-1; failure to suppress serum GH following oral glucose tolerance test. |

| | |
|---|---|
| **Sheehan's syndrome** | Postpartum hypopituitarism. Enlargement of anterior pituitary (↑ lactotrophs) during pregnancy without corresponding ↑ blood supply leads to ↑ risk of infarction of the pituitary gland following severe bleeding and hypoperfusion during delivery. May cause fatigue, anorexia, poor lactation, and loss of pubic and axillary hair. |

**Diabetes insipidus**    Characterized by intense thirst and polyuria together with an inability to concentrate urine owing to lack of ADH (central DI—pituitary tumor, trauma, surgery, histiocytosis X) or to a lack of renal response to ADH (nephrogenic DI—hereditary or 2° to hypercalcemia, lithium, demeclocycline [ADH antagonist]).

Diagnosis    Water deprivation test—urine osmolality doesn't ↑. Response to desmopressin distinguishes between central and nephrogenic.

Findings    Urine specific gravity < 1.006; serum osmolality > 290 mOsm/L.

Treatment    Adequate fluid intake. For central DI—intranasal desmopressin (ADH analog). For nephrogenic DI—hydrochlorothiazide, indomethacin, or amiloride.

---

**SIADH**    Syndrome of inappropriate antidiuretic hormone secretion:

1. Excessive water retention
2. Hyponatremia
3. Urine osmolarity > serum osmolarity

Very low serum sodium levels can lead to seizures (correct slowly).

Treatment: demeclocycline or $H_2O$ restriction.

Causes include:
1. Ectopic ADH (small cell lung cancer)
2. CNS disorders/head trauma
3. Pulmonary disease
4. Drugs (e.g., cyclophosphamide)

---

**Diabetes mellitus**

Acute manifestations    Polydipsia, polyuria, polyphagia, weight loss, DKA (type 1), hyperosmolar coma (type 2), unopposed secretion of GH and epinephrine (exacerbating hyperglycemia).

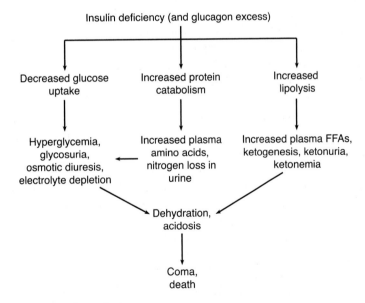

Chronic manifestations    Nonenzymatic glycosylation:
1. Small vessel disease (diffuse thickening of basement membrane) → retinopathy (hemorrhage, exudates, microaneurysms, vessel proliferation), glaucoma, nephropathy (nodular sclerosis, progressive proteinuria, chronic renal failure, arteriosclerosis leading to hypertension, Kimmelstiel-Wilson nodules)
2. Large vessel atherosclerosis, CAD, peripheral vascular occlusive disease and gangrene, cerebrovascular disease

Osmotic damage:
1. Neuropathy (motor, sensory, and autonomic degeneration)
2. Cataracts (sorbitol accumulation)

Tests    Fasting serum glucose, glucose tolerance test, $HbA_{1c}$ (measures long-term diabetic control).

### Type 1 vs. type 2 diabetes mellitus

| Variable | Type 1 (juvenile onset, IDDM) | Type 2 (adult onset, NIDDM) |
|---|---|---|
| 1° defect | Viral or immune destruction of β cells (see Image 67) | ↑ resistance to insulin |
| Insulin necessary in treatment | Always | Sometimes |
| Age (exceptions commonly occur) | < 30 | > 40 |
| Association with obesity | No | Yes |
| Genetic predisposition | Weak, polygenic | Strong, polygenic |
| Association with HLA system | Yes (HLA-DR3 and 4) | No |
| Glucose intolerance | Severe | Mild to moderate |
| Ketoacidosis | Common | Rare |
| β-cell numbers in the islets | ↓ | Variable (with amyloid deposits) |
| Serum insulin level | ↓ | Variable |
| Classic symptoms of polyuria, polydipsia, thirst, weight loss | Common | Sometimes |

| | | |
|---|---|---|
| **Diabetic ketoacidosis** | One of the most important complications of type 1 diabetes. Usually due to ↑ insulin requirements from ↑ stress (e.g., infection). Excess fat breakdown and ↑ ketogenesis from ↑ free fatty acids, which are then made into ketone bodies (β-hydroxybutyrate > acetoacetate). | |
| Signs/symptoms | Kussmaul respirations (rapid/deep breathing), nausea/vomiting, abdominal pain, psychosis/delirium, dehydration. Fruity breath odor (due to exhaled acetone). | |
| Labs | Hyperglycemia, ↑ $H^+$, ↓ $HCO_3^-$ (anion gap metabolic acidosis), ↑ blood ketone levels, leukocytosis. Hyperkalemia, but depleted intracellular $K^+$ due to transcellular shift from ↓ insulin. | |
| Complications | Life-threatening mucormycosis, *Rhizopus* infection, cerebral edema, cardiac arrhythmias, heart failure. | |
| Treatment | Fluids, insulin, and $K^+$ (to replete intracellular stores); glucose if necessary to prevent hypoglycemia. | |

| | | |
|---|---|---|
| **Carcinoid syndrome** | Rare syndrome caused by carcinoid tumors (neuroendocrine cells), especially metastatic small bowel tumors, which secrete high levels of serotonin (5-HT). Not seen if tumor is limited to GI tract (5-HT undergoes first-pass metabolism in liver). Results in recurrent **diarrhea, cutaneous flushing, asthmatic wheezing,** and **right-sided valvular disease.** Most common tumor of appendix. ↑ 5-HIAA in urine. | **Rule of 1/3s:** 1/3 metastasize 1/3 present with 2nd malignancy 1/3 multiple Derived from neuroendocrine cells of GI tract. Treatment: octreotide. |

| | |
|---|---|
| **Zollinger-Ellison syndrome** | Gastrin-secreting tumor of pancreas or duodenum. Causes recurrent ulcers. May be associated with MEN type 1. |

**Multiple endocrine neoplasias (MEN)**

| Subtype | Characteristics | |
|---|---|---|
| MEN 1 (Wermer's syndrome) | Parathyroid tumors<br>Pituitary tumors (prolactin or GH)<br>Pancreatic endocrine tumors—Zollinger-Ellison syndrome, insulinomas, VIPomas, glucagonomas (rare)<br>Commonly presents with kidney stones and stomach ulcers | MEN 1 = **3 P's** (**P**ancreas, **P**ituitary, and **P**arathyroid).<br>MEN 2A = **2 P's** (**P**heochromocytoma and **P**arathyroid).<br>MEN 2B = **1 P** (**P**heochromocytoma). |
| MEN 2A (Sipple's syndrome) | Medullary thyroid carcinoma (secretes calcitonin)<br>Pheochromocytoma<br>Parathyroid tumors | All MEN syndromes have autosomal-dominant inheritance. |
| MEN 2B | Medullary thyroid carcinoma (secretes calcitonin)<br>Pheochromocytoma<br>Oral/intestinal ganglioneuromatosis (associated with marfanoid habitus) | Associated with *ret* gene in MEN types 2A and 2B. |

**Diabetes drugs**   Treatment strategy for type 1 DM—low-sugar diet, insulin replacement.
Treatment strategy for type 2 DM—dietary modification and exercise for weight loss; oral hypoglycemics and insulin replacement.

| Drug Classes | Action | Clinical Use | Toxicities |
|---|---|---|---|
| **Insulin:**<br>Lispro (short-acting)<br>Aspart (short-acting)<br>Regular (short-acting)<br>NPH (intermediate)<br>Glargine (long-acting)<br>Detemir (long-acting) | **Bind insulin receptor**<br>(tyrosine kinase activity).<br>Liver: ↑ glucose stored as glycogen.<br>Muscle: ↑ glycogen and protein synthesis, $K^+$ uptake.<br>Fat: aids TG storage. | Type 1 DM, type 2 DM<br>Also life-threatening hyperkalemia and stress-induced hyperglycemia. | Hypoglycemia, hypersensitivity reaction (very rare). |
| **Sulfonylureas:**<br>First generation:<br>Tolbutamide<br>Chlorpropamide<br>Second generation:<br>Glyburide<br>Glimepiride<br>Glipizide | Close $K^+$ channel in β-cell membrane, so cell depolarizes → **triggering of insulin release** via ↑ $Ca^{2+}$ influx. | Stimulate release of endogenous insulin in type 2 DM. Require some islet function, so useless in type 1 DM. | First generation: disulfiram-like effects.<br>Second generation: hypoglycemia. |
| **Biguanides:**<br>Metformin | Exact mechanism is unknown. Possibly ↓ **gluconeogenesis,** ↑ glycolysis, ↓ serum glucose levels. Overall acts as insulin sensitizer. | Used as oral hypoglycemic. Can be used in patients without islet function. | Most grave adverse effect is lactic acidosis (contraindicated in renal failure). |
| **Glitazones/**<br>**thiazolidinediones:**<br>Pioglitazone<br>Rosiglitazone | ↑ insulin sensitivity in peripheral tissue. | Used as monotherapy in type 2 DM or combined with above agents. | Weight gain, edema. Hepatotoxicity, CV toxicity. |
| **α-glucosidase inhibitors:**<br>Acarbose<br>Miglitol | **Inhibit intestinal brush-border α-glucosidases.** Delayed sugar hydrolysis and glucose absorption lead to ↓ postprandial hyperglycemia. | Used as monotherapy in type 2 DM or in combination with above agents. | GI disturbances. |
| **Mimetics:**<br>Pramlintide | ↓ glucagon. | Type 2 DM. | Hypoglycemia, nausea, diarrhea. |
| **GLP-1 mimetics:**<br>Exenatide | ↑ insulin, ↓ glucagon release. | Type 2 DM. | Nausea, vomiting; pancreatitis. |

**Orlistat**

| | |
|---|---|
| Mechanism | Alters fat metabolism by inhibiting pancreatic lipases.   **Orl**istat gets rid of **fat**. |
| Clinical use | Long-term obesity management (in conjunction with modified diet). |
| Toxicity | Steatorrhea, GI discomfort, reduced absorption of fat-soluble vitamins, headache. |

## Sibutramine

| | |
|---|---|
| Mechanism | Sympathomimetic serotonin and norepinephrine reuptake inhibitor. |
| Clinical use | Short-term and long-term obesity management. |
| Toxicity | Hypertension and tachycardia. |

## Propylthiouracil, methimazole

| | |
|---|---|
| Mechanism | Inhibit organification of iodide and coupling of thyroid hormone synthesis. Propylthiouracil also ↓ peripheral conversion of $T_4$ to $T_3$. |
| Clinical use | Hyperthyroidism. |
| Toxicity | Skin rash, agranulocytosis (rare), aplastic anemia. |

## Levothyroxine, triiodothyronine

| | |
|---|---|
| Mechanism | Thyroxine replacement. |
| Clinical use | Hypothyroidism, myxedema. |
| Toxicity | Tachycardia, heat intolerance, tremors, arrhythmias. |

## Hypothalamic/pituitary drugs

| Drug | Clinical use |
|---|---|
| GH | GH deficiency, Turner's syndrome |
| Somatostatin (octreotide) | Acromegaly, carcinoid, gastrinoma, glucagonoma |
| Oxytocin | Stimulates labor, uterine contractions, milk let-down; controls uterine hemorrhage |
| ADH (desmopressin) | Pituitary (central, not nephrogenic) DI |

## Demeclocycline

| | |
|---|---|
| Mechanism | ADH antagonist (member of the tetracycline family). |
| Clinical use | SIADH. |
| Toxicity | Nephrogenic DI, photosensitivity, abnormalities of bone and teeth. |

## Glucocorticoids

| | |
|---|---|
| | Hydrocortisone, prednisone, triamcinolone, dexamethasone, beclomethasone. |
| Mechanism | ↓ the production of leukotrienes and prostaglandins by inhibiting phospholipase $A_2$ and expression of COX-2. |
| Clinical use | Addison's disease, inflammation, immune suppression, asthma. |
| Toxicity | Iatrogenic Cushing's syndrome—buffalo hump, moon facies, truncal obesity, muscle wasting, thin skin, easy bruisability, osteoporosis, adrenocortical atrophy, peptic ulcers, diabetes (if chronic). |

# Gastrointestinal

*"A good set of bowels is worth more to a man than any quantity of brains."*
— Josh Billings

*"Man should strive to have his intestines relaxed all the days of his life."*
— Moses Maimonides

*"The colon is the playing field for all human emotions."*
— Cyrus Kapadia, MD

▶ Anatomy

▶ Physiology

▶ Pathology

▶ Pharmacology

## Abdominal layers

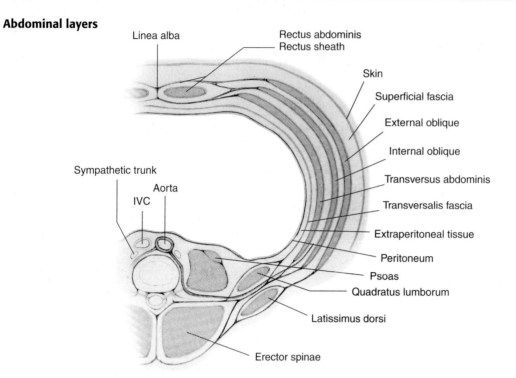

(Reproduced, with permission, from White JS. *USMLE Road Map: Gross Anatomy,* 1st ed. New York: McGraw-Hill, 2003: 67.)

## Retroperitoneal structures

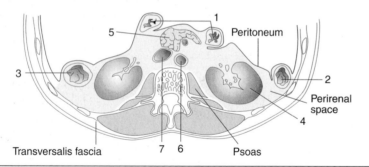

1. Duodenum (2nd, 3rd, 4th parts)
2. Descending colon
3. Ascending colon
4. Kidney and ureters
5. Pancreas (except tail)
6. Aorta
7. IVC

Adrenal glands and rectum (not shown in diagram)

## Important GI ligaments

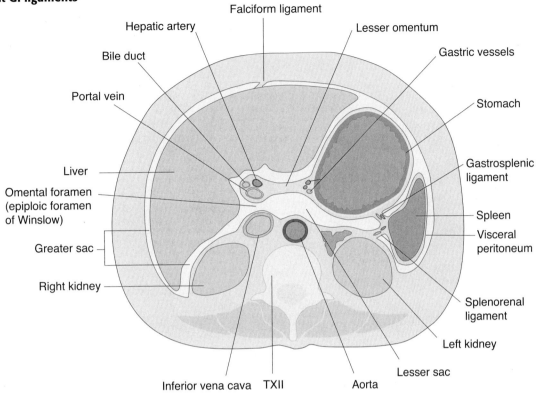

| Ligament | Connects | Structures Contained | Notes |
|---|---|---|---|
| Falciform | Liver to anterior abdominal wall | Ligamentum teres | Derivative of fetal umbilical vein |
| Hepatoduodenal | Liver to duodenum | Portal triad: hepatic artery, portal vein, common bile duct | May be compressed between thumb and index finger placed in omental foramen (epiploic foramen of Winslow) to control bleeding<br>Connects greater and lesser sacs |
| Gastrohepatic (not shown) | Liver to lesser curvature of stomach | Gastric arteries | Separates right greater and lesser sacs<br>May be cut during surgery to access lesser sac |
| Gastrocolic (not shown) | Greater curvature and transverse colon | Gastroepiploic arteries | Part of greater omentum |
| Gastrosplenic | Greater curvature and spleen | Short gastrics | Separates left greater and lesser sacs |
| Splenorenal | Spleen to posterior abdominal wall | Splenic artery and vein | |

## Digestive tract anatomy

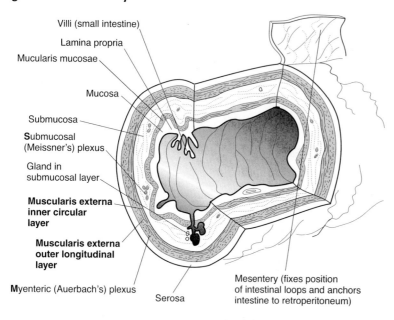

Villi (small intestine)
Lamina propria
Mucularis mucosae
Mucosa
Submucosa
Submucosal (Meissner's) plexus
Gland in submucosal layer
Muscularis externa inner circular layer
Muscularis externa outer longitudinal layer
Myenteric (Auerbach's) plexus
Serosa
Mesentery (fixes position of intestinal loops and anchors intestine to retroperitoneum)

Layers of gut wall (inside to outside):
1. **Mucosa**—epithelium (absorption), lamina propria (support), muscularis mucosae (motility)
2. **Submucosa**—includes Submucosal nerve plexus (Meissner's)
3. **Muscularis externa**—includes **M**yenteric nerve plexus (Auerbach's)
4. **Serosa/adventitia**

Frequencies of basal electric rhythm (slow waves):
Stomach—3 waves/min
Duodenum—12 waves/min
Ileum—8–9 waves/min

(Adapted, with permission, from McPhee S et al. *Pathophysiology of Disease: An Introduction to Clinical Medicine,* 3rd ed. New York: McGraw-Hill, 2000: 296.)

## Digestive tract histology

| Organ | Histology |
|---|---|
| Esophagus | Nonkeratinized stratified squamous epithelium. |
| Stomach | Gastric glands. |
| Duodenum | Villi and microvilli ↑ absorptive surface. Duodenum > jejunum > ileum. |
| | Brunner's glands (submucosa) and crypts of Lieberkühn. |
| Jejunum | Jejunum has largest number of goblet cells in the small intestine. Plicae circulares and crypts of Lieberkühn. |
| Ileum | Peyer's patches (lamina propria, submucosa), plicae circulares (proximal ileum), and crypts of Lieberkühn. |
| Colon | Colon has crypts but no villi. |

## Enteric nerve plexuses

| | |
|---|---|
| Myenteric (Auerbach's) | Coordinates **M**otility along entire gut wall. Contains cell bodies of some parasympathetic terminal effector neurons. Located between inner (circular) and outer (longitudinal) layers of smooth muscle in GI tract wall (**AU**erbach's is on the **AU**tside). |
| Submucosal (Meissner's) | Regulates local Secretions, blood flow, and absorption. Contains cell bodies of some parasympathetic terminal effector neurons. Located between mucosa and inner layer of smooth muscle in GI tract wall. |

## Esophageal anatomy

| | |
|---|---|
| Upper ⅓ | Striated muscle. |
| Middle ⅓ | Striated and smooth muscle. |
| Lower ⅓ | Smooth muscle. |

HIGH-YIELD SYSTEMS

GASTROINTESTINAL

**Aorta and its branches**

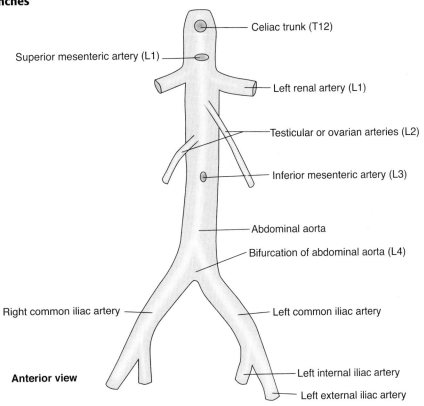

Celiac trunk (T12)

Superior mesenteric artery (L1)

Left renal artery (L1)

Testicular or ovarian arteries (L2)

Inferior mesenteric artery (L3)

Abdominal aorta

Bifurcation of abdominal aorta (L4)

Right common iliac artery

Left common iliac artery

**Anterior view**

Left internal iliac artery

Left external iliac artery

**GI blood supply and innervation**

| Embryonic gut region | Artery | Parasympathetic innervation | Vertebral level | Structures supplied |
|---|---|---|---|---|
| Foregut | Celiac | Vagus | T12/L1 | Stomach to proximal duodenum; liver, gallbladder, pancreas, spleen (mesoderm) |
| Midgut | SMA | Vagus | L1 | Distal duodenum to proximal $2/3$ of transverse colon |
| Hindgut | IMA | Pelvic | L3 | Distal $1/3$ of transverse colon to upper portion of rectum; splenic flexure is a watershed region |

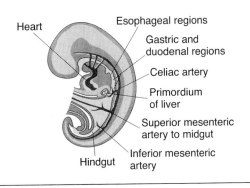

Heart

Esophageal regions

Gastric and duodenal regions

Celiac artery

Primordium of liver

Superior mesenteric artery to midgut

Hindgut

Inferior mesenteric artery

**Celiac trunk**    Branches of celiac trunk: common hepatic, splenic, left gastric. These comprise the main blood supply of the stomach.

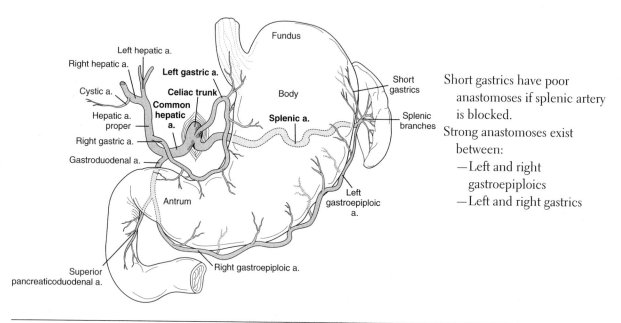

Short gastrics have poor anastomoses if splenic artery is blocked.

Strong anastomoses exist between:
—Left and right gastroepiploics
—Left and right gastrics

**Collateral circulation**    If the abdominal aorta is blocked, these arterial anastomoses (origin) compensate:
1. Internal thoracic/mammary (subclavian) ↔ superior epigastric (internal thoracic) ↔ inferior epigastric (external iliac)
2. Superior pancreaticoduodenal (celiac trunk) ↔ inferior pancreaticoduodenal (SMA)
3. Middle colic (SMA) ↔ left colic (IMA)
4. Superior rectal (IMA) ↔ middle rectal (internal iliac)

## Portosystemic anastomoses

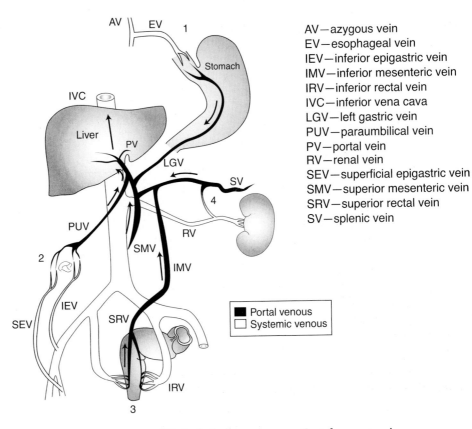

AV—azygous vein
EV—esophageal vein
IEV—inferior epigastric vein
IMV—inferior mesenteric vein
IRV—inferior rectal vein
IVC—inferior vena cava
LGV—left gastric vein
PUV—paraumbilical vein
PV—portal vein
RV—renal vein
SEV—superficial epigastric vein
SMV—superior mesenteric vein
SRV—superior rectal vein
SV—splenic vein

Portal venous
Systemic venous

| Site of anastomosis | Clinical sign | Portal ↔ systemic |
|---|---|---|
| 1. Esophagus | Esophageal varices | Left gastric ↔ esophageal |
| 2. Umbilicus | Caput medusae | Paraumbilical ↔ superficial and inferior epigastric |
| 3. Rectum | Internal hemorrhoids | Superior rectal ↔ middle and inferior rectal |

Varices of **gut, butt,** and **caput** (medusae) are commonly seen with portal hypertension. Inserting a portocaval shunt between the splenic and left renal veins (4 in diagram above) or connecting the portal vein to the IVC (not shown) relieves portal hypertension by shunting blood to the systemic circulation.

## Pectinate line

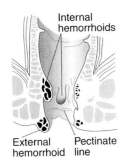

Internal hemorrhoids

External hemorrhoid   Pectinate line

Formed where hindgut meets ectoderm.

**Above pectinate line**—internal hemorrhoids, adenocarcinoma. Arterial supply from superior rectal artery (branch of IMA). Venous drainage is to superior rectal vein → inferior mesenteric vein → portal system.

**Below pectinate line**—external hemorrhoids, squamous cell carcinoma. Arterial supply from inferior rectal artery (branch of internal pudendal artery). Venous drainage to inferior rectal vein → internal pudendal vein → internal iliac vein → IVC.

Internal hemorrhoids receive visceral innervation and are therefore NOT painful. Can be a sign of portal hypertension.

External hemorrhoids receive somatic innervation and are therefore painful. Innervated by inferior rectal nerve (branch of pudendal nerve).

**Liver anatomy**

Apical surface of hepatocytes faces bile canaliculi. Basolateral surface faces sinusoids.

Zone I: periportal zone:
—Affected 1st by viral hepatitis
Zone II: intermediate zone.
Zone III: pericentral vein (centrilobular) zone:
—Affected 1st by ischemia
—Contains P-450 system
—Most sensitive to toxic injury
—Alcoholic hepatitis

Sinusoids draining to central vein
Liver cell plates
Bile canaliculus
Kupffer cell
Bile ductule
Space of Disse (lymphatic drainage)
Branch of portal vein
Central vein (to hepatic veins and systemic circulation)
Branch of hepatic artery
Portal triad
Blood flow
Bile flow
Zone I    Zone II    Zone III

**Sinusoids of liver**

Irregular "capillaries" with fenestrated endothelium (pores 100–200 nm in diameter). No basement membrane. Allow macromolecules of plasma full access to basal surface of hepatocytes through perisinusoidal space (space of Disse).

**Biliary structures**

Central veins, to hepatic veins, to inferior vena cava and systemic circulation

Right hepatic duct
Left hepatic duct
Cystic duct
Common hepatic duct
Gallbladder
Common bile duct
Pancreatic duct
Sphincter of Oddi (around the duct)
Ampulla of Vater (lumen of the duct)
Duodenum

## Femoral region

**Organization**  Lateral to medial: Nerve-Artery-Vein-Empty space-Lymphatics.  You go from lateral to medial to find your **NAVEL**.
**Venous** near the **penis**.

**Femoral triangle**  Contains femoral vein, artery, nerve.

**Femoral sheath**  Fascial tube 3–4 cm below inguinal ligament. Contains femoral vein, artery, and canal (deep inguinal lymph nodes) but **not** femoral nerve.

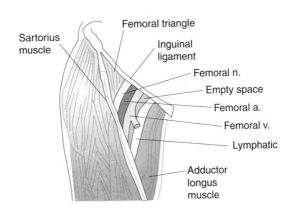

Sartorius muscle
Femoral triangle
Inguinal ligament
Femoral n.
Empty space
Femoral a.
Femoral v.
Lymphatic
Adductor longus muscle

## Inguinal canal

Parietal peritoneum
Internal (deep) inguinal ring: site of protrusion of indirect hernia
Inferior epigastric vessels
Abdominal wall: site of protrusion of direct hernia
Medial umbilical ligament
Median umbilical ligament
Transversalis fascia
Rectus abdominis m.
Transversus abdominis
Pyramidalis m.
Internal oblique
Linea alba
External oblique
Inguinal ligament
External (superficial) inguinal ring
Spermatic cord
External spermatic fascia
Cremasteric muscle and fascia
Internal spermatic fascia

(Adapted, with permission, from White JS. *USMLE Road Map: Gross Anatomy,* 1st ed. New York: McGraw-Hill, 2003: 69.)

**Hernias**  A protrusion of peritoneum through an opening, usually a site of weakness.

Diaphragmatic hernia

Abdominal structures enter the thorax; may occur in infants as a result of defective development of pleuroperitoneal membrane. Most commonly a **hiatal hernia**, in which stomach herniates upward through the esophageal hiatus of the diaphragm.

**Sliding** hiatal hernia is most common. GE junction is displaced; "hourglass stomach."

**Paraesophageal hernia**—GE junction is normal. Cardia moves into the thorax.

Indirect inguinal hernia

Goes through the **IN**ternal (deep) inguinal ring, external (superficial) inguinal ring, and **IN**to the scrotum. Enters internal inguinal ring lateral to inferior epigastric artery. Occurs in **IN**fants owing to failure of processus vaginalis to close. Much more common in males.

An indirect inguinal hernia follows the path of descent of the testes. Covered by all 3 layers of spermatic fascia.

Direct inguinal hernia

Protrudes through the inguinal (Hesselbach's) triangle. Bulges directly through abdominal wall medial to inferior epigastric artery. Goes through the external (superficial) inguinal ring only. Covered by external spermatic fascia. Usually in older men.

**MD**s don't **LI**e:
  **M**edial to inferior epigastric artery = **D**irect hernia.
  **L**ateral to inferior epigastric artery = **I**ndirect hernia.

Femoral hernia

Protrudes below inguinal ligament through femoral canal below and lateral to pubic tubercle. More common in women.

Leading cause of bowel incarceration.

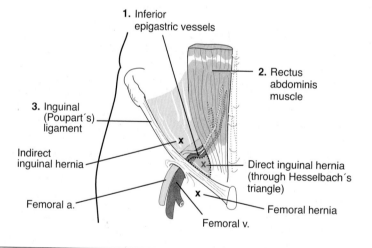

1. Inferior epigastric vessels
2. Rectus abdominis muscle
3. Inguinal (Poupart's) ligament
Indirect inguinal hernia
Femoral a.
Direct inguinal hernia (through Hesselbach's triangle)
Femoral hernia
Femoral v.

Hesselbach's triangle:
  Inferior epigastric artery
  Lateral border of rectus abdominis
  Inguinal ligament

### GI hormones

| Hormone | Source | Action | Regulation | Notes |
|---|---|---|---|---|
| Gastrin | G cells (antrum of stomach) | ↑ gastric $H^+$ secretion<br>↑ growth of gastric mucosa<br>↑ gastric motility | ↑ by stomach distention, amino acids, peptides, vagal stimulation<br>↓ by stomach pH < 1.5 | ↑↑ in Zollinger-Ellison syndrome. Phenylalanine and tryptophan are potent stimulators. |
| Cholecysto-kinin | I cells (duodenum, jejunum) | ↑ pancreatic secretion<br>↑ gallbladder contraction<br>↓ gastric emptying | ↑ by fatty acids, amino acids | In cholelithiasis, pain worsens after fatty food ingestion due to ↑ CCK. |
| Secretin | S cells (duodenum) | ↑ pancreatic $HCO_3^-$ secretion<br>↓ gastric acid secretion<br>↑ bile secretion | ↑ by acid, fatty acids in lumen of duodenum | ↑ $HCO_3^-$ neutralizes gastric acid in duodenum, allowing pancreatic enzymes to function. |
| Somatostatin | D cells (pancreatic islets, GI mucosa) | ↓ gastric acid and pepsinogen secretion<br>↓ pancreatic and small intestine fluid secretion<br>↓ gallbladder contraction<br>↓ insulin and glucagon release | ↑ by acid<br>↓ by vagal stimulation | Inhibitory hormone. Antigrowth hormone effects (digestion and absorption of substances needed for growth). Used to treat VIPoma and carcinoid tumors. |
| Glucose-dependent insulinotropic peptide (GIP) | K cells (duodenum, jejunum) | Exocrine:<br>↓ gastric $H^+$ secretion<br>Endocrine:<br>↑ insulin release | ↑ by fatty acids, amino acids, oral glucose | An oral glucose load is used more rapidly than the equivalent given by IV. |
| Vasoactive intestinal polypeptide (VIP) | Parasympathetic ganglia in sphincters, gallbladder, small intestine | ↑ intestinal water and electrolyte secretion<br>↑ relaxation of intestinal smooth muscle and sphincters | ↑ by distention and vagal stimulation<br>↓ by adrenergic input | **VIPoma**—non-α, non-β islet cell pancreatic tumor that secretes VIP. Copious diarrhea. |
| Nitric oxide | | ↑ smooth muscle relaxation, including lower esophageal sphincter | | Loss of NO secretion is implicated in ↑ lower esophageal tone of achalasia. |
| Motilin | Small intestine | Produces migrating motor complexes (MMCs) | ↑ in fasting state | |
| Ghrelin | P/D1 cells (stomach) | ↑ growth hormone, ACTH, cortisol, and prolactin secretion | ↑ before meals<br>↓ after meals | Regulates hunger, meal initiation. Lost following gastric bypass surgery. Associated with hyperphagia in Prader-Willi. |

### GI secretory products

| Product | Source | Action | Regulation | Notes |
|---|---|---|---|---|
| Intrinsic factor | Parietal cells (stomach) | Vitamin $B_{12}$ binding protein (required for $B_{12}$ uptake in terminal ileum) | | Autoimmune destruction of parietal cells → chronic gastritis and pernicious anemia. |
| Gastric acid | Parietal cells (stomach) | ↓ stomach pH | ↑ by histamine, ACh, gastrin<br>↓ by somatostatin, GIP, prostaglandin, secretin | **Gastrinoma:** gastrin-secreting tumor that causes continuous high levels of acid secretion and ulcers. |
| Pepsin | Chief cells (stomach) | Protein digestion | ↑ by vagal stimulation, local acid | Inactive pepsinogen → pepsin by $H^+$. |
| $HCO_3^-$ | Mucosal cells (stomach, duodenum, salivary glands, pancreas) and Brunner's glands (duodenum) | Neutralizes acid | ↑ pancreatic and biliary secretion with secretin | $HCO_3^-$ is trapped in mucus that covers the gastric epithelium. |

### Locations of GI secretory cells

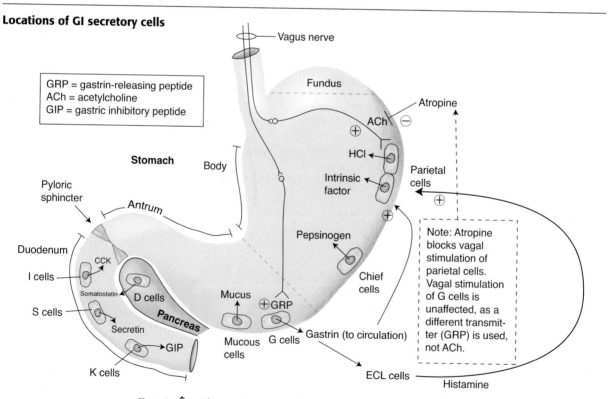

Gastrin ↑ acid secretion primarily through its effects on ECL cells (leading to histamine release) rather than through its direct effect on parietal cells.

## Salivary secretion

| | | |
|---|---|---|
| Source | Parotid (most serous), submandibular, submaxillary, and sublingual (most mucinous) glands. | Serous on the Sides (parotids); Mucinous in the Middle (sublingual). |
| Function | 1. α-amylase (ptyalin) begins starch digestion; inactivated by low pH on reaching stomach<br>2. Bicarbonate neutralizes oral bacterial acids, maintains dental health<br>3. Mucins (glycoproteins) lubricate food<br>4. Antibacterial secretory products<br>5. Growth factors that promote epithelial renewal | Salivary secretion is stimulated by both sympathetic (T1–T3 superior cervical ganglion) and parasympathetic (facial, glossopharyngeal nerve) activity. Low flow rate → hypotonic (more time to reabsorb $Na^+$ and $Cl^-$). High flow rate → closer to isotonic (less time to reabsorb $Na^+$ and $Cl^-$).<br>CN VII runs through parotid gland. Can be damaged during surgery. |

## Gastric parietal cell

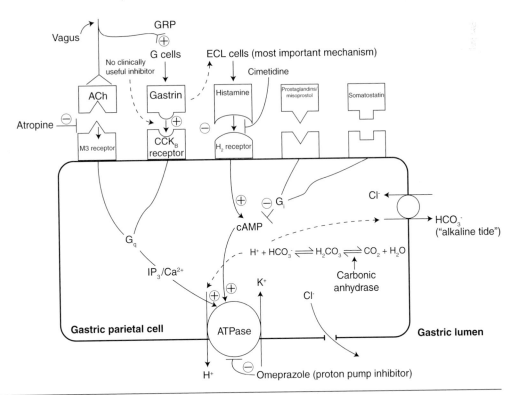

## Brunner's glands

Secrete alkaline mucus to neutralize acid contents entering the duodenum from the stomach. Located in **duodenal submucosa** (the only GI submucosal glands). Hypertrophy of Brunner's glands is seen in peptic ulcer disease.

| | |
|---|---|
| **Pancreatic enzymes** | α-amylase—starch digestion, secreted in active form.<br>Lipase, phospholipase A, colipase—fat digestion.<br>Proteases (trypsin, chymotrypsin, elastase, carboxypeptidases)—protein digestion, secreted as proenzymes also known as "zymogens."<br>Trypsinogen—converted to active enzyme trypsin by **enterokinase/enteropeptidase**, an enzyme secreted from duodenal mucosa. Trypsin activates other proenzymes and more trypsinogen (positive feedback loop). |

### Carbohydrate digestion

| | |
|---|---|
| Salivary amylase | Starts digestion, hydrolyzes α-1,4 linkages to yield disaccharides (maltose, maltotriose, and α-limit dextrans). |
| Pancreatic amylase | Highest concentration in duodenal lumen, hydrolyzes starch to oligosaccharides and disaccharides. |
| Oligosaccharide hydrolases | At brush border of intestine, the rate-limiting step in carbohydrate digestion, produce monosaccharides from oligo- and disaccharides. |

| | |
|---|---|
| **Carbohydrate absorption** | Only monosaccharides (glucose, galactose, fructose) are absorbed by enterocytes. Glucose and galactose are taken up by SGLT1 ($Na^+$ dependent). Fructose is taken up by facilitated diffusion by GLUT-5. All are transported to blood by GLUT-2. |

### Vitamin/mineral absorption

| | |
|---|---|
| Iron | Absorbed as $Fe^{2+}$ in duodenum. |
| Folate | Absorbed in jejunum. |
| $B_{12}$ | Absorbed in ileum along with bile acids. |

| | | |
|---|---|---|
| **Peyer's patches** | Unencapsulated lymphoid tissue found in lamina propria and submucosa of small intestine. Contain specialized M cells that take up antigen.<br>B cells stimulated in germinal centers of Peyer's patches differentiate into IgA-secreting plasma cells, which ultimately reside in lamina propria. IgA receives protective secretory component and is then transported across epithelium to gut to deal with intraluminal antigen. | Think of **IgA**, the Intra-gut Antibody. And always say "secretory IgA." |

| | |
|---|---|
| **Bile** | Composed of bile salts (bile acids conjugated to glycine or taurine, making them water soluble), phospholipids, cholesterol, bilirubin, water, and ions. The only significant mechanism for cholesterol excretion. Needed for digestion of triglycerides and micelle formation in small intestine. |

| **Bilirubin** | Product of heme metabolism. Bilirubin is removed from blood by liver, conjugated with glucuronate, and excreted in bile. Jaundice (yellow skin/sclerae) results from elevated bilirubin levels.<br>Direct bilirubin—conjugated with glucuronic acid; water soluble.<br>Indirect bilirubin—unconjugated; water insoluble. |
|---|---|

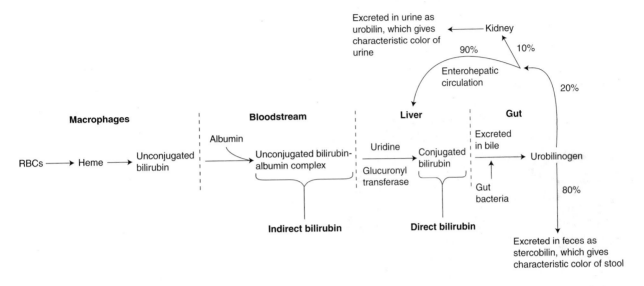

► GASTROINTESTINAL–PATHOLOGY

| **Salivary gland tumors** | Generally benign and occur in parotid gland. Types include pleomorphic adenoma (most common tumor; painless, movable mass; benign with high rate of recurrence), Warthin's tumor (benign; heterotopic salivary gland tissue trapped in a lymph node, surrounded by lymphatic tissue), and mucoepidermoid carcinoma (most common malignant tumor). |
|---|---|

**Achalasia**

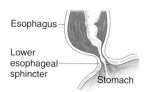

Failure of relaxation of lower esophageal sphincter (LES) due to loss of **myenteric (Auerbach's) plexus**. High LES opening pressure and uncoordinated peristalsis → progressive dysphagia. Barium swallow shows dilated esophagus with an area of distal stenosis. Associated with an ↑ risk of esophageal carcinoma.

*A-chalasia* = absence of relaxation.
"Bird's beak" on barium swallow.
2° achalasia may arise from Chagas' disease.
Scleroderma (CREST syndrome) is associated with esophageal dysmotility involving low pressure proximal to LES.

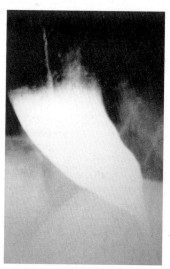

(Reproduced, with permission, from Lalwani AK. *Current Diagnosis & Treatment in Otolaryngology: Head & Neck Surgery,* 2nd ed. New York: McGraw-Hill, 2007, Fig. 35-3.)

**Esophageal pathologies**

| | |
|---|---|
| Gastroesophageal reflux disease (GERD) | Commonly presents as heartburn and regurgitation upon lying down. May also present with nocturnal cough and dyspnea. |
| Esophageal varices | **Painless** bleeding of submucosal veins in lower ⅓ of esophagus (see Image 34). |
| Mallory-Weiss syndrome | **Painful** mucosal lacerations at the gastroesophageal junction due to severe vomiting. Leads to hematemesis. Usually found in alcoholics and bulimics. |
| Boerhaave syndrome | Transmural esophageal rupture due to violent retching. "Been-heaving syndrome." |
| Esophageal strictures | Associated with lye ingestion and acid reflux. |
| Esophagitis | Associated with reflux, infection (HSV-1, CMV, *Candida*), or chemical ingestion. |
| Plummer-Vinson syndrome | Triad of: 1. Dysphagia (due to esophageal webs) 2. Glossitis 3. Iron deficiency anemia |

| **Barrett's esophagus** | Glandular metaplasia—replacement of nonkeratinized (stratified) squamous epithelium with intestinal (columnar) epithelium in the distal esophagus. Due to chronic acid reflux (GERD). | **BARR**ett's = **B**ecomes **A**denocarcinoma, **R**esults from **R**eflux. |

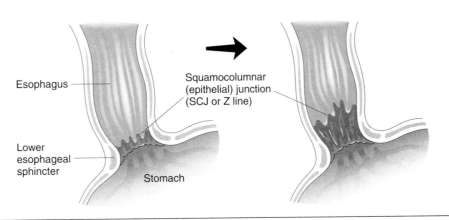

Esophagus

Squamocolumnar (epithelial) junction (SCJ or Z line)

Lower esophageal sphincter

Stomach

| **Esophageal cancer** | Progressive dysphagia (solids → liquids) → weight loss. Risk factors for esophageal cancer are: | |
| | Alcohol/Achalasia | **ABCDEF.** |
| | Barrett's esophagus | Worldwide, squamous cell is |
| | Cigarettes | most common. |
| | Diverticuli (e.g., Zenker's diverticulum) | In the United States, squamous |
| | Esophageal web (e.g., Plummer-Vinson)/ | and adenocarcinoma are |
| | Esophagitis | equal in incidence. |
| | Familial | Squamous cell—upper and |
| | | middle ⅓. |
| | | Adenocarcinoma—lower ⅓. |

| **Malabsorption syndromes** | Can cause diarrhea, steatorrhea, weight loss, weakness. |
| Celiac sprue | Autoantibodies to gluten (gliadin) in wheat and other grains. Proximal small bowel primarily. |
| Tropical sprue | Probably infectious; responds to antibiotics. Similar to celiac sprue, but can affect entire small bowel. |
| Whipple's disease | Infection with *Tropheryma whippelii* (gram positive); PAS-positive macrophages in intestinal lamina propria, mesenteric nodes. Arthralgias, cardiac and neurologic symptoms are common. Most often occurs in older men. |
| Disaccharidase deficiency | Most common is lactase deficiency → milk intolerance. Normal-appearing villi. Osmotic diarrhea. Since lactase is located at tips of intestinal villi, self-limited lactase deficiency can occur following injury (e.g., viral diarrhea). |
| Pancreatic insufficiency | Due to cystic fibrosis, obstructing cancer, and chronic pancreatitis. Causes malabsorption of fat and fat-soluble vitamins (vitamins A, D, E, K). |
| Abeta-lipoproteinemia | ↓ synthesis of apo B → inability to generate chylomicrons → ↓ secretion of cholesterol, VLDL into bloodstream → fat accumulation in enterocytes. Presents in early childhood with malabsorption and neurologic manifestations. |

HIGH-YIELD SYSTEMS

GASTROINTESTINAL

**Celiac sprue**

Autoimmune-mediated intolerance of gliadin (wheat) leading to steatorrhea. Associated with people of northern European descent. Findings include antibodies to **gliadin** and **tissue transglutaminase**, blunting of villi (see Image 33), and lymphocytes in the lamina propria. ↓ mucosal absorption that primarily affects jejunum. Serum levels of tissue transglutaminase antibodies are used for screening. Associated with dermatitis herpetiformis. Moderately ↑ risk of malignancy (e.g., T-cell lymphoma).

**Gastritis**

Acute gastritis (erosive)

Disruption of mucosal barrier → inflammation. Can be caused by stress, NSAIDs (↓ $PGE_2$ → ↓ gastric mucosa production), alcohol, uremia, burns (**Curling's** ulcer—↓ plasma volume → sloughing of gastric mucosa), and brain injury (**Cush**ing's ulcer— ↑ vagal stimulation → ↑ ACh → ↑ $H^+$ production).

Burned by the **Curling** iron. Always **Cush**ion the brain. Especially common among alcoholics and patients taking daily NSAIDs (e.g., patients with rheumatoid arthritis).

Chronic gastritis (nonerosive)

Type A (fundus/ body)

Autoimmune disorder characterized by **A**utoantibodies to parietal cells, pernicious **A**nemia, and **A**chlorhydria. Associated with other autoimmune disorders.

**AB pairing**—pernicious **A**nemia affects gastric **B**ody.

Type B (antrum)

Most common type. Caused by *H. pylori* infection. ↑ risk of MALT lymphoma.

*H. pylori* **B**acterium affects **A**ntrum.

**Ménétrier's disease**

Gastric hypertrophy with protein loss, parietal cell atrophy, and ↑ mucous cells. Precancerous. Rugae of stomach are so hypertrophied that they look like brain gyri.

**Stomach cancer**

Almost always adenocarcinoma. Early aggressive local spread and node/liver mets. Associated with dietary nitrosamines (smoked foods), achlorhydria, chronic gastritis, type A blood. Signet ring cells, acanthosis nigricans are common features. Termed linitis plastica when diffusely infiltrative (thickened, rigid appearance, "leather bottle").

Virchow's node—involvement of left supraclavicular node by mets from stomach.
Krukenberg's tumor—bilateral mets to ovaries. Abundant mucus, signet ring cells.
Sister Mary Joseph's nodule—subcutaneous periumbilical metastasis.

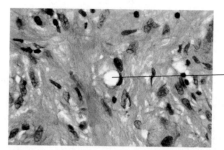

— Signet ring cell

(Reproduced, with permission, from USMLERx.com.)

## Peptic ulcer disease

| | |
|---|---|
| Gastric ulcer | Pain can be **G**reater with meals—weight loss. Often occurs in older patients. *H. pylori* infection in 70%; chronic NSAID use also implicated. Due to ↓ mucosal protection against gastric acid. |
| Duodenal ulcer | Pain **D**ecreases with meals—weight gain. Almost 100% have *H. pylori* infection. Due to ↑ gastric acid secretion (e.g., Zollinger-Ellison syndrome) or ↓ mucosal protection. Hypertrophy of Brunner's glands. Tend to have clean, "punched-out" margins unlike the raised/irregular margins of carcinoma. Potential complications include bleeding, penetration into pancreas, perforation, and obstruction (not intrinsically precancerous). |

### Inflammatory bowel disease (IBD)

| | Crohn's disease | Ulcerative colitis |
|---|---|---|
| Possible etiology | Disordered response to intestinal bacteria. | Autoimmune. |
| Location | Any portion of the GI tract, usually the terminal ileum and colon. **Skip** lesions, **rec**tal sparing. | *Colitis* = colon inflammation. Continuous colonic lesions, always with rectal involvement. |
| Gross morphology | Transmural inflammation. **Cobblestone** mucosa, creeping **fat**, bowel wall thickening ("string sign" on barium swallow x-ray), linear ulcers, fissures, fistulas. | Mucosal and submucosal inflammation only. Friable mucosal pseudopolyps with freely hanging mesentery. Loss of haustra → "lead pipe" appearance on imaging. |
| Microscopic morphology | Noncaseating **gran**ulomas and lymphoid aggregates. | Crypt abscesses and ulcers, bleeding, no granulomas. |
| Complications | Strictures, fistulas, perianal disease, malabsorption, nutritional depletion. | Malnutrition, toxic megacolon, **colorectal carcinoma.** |
| Intestinal manifestation | Diarrhea that may or may not be bloody. | Bloody diarrhea. |
| Extraintestinal manifestations | Migratory polyarthritis, erythema nodosum, ankylosing spondylitis, uveitis, immunologic disorders. | Pyoderma gangrenosum, 1° sclerosing cholangitis. |
| Treatment | Corticosteroids, infliximab. | ASA preparations (sulfasalazine), infliximab, colectomy. |

For **Crohn's**, think of a **fat gran**ny and an old **crone skipping** down a **cobblestone** road away from the **wreck** (rectal sparing).

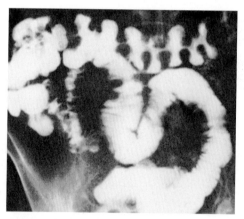

Crohn's disease (note multiple "string sign" lesions)

(Reproduced, with permission, from Way LW, Doherty GM. *Current Surgical Diagnosis & Treatment*, 11th ed. New York: McGraw-Hill, 2003: 691.)

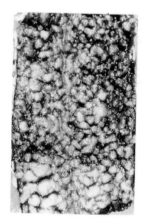

Ulcerative colitis (note pseudopolyps)

---

**Irritable bowel syndrome (IBS)**

Recurrent abdominal pain associated with ≥ 2 of the following:
1. Pain improves with defecation
2. Change in stool frequency
3. Change in appearance of stool

No structural abnormalities. May present with diarrhea, constipation, or alternating. Pathophysiology is multifaceted. Treat symptoms.

| **Appendicitis** | All age groups; most common indication for emergent abdominal surgery in children. Initial diffuse periumbilical pain → localized pain at McBurney's point (⅓ the distance from iliac crest to umbilicus). Nausea, fever; may perforate → peritonitis. Differential: diverticulitis (elderly), ectopic pregnancy (use β-hCG to rule out). | |

**Diverticular disease**

| Diverticulum | Blind pouch protruding from the alimentary tract that communicates with the lumen of the gut. Most diverticula (esophagus, stomach, duodenum, colon) are acquired and are termed "false" in that they lack or have an attenuated muscularis externa. Most often in sigmoid colon. | "**True**" diverticulum—all 3 gut wall layers outpouch. "**False**" diverticulum or pseudodiverticulum—only mucosa and submucosa outpouch. Occur especially where vasa recta perforate muscularis externa. |
|---|---|---|
| Diverticulosis | Many diverticula. Common (in ~50% of people > 60 years). Caused by ↑ intraluminal pressure and focal weakness in colonic wall. Associated with low-fiber diets. Most often in sigmoid colon. | Often asymptomatic or associated with vague discomfort and/or painless rectal bleeding. |
| Diverticulitis | Inflammation of diverticula classically causing LLQ pain, fever, leukocytosis. May perforate → peritonitis, abscess formation, or bowel stenosis (see Image 32). Give antibiotics. | May cause bright red rectal bleeding. May also cause colovesical fistula (fistula with bladder) → pneumaturia. Sometimes called "left-sided appendicitis" due to clinical presentation. |

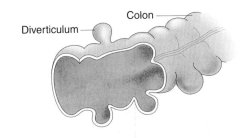

Colon
Diverticulum

| **Zenker's diverticulum** | False diverticulum. Herniation of mucosal tissue at junction of pharynx and esophagus. Presenting symptoms: halitosis (due to trapped food particles), dysphagia, obstruction. | |

| **Meckel's diverticulum** | Persistence of the vitelline duct or yolk stalk. May contain ectopic acid–secreting gastric mucosa and/or pancreatic tissue. **Most common congenital anomaly of the GI tract.** Can cause bleeding, intussusception, volvulus, or obstruction near the terminal ileum. Contrast with omphalomesenteric cyst = cystic dilatation of vitelline duct. | The five 2's: 2 inches long. 2 feet from the ileocecal valve. 2% of population. Commonly presents in first 2 years of life. May have 2 types of epithelia (gastric/ pancreatic). |

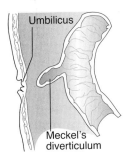

Umbilicus

Meckel's diverticulum

**Intussusception and volvulus**

Intussusception—"telescoping" of 1 bowel segment into distal segment; can compromise blood supply (see Image 35). Unusual in adults (associated with intraluminal mass or tumor). Majority of cases occur in children (usually idiopathic; may be viral [adenovirus]). Abdominal emergency in early childhood.

Volvulus—twisting of portion of bowel around its mesentery; can lead to obstruction and infarction. May occur at cecum and sigmoid colon, where there is redundant mesentery. Usually in elderly.

Intussusception

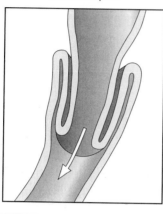

Volvulus

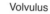
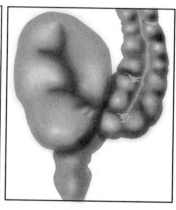

**Hirschsprung's disease**

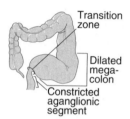

Transition zone

Dilated mega-colon

Constricted aganglionic segment

Congenital megacolon characterized by lack of ganglion cells/enteric nervous plexuses (Auerbach's and Meissner's plexuses) in segment on intestinal biopsy. Due to **failure of neural crest cell migration.**

Presents as chronic constipation early in life. Dilated portion of the colon proximal to the aganglionic segment, resulting in a "transition zone." Involves rectum. Usually failure to pass meconium.

Think of a giant spring that has **sprung** in the colon.
Risk ↑ with Down syndrome.

**Other intestinal disorders**

| | |
|---|---|
| Duodenal atresia | Causes early bilious vomiting with proximal stomach distention ("double bubble") due to failure of recanalization of small bowel. Associated with Down syndrome. |
| Meconium ileus | In cystic fibrosis, meconium plug obstructs intestine, preventing stool passage at birth. |
| Necrotizing enterocolitis | Necrosis of intestinal mucosa and possible perforation. Colon is usually involved, but can involve entire GI tract. In neonates, more common in preemies (↓ immunity). |
| Ischemic colitis | Reduction in intestinal blood causes ischemia. Pain after eating → weight loss. Commonly occurs at splenic flexure and distal colon. Typically affects elderly. |
| Adhesion | Acute bowel obstruction, commonly from a recent surgery. Can have well-demarcated necrotic zones. |
| Angiodysplasia | Tortuous dilation of vessels → bleeding. Most often found in cecum, terminal ileum, and ascending colon. More common in older patients. Confirmed by angiography. |

| **Colonic polyps** | Masses protruding into gut lumen → sawtooth appearance. 90% are non-neoplastic. Often rectosigmoid. |
| | Adenomatous polyps are precancerous. Malignant risk is associated with ↑ size, villous histology, ↑ epithelial dysplasia (see Image 31). Precursor to colorectal cancer (CRC). The more villous the polyp, the more likely it is to be malignant (**VILL**ous = **VILL**ain**OUS**). |
| Hyperplastic | Most common non-neoplastic polyp in colon (> 50% found in rectosigmoid colon). |
| Juvenile | Mostly sporadic lesions in children < 5 years of age. 80% in rectum. If single, no malignant potential. |
| | Juvenile polyposis syndrome—multiple juvenile polyps in GI tract, ↑ risk of adenocarcinoma. |
| Peutz-Jeghers | Single polyps are not malignant. |
| | Peutz-Jeghers syndrome—autosomal-dominant syndrome featuring multiple nonmalignant hamartomas throughout GI tract, along with hyperpigmented mouth, lips, hands, genitalia. Associated with ↑ risk of CRC and other visceral malignancies. |

| **Colorectal cancer (CRC)** | |
| Epidemiology | 3rd most common cancer; 3rd most deadly in United States. Most patients are > 50 years of age. ~ 25% have a family history. |
| Genetics | **Familial adenomatous polyposis (FAP)**—autosomal-dominant mutation of *APC* gene on chromosome 5q. Two-hit hypothesis. 100% progress to CRC. Thousands of polyps; pancolonic; always involves rectum. |
| | **Gardner's syndrome**—FAP + osseous and soft tissue tumors, retinal hyperplasia. |
| | **Turcot's syndrome**—FAP + malignant CNS tumor. **TUR**cot = **TUR**ban. |
| | **Hereditary nonpolyposis colorectal cancer (HNPCC/Lynch syndrome)**—autosomal-dominant mutation of DNA mismatch repair genes. ~ 80% progress to CRC. Proximal colon is always involved. |
| Additional risk factors | IBD, *Streptococcus bovis* bacteremia, tobacco use, large villous adenomas, juvenile polyposis syndrome, Peutz-Jeghers syndrome. |
| Presentation | Distal colon—obstruction, colicky pain, hematochezia. |
| | Proximal colon—dull pain, iron deficiency anemia, fatigue. |
| Diagnosis | Iron deficiency anemia in older males. |
| | Screen patients > 50 years of age with stool occult blood test and colonoscopy. |
| | "Apple core" lesion seen on barium enema x-ray. |
| | CEA tumor marker. |

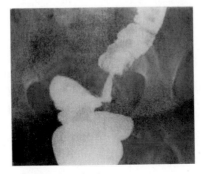

"Apple core" lesion

(Reproduced, with permission, from USMLERx.com.)

**Molecular pathogenesis of CRC**

There are 2 molecular pathways that lead to CRC:

1. Microsatellite instability pathway (15%): DNA mismatch repair gene mutations → sporadic and HNPCC syndrome. Mutations accumulate, but no defined morphologic correlates.
2. APC/β-catenin (chromosomal instability) pathway (85%):

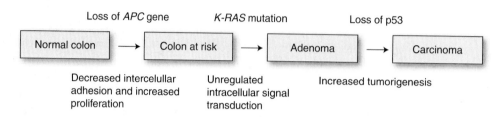

Loss of *APC* gene   *K-RAS* mutation   Loss of p53

Normal colon → Colon at risk → Adenoma → Carcinoma

Decreased intercelullar adhesion and increased proliferation   Unregulated intracellular signal transduction   Increased tumorigenesis

**Carcinoid tumor**

Tumor of endocrine cells. Comprise 50% of small bowel tumors. Most common site is in small intestine. "Dense core bodies" seen on EM. Often produce 5-HT, which can lead to carcinoid syndrome. Classic symptoms: wheezing, right-sided heart murmurs, diarrhea, flushing. If tumor is confined to GI system, no carcinoid syndrome is observed, since liver metabolizes 5-HT. If tumor or metastases (usually to liver) exist outside GI system, carcinoid syndrome is observed. Thus, tumor location determines whether or not the syndrome appears.

**Cirrhosis and portal hypertension**

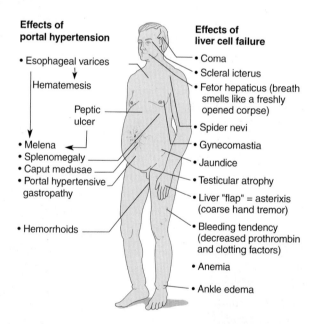

**Effects of portal hypertension**

• Esophageal varices
↓
Hematemesis

Peptic ulcer

• Melena
• Splenomegaly
• Caput medusae
• Portal hypertensive gastropathy

• Hemorrhoids

**Effects of liver cell failure**

• Coma
• Scleral icterus
• Fetor hepaticus (breath smells like a freshly opened corpse)
• Spider nevi
• Gynecomastia
• Jaundice
• Testicular atrophy
• Liver "flap" = asterixis (coarse hand tremor)
• Bleeding tendency (decreased prothrombin and clotting factors)
• Anemia
• Ankle edema

(Adapted, with permission, from Chandrasoma P, Taylor CE. *Concise Pathology*, 3rd ed. Stamford, CT: Appleton & Lange, 1998: 654.)

*Cirrho* (Greek) = tawny yellow. Diffuse fibrosis of liver, destroys normal architecture. Nodular regeneration.

**Micronodular**—nodules < 3 mm, uniform size. Due to metabolic insult (e.g., alcohol, hemochromatosis, Wilson's disease).

**Macronodular**—nodules > 3 mm, varied size. Usually due to significant liver injury leading to hepatic necrosis (e.g., postinfectious or drug-induced hepatitis). ↑ risk of hepatocellular carcinoma.

Shunt between portal and systemic circulation can relieve portal hypertension (see Image 30).

HIGH-YIELD SYSTEMS

GASTROINTESTINAL

| Markers of GI pathology | Serum enzyme | Major diagnostic use |
|---|---|---|
| | Aminotransferases (AST and ALT) | Viral hepatitis (ALT > AST)<br>Alcoholic hepatitis (AST > ALT)<br>Myocardial infarction (AST) |
| | GGT (γ-glutamyl transpeptidase) | Various liver diseases; ↑ with heavy alcohol consumption |
| | Alkaline phosphatase | Obstructive liver disease (hepatocellular carcinoma), bone disease, bile duct disease |
| | Amylase | Acute pancreatitis, mumps |
| | Lipase | Acute pancreatitis |
| | Ceruloplasmin (↓) | Wilson's disease |

**Reye's syndrome**

Rare, often fatal childhood hepatoencephalopathy. Findings: mitochondrial abnormalities, fatty liver (microvesicular fatty change), hypoglycemia, coma. Associated with viral infection (especially VZV and influenza B) that has been treated with salicylates. Mechanism: aspirin metabolites ↓ β-oxidation by reversible inhibition of mitochondrial enzyme. **Aspirin is not recommended for children** (use acetaminophen, with caution).

**Alcoholic liver disease**

| | | |
|---|---|---|
| Hepatic steatosis | Short-term change with moderate alcohol intake. Macrovesicular fatty change that may be reversible with alcohol cessation (see Image 29). | |
| Alcoholic hepatitis | Requires sustained, long-term consumption. Swollen and necrotic hepatocytes with neutrophilic infiltration. **Mallory bodies** (intracytoplasmic eosinophilic inclusions) are present. | You're toASTed with alcoholic hepatitis: AST > ALT (ratio usually > 1.5). |
| Alcoholic cirrhosis | Final and irreversible form. Micronodular, irregularly shrunken liver with "hobnail" appearance (see Image 30). Sclerosis around central vein (zone III). Has manifestations of chronic liver disease (e.g., jaundice, hypoalbuminemia). | |

**Hepatocellular carcinoma/hepatoma**

Most common 1° malignant tumor of the liver in adults. ↑ incidence is associated with hepatitis B and C, Wilson's disease, hemochromatosis, $\alpha_1$-antitrypsin deficiency, alcoholic cirrhosis, and carcinogens (e.g., aflatoxin in peanuts). Findings: jaundice, tender hepatomegaly, ascites, polycythemia, and hypoglycemia.

Commonly spread by hematogenous dissemination.
↑ α-fetoprotein. May lead to Budd-Chiari syndrome.

**Nutmeg liver**

Due to backup of blood into liver. Commonly caused by right-sided heart failure and Budd-Chiari syndrome. The liver appears mottled like a nutmeg. If the condition persists, centrilobular congestion and necrosis can result in cardiac cirrhosis.

| | |
|---|---|
| **Budd-Chiari syndrome** | Occlusion of IVC or hepatic veins with centrilobular congestion and necrosis, leading to congestive liver disease (hepatomegaly, ascites, abdominal pain, and eventual liver failure). May develop varices and have visible abdominal and back veins. Absence of JVD. Associated with polycythemia vera, pregnancy, and hepatocellular carcinoma. |
| **$\alpha_1$-antitrypsin deficiency** | Misfolded gene product protein accumulates in hepatocellular ER. ↓ elastic tissue in lungs → panacinar emphysema. PAS-positive globules in liver. Codominant trait. |
| **Physiologic neonatal jaundice** | At birth, immature UDP-glucuronyl transferase → unconjugated hyperbilirubinemia → jaundice/kernicterus.<br>Treatment: phototherapy (converts UCB to water-soluble form). |
| **Jaundice** | Normally, liver cells convert unconjugated (indirect) bilirubin into conjugated (direct) bilirubin. Direct bilirubin is water soluble and can be excreted into urine and by the liver into bile to be converted by gut bacteria to urobilinogen (some of which is reabsorbed). Some urobilinogen is also formed directly from heme metabolism. |

| Jaundice type | Hyperbilirubinemia | Urine bilirubin | Urine urobilinogen |
|---|---|---|---|
| Hepatocellular | Conjugated/unconjugated | ↑ | Normal/↓ |
| Obstructive | Conjugated | ↑ | ↓ |
| Hemolytic | Unconjugated | Absent (acholuria) | ↑ |

## Hereditary hyperbilirubinemias

| | | |
|---|---|---|
| Gilbert's syndrome | Mildly ↓ UDP-glucuronyl transferase or ↓ bilirubin uptake. Asymptomatic. Elevated unconjugated bilirubin without overt hemolysis. Associated with stress. | No clinical consequences. |
| Crigler-Najjar syndrome, type I | Absent UDP-glucuronyl transferase. Presents early in life; patients die within a few years.<br>Findings: jaundice, kernicterus (bilirubin deposition in brain), ↑ unconjugated bilirubin.<br>Treatment: plasmapheresis and phototherapy. | Type II is less severe and responds to phenobarbital, which ↑ liver enzyme synthesis. |
| Dubin-Johnson syndrome | Conjugated hyperbilirubinemia due to defective liver excretion. Grossly black liver. Benign. | **Rotor's syndrome** is similar but even milder and does not cause black liver. |

1. Gilbert's = problem with bilirubin uptake → unconjugated bilirubinemia
2. Crigler-Najjar = problem with bilirubin conjugation → unconjugated bilirubinemia
3. Dubin-Johnson = problem with excretion of conjugated bilirubin → conjugated bilirubinemia

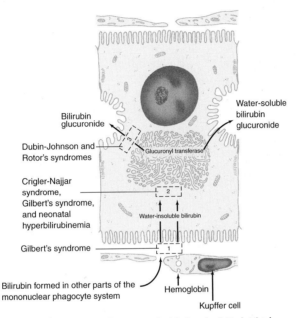

(Adapted, with permission, from Junqueira LC, Carneiro J. *Basic Histology*, 11th ed. New York: McGraw-Hill, 2005: 335.)

| | | |
|---|---|---|
| **Wilson's disease (hepatolenticular degeneration)** | Inadequate hepatic copper excretion and failure of copper to enter circulation as ceruloplasmin. Leads to copper accumulation, especially in liver, brain, cornea, kidneys, and joints.<br>Characterized by:<br>  **A**sterixis<br>  **B**asal ganglia degeneration (parkinsonian symptoms)<br>  **C**eruloplasmin ↓, **C**irrhosis, **C**orneal deposits (Kayser-Fleischer rings—see Image 51), **C**opper accumulation, **C**arcinoma (hepatocellular), **C**horeiform movements<br>  **D**ementia<br>  Hemolytic anemia | Treat with penicillamine. Autosomal-recessive inheritance.<br><br>**ABCD.** |

**Hemochromatosis**

Hemosiderosis is the deposition of hemosiderin (iron); hemochromatosis is the disease caused by this iron deposition (see Image 28). Classic triad of micronodular Cirrhosis, Diabetes mellitus, and skin pigmentation → "bronze" diabetes. Results in CHF and ↑ risk of hepatocellular carcinoma. Disease may be 1° (autosomal recessive) or 2° to chronic transfusion therapy (e.g., β-thalassemia major). ↑ ferritin, ↑ iron, ↓ TIBC → ↑ transferrin saturation.

Hemochromatosis Can Cause Deposits.
Total body iron may reach 50 g, enough to set off metal detectors at airports.
Treatment of hereditary hemochromatosis: repeated phlebotomy, deferoxamine.
Associated with HLA-A3.

**Biliary tract disease**

| | Secondary Biliary Cirrhosis | Primary Biliary Cirrhosis | Primary Sclerosing Cholangitis |
|---|---|---|---|
| Pathophysiology/ pathology | Extrahepatic biliary obstruction (gallstone, biliary stricture, chronic pancreatitis, carcinoma of the pancreatic head) → ↑ pressure in intrahepatic ducts → injury/fibrosis and bile stasis. | Autoimmune reaction → lymphocytic infiltrate + granulomas. ↑ serum mitochondrial antibody. | Unknown cause of concentric "onion skin" bile duct fibrosis → alternating strictures and dilation with "beading" of intra- and extrahepatic bile ducts on ERCP. |
| Presentation | Pruritus, jaundice, dark urine, light stools, hepatosplenomegaly. | Same. | Same. |
| Labs | ↑ conjugated bilirubin, ↑ cholesterol, ↑ alkaline phosphatase. | Same. | Same. |
| Additional information | Complicated by ascending cholangitis. | ↑ **serum mitochondrial antibodies.** Associated with other autoimmune conditions (e.g., CREST, rheumatoid arthritis, celiac disease). | Hypergammaglobulinemia (IgM). Associated with ulcerative colitis. Can lead to 2° biliary cirrhosis. |

## Gallstones (cholelithiasis)

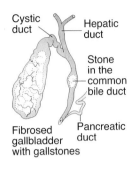

Cystic duct
Hepatic duct
Stone in the common bile duct
Fibrosed gallbladder with gallstones
Pancreatic duct

Form when solubilizing bile acids and lecithin are overwhelmed by ↑ cholesterol and/or bilirubin or gallbladder stasis.

2 types of stones:

1. **Cholesterol stones** (radiolucent with 10–20% opaque due to calcifications)—80% of stones. Associated with obesity, Crohn's disease, cystic fibrosis, advanced age, clofibrate, estrogens, multiparity, rapid weight loss, and Native American origin.

2. **Pigment stones** (radiopaque)—seen in patients with chronic hemolysis, alcoholic cirrhosis, advanced age, and biliary infection.

Can cause ascending cholangitis, acute pancreatitis, bile stasis, cholecystitis.

Can also → **biliary colic**—gallstones interfere with bile flow, causing bile duct contraction. May present without pain (e.g., in diabetics).

Can cause fistula between gallbladder and small intestine. If gallstone obstructs ileocecal valve (gallstone ileus), air can be seen in biliary tree on imaging.

Diagnose with ultrasound. Treat with cholecystectomy.

Risk factors (4 F's):
1. Female
2. Fat
3. Fertile
4. Forty

Charcot's triad of cholangitis:
1. Jaundice
2. Fever
3. RUQ pain

Positive Murphy's sign—inspiratory arrest on deep palpation.

---

## Cholecystitis

Inflammation of gallbladder. Usually from gallstones; rarely ischemia or infectious (CMV). ↑ alkaline phosphatase if bile duct becomes involved (e.g., ascending cholangitis).

---

## Acute pancreatitis

Autodigestion of pancreas by pancreatic enzymes.

Causes: Gallstones, Ethanol, Trauma, Steroids, Mumps, Autoimmune disease, Scorpion sting, Hypercalcemia/Hyperlipidemia, ERCP, Drugs (e.g., sulfa drugs).

Clinical presentation: epigastric abdominal pain radiating to back, anorexia, nausea.

Labs: elevated amylase, lipase (higher specificity).

Can lead to DIC, ARDS, diffuse fat necrosis, hypocalcemia ($Ca^{2+}$ collects in pancreatic calcium soap deposits), pseudocyst formation, hemorrhage, infection, and multiorgan failure.

Chronic pancreatitis can lead to pancreatic insufficiency → steatorrhea, fat-soluble vitamin deficiency, and diabetes mellitus.

Chronic calcifying pancreatitis is strongly associated with alcoholism, ↑ risk of pancreatic cancer.

**GET SMASHED.**

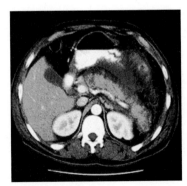

(Reproduced, with permission, from the PEIR Digital Library.)

**Pancreatic adenocarcinoma**

Prognosis averages 6 months or less; very aggressive; usually already metastasized at presentation; tumors more common in pancreatic head (→ obstructive jaundice). ↑ risk in Jewish and African-American males. CEA and CA-19-9 tumor markers. Associated with cigarettes but not EtOH.

Often presents with:
1. Abdominal pain radiating to back
2. Weight loss (due to malabsorption and anorexia)
3. Migratory thrombophlebitis—redness and tenderness on palpation of extremities (Trousseau's syndrome)
4. Obstructive jaundice with palpable gallbladder (Courvoisier's sign)

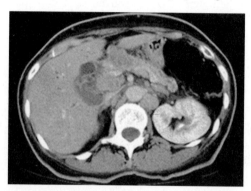

Pancreatic adenocarcinoma (note the large, heterogeneously enhancing mass visible at the neck of the pancreas).

(Reproduced, with permission, from the PEIR Digital Library.)

## GI therapy

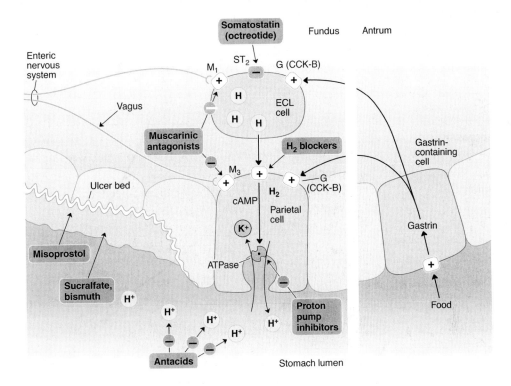

(Adapted, with permission, from Katzung BG, Trevor AJ. *USMLE Road Map: Pharmacology*, 1st ed. New York: McGraw-Hill, 2003: 159.)

| **H$_2$ blockers** | Cimeti**dine**, raniti**dine**, famoti**dine**, nizati**dine**. | Take H$_2$ blockers before you |
|---|---|---|
| Mechanism | Reversible block of histamine H$_2$ receptors → ↓ H$^+$ secretion by parietal cells. | **DINE**. Think **"table for 2"** to remember H$_2$. |
| Clinical use | Peptic ulcer, gastritis, mild esophageal reflux. | |
| Toxicity | Cimetidine is a potent inhibitor of P-450; it also has antiandrogenic effects (prolactin release, gynecomastia, impotence, ↓ libido in males); can cross blood-brain barrier (confusion, dizziness, headaches) and placenta. Both cimetidine and ranitidine ↓ renal excretion of creatinine. Other H$_2$ blockers are relatively free of these effects. | |

| **Proton pump inhibitors** | Omeprazole, lansoprazole. |
|---|---|
| Mechanism | Irreversibly inhibit H$^+$/K$^+$-ATPase in stomach parietal cells. |
| Clinical use | Peptic ulcer, gastritis, esophageal reflux, Zollinger-Ellison syndrome. |

### Bismuth, sucralfate

| | | |
|---|---|---|
| Mechanism | Bind to ulcer base, providing physical protection, and allow $HCO_3^-$ secretion to reestablish pH gradient in the mucous layer. | Triple therapy of *H. pylori* ulcers—**M**etronidazole, **A**moxicillin (or **T**etracycline), **B**ismuth. |
| Clinical use | ↑ ulcer healing, traveler's diarrhea. | Can also use PPI—Please **MA**ke Tummy **B**etter. |

### Misoprostol

| | |
|---|---|
| Mechanism | A $PGE_1$ analog. ↑ production and secretion of gastric mucous barrier, ↓ acid production. |
| Clinical use | Prevention of NSAID-induced peptic ulcers; maintenance of a patent ductus arteriosus. Also used to induce labor. |
| Toxicity | Diarrhea. Contraindicated in women of childbearing potential (abortifacient). |

### Muscarinic antagonists
Pirenzepine, propantheline.

| | |
|---|---|
| Mechanism | Block M1 receptors on ECL cells (↓ histamine secretion) and M3 receptors on parietal cells (↓ $H^+$ secretion). |
| Clinical use | Peptic ulcer (rarely used). |
| Toxicity | Tachycardia, dry mouth, difficulty focusing eyes. |

### Antacid use

| | |
|---|---|
| | Can affect absorption, bioavailability, or urinary excretion of other drugs by altering gastric and urinary pH or by delaying gastric emptying. Overuse can also cause the following problems: |

1. **Aluminum hydroxide**—constipation and hypophosphatemia; proximal muscle weakness, osteodystrophy, seizures — **Alu**mi**nimum** amount of feces.
2. **Magnesium hydroxide**—diarrhea, hyporeflexia, hypotension, cardiac arrest — **Mg** = **M**ust **g**o to the bathroom.
3. **Calcium carbonate**—hypercalcemia, rebound acid ↑

All can cause hypokalemia. — Can chelate and ↓ effectiveness of other drugs (e.g., tetracycline).

### Infliximab

| | | |
|---|---|---|
| Mechanism | A monoclonal antibody to TNF, proinflammatory cytokine. | **INFLIX**imab **INFLIX** pain on TNF. |
| Clinical use | Crohn's disease, rheumatoid arthritis. | |
| Toxicity | Respiratory infection (including reactivation of latent TB), fever, hypotension. | |

### Sulfasalazine

| | |
|---|---|
| Mechanism | A combination of sulfapyridine (antibacterial) and 5-aminosalicylic acid (anti-inflammatory). Activated by colonic bacteria. |
| Clinical use | Ulcerative colitis, Crohn's disease. |
| Toxicity | Malaise, nausea, sulfonamide toxicity, reversible oligospermia. |

### Ondansetron

| | |
|---|---|
| Mechanism | 5-HT$_3$ antagonist. Powerful central-acting antiemetic. |
| Clinical use | Control vomiting postoperatively and in patients undergoing cancer chemotherapy. |
| Toxicity | Headache, constipation. |

You will not vomit with **ONDANS**etron, so you can go **ON DANC**ing.

### Metoclopramide

| | |
|---|---|
| Mechanism | D$_2$ receptor antagonist. ↑ resting tone, contractility, LES tone, motility. Does not influence colon transport time. |
| Clinical use | Diabetic and post-surgery gastroparesis. |
| Toxicity | ↑ parkinsonian effects. Restlessness, drowsiness, fatigue, depression, nausea, diarrhea. Drug interaction with digoxin and diabetic agents. Contraindicated in patients with small bowel obstruction. |

# Hematology and Oncology

▶ Anatomy

▶ Physiology

▶ Pathology

▶ Pharmacology

*"The best blood will at some time get into a fool or a mosquito."*
—Austin O'Malley

*"A day without blood is like a day without sunshine."*
—Joker in *Full Metal Jacket*

Study tip: When reviewing oncologic drugs, focus on mechanisms and side effects. Memorizing clinical uses is lower yield.

## Blood cell differentiation

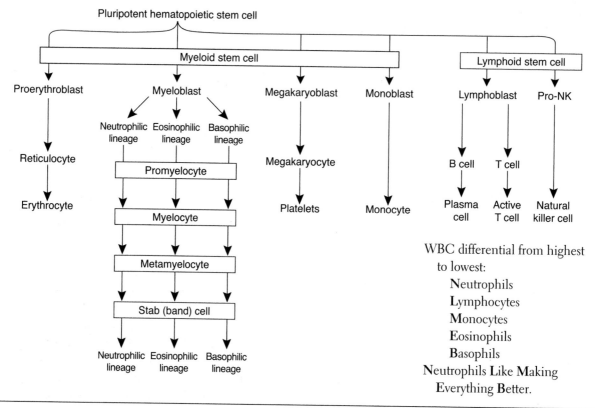

WBC differential from highest to lowest:
  Neutrophils
  Lymphocytes
  Monocytes
  Eosinophils
  Basophils
**N**eutrophils **L**ike **M**aking **E**verything **B**etter.

| | | |
|---|---|---|
| **Erythrocyte** 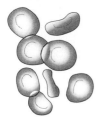 | Anucleate, biconcave → large surface area: volume ratio → easy gas exchange ($O_2$ and $CO_2$). Source of energy—glucose (90% anaerobically degraded to lactate, 10% by HMP shunt). Survival time—120 days. Membrane contains the chloride-bicarbonate antiport important in the "physiologic chloride shift," which allows the RBC to transport $CO_2$ from the periphery to the lungs for elimination. | *Eryth* = red; *cyte* = cell. Erythrocytosis = polycythemia = ↑ number of red cells. Anisocytosis = varying sizes. Poikilocytosis = varying shapes. Reticulocyte = immature erythrocyte. |
| **Platelet (thrombocyte)** | Small cytoplasmic fragment derived from megakaryocytes. Involved in 1° hemostasis. When activated by endothelial injury, aggregates with other platelets and interacts with fibrinogen to form hemostatic plug. Contains dense granules (ADP, calcium) and α-granules (vWF, fibrinogen). Approximately ⅓ of platelet pool is stored in the spleen. Life span of 8–10 days. | Promotes blood clotting and prevents leakage of RBCs from damaged vessels. Thrombocytopenia or platelet dysfunction results in petechiae. |
| **Leukocyte** | Types: granulocytes (basophils, eosinophils, neutrophils) and mononuclear cells (monocytes, lymphocytes). Responsible for defense against infections. Normally 4000–10,000 per microliter. | *Leuk* = white; *cyte* = cell. |

| | | |
|---|---|---|
| **Basophil**<br> | Mediates allergic reaction. < 1% of all leukocytes. Bilobate nucleus. Densely basophilic granules containing heparin (anticoagulant), histamine (vasodilator) and other vasoactive amines, and leukotrienes (LTD-4). Found in the blood. | **Baso**philic—staining readily with **basic** stains. |
| **Mast cell**<br>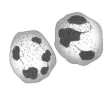 | Mediates allergic reaction. Degranulation— histamine, heparin, and eosinophil chemotactic factors. Can bind IgE to membrane. Mast cells resemble basophils structurally and functionally but are not the same cell type. Found in tissue. | Involved in type I hypersensitivity reactions. Cromolyn sodium prevents mast cell degranulation (used to treat asthma). |
| **Eosinophil**<br>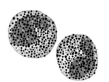 | 1–6% of all leukocytes. Bilobate nucleus. Packed with large eosinophilic granules of uniform size. Defends against helminthic and protozoan infections (major basic protein). Highly phagocytic for antigen-antibody complexes. Produces histaminase and arylsulfatase (help limit reaction following mast cell degranulation). | *Eosin* = a dye; *philic* = loving. Causes of eosinophilia = **NAACP:** **N**eoplastic **A**sthma **A**llergic processes **C**ollagen vascular diseases **P**arasites (invasive) |
| **Neutrophil**<br> | Acute inflammatory response cell. 40–75% WBCs. Phagocytic. Multilobed nucleus. Large, spherical, azurophilic granules (lysosomes) contain hydrolytic enzymes, lysozyme, myeloperoxidase, and lactoferrin. | Hypersegmented polys are seen in vitamin $B_{12}$/ folate deficiency. |
| **Monocyte**<br>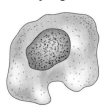 | 2–10% of leukocytes. Large. Kidney-shaped nucleus. Extensive "frosted glass" cytoplasm. Differentiates into macrophages in tissues. | *Mono* = one (nucleus); *cyte* = cell. |
| **Macrophage** | Phagocytoses bacteria, cell debris, and senescent red cells and scavenges damaged cells and tissues. Long life in tissues. Macrophages differentiate from circulating blood monocytes. Activated by γ-interferon. Can function as antigen-presenting cell (APC) via MHC II. | *Macro* = large; *phage* = eater. |

**Dendritic cells**

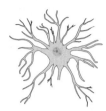

Professional antigen-presenting cells (APCs). Express MHC II and Fc receptor (FcR) on surface. Main inducers of 1° antibody response. Called Langerhans cells on skin.

**Lymphocyte**

Round, densely staining nucleus. Small amount of pale cytoplasm. B lymphocytes produce antibodies. T lymphocytes manifest the cellular immune response as well as regulate B lymphocytes and macrophages.

**B lymphocyte**

Part of humoral immune response. Arises from stem cells in bone marrow. Matures in marrow. Migrates to peripheral lymphoid tissue (follicles of lymph nodes, white pulp of spleen, unencapsulated lymphoid tissue). When antigen is encountered, B cells differentiate into plasma cells and produce antibodies. Has memory. Can function as an APC via MHC II.

B = **B**one marrow.

**Plasma cell**

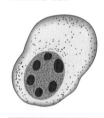

Off-center nucleus, clock-face chromatin distribution, abundant RER and well-developed Golgi apparatus. B cells differentiate into plasma cells, which produce large amounts of antibody specific to a particular antigen.

Multiple myeloma is a plasma cell neoplasm.

**T lymphocyte**

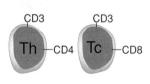

Mediates cellular immune response. Originates from stem cells in the bone marrow, but matures in the thymus. T cells differentiate into cytotoxic T cells (MHC I, CD8), helper T cells (MHC II, CD4), and suppressor T cells. The majority of circulating lymphocytes are T cells (80%).

**T** is for **T**hymus. **CD** is for **C**luster of **D**ifferentiation. **MHC** × **CD** = 8 (e.g., MHC 2 × CD4 = 8, and MHC 1 × CD8 = 8).

## Blood groups

| | | |
|---|---|---|
| A | A antigen on RBC surface and B antibody in plasma. | Incompatible blood transfusions can cause immunologic response, hemolysis, renal failure, shock, and death. Note: anti-AB antibodies—IgM (do not cross placenta); anti-Rh—IgG (cross placenta). |
| B | B antigen on RBC surface and A antibody in plasma. | |
| AB | A and B antigens on RBC surface; no antibodies in plasma; "universal recipient." | |
| O | Neither A nor B antigen on RBC surface; both antibodies in plasma; "universal donor." | |
| Rh | Rh+ indicates presence of antigen; Rh− indicates absence. Rh− mothers exposed to Rh+ blood (often during birth) may make anti-Rh IgG that can cross placenta during subsequent pregnancy, causing hemolytic disease of the newborn (erythroblastosis fetalis). Rh antigen immunoglobulin is given to mother after delivery to prevent future erythroblastosis. | |

## Convergence of coagulation, complement, and kinin pathways

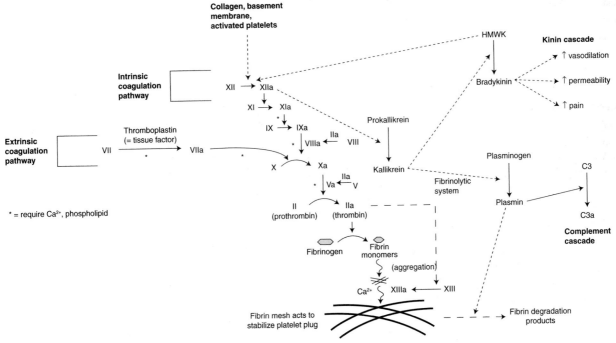

Note: Kallikrein activates bradykinin; ACE inactivates bradykinin.

Hemophilia A: deficiency of factor VIII.

Hemophilia B: deficiency of factor IX.

Vitamin K deficiency: ↓ synthesis of factors II, VII, IX, X, protein C, protein S.

Antithrombin: inhibits thrombin and factors IXa, Xa, XIa, and XIIa. Activated by heparin.

## Thrombogenesis (formation of insoluble fibrin mesh)

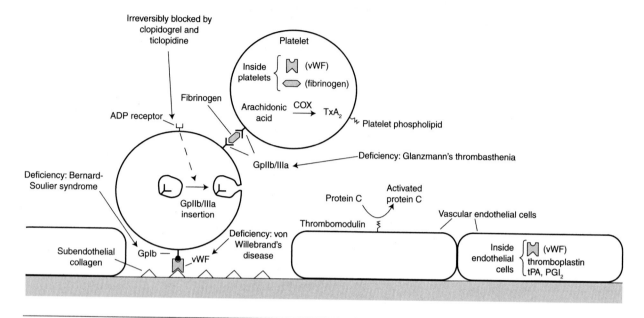

## Coagulation cascade and platelet plug formation

Components of platelet plug formation

1. **Adhesion**—vWF mediates linking of platelet Gp1b receptor to subendothelial collagen
2. **Aggregation**—represents a balance between pro-aggregation and anti-aggregation factors:
   —$TxA_2$ released by platelets ↑ aggregation
   —$PGI_2$ and NO released by endothelial cells ↓ aggregation
3. **Swelling**—binding of ADP on platelet receptors → insertion of GpIIb/IIIa on platelet membrane, allowing platelet cohesion; $Ca^{2+}$ also strengthens platelet plug

Aspirin inhibits cyclooxygenase, inhibiting $TxA_2$ synthesis.
Ticlopidine and clopidogrel inhibit ADP-induced expression of GpIIb/IIIa.
Abciximab inhibits GpIIb/IIIa directly.

Components of coagulation cascade

1. **Pro-coagulation:**

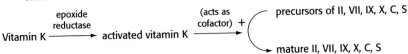

Warfarin inhibits reductase.
Neonates lack enteric bacteria, which produce vitamin K.

von Willebrand's factor carries/protects VIII.

2. **Anti-coagulation:**
   Antithrombin inactivates factors II, VII, IX, X, XI.

Heparin-activated antithrombin.

Protein C $\xrightarrow{\text{protein S; thrombomodulin (endothelial cells)}}$ activated protein C (APC) ⟶ cleaves and inactivates Va, VIIIa

Factor V Leiden mutation produces a factor V resistant to APC's inhibition.
tPA is used clinically as a thrombolytic.

Plasminogen $\xrightarrow{\text{tPA}}$ plasmin ⟶ cleavage of fibrin mesh

**Pathologic RBC forms**

| Type | Example | Associated pathology | Mnemonic |
|---|---|---|---|
| Acanthocyte (spur cell) | | Liver disease, abetalipoproteinemia. | |
| **Bas**ophilic stippling | | **T**halassemias, **A**nemia of chronic disease, **I**ron deficiency, **L**ead poisoning. | **Bas**te the ox **TAIL**. |
| Bite cell | | G6PD deficiency. | |
| Elliptocyte | | Hereditary elliptocytosis. | |
| Macro-ovalocyte | | Megaloblastic anemia (also hypersegmented PMNs), marrow failure. | |
| Ringed sideroblasts | | Sideroblastic anemia. | |
| Schistocyte, helmet cell | | DIC, TTP/HUS, traumatic hemolysis. | |
| Sickle cell | | Sickle cell anemia. | |
| Spherocyte | | Hereditary spherocytosis, autoimmune hemolysis. | |
| Teardrop cell | | Bone marrow infiltration (e.g., myelofibrosis). | |
| Target cell | | **H**bC disease, **A**splenia, **L**iver disease, **T**halassemia. | "**HALT**," said the hunter to his **target**. |

## Other RBC pathologies

| Type | Example | Process | Associated pathology |
|------|---------|---------|---------------------|
| Heinz bodies |  | Oxidation of iron from ferrous to ferric form leads to denatured hemoglobin precipitation and damage to RBC membrane. Leads to formation of bite cells. | Seen with α-thalassemia, G6PD deficiency. |
| Howell-Jolly bodies |  | Basophilic nuclear remnants found in RBCs. | Seen in patients with functional hyposplenia or asplenia. |

## Microcytic, hypochromic (MCV < 80) anemia

| | |
|---|---|
| Iron deficiency | ↓ iron due to chronic bleeding, malnutrition/absorption disorders or ↑ demand (e.g., pregnancy) → ↓ heme synthesis (see Image 22). May manifest as Plummer-Vinson syndrome (triad of iron deficiency anemia, esophageal web, and atrophic glossitis). |
| α-thalassemia | Prevalent in Asia and Africa. **Defect:** α-globin gene mutations → ↓ α-globin synthesis. Deletion of 4 genes is incompatible with life → Hb Barts ($\gamma_4$), which causes hydrops fetalis. Deletion of 3 genes → HbH disease ($\beta_4$). Deletion of 1–2 genes is not associated with anemia. |
| β-thalassemia | Prevalent in Mediterranean populations. **Defect:** point mutations in splicing sites and promoter sequences. **β-thalassemia minor (heterozygote):** 1. β chain is underproduced. 2. Usually asymptomatic. 3. Diagnosis confirmed by ↑ $HbA_2$ (> 3.5%). **β-thalassemia major (homozygote):** 1. β chain is absent → severe anemia requiring blood transfusion (2° hemochromatosis). 2. Marrow expansion ("crew cut" on skull x-ray) → skeletal deformities. Chipmunk facies. Both major and minor → ↑ HbF ($\alpha_2\gamma_2$). **HbS/β-thalassemia heterozygote:** mild to moderate sickle cell disease depending on amount of β-globin production (see Image 21). |
| Lead poisoning | Lead inhibits ferrochelatase and ALA dehydratase → ↓ heme synthesis. Also inhibits RNA degradation → basophilic stippling. |
| Sideroblastic anemia | **Defect in heme synthesis.** Hereditary: X-linked defect in δ-aminolevulinic acid synthase gene. Treatment: pyridoxine ($B_6$) therapy. Reversible etiologies: alcohol, lead. ↑ iron, normal TIBC, ↑ ferritin. Ringed sideroblasts (with iron-laden mitochondria). |

| | |
|---|---|
| **Macrocytic (MCV > 100) anemia** | Impaired DNA synthesis → maturation of nucleus delayed relative to maturation of cytoplasm. |
| Megaloblastic anemia caused by folate deficiency | Findings: hypersegmented neutrophils, glossitis, ↓ folate, ↑ homocysteine but normal methylmalonic acid. |
| | Etiologies: malnutrition (e.g., alcoholics), malabsorption, impaired metabolism (e.g., methotrexate, trimethoprim), ↑ requirement (e.g., hemolytic anemia, pregnancy). |
| Megaloblastic anemia caused by $B_{12}$ deficiency | Findings: hypersegmented neutrophils, glossitis, ↓ $B_{12}$, ↑ homocysteine, ↑ methylmalonic acid. |
| | Etiologies: malnutrition (e.g., alcoholics), malabsorption (e.g., Crohn's disease), pernicious anemia, *Diphyllobothrium latum* (fish tapeworm). |
| | Neurologic symptoms: subacute combined degeneration (due to involvement of $B_{12}$ in fatty acid pathways). |
| Nonmegaloblastic macrocytic anemias | 1. Liver disease |
| | 2. Alcoholism: macrocytosis and bone marrow suppression can occur in the absence of folate/$B_{12}$ deficiency |
| | 3. Reticulocytosis: reticulocytes are bigger than mature RBCs → ↑ MCV |
| | 4. Metabolic disorder (e.g., orotic aciduria): congenital deficiencies of purine or pyrimidine synthesis |
| | 5. Drugs: 5-FU, AZT, hydroxyurea |
| **Normocytic, normochromic anemia** | Normocytic, normochromic anemia may be classified as nonhemolytic vs. hemolytic. The hemolytic anemias are further classified according to the cause of the hemolysis (intrinsic vs. extrinsic to the RBC) and by the location of the hemolysis (intravascular vs. extravascular). |
| Nonhemolytic | Anemia of chronic disease (ACD), aplastic anemia, kidney disease. |
| Intrinsic hemolytic | Hereditary spherocytosis, G6PD deficiency, pyruvate kinase deficiency, sickle cell anemia, HbC defect, paroxysmal nocturnal hemoglobinuria. |
| Extrinsic hemolytic | Autoimmune, microangiopathic (e.g., DIC, TTP-HUS), infectious. |
| Intravascular hemolysis | Paroxysmal nocturnal hemoglobinuria, autoimmune (cold agglutinins), mechanical destruction (e.g., aortic stenosis, prosthetic valve). |
| Extravascular hemolysis | Hereditary spherocytosis, G6PD deficiency, pyruvate kinase deficiency, sickle cell anemia, HbC defect, autoimmune (warm agglutinins), microangiopathic (e.g., DIC, TTP-HUS). |

## Nonhemolytic, normocytic anemia

| | |
|---|---|
| Anemia of chronic disease (ACD) | Inflammation → ↑ hepcidin → ↓ release of iron from macrophages. <br> ↓ iron, ↓ TIBC, ↑ ferritin. <br> Can become microcytic, hypochromic in long-standing disease. |
| Aplastic anemia | Pathologic features: pancytopenia characterized by severe anemia, neutropenia, and thrombocytopenia. Normal cell morphology, but hypocellular bone marrow with fatty infiltration. <br> Causes: failure or destruction of myeloid stem cells due to: <br> 1. Radiation and drugs (benzene, chloramphenicol, alkylating agents, antimetabolites) <br> 2. Viral agents (parvovirus B19, EBV, HIV) <br> 3. Fanconi's anemia (inherited defect in DNA repair) <br> 4. Idiopathic (immune mediated, 1° stem cell defect); may follow acute hepatitis <br> Symptoms: fatigue, malaise, pallor, purpura, mucosal bleeding, petechiae, infection. <br> Treatment: withdrawal of offending agent, immunosuppressive regimens (antithymocyte globulin, cyclosporine), allogeneic bone marrow transplantation, RBC and platelet transfusion, G-CSF or GM-CSF. |
| Kidney disease | ↓ erythropoietin → ↓ hematopoiesis. |

## Intrinsic hemolytic normocytic anemia

| | |
|---|---|
| Hereditary spherocytosis | Defect in proteins interacting with RBC membrane skeleton and plasma membrane (e.g., ankyrin, band 3.1, or spectrin). |
| | Pathogenesis: less membrane causes small and round RBCs with no central pallor ($\uparrow$ MCHC, $\uparrow$ RDW) → premature removal of RBCs by spleen. |
| | Findings: splenomegaly, aplastic crisis (B19 infection). Howell-Jolly bodies present after splenectomy. |
| | Labs: positive osmotic fragility test. |
| G6PD deficiency | X-linked. Defect in G6PD → $\downarrow$ glutathione → $\uparrow$ RBC susceptibility to oxidant stress. |
| | Findings: hemolytic anemia following oxidant stress (e.g., sulfa drugs, infections, fava beans). |
| | Labs: blood smear shows RBCs with Heinz bodies and bite cells. |
| Pyruvate kinase deficiency | Autosomal recessive. Defect in pyruvate kinase → $\downarrow$ ATP → rigid RBCs. |
| | Presentation: hemolytic anemia in a newborn. |
| Sickle cell anemia | 8% of African-Americans carry the HbS trait; 0.2% have the disease. |
| | Sickled cells are crescent-shaped RBCs. |
| | "Crew cut" on skull x-ray due to marrow expansion from $\uparrow$ erythropoiesis (also in thalassemias). |
| | Newborns are initially asymptomatic owing to $\uparrow$ HbF and $\downarrow$ HbS. |
| | Mutation: HbS mutation is a single amino acid replacement in $\beta$ chain (substitution of normal glutamic acid with valine). |
| | Pathogenesis: deoxygenated HbS polymerizes. Low $O_2$ or dehydration precipitates sickling. |
| | Heterozygotes (sickle cell trait) have resistance to malaria. |
| | Complications in homozygotes (sickle cell disease): |
| |   1. Aplastic crisis (due to parvovirus B19 infection) |
| |   2. Autosplenectomy → $\uparrow$ risk of infection with encapsulated organisms |
| |   3. *Salmonella* osteomyelitis |
| |   4. Painful crisis (vaso-occlusive) |
| |   5. Renal papillary necrosis (due to low $O_2$ in papilla) |
| |   6. Splenic sequestration crisis (see Image 23) |
| | Treatment: hydroxyurea ($\uparrow$ HbF) and bone marrow transplantation. |
| HbC defect | A different $\beta$-chain mutation; patients with HbC or HbSC (1 of each mutant gene) have milder disease than do HbSS patients. |
| Paroxysmal nocturnal hemoglobinuria | Pathogenesis: intravascular hemolysis due to $\uparrow$ complement-mediated RBC lysis (impaired synthesis of GPI anchor/decay-accelerating factor in RBC membrane). |
| | Labs: $\uparrow$ urine hemosiderin. |

## Extrinsic hemolytic normocytic anemia

| | | |
|---|---|---|
| Autoimmune hemolytic anemia | **Warm** agglutinin (Ig**G**)—chronic anemia seen in SLE, in CLL, or with certain drugs (e.g., α-methyldopa). | **Warm** weather is **GGG**reat. |
| | **Cold** agglutinin (Ig**M**)—acute anemia triggered by cold; seen with *Mycoplasma pneumoniae* infections or infectious mononucleosis. | **Cold** ice cream—**MMM.** |
| | Erythroblastosis fetalis—seen in newborns due to Rh or other blood antigen incompatibility → mother's antibodies attack fetal RBCs. | |
| | Autoimmune hemolytic anemias are usually Coombs positive. | |
| | • Direct Coombs' test—anti-Ig antibody added to patient's RBCs agglutinate if RBCs are coated with Ig. | |
| | • Indirect Coombs' test—normal RBCs added to patient's serum agglutinate if serum has anti-RBC surface Ig. | |
| Microangiopathic anemia | Pathogenesis: RBCs are damaged when passing through obstructed or narrowed vessel lumina. Seen in DIC, TTP-HUS, SLE, and malignant hypertension. | |
| | **Schistocytes** (helmet cells) are seen on blood smear due to mechanical destruction of RBCs. | |
| | **Prosthetic heart valves** and aortic stenosis may also cause hemolytic anemia 2° to mechanical destruction. | |
| Infections | ↑ destruction of RBCs (e.g., malaria, *Babesia*). | |

## Lab values in anemia

| | Iron Deficiency | Chronic Disease | Hemo-chromatosis | Pregnancy/ OCP Use |
|---|---|---|---|---|
| Serum iron | ↓ (1°) | ↓ | ↑ (1°) | — |
| Transferrin/ TIBC (indirectly measures transferrin) | ↑ | ↓* | ↓ | ↑ (1°) |
| Ferritin | ↓ | ↑ (1°) | ↑ | — |
| % transferrin saturation (serum Fe/TIBC) | ↓↓ | — | ↑↑ | ↓ |

Ferritin—1° iron storage protein of body.
Transferrin—transports iron in blood.
*Evolutionary reasoning—pathogens use circulating iron to thrive. The body has adapted a system in which iron is stored within the cells of the body and prevents pathogens from acquiring circulating iron.

**Heme synthesis, porphyrias, and lead poisoning**

The porphyrias are conditions of defective heme synthesis that lead to the accumulation of heme precursors. Lead inhibits specific enzymes needed in heme synthesis, leading to a similar condition.

| Condition | Affected Enzyme | Accumulated Substrate | Presenting Symptoms |
|---|---|---|---|
| Lead poisoning | Ferrochelatase and ALA dehydratase | Protoporphyrin (blood) | Microcytic anemia, GI and kidney disease. Children—exposure to lead paint → mental deterioration. Adults—environmental exposure (battery/ammunition/radiator factory) → headache, memory loss, demyelination. |
| Acute intermittent porphyria | Porphobilinogen deaminase (aka uroporphyrinogen-I-synthase) | Porphobilinogen, δ-ALA, uroporphyrin (urine) | Symptoms = 5 P's:<br>Painful abdomen<br>Pink urine<br>Polyneuropathy<br>Psychological disturbances<br>Precipitated by drugs<br>Treatment: glucose and heme, which inhibit ALA synthase. |
| Porphyria cutanea tarda | Uroporphyrinogen decarboxylase | Uroporphyrin (tea-colored urine) | Blistering cutaneous photosensitivity. Most common porphyria. |

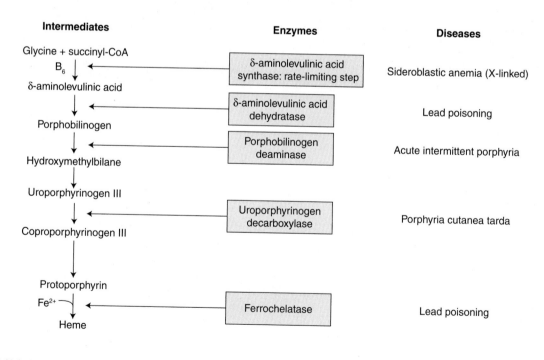

| Intermediates | Enzymes | Diseases |
|---|---|---|
| Glycine + succinyl-CoA | | |
| ↓ B$_6$ | δ-aminolevulinic acid synthase: rate-limiting step | Sideroblastic anemia (X-linked) |
| δ-aminolevulinic acid | | |
| ↓ | δ-aminolevulinic acid dehydratase | Lead poisoning |
| Porphobilinogen | | |
| ↓ | Porphobilinogen deaminase | Acute intermittent porphyria |
| Hydroxymethylbilane | | |
| ↓ | | |
| Uroporphyrinogen III | | |
| ↓ | Uroporphyrinogen decarboxylase | Porphyria cutanea tarda |
| Coproporphyrinogen III | | |
| ↓ | | |
| Protoporphyrin | | |
| ↓ Fe$^{2+}$ | Ferrochelatase | Lead poisoning |
| Heme | | |

↓ heme → ↑ ALA dehydratase activity
↑ heme → ↓ ALA dehydratase activity

| | | | | |
|---|---|---|---|---|
| **Lead poisoning** | Lead **L**ines on gingivae (Burton's lines) and on epiphyses of long bones on x-ray. | | **LEAD.** High risk in houses with chipped paint. | |

**Lead poisoning**

Lead **L**ines on gingivae (Burton's lines) and on epiphyses of long bones on x-ray.

**E**ncephalopathy and **E**rythrocyte basophilic stippling.

**A**bdominal colic and sideroblastic **A**nemia.

**D**rops—wrist and foot drop. **D**imercaprol and EDTA 1st line of treatment. **Succ**imer for kids.

**LEAD.**
High risk in houses with chipped paint.

It "**sucks**" to be a kid who eats lead.

**Platelet disorders**

Defects in platelet plug formation → ↑ bleeding time (BT).

Platelet abnormalities → microhemorrhage: mucous membrane bleeding, epistaxis, petechiae, purpura, ↑ bleeding time, possible ↓ platelet count (PC).

| Disorder | PC | BT | Mechanism and Comments |
|---|:---:|:---:|---|
| Bernard-Soulier disease | ↓ | ↑ | Defect in platelet plug formation.<br>↓ Gp1b → defect in platelet-to-collagen adhesion. |
| Glanzmann's thrombasthenia | – | ↑ | Defect in platelet plug formation.<br>↓ GpIIb/IIIa → defect in platelet-to-platelet aggregation.<br>Labs: blood smear shows no platelet clumping. |
| Idiopathic thrombocytopenic purpura (ITP) | ↓ | ↑ | ↓ platelet survival.<br>Defect: anti-GpIIb/IIIa antibodies → peripheral platelet destruction.<br>Labs: ↑ megakaryocytes. |
| Thrombotic thrombocytopenic purpura (TTP) | ↓ | ↑ | ↓ platelet survival.<br>Deficiency of ADAMTS 13 (vWF metalloprotease) → ↓ degradation of vWF multimers.<br>Pathogenesis: ↑ large vWF multimers → ↑ platelet aggregation and thrombosis.<br>Labs: schistocytes, ↑ LDH.<br>Symptoms: pentad of neurologic and renal symptoms, fever, thrombocytopenia, and microangiopathic hemolytic anemia. |

**Coagulation disorders**

PT—tests function of factors I, II, V, VII, and X (extrinsic pathway). Defect → ↑ PT.

PTT—tests function of all factors except VII and XIII (intrinsic pathway). Defect → ↑ PTT.

| Disorder | PT | PTT | Mechanism and Comments |
|---|:---:|:---:|---|
| Hemophilia A or B | – | ↑ | Intrinsic pathway coagulation defect.<br>A: deficiency of factor VIII → ↑ PTT.<br>B: deficiency of factor IX → ↑ PTT.<br>Macrohemorrhage in hemophilia—hemarthroses (bleeding into joints), easy bruising, ↑ PT and/or PTT. |
| Vitamin K deficiency | ↑ | ↑ | General coagulation defect.<br>↓ synthesis of factors II, VII, IX, X, protein C, protein S. |

## Mixed platelet and coagulation disorders

| Disorder | PC | BT | PT | PTT | Mechanism and Comments |
|---|---|---|---|---|---|
| von Willebrand's disease | — | ↑ | — | — or ↑ | Intrinsic pathway coagulation defect: ↓ vWF → normal or ↑ PTT (depends on severity; vWF acts to carry/protect factor VIII). Defect in platelet plug formation: ↓ vWF → defect in platelet-to-collagen adhesion. Mild but most common inherited bleeding disorder (AD). |
| DIC | ↓ | ↑ | ↑ | ↑ | Widespread activation of clotting leads to a deficiency in clotting factors, which creates a bleeding state. Causes: Sepsis (gram-negative), Trauma, Obstetric complications, acute Pancreatitis, Malignancy, Nephrotic syndrome, Transfusion (STOP Making New Thrombi). Labs: schistocytes, ↑ fibrin split products (D-dimers), ↓ fibrinogen, ↓ factors V and VIII. |

## Hereditary thrombosis syndromes leading to hypercoagulability

| Disease | Description |
|---|---|
| Factor V Leiden | Production of mutant factor V that cannot be degraded by protein C. Most common cause of inherited hypercoagulability. |
| Prothrombin gene mutation | Mutation in 3′ untranslated region associated with venous clots. |
| ATIII deficiency | Inherited deficiency of antithrombin III; reduced ↑ in PTT after administration of heparin. |
| Protein C or S deficiency | ↓ ability to inactivate factors V and VIII. ↑ risk of hemorrhagic skin necrosis following administration of warfarin. |

| **Leukemia vs. lymphoma** | Leukemia—lymphoid neoplasms with widespread involvement of bone marrow. Tumor cells are usually found in peripheral blood. Lymphoma—discrete tumor masses. Presentations often blur definitions. |
|---|---|

## Hodgkin's vs. Non-Hodgkin's lymphoma

### Hodgkin's

Presence of Reed-Sternberg cells

Localized, single group of nodes; extranodal rare; contiguous spread (stage is strongest predictor of prognosis)

Constitutional ("B") signs/symptoms—low-grade fever, night sweats, weight loss

Mediastinal lymphadenopathy (nontender)

50% of cases associated with EBV; bimodal distribution —young and old; more common in men except for nodular sclerosing type

Good prognosis = ↑ lymphocytes, ↓ RS

### Non-Hodgkin's

May be associated with HIV and immunosuppression

Multiple, peripheral nodes; extranodal involvement common; noncontiguous spread

Majority involve B cells (except those of lymphoblastic T-cell origin)

Fewer constitutional signs/symptoms

Peak incidence for certain subtypes at 20–40 years of age

---

**Reed-Sternberg cells**

Distinctive tumor giant cell seen in Hodgkin's disease (see Image 27); binucleate or bilobed with the 2 halves as mirror images ("owl's eyes"). RS cells are CD30+ and CD15+ B-cell origin. Necessary but not sufficient for a diagnosis of Hodgkin's disease. Variants include lacunar cells in nodular sclerosis variant.

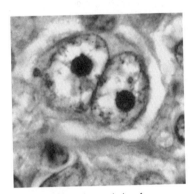

(Reproduced, with permission, from the PEIR Digital Library.)

---

### Hodgkin's lymphoma

| Type | RS | Lymphocyte | Prognosis | Comments |
|---|---|---|---|---|
| Nodular sclerosing (65–75%) | + | +++ | Excellent | Most common; collagen banding; lacunar cells; women > men; primarily young adults. |
| Mixed cellularity (25%) | ++++ | +++ | Intermediate | Numerous RS cells. |
| Lymphocyte predominant (6%) | + | ++++ | Excellent | < 35-year-old males. |
| Lymphocyte depleted (rare) | * | + | Poor | Older males with disseminated disease. |

*RS high relative to lymphocytes. Note: ↑ lymphocyte-to-RS ratio roughly correlates with good prognosis.

**Non-Hodgkin's lymphoma**

| Type | Occurs in | Genetics | Comments |
|---|---|---|---|
| **Neoplasms of mature B cells** | | | |
| Burkitt's lymphoma | Adolescents or young adults | t(8;14) c-*myc* gene moves next to heavy-chain Ig gene (14) | "Starry-sky" appearance (sheets of lymphocytes with interspersed macrophages); associated with EBV; jaw lesion in endemic form in Africa; pelvis or abdomen in sporadic form (see Image 26). |
| Diffuse large B-cell lymphoma | Usually older adults, but 20% in children | | Most common adult NHL. May be mature T cell in origin (20%). |
| Mantle cell lymphoma | Older males | t(11;14) | Poor prognosis, CD5+. |
| Follicular lymphoma | Adults | t(14;18) *bcl*-2 expression | Difficult to cure; indolent course; *bcl*-2 inhibits apoptosis. |
| **Neoplasms of mature T cells** | | | |
| Adult T-cell lymphoma | Adults | Caused by HTLV-1 | Adults present with cutaneous lesions; especially affects populations in Japan, West Africa, and the Caribbean. Aggressive. |
| Mycosis fungoides/ Sézary syndrome | Adults | | Adults present with cutaneous patches/ nodules. Indolent. |

**Multiple myeloma**

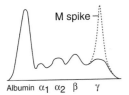

Monoclonal plasma cell ("fried-egg" appearance) cancer that arises in the marrow and produces large amounts of IgG (55%) or IgA (25%). Most common 1° tumor arising within bone in the elderly (> 40–50 years of age). Destructive bone lesions and consequent hypercalcemia. Renal insufficiency, ↑ susceptibility to infection, and anemia. Associated with 1° amyloidosis (AL) and punched-out lytic bone lesions on x-ray (see Image 25). Characterized by monoclonal immunoglobulin spike (M protein) on serum protein electrophoresis and Ig light chains in urine (Bence Jones protein). Blood smear shows RBCs stacked like poker chips (rouleaux formation). Compare with Waldenström's macroglobulinemia → M spike = IgM (→ hyperviscosity symptoms); no lytic bone lesions.

If asymptomatic, called monoclonal gammopathy of undetermined significance (MGUS).

Think **CRAB**:
hyper**C**alcemia
**R**enal insufficiency
**A**nemia
**B**one/**B**ack pain

**Leukemias**

Unregulated growth of leukocytes in bone marrow → ↑ or ↓ number of circulating leukocytes in blood and marrow failure → anemia (↓ RBCs), infections (↓ mature WBCs), and hemorrhage (↓ platelets); leukemic cell infiltrates in liver, spleen, and lymph nodes are possible (see Image 24).

| Type | Occurs in | Comments |
|---|---|---|
| Lymphoid neoplasms | | |
| Acute lymphoblastic leukemia/ lymphoma (ALL) | Children | May present with bone marrow involvement in childhood or mediastinal mass in adolescent males. Bone marrow replaced by ↑↑↑ lymphoblasts. TdT+ (marker of pre-T and pre-B cells), CALLA+. Most responsive to therapy. May spread to CNS and testes. t(12;21) → better prognosis. |
| Small lymphocytic lymphoma (SLL)/ chronic lymphocytic leukemia (CLL) | Older adults (> 60 years of age) | Often asymptomatic; smudge cells in peripheral blood smear; warm antibody autoimmune hemolytic anemia. SLL same as CLL except CLL has ↑ peripheral blood lymphocytosis. |
| Hairy cell leukemia | Elderly | Mature B-cell tumor in the elderly. Cells have filamentous, hairlike projections. Stains TRAP (tartrate-resistant acid phosphatase) positive. |
| Myeloid neoplasms | | |
| Acute myelogenous leukemia (AML) | Adults | Auer rods; ↑↑↑ circulating myeloblasts on peripheral smear; adults. M3 responds to all-*trans* retinoic acid (vitamin A), inducing differentiation of myeloblasts. |
| Chronic myelogenous leukemia (CML) | | Defined by the Philadelphia chromosome (t[9;22], *bcr-abl*); myeloid stem cell proliferation; presents with ↑ neutrophils, metamyelocytes, basophils; splenomegaly; may accelerate and transform to AML or ALL ("blast crisis"). Very low leukocyte alkaline phosphatase (vs. leukemoid reaction). Responds to imatinib (anti-*bcr-abl* antibody). |

**Leukemias** *(continued)*

**LEUKEMIA**
Abnormal stem cells
in bone marrow

Approximate ages:
ALL = < 15.
AML = median onset ~ 60.
CML = 30–60.
CLL = > 60.

**ACUTE LEUKEMIAS**
Blasts predominate
Children or elderly
Short and drastic course

**CHRONIC LEUKEMIAS**
More mature cells
Midlife age range
Longer, less devastating course

**ALL**
Lymphoblasts
(pre-B or pre-T)

**AML**
Myeloblasts

**CLL**
Lymphocytes
Non-antibody-
producing B cells

**CML**
Myeloid stem cells
"Blast crisis"

| | |
|---|---|
| **Leukemoid reaction** | ↑ WBC count with left shift (e.g., 80% bands) and ↑ leukocyte alkaline phosphatase. |
| **Auer bodies (rods)** | Peroxidase-positive cytoplasmic inclusions in granulocytes and myeloblasts. Commonly seen in acute promyelocytic leukemia (M3). Treatment of AML M3 can release Auer rods → DIC. |

**Chromosomal translocations**

| Translocation | Associated disorder | |
|---|---|---|
| t(9;22) (**Philadelphia** chromosome) | CML (*bcr-abl* hybrid) | Philadelphia Crea**ML** cheese. |
| t(8;14) | Burkitt's lymphoma (c-*myc* activation) | |
| t(14;18) | Follicular lymphomas (*bcl-2* activation) | |
| t(15;17) | M3 type of AML (responsive to all-*trans* retinoic acid) | |
| t(11;22) | Ewing's sarcoma | |
| t(11;14) | Mantle cell lymphoma | |

| | |
|---|---|
| **Langerhans cell histiocytoses (histiocytosis X)** | Proliferative disorders of dendritic (Langerhans) cells from the monocyte lineage. Defective cells express S-100 and CD1a. Birbeck granules ("tennis rackets" on EM) are characteristic. Older terms for 3 different clinical expressions of the same basic disorder: Letterer-Siwe disease, Hand-Schüller-Christian disease, eosinophilic granulomas. |

**Chronic myeloproliferative disorders**

| | RBCs | WBCs | Platelets | Philadelphia chromosome | JAK2 mutations |
|---|---|---|---|---|---|
| Polycythemia vera | ↑ | ↑ | ↑ | Negative | Positive |
| Essential thrombocytosis | – | – | ↑ | Negative | Positive (30–50%) |
| Myelofibrosis | ↓ | Variable | Variable | Negative | Positive (30–50%) |
| CML | ↓ | ↑ | ↑ | Positive | Negative |

| | |
|---|---|
| | The myelofibroproliferative disorders represent an often-overlapping spectrum, but the classic findings are described below. |
| Polycythemia vera | Abnormal clone of hematopoietic stem cells are increasingly sensitive to growth factors. |
| Essential thrombocytosis | Similar to polycythemia vera, but specific for megakaryocytes. |
| Myelofibrosis | Fibrotic obliteration of bone marrow. |
| CML | *bcr-abl* transformation leads to ↑ cell division and inhibition of apoptosis. |
| | *JAK2* is involved in hematopoietic growth factor signaling. Mutations are implicated in myeloproliferative disorders other than CML. |

## ▶ HEMATOLOGY AND ONCOLOGY–PHARMACOLOGY

**Heparin**

| | |
|---|---|
| Mechanism | Cofactor for the activation of antithrombin, ↓ thrombin and Xa. Short half-life. |
| Clinical use | Immediate anticoagulation for pulmonary embolism, stroke, acute coronary syndrome, MI, DVT. Used during pregnancy (does not cross placenta). Follow PTT. |
| Toxicity | Bleeding, thrombocytopenia (HIT), osteoporosis, drug-drug interactions. For rapid reversal of heparinization, use **protamine sulfate** (positively charged molecule that acts by binding negatively charged heparin). |
| Notes | Newer **low-molecular-weight heparins** (e.g., enoxaparin) act more on Xa, have better bioavailability and 2–4 times longer half-life. Can be administered subcutaneously and without laboratory monitoring. Not easily reversible. |
| | Heparin-induced thrombocytopenia (HIT)—heparin binds to platelets, causing autoantibody production that destroys platelets and overactivates the remaining ones, resulting in a thrombocytopenic, hypercoagulable state. |

| | |
|---|---|
| **Lepirudin, bivalirudin** | Hirudin derivatives; directly inhibit thrombin. Used as an alternative to heparin for anticoagulating patients with HIT. |

HIGH-YIELD SYSTEMS

HEMATOLOGY AND ONCOLOGY

## Warfarin (Coumadin)

**Mechanism**  Interferes with normal synthesis and γ-carboxylation of vitamin K–dependent clotting factors II, VII, IX, and X and protein C and S. Metabolized by the cytochrome P-450 pathway. In laboratory assay, has effect on **EX**trinsic pathway and ↑ **PT.** Long half-life.

The **EX**-Presiden**T** went to **WAR**(farin).

**Clinical use**  Chronic anticoagulation. Not used in pregnant women (because warfarin, unlike heparin, can cross the placenta). Follow PT/INR values.

**Toxicity**  Bleeding, teratogenic, skin/tissue necrosis, drug-drug interactions.

## Heparin vs. warfarin

|  | Heparin | Warfarin |
|---|---|---|
| Structure | Large anionic, acidic polymer | Small lipid-soluble molecule |
| Route of administration | Parenteral (IV, SC) | Oral |
| Site of action | Blood | Liver |
| Onset of action | Rapid (seconds) | Slow, limited by half-lives of normal clotting factors |
| Mechanism of action | Activates antithrombin, which ↓ the action of IIa (thrombin) and Xa | Impairs the synthesis of vitamin K–dependent clotting factors II, VII, IX, and X (vitamin K antagonist) |
| Duration of action | Acute (hours) | Chronic (days) |
| Inhibits coagulation in vitro | Yes | No |
| Treatment of acute overdose | Protamine sulfate | IV vitamin K and fresh frozen plasma |
| Monitoring | PTT (intrinsic pathway) | PT/INR (extrinsic pathway) |
| Crosses placenta | No | Yes (teratogenic) |

| | |
|---|---|
| **Thrombolytics** | Streptokinase, urokinase, tPA (alteplase), APSAC (anistreplase). |
| Mechanism | Directly or indirectly aid conversion of plasminogen to plasmin, which cleaves thrombin and fibrin clots. ↑ PT, ↑ PTT, no change in platelet count. |
| Clinical use | Early MI, early ischemic stroke. |
| Toxicity | Bleeding. Contraindicated in patients with active bleeding, history of intracranial bleeding, recent surgery, known bleeding diatheses, or severe hypertension. Treat toxicity with aminocaproic acid, an inhibitor of fibrinolysis. |

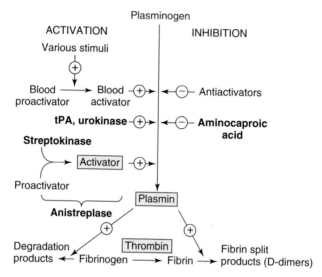

(Adapted, with permission, from Katzung BG. *Basic and Clinical Pharmacology,* 7th ed. Stamford, CT: Appleton & Lange, 1997: 550.)

### Mechanism of antiplatelet interaction

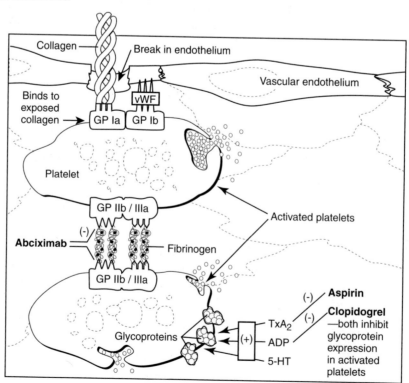

## Aspirin (ASA)

Mechanism  Acetylates and irreversibly inhibits cyclooxygenase (both COX-1 and COX-2) to prevent conversion of arachidonic acid to thromboxane $A_2$ ($TxA_2$). ↑ bleeding time. No effect on PT, PTT.

Clinical use  Antipyretic, analgesic, anti-inflammatory, antiplatelet drug.

Toxicity  Gastric ulceration, bleeding, hyperventilation, Reye's syndrome, tinnitus (CN VIII).

## Clopidogrel, ticlopidine

Mechanism  Inhibit platelet aggregation by irreversibly blocking ADP receptors. Inhibit fibrinogen binding by preventing glycoprotein IIb/IIIa expression.

Clinical use  Acute coronary syndrome; coronary stenting. ↓ incidence or recurrence of thrombotic stroke.

Toxicity  Neutropenia (ticlopidine).

## Abciximab

Mechanism  Monoclonal antibody that binds to the glycoprotein receptor IIb/IIIa on activated platelets, preventing aggregation.

Clinical use  Acute coronary syndromes, percutaneous transluminal coronary angioplasty.

Toxicity  Bleeding, thrombocytopenia.

## Cancer drugs—cell cycle

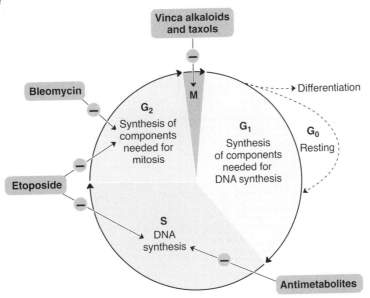

(Adapted, with permission, from Katzung BG, Trevor AJ. *USMLE Road Map: Pharmacology*, 1st ed. New York: McGraw-Hill, 2003: 133.)

## Antineoplastics

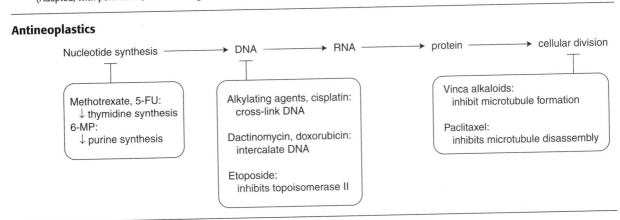

## Antimetabolites

| Drug | Mechanism* | Clinical use | Toxicity |
|---|---|---|---|
| Methotrexate (MTX) | **Folic acid analog** that inhibits dihydrofolate reductase → ↓ dTMP → ↓ DNA and ↓ protein synthesis. | **Cancers:** Leukemias, lymphomas, choriocarcinoma, sarcomas. **Non-neoplastic:** Abortion, ectopic pregnancy, rheumatoid arthritis, psoriasis. | Myelosuppression, which is reversible with **leucovorin** (folinic acid) "rescue." Macrovesicular fatty change in liver; mucositis; teratogenic. |
| 5-fluorouracil (5-FU) | **Pyrimidine analog** bioactivated to 5F-dUMP, which covalently complexes folic acid. This complex **inhibits thymidylate synthase** → ↓ dTMP → ↓ DNA and ↓ protein synthesis. | Colon cancer and other solid tumors, basal cell carcinoma (topical). Synergy with MTX. | Myelosuppression, which is **not** reversible with leucovorin. Overdose: "rescue" with **thymidine.** Photosensitivity. |
| 6-mercaptopurine (6-MP) | **Purine** (thiol) analog → ↓ de novo purine synthesis. Activated by HGPRTase. | Leukemias, lymphomas (not CLL or Hodgkin's). | Bone marrow, GI, liver. Metabolized by xanthine oxidase; thus ↑ toxicity with allopurinol. |
| 6-thioguanine (6-TG) | Same as 6-MP. | Acute lymphoid leukemia. | Bone marrow depression, liver. Can be given with allopurinol. |
| Cytarabine (ara-C) | Pyrimidine antagonist → inhibition of DNA polymerase. | AML, ALL, high-grade non-Hodgkin's lymphoma. | Leukopenia, thrombocytopenia, megaloblastic anemia. |

*All are S-phase specific.

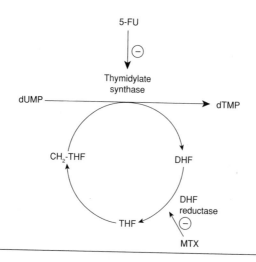

## Antitumor antibiotics

| Drug | Mechanism | Clinical use | Toxicity |
|------|-----------|--------------|----------|
| Dactinomycin (**ACT**inomycin D) | Intercalates in DNA. | Wilms' tumor, Ewing's sarcoma, rhabdomyosarcoma. Used for childhood tumors (children **ACT** out). | Myelosuppression. |
| Doxorubicin (**A**driamycin), daunorubicin | Generate free radicals. Noncovalently intercalate in DNA → breaks in DNA → ↓ replication. | Part of the **ABVD** combination regimen for Hodgkin's lymphomas; also for myelomas, sarcomas, and solid tumors (breast, ovary, lung). | Cardiotoxicity; also myelosuppression and marked alopecia. Toxic to tissues with extravasation. |
| **B**leomycin | $G_2$-phase specific. Induces formation of free radicals, which cause breaks in DNA strands. | Testicular cancer, Hodgkin's lymphoma (part of the **ABVD** regimen for Hodgkin's). | Pulmonary fibrosis, skin changes, but minimal myelosuppression. |
| Etoposide (VP-16), teniposide | Late S- to $G_2$-phase specific. Inhibits topoisomerase II → ↑ DNA degradation. | Small cell carcinoma of the lung and prostate, testicular carcinoma. | Myelosuppression, GI irritation, alopecia. |

## Alkylating agents

| Drug | Mechanism | Clinical Use | Toxicity |
|------|-----------|--------------|----------|
| Cyclophosphamide, ifosfamide | Covalently X-link (interstrand) DNA at guanine N-7. Require bioactivation by liver. | Non-Hodgkin's lymphoma, breast and ovarian carcinomas. Also immuno-suppressants. | Myelosuppression; hemorrhagic cystitis, which can be partially prevented with mesna. |
| Nitrosoureas (carmustine, lomustine, semustine, streptozocin) | Require bioactivation. Cross blood-brain barrier → CNS. | Brain tumors (including glioblastoma multiforme). | CNS toxicity (dizziness, ataxia). |
| Busulfan | Alkylates DNA. | CML. Also used for ablating bone marrow in hematopoietic stem cell transplants. | Pulmonary fibrosis, hyperpigmentation. |

**Microtubule inhibitors**

| Drug | Mechanism | Clinical Use | Toxicity |
|---|---|---|---|
| Vincristine, vinblastine | Alkaloids that bind to tubulin in M phase and block polymerization of microtubules so that mitotic spindle cannot form. Microtubules are the **vines** of your cells. | Part of the MOPP (**O**ncovin [vincristine]) regimen for Hodgkin's lymphoma, Wilms' tumor, choriocarcinoma. | Vincristine—neurotoxicity (areflexia, peripheral neuritis), paralytic ileus. Vin**BLAST**ine **BLAST**s **B**one marrow (suppression). |
| Pacli**TAX**el, other **TAX**ols | Hyperstabilize polymerized microtubules in M phase so that mitotic spindle cannot break down (anaphase cannot occur). It is **TAX**ing to stay polymerized. | Ovarian and breast carcinomas. | Myelosuppression and hypersensitivity. |

**Cisplatin, carboplatin**

| | |
|---|---|
| Mechanism | Cross-link DNA. |
| Clinical use | Testicular, bladder, ovary, and lung carcinomas. |
| Toxicity | Nephrotoxicity and acoustic nerve damage. |

**Hydroxyurea**

| | |
|---|---|
| Mechanism | Inhibits **R**ibonucleotide **R**eductase → ↓ DNA **S**ynthesis (**S**-phase specific). |
| Clinical use | Melanoma, CML, sickle cell disease (↑ HbF). |
| Toxicity | Bone marrow suppression, GI upset. |

**Prednisone**

| | |
|---|---|
| Mechanism | May trigger apoptosis. May even work on nondividing cells. |
| Clinical use | Most commonly used glucocorticoid in cancer chemotherapy. Used in CLL, Hodgkin's lymphomas (part of the MOPP regimen). Also an immunosuppressant used in autoimmune diseases. |
| Toxicity | Cushing-like symptoms; immunosuppression, cataracts, acne, osteoporosis, hypertension, peptic ulcers, hyperglycemia, psychosis. |

**Tamoxifen, raloxifene**

| | |
|---|---|
| Mechanism | SERMs—receptor antagonists in breast, agonists in bone; block the binding of estrogen to estrogen receptor–positive cells. |
| Clinical use | Breast cancer. Also useful to prevent osteoporosis. |
| Toxicity | Tamoxifen may ↑ the risk of endometrial carcinoma via partial agonist effects; "hot flashes." Raloxifene does not cause endometrial carcinoma because it is an endometrial antagonist. |

### Trastuzumab (Herceptin)

| | |
|---|---|
| Mechanism | Monoclonal antibody against HER-2 (*erb*-B2). Helps kill breast cancer cells that overexpress HER-2, possibly through antibody-dependent cytotoxicity. |
| Clinical use | Metastatic breast cancer. |
| Toxicity | Cardiotoxicity. |

### Imatinib (Gleevec)

| | |
|---|---|
| Mechanism | Philadelphia chromosome *bcr-abl* tyrosine kinase inhibitor. |
| Clinical use | CML, GI stromal tumors. |
| Toxicity | Fluid retention. |

# Musculoskeletal and Connective Tissue

*"I just use my muscles like a conversation piece, like someone walking a cheetah down 42nd Street."*

—Arnold Schwarzenegger

*"Beauty may be skin deep, but ugly goes clear to the bone."*

—Redd Foxx

*"I try to catch him right on the tip of his nose because I try to punch the bone into the brain."*

—Mike Tyson

*"The function of muscle is to pull and not to push, except in the case of the genitals and the tongue."*

—Leonardo da Vinci

▶ Anatomy and Physiology

▶ Pathology

▶ Pharmacology

HIGH-YIELD SYSTEMS

MUSCULOSKELETAL

**Epidermis layers**

From surface to base: stratum Corneum, stratum Lucidum, stratum Granulosum, stratum Spinosum, stratum Basalis.

Californians Like Girls in String Bikinis.

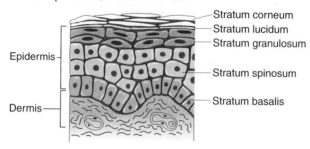

**Epithelial cell junctions**

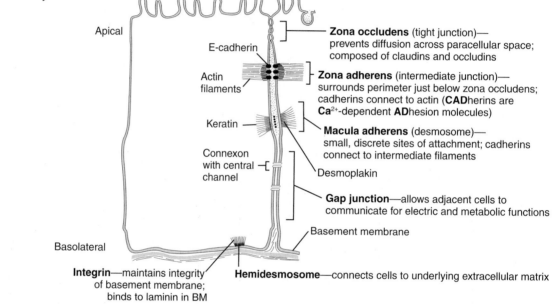

Apical

E-cadherin

Actin filaments

Keratin

Connexon with central channel

Basolateral

**Zona occludens** (tight junction)— prevents diffusion across paracellular space; composed of claudins and occludins

**Zona adherens** (intermediate junction)— surrounds perimeter just below zona occludens; cadherins connect to actin (**CAD**herins are Ca²⁺-dependent **AD**hesion molecules)

**Macula adherens** (desmosome)— small, discrete sites of attachment; cadherins connect to intermediate filaments

Desmoplakin

**Gap junction**—allows adjacent cells to communicate for electric and metabolic functions

Basement membrane

**Integrin**—maintains integrity of basement membrane; binds to laminin in BM

**Hemidesmosome**—connects cells to underlying extracellular matrix

**Unhappy triad/ knee injury**

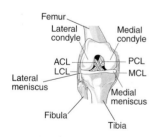

This common football injury (caused by clipping from the lateral side) consists of damage to medial collateral ligament (MCL), anterior cruciate ligament (ACL), and lateral (**not** medial) meniscus.

PCL = posterior cruciate ligament. LCL = lateral collateral ligament.

"Anterior" and "posterior" in ACL and PCL refer to sites of **tibial** attachment.

Positive anterior drawer sign indicates tearing of the ACL.

Abnormal passive abduction indicates a torn MCL.

| | | |
|---|---|---|
| **Clinically important landmarks** | Pudendal nerve block (to relieve pain of pregnancy)—ischial spine.<br>Appendix—$2/3$ of the way from the umbilicus to the anterior superior iliac spine (McBurney's point).<br>Lumbar puncture—iliac crest. | |
| **Rotator cuff muscles**<br><br>Acromion  Supraspinatus<br>Coracoid<br>Infra-spinatus  Biceps tendon<br>Teres minor  Sub-scapularis<br><br>**Posterior ⟶ Anterior** | Shoulder muscles that form the rotator cuff:<br>**S**upraspinatus—helps deltoid abduct arm.<br>**I**nfraspinatus—laterally rotates arm.<br>**T**eres minor—adducts and laterally rotates arm.<br>**S**ubscapularis—medially rotates and adducts arm. | **SItS** (small t is for teres minor). |

## Upper extremity innervation

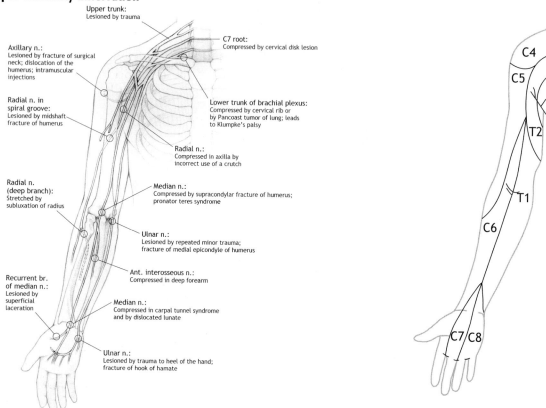

**Upper trunk:**
Lesioned by trauma

**C7 root:**
Compressed by cervical disk lesion

**Axillary n.:**
Lesioned by fracture of surgical neck; dislocation of the humerus; intramuscular injections

**Lower trunk of brachial plexus:**
Compressed by cervical rib or by Pancoast tumor of lung; leads to Klumpke's palsy

**Radial n. in spiral groove:**
Lesioned by midshaft fracture of humerus

**Radial n.:**
Compressed in axilla by incorrect use of a crutch

**Radial n. (deep branch):**
Stretched by subluxation of radius

**Median n.:**
Compressed by supracondylar fracture of humerus; pronator teres syndrome

**Ulnar n.:**
Lesioned by repeated minor trauma; fracture of medial epicondyle of humerus

**Ant. interosseous n.:**
Compressed in deep forearm

**Recurrent br. of median n.:**
Lesioned by superficial laceration

**Median n.:**
Compressed in carpal tunnel syndrome and by dislocated lunate

**Ulnar n.:**
Lesioned by trauma to heel of the hand; fracture of hook of hamate

### A. Upper limb nerve routes and common lesions

C4, C5, T2, T1, C6, C7, C8

### B. Dermatomes of the upper limb

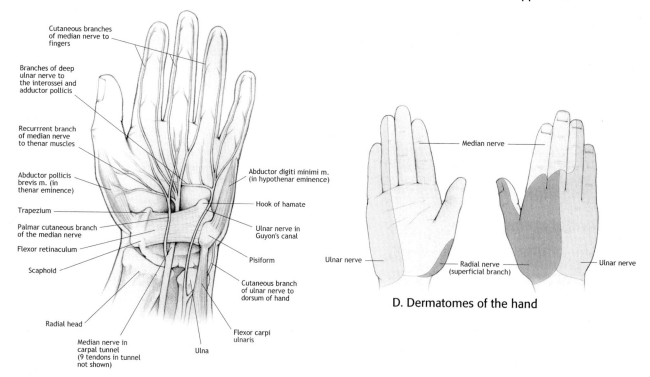

Cutaneous branches of median nerve to fingers

Branches of deep ulnar nerve to the interossei and adductor pollicis

Recurrrent branch of median nerve to thenar muscles

Abductor pollicis brevis m. (in thenar eminence)

Trapezium

Palmar cutaneous branch of the median nerve

Flexor retinaculum

Scaphoid

Radial head

Median nerve in carpal tunnel (9 tendons in tunnel not shown)

Abductor digiti minimi m. (in hypothenar eminence)

Hook of hamate

Ulnar nerve in Guyon's canal

Pisiform

Cutaneous branch of ulnar nerve to dorsum of hand

Flexor carpi ulnaris

Ulna

### C. Innervation of the hand

Median nerve

Ulnar nerve

Radial nerve (superficial branch)

Ulnar nerve

### D. Dermatomes of the hand

(Reproduced, with permission, from White JS. *USMLE Road Map: Gross Anatomy,* 2nd ed. New York: McGraw-Hill, 2005: 145–147.)

## Brachial plexus lesions

1. Waiter's tip (Erb's palsy)
2. Total claw hand (Klumpke's palsy)
3. Wrist drop
4. Winged scapula
5. Deltoid paralysis
6. Saturday night palsy (wrist drop)
7. Difficulty flexing elbow, variable sensory loss
8. ↓ thumb function ("ape hand")
9. Intrinsic muscles of hand, claw hand ("Pope's blessing")

**LT** = long thoracic nerve
**Rad** = radial nerve
**Ax** = axillary nerve
**MC** = musculocutaneous nerve
**Med** = median nerve
**Uln** = ulnar nerve

Clavicle fracture is relatively common—brachial plexus is protected from injury by subclavius muscle.

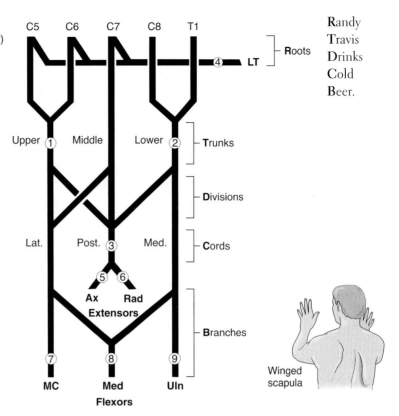

**R**andy **T**ravis **D**rinks **C**old **B**eer.

Winged scapula

**Upper extremity nerves**

| Nerve | Cause of Injury | Motor Deficit | Sensory Deficit | Sign |
|-------|-----------------|---------------|-----------------|------|
| Axillary (C5, C6) | Fractured surgical neck of humerus, dislocation of humeral head | Arm abduction at shoulder | Over deltoid muscle | Flattened deltoid |
| Radial (C5–C8) | Fracture at midshaft of humerus; "Saturday night palsy" (extended compression of axilla by back of chair or crutches) | Wrist extension Finger extension at MCP joints Supination Thumb extension and abduction | Posterior arm and dorsal hand and dorsal thumb | Wrist drop |
| Median (C6–C8, T1) | **Proximal lesion:** Fracture of supracondylar humerus **Distal lesion:** Carpal tunnel syndrome; dislocated lunate | Opposition of thumb Lateral finger flexion Wrist flexion | Dorsal and palmar aspects of lateral 3½ fingers, thenar eminence Dorsal and palmar aspects of lateral 3½ fingers | "Ape hand" Ulnar deviation of wrist upon wrist flexion |
| Ulnar (C8, T1) | **Proximal lesion:** Fracture of medial epicondyle of humerus **Distal lesion:** Fracture of hook of hamate (falling onto outstretched hand) | Medial finger flexion Wrist flexion Abduction and adduction of fingers (interossei) Adduction of thumb Extension of 4th and 5th fingers (lumbricals) | Medial 1½ fingers, hypothenar eminence | Radial deviation of wrist upon wrist flexion Ulnar claw hand (when asked to straighten fingers) —"Pope's blessing/ hand of benediction" |
| Musculo-cutaneous (C5–C7) | Upper trunk compression | Flexion of arm at elbow | Lateral forearm | |

**Causes of mononeuropathy**    Compression, trauma, diabetes, vasculitis, radiation, inflammation (e.g., VZV).

| | | |
|---|---|---|
| **Erb-Duchenne palsy ("waiter's tip")** 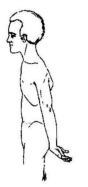 | Traction or tear of the upper trunk of the brachial plexus (C5 and C6 roots); follows blow to shoulder or trauma during delivery.<br>Findings: limb hangs by side (paralysis of abductors), medially rotated (paralysis of lateral rotators), forearm is pronated (loss of biceps). | "Waiter's tip" owing to appearance of arm. |

**Klumpke's palsy and thoracic outlet syndrome**

An embryologic or childbirth defect affecting inferior trunk of brachial plexus (C8, T1); a cervical rib can compress subclavian artery and inferior trunk, resulting in thoracic outlet syndrome:

1. Atrophy of the thenar and hypothenar eminences
2. Atrophy of the interosseous muscles
3. Sensory deficits on the medial side of the forearm and hand
4. Disappearance of the radial pulse upon moving the head toward the opposite side

**Distortions of the hand**

Multiple types: ulnar claw, median claw, "ape hand," and Klumpke's total claw (clawing of all digits). To keep things straight, just remember it's all about the lumbricals, which flex the MCP joints and extend both the DIP and PIP joints.

Ulnar claw

Distal ulnar nerve lesion → loss of medial lumbrical function; 4th and 5th digits are clawed ("Pope's blessing").

Median claw

Distal median nerve lesion (after branch containing C5–C7 branches off to feed forearm flexors) → loss of lateral lumbrical function; 2nd and 3rd digits are clawed.

"Ape hand"

Proximal median nerve lesion → loss of opponens pollicis muscle function → unopposable thumb (inability to abduct thumb), hence "ape hand."

Klumpke's total claw

Lesion of lower trunk (C8, T1) of brachial plexus → loss of function of all lumbricals; forearm finger flexors (fed by part of median nerve with C5–C7) and finger extensors (fed by radial nerve) are unopposed → clawing of all digits.

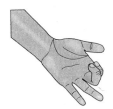

Claw hand of 2nd and 3rd digits
Median nerve

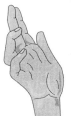

Claw hand of 4th and 5th digits ("Pope's blessing")
Distal ulnar nerve lesion

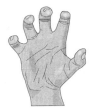

Klumpke's total claw hand
Lower trunk (C8, T1)

**Radial nerve**

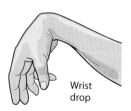

Wrist drop

Known as the "great extensor nerve." Provides innervation of the **B**rachioradialis, **E**xtensors of the wrist and fingers, **S**upinator, and **T**riceps.

Radial nerve innervates the **BEST**!
To **SUP**inate is to move as if carrying a bowl of **SOUP.**

---

**Hand muscles**

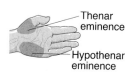

Thenar eminence

Hypothenar eminence

Thenar—**O**pponens pollicis, **A**bductor pollicis brevis, **F**lexor pollicis brevis.
Hypothenar—**O**pponens digiti minimi, **A**bductor digiti minimi, **F**lexor digiti minimi.
Dorsal interosseous muscles—abduct the fingers.
Palmar interosseous muscles—adduct the fingers.
Lumbrical muscles—flex at the MP joint.

Both groups perform the same functions: **O**ppose, **A**bduct, and **F**lex (**OAF**).

**DAB** = **D**orsals **AB**duct.
**PAD** = **P**almars **AD**duct.

---

**Repetitive elbow trauma**

Degenerative injury due to repeated use; leads to tiny tears in tendons and muscles. May be inflammatory—e.g., lateral epicondylitis (tennis elbow), medial epicondylitis (golf elbow).

---

**Lower extremity nerves**

| Nerve | Cause of Injury | Motor Deficit | Sensory Deficit |
|---|---|---|---|
| Obturator | Anterior hip dislocation | Thigh adduction | Medial thigh |
| Femoral | Pelvic fracture | Thigh flexion and leg extension | Anterior thigh and medial leg |
| Common peroneal | Trauma to lateral aspect of leg or fibula neck fracture | Foot eversion and dorsiflexion; toe extension | Anterolateral leg and dorsal aspect of foot |
| Tibial | Knee trauma | Foot inversion and plantarflexion; toe flexion | Sole of foot |
| Superior gluteal | Posterior hip dislocation or polio | Thigh abduction (positive Trendelenburg sign) | |
| Inferior gluteal | Posterior hip dislocation | Can't jump, climb stairs, or rise from seated position | |

**PED** = **P**eroneal **E**verts and **D**orsiflexes; if injured, foot drop**PED** (dorsiflex = extend foot).
**TIP** = **T**ibial **I**nverts and **P**lantarflexes; if injured, can't stand on **TIP**toes.

## Muscle conduction to contraction

**A.**

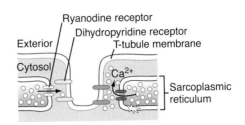

**B.**

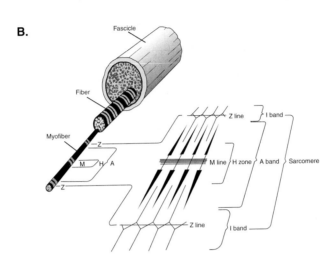

Thin lines along Z line = actin

Triangular structures emanating from M line = myosin

**C.**

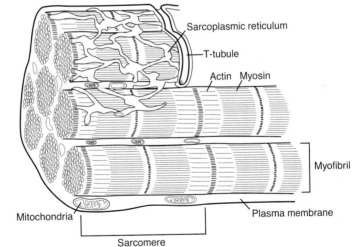

### Muscle contraction:

1. Action potential depolarization opens voltage-gated $Ca^{2+}$ channels, inducing neurotransmitter release.
2. Postsynaptic ligand binding leads to muscle cell depolarization in the motor end plate.
3. Depolarization travels along muscle cell and down the T-tubule.
4. Depolarization of the voltage-sensitive dihydropyridine receptor, coupled to the ryanodine receptor on the sarcoplasmic reticulum, induces a conformational change causing $Ca^{2+}$ release from sarcoplasmic reticulum (calcium-induced calcium release).
5. Released $Ca^{2+}$ binds to troponin C, causing a conformational change that moves tropomyosin out of the myosin-binding groove on actin filaments.
6. Myosin releases bound ADP and is displaced on the actin filament (power stroke). Contraction results in H- and I-band shortening, but the A band remains the same length (**A** band is **A**lways the same length; **HIZ** shrinkage).

### Types of muscle fibers

| | | |
|---|---|---|
| Type 1 muscle | Slow twitch; red fibers due to ↑ mitochondria and myoglobin concentration (↑ oxidative phosphorylation) → sustained contraction. | Think "one slow red ox." |
| Type 2 muscle | Fast twitch; white fibers due to ↓ mitochondria and myoglobin concentration (↑ anaerobic glycolysis); weight training results in hypertrophy of fast-twitch muscle fibers. | |

### Skeletal and cardiac muscle contraction

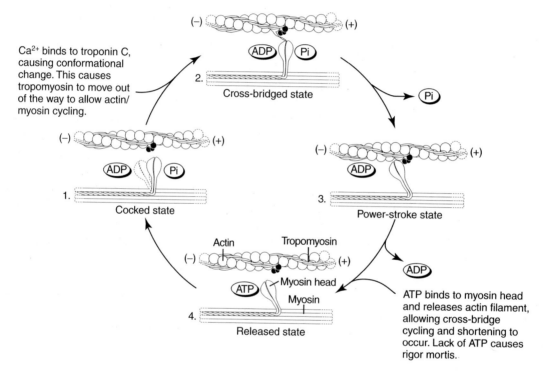

Ca²⁺ binds to troponin C, causing conformational change. This causes tropomyosin to move out of the way to allow actin/myosin cycling.

2. Cross-bridged state

1. Cocked state

3. Power-stroke state

4. Released state

ATP binds to myosin head and releases actin filament, allowing cross-bridge cycling and shortening to occur. Lack of ATP causes rigor mortis.

### Smooth muscle contraction

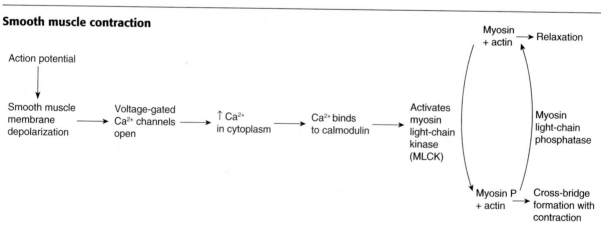

## Bone formation

| | | |
|---|---|---|
| Endochondral ossification | Longitudinal bone growth. Cartilaginous model of bone is first made by chondrocytes. Osteoclasts and osteoblasts later replace with woven bone and remodel to lamellar bone. | Osteoblast source— mesenchymal stem cells in periosteum. |
| Membranous ossification | Flat bone growth (skull, facial bones, and axial skeleton). Woven bone formed directly without cartilage. Later remodeled to lamellar bone. | |

**Achondroplasia** — Failure of longitudinal bone growth → short limbs. Membranous ossification is not affected → normal-sized head. Constitutive activation of fibroblast growth factor receptor (FGFR3) actually inhibits chondrocyte proliferation. > 85% of mutations occur sporadically and are associated with advanced paternal age, but the condition also demonstrates autosomal-dominant inheritance. Common cause of dwarfism. Normal life span and fertility.

**Osteoporosis**

| | | |
|---|---|---|
| | Reduction of primarily trabecular (spongy) bone mass in spite of normal bone mineralization. | Vertebral crush fractures— acute back pain, loss of height, kyphosis. |
| Type I | Postmenopausal; ↑ bone resorption due to ↓ estrogen levels. Estrogen replacement is controversial as prophylaxis (side effects). | Femoral neck fracture, distal radius (Colles') fractures. Prophylaxis: exercise and calcium ingestion before age 30. |
| Type II | Senile osteoporosis—affects men and women > 70 years of age. | Treatment: estrogen and/or calcitonin; bisphosphonates or pulsatile PTH for severe cases. Glucocorticoids are contra-indicated. |

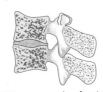 

Mild compression fracture          Normal vertebra

**Osteopetrosis (marble bone disease)** — Failure of normal bone resorption → thickened, dense bones that are prone to fracture. Bone defect is due to abnormal function of osteoclasts. Serum calcium, phosphate, and **alkaline phosphatase (ALP)** are **normal**. ↓ marrow space leads to anemia, thrombocytopenia, infection. Genetic deficiency of carbonic anhydrase II. X-rays show "Erlenmeyer flask" bones that flare out. Can result in cranial nerve impingement and palsies due to narrowed foramina.

**Osteomalacia/rickets** — Defective mineralization/calcification of osteoid → soft bones. Vitamin D deficiency in adults → ↓ calcium levels → ↑ secretion of PTH, ↓ in serum phosphate. Reversible when vitamin D is replaced. Vitamin D deficiency in childhood causes rickets.

**Osteitis fibrosa cystica**  
Caused by hyperparathyroidism. Characterized by "brown tumors" (cystic spaces lined by osteoclasts, filled with fibrous stroma and sometimes blood). High serum calcium, low serum phosphorus, and high ALP.

**Paget's disease (osteitis deformans)**  
Abnormal bone architecture caused by ↑ in both osteoblastic and osteoclastic activity. Possibly viral in origin (paramyxovirus is suspected). Serum calcium, phosphorus, and PTH levels are normal. ↑ **ALP.** Mosaic bone pattern; long bone chalk-stick fractures. ↑ blood flow from ↑ arteriovenous shunts may cause high-output heart failure. Can lead to osteogenic sarcoma.

Hat size can be ↑; hearing loss is common due to auditory foramen narrowing.

### Lab values in bone disorders

| | Serum Ca$^{2+}$ | Phosphate | ALP | PTH | Comments |
|---|---|---|---|---|---|
| Osteoporosis | — | — | — | — | ↓ bone mass |
| Osteopetrosis | — | — | — | — | Thickened, dense bones |
| Osteomalacia/rickets | ↓ | ↓ | — | ↑ | Soft bones |
| Osteitis fibrosa cystica | ↑ | ↓ | ↑ | ↑ | "Brown tumors" |
| Paget's disease | — | — | ↑ | — | Abnormal bone architecture |

**Polyostotic fibrous dysplasia**  
Bone is replaced by fibroblasts, collagen, and irregular bony trabeculae. Affects many bones. **McCune-Albright syndrome** is a form of polyostotic fibrous dysplasia characterized by multiple unilateral bone lesions associated with endocrine abnormalities (precocious puberty) and unilateral pigmented skin lesions (café-au-lait spots/"coast of Maine" spots).

## Primary bone tumors

### Benign tumors

| | |
|---|---|
| Osteoma | Associated with Gardner's syndrome (FAP). New piece of bone grows on another piece of bone, often in the skull. |
| Osteoid osteoma | Interlacing trabeculae of woven bone surrounded by osteoblasts. < 2 cm and found in proximal tibia and femur. Most common in men < 25 years of age. |
| Osteoblastoma | Same morphologically as osteoid osteoma, but larger and found in vertebral column. |
| Giant cell tumor (osteoclastoma) | Occurs most commonly at epiphyseal end of long bones. Peak incidence 20–40 years of age. Locally aggressive benign tumor often around the distal femur, proximal tibial region (knee). Characteristic "double bubble" or "soap bubble" appearance on x-ray. Spindle-shaped cells with multinucleated giant cells. |
| Osteochondroma (exostosis) | Most common benign bone tumor. Mature bone with cartilaginous cap. Usually in men < 25 years of age. Commonly originates from long metaphysis. Malignant transformation to chondrosarcoma is rare. |
| Enchondroma | Benign cartilaginous neoplasm found in intramedullary bone. Usually distal extremities (vs. chondrosarcoma). |

### Malignant tumors

| | |
|---|---|
| Osteosarcoma (osteogenic sarcoma) | 2nd most common 1° malignant tumor of bone (after multiple myeloma). Peak incidence in men 10–20 years of age. Commonly found in the metaphysis of long bones, often around distal femur, proximal tibial region (knee). Predisposing factors include Paget's disease of bone, bone infarcts, radiation, and familial retinoblastoma. Codman's triangle or sunburst pattern (from elevation of periosteum) on x-ray. Poor prognosis. |
| Ewing's sarcoma | Anaplastic small blue cell malignant tumor. Most common in boys < 15. Extremely aggressive with early mets, but responsive to chemotherapy. Characteristic "onion-skin" appearance in bone ("going out for Ewings and onion rings"). Commonly appears in diaphysis of long bones, pelvis, scapula, and ribs. 11;22 translocation. 11 + 22 = 33 (Patrick Ewing's jersey number). |
| Chondrosarcoma | Malignant cartilaginous tumor. Most common in men aged 30–60. Usually located in pelvis, spine, scapula, humerus, tibia, or femur. May be of 1° origin or from osteochondroma. Expansile glistening mass within the medullary cavity. |

### Primary bone tumor locations

| | Benign | Malignant |
|---|---|---|
| Epiphysis | Giant cell tumor (osteoclastoma) | — |
| Metaphysis | Osteochondroma | Osteosarcoma |
| Diaphysis | Osteoid osteoma | Ewing's sarcoma |
| Intramedullary | Enchondroma | Chondrosarcoma |

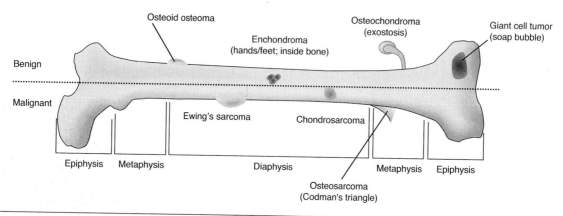

### Osteoarthritis

Mechanical—wear and tear of joints leads to destruction of articular cartilage (see Image 119), subchondral cysts, sclerosis, osteophytes (bone spurs), eburnation (polished, ivory-like appearance of bone), Heberden's nodes (DIP), and Bouchard's nodes (PIP). Predisposing factors: age, obesity, joint deformity.

Classic presentation: pain in weight-bearing joints after use (e.g., at the end of the day), improving with rest. In knees, cartilage loss begins on medial aspect ("bowlegged"). Noninflammatory. No systemic symptoms.

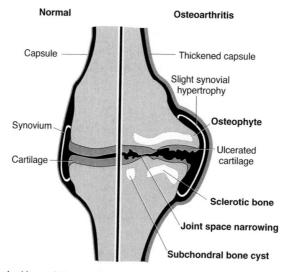

(Adapted, with permission, from Stobo J et al. *The Principles and Practice of Medicine*, 23rd ed. Stamford, CT: Appleton & Lange, 1996: 241.)

**Rheumatoid arthritis**

Autoimmune—inflammatory disorder affecting synovial joints, with pannus formation in joints (MCP, PIP), subcutaneous rheumatoid nodules (fibrinoid necrosis surrounded by palisading histiocytes), ulnar deviation, subluxation, Baker's cyst (behind the knee) (see Image 56). No DIP involvement.

Females > males. Type III hypersensitivity. 80% of RA patients have **positive rheumatoid factor** (anti-IgG antibody); anti-CCP antibody is less sensitive but more specific. Strong association with HLA-DR4.

Classic presentation: morning stiffness lasting > 30 minutes and improving with use, symmetric joint involvement, systemic symptoms (fever, fatigue, pleuritis, pericarditis).

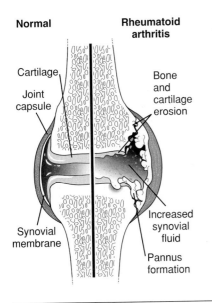

Normal | Rheumatoid arthritis

Cartilage
Joint capsule
Synovial membrane

Bone and cartilage erosion
Increased synovial fluid
Pannus formation

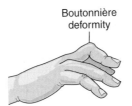

Boutonnière deformity

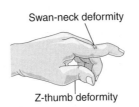

Swan-neck deformity

Z-thumb deformity

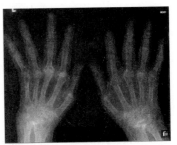

Rheumatoid arthritis (note joint space narrowing of MCP)

(Reproduced, with permission, from USMLERx.com.)

**Sjögren's syndrome**

Classic triad:
1. Xerophthalmia (dry eyes, conjunctivitis, "sand in my eyes")
2. Xerostomia (dry mouth, dysphagia)
3. Arthritis

Parotid enlargement, ↑ risk of B-cell lymphoma, dental caries. Autoantibodies to ribonucleoprotein antigens, **SS-A (Ro), SS-B (La)**.

Predominantly affects females between 40 and 60 years of age.

Associated with rheumatoid arthritis.

**Sicca syndrome**—dry eyes, dry mouth, nasal and vaginal dryness, chronic bronchitis, reflux esophagitis. No arthritis.

**Gout**

| | |
|---|---|
| Symptoms | Asymmetric joint distribution. Joint is swollen, red, and painful. Classic manifestation is painful MTP joint of the big toe (podagra). Tophus formation (often on external ear, olecranon bursa, or Achilles tendon). Acute attack tends to occur after a large meal or alcohol consumption (alcohol metabolites compete for same excretion sites in kidney as uric acid, causing ↓ uric acid secretion and subsequent buildup in blood). |
| Findings | Precipitation of monosodium urate crystals into joints due to hyperuricemia, which can be caused by Lesch-Nyhan syndrome, PRPP excess, ↓ excretion of uric acid (e.g., thiazide diuretics), ↑ cell turnover, or von Gierke's disease. 90% due to underexcretion; 10% due to overproduction. Crystals are needle shaped and **negatively birefringent** = yellow crystals under parallel light (see Image 54). More common in men. |
| Treatment | Colchicine, NSAIDs (e.g., indomethacin), probenecid, allopurinol. |

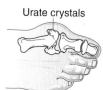
Urate crystals

**Pseudogout**

Caused by deposition of calcium pyrophosphate crystals within the joint space. Forms basophilic, rhomboid crystals that are **weakly positively birefringent.** Usually affects large joints (classically the knee). > 50 years old; both sexes affected equally. No treatment.

Gout—crystals are yellow when parallel (∥) and blue when perpendicular (⊥) to the light.
Pseudogout—crystals are yellow when perpendicular (⊥) and blue when parallel (∥) to the light.

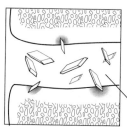
Calcium pyrophosphate crystals

**Infectious arthritis**

| | |
|---|---|
| Septic | *S. aureus*, *Streptococcus*, and *Neisseria gonorrhoeae* are common. Gonococcal arthritis is an **STD** that presents as a monoarticular, migratory arthritis with an asymmetrical pattern. Affected joint is swollen, red, and painful. **STD** = **S**ynovitis (e.g., knee), **T**enosynovitis (e.g., hand), and **D**ermatitis (e.g., pustules). |
| Chronic | TB (from mycobacterial dissemination), Lyme disease. |

| | | |
|---|---|---|
| **Seronegative spondylo-arthropathies** | Arthritis without rheumatoid factor (no anti-IgG antibody). Strong association with **HLA-B27** (gene that codes for HLA MHC I). Occurs more often in males. | |
| Ankylosing spondylitis | Chronic inflammatory disease of spine and sacroiliac joints → ankylosis (stiff spine due to fusion of joints), uveitis, and aortic regurgitation. | Bamboo spine. |
| Reactive arthritis (Reiter's syndrome) | Classic triad:<br>1. Conjunctivitis and anterior uveitis<br>2. Urethritis<br>3. Arthritis | "Can't **see**,<br>    can't **pee**,<br>    can't climb a **tree**."<br>Post-GI or chlamydia<br>    infections. |
| Psoriatic arthritis | Joint pain and stiffness associated with psoriasis. Asymmetric and patchy involvement. Dactylitis ("sausage fingers"), "pencil-in-cup" deformity on x-ray. Seen in fewer than ⅓ of patients with psoriasis. | 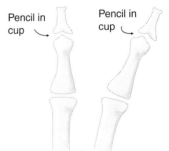 |

| | | |
|---|---|---|
| **Systemic lupus erythematosus** | 90% are female and between ages 14 and 45. Most common and severe in black females. Symptoms include fever, fatigue, weight loss, nonbacterial verrucous endocarditis, hilar adenopathy, and Raynaud's phenomenon (see Image 52).<br>Wire-loop lesions in kidney with immune complex deposition (usually nephritic syndrome); death from renal failure and infections. False positives on syphilis tests (RPR/VDRL) due to antiphospholipid antibodies, which cross-react with cardiolipin used in tests. Lab tests detect presence of:<br>1. Antinuclear antibodies (ANA)—sensitive, but not specific for SLE<br>2. Antibodies to double-stranded DNA (anti-dsDNA)—very specific, poor prognosis<br>3. Anti-Smith antibodies (anti-Sm)—very specific, but not prognostic<br>4. Antihistone antibodies—drug-induced lupus | **I'M DAMN SHARP:**<br>Immunoglobulins<br>    (anti-dsDNA, anti-Sm,<br>    antiphospholipid)<br>Malar rash<br>Discoid rash<br>Antinuclear antibody<br>Mucositis (oropharyngeal<br>    ulcers)<br>Neurologic disorders<br>Serositis (pleuritis,<br>    pericarditis)<br>Hematologic disorders<br>Arthritis<br>Renal disorders<br>Photosensitivity |

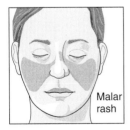

| | |
|---|---|
| **Positive antinuclear antibodies** | SLE, Sjögren's (and sicca), scleroderma, polymyositis, dermatomyositis, rheumatoid arthritis, juvenile arthritis, mixed connective tissue disease. |

| | | |
|---|---|---|
| **Sarcoidosis** | Characterized by immune-mediated, widespread **noncaseating granulomas** and elevated serum ACE levels. Common in black females. Associated with restrictive lung disease, bilateral hilar lymphadenopathy, erythema nodosum, Bell's palsy, epithelial granulomas containing microscopic Schaumann and asteroid bodies, uveoparotitis, and hypercalcemia (due to elevated conversion of vitamin D to its active form in epithelioid macrophages) (see Image 95). Treatment: steroids. | **GRAIN:** Gammaglobulinemia Rheumatoid arthritis ACE increase Interstitial fibrosis Noncaseating granulomas |

**Polymyalgia rheumatica**

| | |
|---|---|
| Symptoms | Pain and stiffness in shoulders and hips, often with fever, malaise, and weight loss. Does not cause muscular weakness. Occurs in patients > 50 years of age; associated with temporal (giant cell) arteritis. |
| Findings | ↑ ESR, normal CK. |
| Treatment | Prednisone. |

**Polymyositis/dermatomyositis**

| | |
|---|---|
| Symptoms | **Polymyositis**—progressive symmetric proximal muscle weakness caused by CD8+ T-cell-induced injury to myofibers. Most often involves shoulders. Muscle biopsy with evidence of inflammation is diagnostic. |
| | **Dermatomyositis**—similar to polymyositis, but also involves malar rash (similar to SLE), heliotrope rash, "shawl and face" rash, Gottron's papules, "mechanic's hands." ↑ risk of malignancy. |
| Findings | ↑ CK, ↑ aldolase, and **positive ANA, anti-Jo-1.** |
| Treatment | Steroids. |

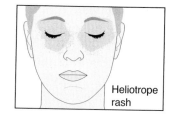

Heliotrope rash

**Neuromuscular junction diseases**

| | |
|---|---|
| Myasthenia gravis | Most common NMJ disorder. Autoantibodies to postsynaptic AChR cause ptosis, diplopia, and general weakness. Associated with thymoma. Symptoms worsen with muscle use. Reversal of symptoms occurs with AChE inhibitors. |
| Lambert-Eaton syndrome | Autoantibodies to presynaptic $Ca^{2+}$ channel results in ↓ ACh release leading to proximal muscle weakness. In contrast to myasthenia gravis, extraocular muscles are spared. Associated with paraneoplastic diseases (small cell lung cancer). Symptoms improve with muscle use. No reversal of symptoms with AChE inhibitors alone. |

| | | |
|---|---|---|
| **Mixed connective tissue disease** | **R**aynaud's phenomenon, **F**atigue, **A**rthralgias, **M**yalgias, and **E**sophageal hypomotility. Antibodies to U1RNP. Responds to steroids. | Raynaud's FAME. Remember there are antibodies against a "**mix**" of macromolecules: ribo-nucleo-protein. |

| | | |
|---|---|---|
| **Scleroderma (progressive systemic sclerosis—PSS)** | Excessive fibrosis and collagen deposition throughout the body. Commonly sclerosis of skin, manifesting as puffy and taut skin with absence of wrinkles (see Image 53). Also sclerosis of renal, pulmonary, cardiovascular, and GI systems. 75% female. 2 major types: | |

1. Diffuse scleroderma—widespread skin involvement, rapid progression, early visceral involvement. Associated with anti-Scl-70 antibody (anti-DNA topoisomerase I antibody).
2. **CREST** syndrome—**C**alcinosis, **R**aynaud's phenomenon, **E**sophageal dysmotility, **S**clerodactyly, and **T**elangiectasia. Limited skin involvement, often confined to fingers and face. More benign clinical course. Associated with **antiCentromere antibody (C for CREST)**.

### Soft tissue tumors

| | |
|---|---|
| Lipoma | Soft, well-encapsulated fat tumor. Benign. Simple excision is usually curative. |
| Liposarcoma | Malignant fat tumor that can be quite large. Will recur unless adequately excised. |
| Rhabdomyoma | Benign tumor derived from striated muscle (skeletal or cardiac). Rhabdomyoma of the heart occurs in tuberous sclerosis. |
| Rhabdomyosarcoma | Most common soft tissue tumor of childhood. Malignant. Arises from skeletal muscle, most often in head/neck. |

### Dermatologic terminology

| Lesion | Characteristics | Examples |
|---|---|---|
| Macule | Flat discoloration < 1 cm | Tinea versicolor |
| Patch | Macule > 1 cm | |
| Papule | Elevated skin lesion < 1 cm | Acne vulgaris |
| Plaque | Papule > 1 cm | Psoriasis |
| Vesicle | Small fluid-containing blister | Chickenpox |
| Wheal | Transient vesicle | Hives |
| Bulla | Large fluid-containing blister | Bullous pemphigoid |
| Keloid | Irregular, raised lesion resulting from scar tissue hypertrophy (follows trauma to skin, especially in African-Americans) | *T. pertenue* (yaws) |
| Pustule | Blister containing pus | Impetigo |
| Crust | Dried exudates from a vesicle, bulla, or pustule | |
| Hyperkeratosis | ↑ thickness of stratum corneum | Psoriasis |
| Parakeratosis | Hyperkeratosis with retention of nuclei in stratum corneum | Psoriasis |
| Acantholysis | Separation of epidermal cells | Pemphigus vulgaris |
| Acanthosis | Epidermal hyperplasia (↑ spinosum) | |
| Dermatitis | Inflammation of the skin | |

## Skin disorders

### Common disorders

| | |
|---|---|
| Verrucae | Warts. Soft, tan-colored, cauliflower-like lesions. Epidermal hyperplasia, hyperkeratosis, koilocytosis. Verruca vulgaris on hands; condyloma acuminatum on genitals (caused by HPV). |
| Nevocellular nevus | Common mole. Benign. |
| Urticaria | Hives. Intensely pruritic wheals that form after mast cell degranulation. |
| Ephelis | Freckle. Normal number of melanocytes, ↑ melanin pigment. |
| Atopic dermatitis (eczema) | Pruritic eruption, commonly on skin flexures. Often associated with other atopic diseases (asthma, allergic rhinitis). |
| Allergic contact dermatitis | Type IV hypersensitivity reaction that follows exposure to allergen. Lesions occur at site of contact. |
| Psoriasis | Papules and plaques with silvery scaling, especially on knees and elbows (see Image 65). Acanthosis with parakeratotic scaling (nuclei still in stratum corneum). ↑ stratum spinosum, ↓ stratum granulosum. **Auspitz sign** (bleeding spots when scales are scraped off). Can be associated with nail pitting and psoriatic arthritis. |
| Seborrheic keratosis | Flat, greasy, pigmented squamous epithelial proliferation with keratin-filled cysts (horn cysts). Looks "pasted on." Lesions occur on head, trunk, and extremities. Common benign neoplasm of older persons. Sign of Leser-Trélat—sudden appearance of multiple seborrheic keratoses indicating an underlying malignancy (e.g., GI, lymphoid). |

### Pigmentation disorders

| | |
|---|---|
| Albinism | Normal melanocyte number with ↓ melanin production due to ↓ activity of tyrosinase. Can also be caused by failure of neural crest cell migration during development. |
| Vitiligo | Irregular areas of complete depigmentation. Caused by a ↓ in melanocytes. |
| Melasma | Hyperpigmentation associated with pregnancy ("mask of pregnancy") or OCP use. |

### Infectious disorders

| | |
|---|---|
| Impetigo | Very superficial skin infection. Usually from *S. aureus* or *S. pyogenes*. Highly contagious. **Honey-colored crusting.** |
| Cellulitis | Acute, painful spreading infection of dermis and subcutaneous tissues. Usually from *S. pyogenes* or *S. aureus*. |
| Necrotizing fasciitis | Deeper tissue injury, usually from anaerobic bacteria and *S. pyogenes*. Results in crepitus from methane and $CO_2$ production. "Flesh-eating bacteria." |
| Staphylococcal scalded skin syndrome (SSSS) | Exotoxin destroys keratinocyte attachments in the stratum granulosum only. Characterized by fever and generalized erythematous rash with sloughing of the upper layers of the epidermis. Seen in newborns and children. |
| Hairy leukoplakia | White, painless plaques on the tongue that cannot be scraped off. EBV mediated. Occurs in HIV-positive patients. |

### Blistering disorders

| | |
|---|---|
| Pemphigus vulgaris | Potentially fatal autoimmune skin disorder with IgG antibody against **desmosomes** (anti-epithelial cell antibody); immunofluorescence reveals antibodies around cells of epidermis in a reticular or netlike pattern. Acantholysis—intraepidermal bullae involving the skin and oral mucosa (see Image 63). Positive Nikolsky's sign (separation of epidermis upon manual stroking of skin). |

## Skin disorders (continued)

**Bullous pemphigoid**
Autoimmune disorder with IgG antibody against **hemidesmosomes** (epidermal basement membrane; antibodies are "**bullow**" the epidermis); shows linear immunofluorescence. Eosinophils within blisters. Similar to but less severe than pemphigus vulgaris—affects skin but spares oral mucosa (see Image 64). Negative Nikolsky's sign.

**Dermatitis herpetiformis**
Pruritic papules and vesicles. Deposits of IgA at the tips of dermal papillae. Associated with celiac disease.

**Erythema multiforme**
Associated with infections (e.g., *Mycoplasma pneumoniae*, HSV), drugs (e.g., sulfa drugs, β-lactams, phenytoin), cancers, and autoimmune disease. Presents with multiple types of lesions—macules, papules, vesicles, and target lesions (red papules with a pale central area).

**Stevens-Johnson syndrome**
Characterized by fever, bulla formation and necrosis, sloughing of skin, and a high mortality rate. Usually associated with adverse drug reaction. A more severe form of Stevens-Johnson syndrome is known as toxic epidermal necrolysis.

## Miscellaneous disorders

**Lichen planus**
Pruritic, Purple, Polygonal Papules. Sawtooth infiltrate of lymphocytes at dermal-epidermal junction. Associated with hepatitis C.

**Actinic keratosis**
Premalignant lesions caused by sun exposure. Small, rough, erythematous or brownish papules. "Cutaneous horn." Risk of carcinoma is proportional to epithelial dysplasia.

**Acanthosis nigricans**
Hyperplasia of stratum spinosum. Associated with hyperinsulinemia (e.g., from Cushing's disease, diabetes) and visceral malignancy.

**Erythema nodosum**
Inflammatory lesions of subcutaneous fat, usually on anterior shins. Associated with coccidioidomycosis, histoplasmosis, TB, leprosy, streptococcal infections, sarcoidosis.

**Pityriasis rosea**
"Herald patch" followed days later by "Christmas tree" distribution. Multiple papular eruptions; remits spontaneously.

**Strawberry hemangioma**
First few weeks of life (1/200 births); grows rapidly and regresses spontaneously at 5–8 years of age.

**Cherry hemangioma**
Appears in 30s–40s; does not regress.

**Skin cancer**

| | | |
|---|---|---|
| Squamous cell carcinoma | Very common. Associated with excessive exposure to sunlight and arsenic exposure. Commonly appear on hands and face. Locally invasive, but rarely metastasizes. Ulcerative red lesion. Associated with chronic draining sinuses. Histopathology: keratin "pearls" (see Image 60). | **Actinic keratosis** is a precursor to squamous cell carcinoma. Keratoacanthoma is a variant that grows rapidly (4–6 weeks) and regresses spontaneously (4–8 weeks). |
| Basal cell carcinoma | Most common in sun-exposed areas of body. Locally invasive, but almost never metastasizes. Rolled edges with central ulceration. Gross pathology: pearly papules, commonly with telangiectasias (see Image 62). | Basal cell tumors have "palisading" nuclei. |
| Melanoma | Common tumor with significant risk of metastasis. S-100 tumor marker. Associated with sunlight exposure; fair-skinned persons are at ↑ risk. **Depth** of tumor correlates with risk of metastasis. Dark with irregular borders (see Image 61). | Dysplastic nevus (atypical mole) is a precursor to melanoma. |

**Arachidonic acid products**

Lipoxygenase pathway yields Leukotrienes.
$LTB_4$ is a neutrophil chemotactic agent.
$LTC_4$, $D_4$, and $E_4$ function in bronchoconstriction, vasoconstriction, contraction of smooth muscle, and ↑ vascular permeability.
$PGI_2$ inhibits platelet aggregation and promotes vasodilation.

**L** for **L**ipoxygenase and **L**eukotriene.
Neutrophils arrive "**B4**" others.

**P**latelet-**G**athering **I**nhibitor.

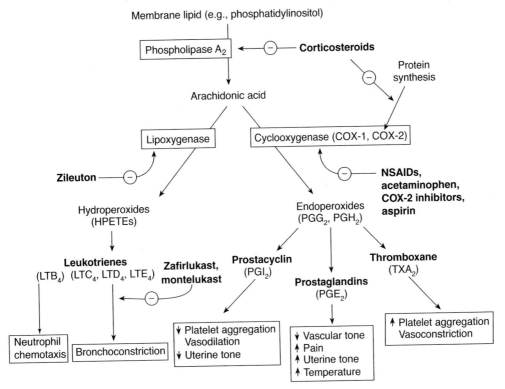

(Adapted, with permission, from Katzung BG, Trevor AJ. *Pharmacology: Examination & Board Review,* 5th ed. Stamford, CT: Appleton & Lange, 1998: 150.)

**Aspirin**

| | |
|---|---|
| Mechanism | Irreversibly inhibits cyclooxygenase by covalent binding, which ↓ synthesis of both thromboxane and prostaglandins. |
| Clinical use | Low dose (< 300 mg/day): ↓ platelet aggregation. Intermediate dose (300–2400 mg/day): antipyretic and analgesic. High dose (2400–4000 mg/day): anti-inflammatory. |
| Toxicity | Gastric upset. Chronic use can lead to acute renal failure, interstitial nephritis, and upper GI bleeding. Reye's syndrome in children with viral infection. |

**NSAIDs**

| | |
|---|---|
| | Ibuprofen, naproxen, indomethacin, ketorolac. |
| Mechanism | Reversibly inhibit cyclooxygenase (both COX-1 and COX-2). Block prostaglandin synthesis. |
| Clinical use | Antipyretic, analgesic, anti-inflammatory. Indomethacin is used to close a PDA. |
| Toxicity | Renal damage, fluid retention, aplastic anemia, GI distress, ulcers. |

### COX-2 inhibitors (celecoxib)

| | |
|---|---|
| Mechanism | Reversibly inhibit specifically the cyclooxygenase (COX) isoform 2, which is found in inflammatory cells and vascular endothelium and mediates inflammation and pain; spares COX-1, which helps maintain the gastric mucosa. Thus, should not have the corrosive effects of other NSAIDs on the GI lining. |
| Clinical use | Rheumatoid and osteoarthritis. |
| Toxicity | ↑ risk of thrombosis. Sulfa allergy. Less toxicity to GI mucosa (lower incidence of ulcers, bleeding than NSAIDs). |

### Acetaminophen

| | |
|---|---|
| Mechanism | Reversibly inhibits cyclooxygenase, mostly in CNS. Inactivated peripherally. |
| Clinical use | Antipyretic, analgesic, but lacking anti-inflammatory properties. Used instead of aspirin to prevent Reye's syndrome in children with viral infection. |
| Toxicity | Overdose produces hepatic necrosis; acetaminophen metabolite depletes glutathione and forms toxic tissue adducts in liver. N-acetylcysteine is antidote—regenerates glutathione. |

### Comparison of OTC analgesics

Acetaminophen = NSAID without anti-inflammatory activity.
Aspirin = NSAID with antiplatelet activity.

### Bisphosphonates

| | |
|---|---|
| | Etidronate, pamidronate, alendronate, risedronate. |
| Mechanism | Inhibit osteoclastic activity; reduce both formation and resorption of hydroxyapatite. |
| Clinical use | Malignancy-associated hypercalcemia, Paget's disease of bone, postmenopausal osteoporosis. |
| Toxicity | Corrosive esophagitis, nausea, diarrhea. |

### Gout drugs

| | |
|---|---|
| Colchicine | Acute gout. Binds and stabilizes tubulin to inhibit polymerization, impairing leukocyte chemotaxis and degranulation. GI side effects, especially if given orally. (Note: **indomethacin** is less toxic, also used in acute gout.) |
| Probenecid | Chronic gout. Inhibits reabsorption of uric acid in PCT (also inhibits secretion of penicillin). |
| Allopurinol | Chronic gout. Inhibits xanthine oxidase, ↓ conversion of xanthine to uric acid. Also used in lymphoma and leukemia to prevent tumor lysis–associated urate nephropathy. ↑ concentrations of azathioprine and 6-MP (both normally metabolized by xanthine oxidase). |

Probenecid and allopurinol should not be used to treat an acute episode of gout.

Do not give salicylates. All but the highest doses depress uric acid clearance. Even high doses (5–6 g/day) have only minor uricosuric activity.

**TNF-α inhibitors**

| Drug | Mechanism | Clinical Use | Toxicity | Notes |
|---|---|---|---|---|
| Etanercept | Recombinant form of human TNF receptor that binds TNF | Rheumatoid arthritis, psoriasis, ankylosing spondylitis | — | Etaner**CEPT** is a TNF decoy re**CEPT**or. |
| Infliximab | Anti-TNF antibody | Crohn's disease, rheumatoid arthritis, ankylosing spondylitis | Predisposes to infections (reactivation of latent TB) | **INFLIX**imab **INFLIX** pain on TNF. |
| Adalimumab | Directly binds TNF-α receptor sites | Rheumatoid arthritis, psoriasis, ankylosing spondylitis | — | — |

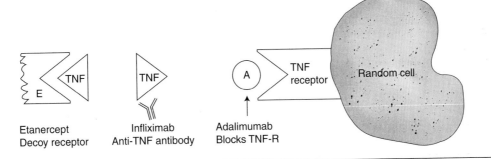

Etanercept
Decoy receptor

Infliximab
Anti-TNF antibody

Adalimumab
Blocks TNF-R

TNF receptor

Random cell

# Neurology

*"Estimated amount of glucose used by an adult human brain each day, expressed in M&Ms: 250."*

—Harper's Index

*"He has two neurons held together by a spirochete."*

—Anonymous

*"I never came upon any of my discoveries through the process of rational thinking."*

—Albert Einstein

*"I like nonsense; it wakes up the brain cells."*

—Dr. Seuss

| | | |
|---|---|---|
| **CNS/PNS origins** | Neuroectoderm—CNS neurons, ependymal cells (inner lining of ventricles, make CSF), oligodendroglia, astrocytes.<br>Neural crest—Schwann cells, PNS neurons.<br>Mesoderm—**M**icroglia, like **M**acrophages, originate from **M**esoderm. | |
| **Neurons** | Comprise nervous system. Permanent cells—do not divide in adulthood.<br>Large cells with prominent nucleoli. Nissl substance (RER) in cell body, dendrites, **not** axon. | |
| **Astrocytes**<br> | Physical support, repair, K⁺ metabolism, removal of excess neurotransmitter, maintenance of blood-brain barrier. Reactive gliosis in response to injury. Astrocyte marker—GFAP. | |
| **Microglia**<br>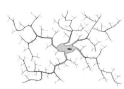 | CNS phagocytes. Mesodermal origin. Not readily discernible in Nissl stains. Have small irregular nuclei and relatively little cytoplasm.<br>Microglia $\xrightarrow{\text{tissue damage}}$ large ameboid phagocytic cells. | HIV-infected microglia fuse to form multinucleated giant cells in the CNS. |
| **Oligodendroglia**<br>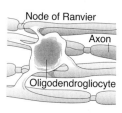 | Each oligodendrocyte myelinates multiple CNS axons (up to 30 each). In Nissl stains, they appear as small nuclei with dark chromatin and little cytoplasm. Predominant type of glial cell in white matter. | These cells are destroyed in multiple sclerosis.<br>Look like fried eggs on H&E staining (see Image 49). |
| **Schwann cells** | Each Schwann cell myelinates only 1 PNS axon. Also promote axonal regeneration. Derived from neural crest. | These cells are destroyed in Guillain-Barré syndrome.<br>Acoustic neuroma—type of schwannoma. Typically located in internal acoustic meatus (CN VIII). |

## Sensory corpuscles

| Receptor type | Location | Senses | |
|---|---|---|---|
| Free nerve endings (C—slow, unmyelinated fibers; Aδ—fast, myelinated fibers) | All skin, epidermis, some viscera | Pain and temperature | 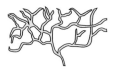 |
| Meissner's corpuscles (large, myelinated fibers) | Glabrous (hairless) skin | Position sense, dynamic fine touch (e.g., manipulation), adapt quickly |  |
| Pacinian corpuscles (large, myelinated fibers) | Deep skin layers, ligaments, and joints | Vibration, pressure |  |
| Merkel's disks (large, myelinated fibers) | Hair follicles | Position sense, static touch (e.g., shapes, edges, textures), adapt slowly |  |

## Peripheral nerve layers

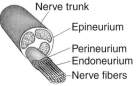

Nerve trunk
Epineurium
Perineurium
Endoneurium
Nerve fibers

Endoneurium—invests single nerve fiber (inflammatory infiltrate in Guillain-Barré)

Perineurium (Permeability barrier)—surrounds a fascicle of nerve fibers. Must be rejoined in microsurgery for limb reattachment.

Epineurium—dense connective tissue that surrounds entire nerve (fascicles and blood vessels).

*Endo* = inner.
*Peri* = around.
*Epi* = outer.

## Neurotransmitters

| Type | Change in disease | Locations of synthesis* |
|---|---|---|
| NE | ↑ in anxiety, ↓ in depression | Locus ceruleus |
| Dopamine | ↑ in schizophrenia, ↓ in Parkinson's and depression | Ventral tegmentum and SNc |
| 5-HT | ↓ in anxiety, depression | Raphe nucleus |
| ACh | ↓ in Alzheimer's, Huntington's, REM sleep | Basal nucleus of Meynert |
| GABA | ↓ in anxiety, Huntington's | Nucleus accumbens |

*Locus ceruleus—stress and panic. Nucleus accumbens and septal nucleus—reward center, pleasure, addiction, fear.

**Blood-brain barrier**

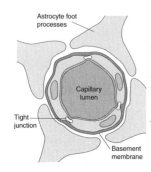

Labels: Astrocyte foot processes; Capillary lumen; Tight junction; Basement membrane

Formed by 3 structures:
1. Tight junctions between nonfenestrated capillary endothelial cells
2. Basement membrane
3. Astrocyte processes

Glucose and amino acids cross slowly by carrier-mediated transport mechanism.

Nonpolar/lipid-soluble substances cross rapidly via diffusion.

A few specialized brain regions with fenestrated capillaries and no blood-brain barrier allow molecules in the blood to affect brain function (e.g., area postrema—vomiting after chemo, OVLT—osmotic sensing) or neurosecretory products to enter circulation (e.g., neurohypophysis—ADH release).

Other barriers include:
1. Blood-testis barrier
2. Maternal-fetal blood barrier of placenta

Infarction destroys endothelial cell tight junctions → vasogenic edema.

---

**Hypothalamus**

The hypothalamus wears **TAN HATS**—Thirst and water balance, Adenohypophysis control, Neurohypophysis releases hormones from hypothalamus, Hunger, Autonomic regulation, Temperature regulation, Sexual urges. Inputs: OVLT (senses change in osmolarity), area postrema (responds to emetics).

Supraoptic nucleus makes ADH.

Paraventricular nucleus makes oxytocin.

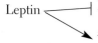

Leptin

Lateral area—hunger. Destruction → anorexia, failure to thrive (infants). Inhibited by leptin.

Ventromedial area—satiety. Destruction (e.g., craniopharyngioma) → hyperphagia. Stimulated by leptin.

Anterior hypothalamus—cooling, pArasympathetic.

Posterior hypothalamus—heating, sympathetic.

Septal nucleus—Sexual urges.

Suprachiasmatic nucleus—circadian rhythm.

If you zap your **lateral** nucleus, you shrink **laterally.**

If you zap your **ventromedial** nucleus, you grow **ventrally** and **medially.**

Anterior nucleus = cool off (cooling, parasympathetic). A/C = anterior cooling.

Posterior nucleus = get fired up (heating, sympathetic). If you zap your Posterior hypothalamus, you become a **P**oikilotherm (cold-blooded, like a snake).

You need **sleep** to be **charismatic** (chiasmatic).

---

**Posterior pituitary (neurohypophysis)**

Receives hypothalamic axonal projections from supraoptic (ADH) and paraventricular (oxytocin) nuclei.

Oxytocin: *oxys* = quick; *tocos* = birth.

Adenohypophysis = Anterior pituitary.

| | | |
|---|---|---|
| **Thalamus** | Major relay for ascending sensory information that ultimately reaches the cortex. | |
| | Lateral geniculate nucleus (LGN)—visual. Projects via optic radiations to occipital cortex. | Lateral for Light. |
| | Medial geniculate nucleus (MGN)—auditory. | Medial for Music. |
| | Ventral posterior nucleus, lateral part (VPL) —body sensation (proprioception, pressure, pain, touch, vibration via dorsal columns, spinothalamic tract). | |
| | Ventral posterior nucleus, medial part (VPM) —facial sensation (via CN V). | You put Makeup on your face, and the sensory info is relayed through the VPM. |
| | Ventral anterior/lateral (VA/VL) nuclei —motor. | Motor is anterior to sensation in the thalamus, just like the cortex. |
| | | Blood supply—posterior communicating, posterior cerebral, and ICA (anterior choroidal arteries). |

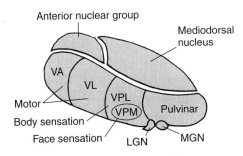

| | | |
|---|---|---|
| **Limbic system** | Includes cingulate gyrus, hippocampus, fornix, and mammillary bodies. Responsible for Feeding, Fleeing, Fighting, Feeling, and sex. | The famous 5 F's. |
| **Cerebellum** | Receives contralateral cortical input via middle cerebellar peduncle and ipsilateral proprioceptive information via inferior cerebellar peduncle. Input nerves = climbing and mossy fibers. | |
| | Provides stimulatory feedback to contralateral cortex to modulate movement. Output nerves = Purkinje fibers output to deep nuclei of cerebellum, which in turn output to cortex via superior cerebellar peduncle. | |
| | Deep nuclei (L → M)—Dentate, Emboliform, Globose, Fastigial ("Don't Eat Greasy Foods"). | |
| | Lateral—voluntary movement of extremities. | |
| | Medial—balance, truncal coordination, ataxia, propensity to fall toward injured (ipsilateral) side. | |

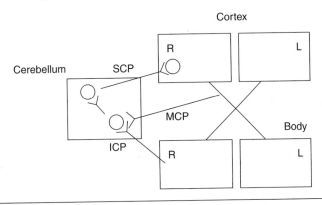

**Basal ganglia**
Important in voluntary movements and making postural adjustments.
Receives cortical input, provides negative feedback to cortex to modulate movement.

■ stimulatory
■ inhibitory
SNc  Substantia nigra pars compacta
SNr  Substantia nigra pars reticulata
GPe  Globus pallidus externus
GPi  Globus pallidus internus
STN  Subthalamic nucleus
D1  Dopamine D1 receptor (excitatory)
D2  Dopamine D2 receptor (inhibitory)

**D1-R = D1Rect pathway.**
Indirect = Inhibitory.

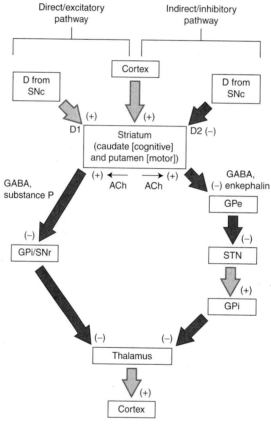

D1 (+) = excitatory
D2 (+) = inhibit inhibitory = excitatory

Excitatory pathway—SNc's dopamine binds to D1 receptors in the excitatory pathway, stimulating the
   excitatory pathway (↑ motion). Therefore, loss of dopamine in Parkinson's inhibits the excitatory pathway
   (↓ motion).
Inhibitory pathway—SNc's dopamine binds to D2 receptors in the inhibitory pathway, inhibiting the
   inhibitory pathway (↑ motion). Therefore, loss of dopamine in Parkinson's excites (i.e., disinhibits) the inhibitory
   pathway (↓ motion).

| | | |
|---|---|---|
| **Parkinson's disease** | Degenerative disorder of CNS associated with Lewy bodies (composed of α-synuclein— intracellular inclusion) and depigmentation of the substantia nigra pars compacta (loss of dopaminergic neurons). Rare cases have been linked to exposure to MPTP, a contaminant in illicit street drugs. | **TRAP** = **T**remor (at rest—e.g., pill-rolling tremor), cogwheel **R**igidity, **A**kinesia, and **P**ostural instability (you are **TRAP**ped in your body). |
| **Hemiballismus** | Sudden, wild flailing of 1 arm +/– leg. Characteristic of contralateral subthalamic nucleus lesion (e.g., lacunar stroke in a patient with a history of hypertension). Loss of inhibition of thalamus through globus pallidus. | Half ballistic (as in throwing a baseball). |
| **Huntington's disease** | Autosomal-dominant trinucleotide repeat disorder. Chromosome 4. Neuronal death via NMDA-R binding and glutamate toxicity. Chorea, depression, progressive dementia. Symptoms manifest in affected individuals between the ages of 20 and 50. | Expansion of **CAG** repeats (anticipation). Caudate loses **ACh** and **GABA**. |

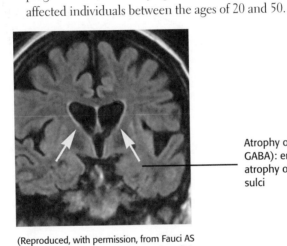

Atrophy of caudate nucleus (loss of GABA): enlarged lateral ventricles, atrophy of putamen, and defined sulci

(Reproduced, with permission, from Fauci AS et al. *Harrison's Principles of Internal Medicine,* 17th ed. New York: McGraw-Hill, 2008, Fig. 367-1.)

| | | |
|---|---|---|
| **Chorea** | Sudden, jerky, purposeless movements. Characteristic of basal ganglia lesion (e.g., Huntington's disease). | *Chorea* = dancing (Greek). Think choral dancing or choreography. |
| **Athetosis** | Slow, writhing movements, especially of fingers. Characteristic of basal ganglia lesion (e.g., Huntington's disease). | *Athetos* = not fixed (Greek). Think snakelike. |
| **Myoclonus** | Sudden, brief muscle contraction. | Jerks, hiccups. |
| **Dystonia** | Sustained, involuntary muscle contractions. | Writer's cramp. |

**Tremor**

Essential/postural tremor—action tremor (worsens when holding posture), autosomal dominant. Essential tremor patients often self-medicate with alcohol, which ↓ tremor. Treatment: β-blockers.

Resting tremor—most noticeable distally. Seen in Parkinson's (pill-rolling tremor).

Intention tremor—slow, zigzag motion when pointing toward a target; associated with cerebellar dysfunction.

**Cerebral cortex functions**

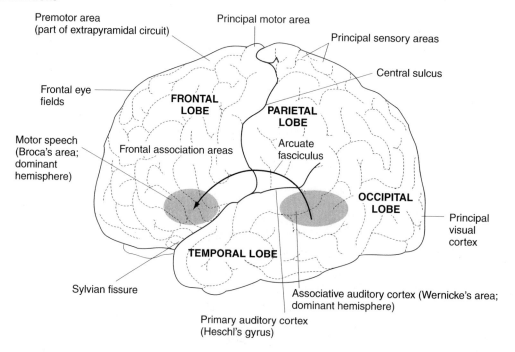

**Frontal lobe functions**

"Executive functions"—planning, inhibition, concentration, orientation, language, abstraction, judgment, motor regulation, mood. Lack of social judgment is most notable in frontal lobe lesion.

Damage = Disinhibition (e.g., Phineas Gage).

| Homunculus | Topographical representation of sensory and motor areas in the cerebral cortex. Used to localize lesion (e.g., in blood supply) leading to specific defects. For example, lower extremity deficit in sensation or movement may indicate involvement of the anterior cerebral artery. | 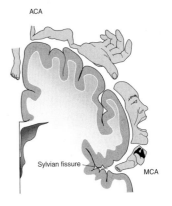 ACA Sylvian fissure MCA |
|---|---|---|

Motor homunculus

## Brain lesions

| Area of lesion | Consequence | Notes |
|---|---|---|
| Amygdala (bilateral) | Klüver-Bucy syndrome (hyperorality, hypersexuality, disinhibited behavior) | |
| Frontal lobe | Disinhibition and deficits in concentration, orientation, and judgment; may have reemergence of primitive reflexes | |
| Right parietal lobe | Spatial neglect syndrome (agnosia of the contralateral side of the world) | |
| Reticular activating system (midbrain) | Reduced levels of arousal and wakefulness (e.g., coma) | |
| Mammillary bodies (bilateral) | Wernicke-Korsakoff syndrome (Wernicke—confusion, ophthalmoplegia, ataxia; Korsakoff—memory loss, confabulation, personality changes) | |
| Basal ganglia | May result in tremor at rest, chorea, or athetosis | |
| Cerebellar hemisphere | Intention tremor, limb ataxia; damage to the cerebellum results in ipsilateral deficits; fall toward side of lesion (cerebellum → SCP → contralateral cortex → corticospinal decussation = ipsilateral) | Cerebellar hemispheres are **laterally** located—affect **lateral** limbs. |
| Cerebellar vermis | Truncal ataxia, dysarthria | Vermis is **centrally** located—affects **central** body. |
| Subthalamic nucleus | Contralateral hemiballismus | |
| Hippocampus | Anterograde amnesia—inability to make new memories | |
| Paramedian pontine reticular formation (PPRF) | Eyes look away from side of lesion | |
| Frontal eye fields | Eyes look toward lesion | |

| Central pontine myelinolysis | Acute paralysis, dysarthria, dysphagia, diplopia, and loss of consciousness. Commonly caused by very rapid correction of hyponatremia. |
|---|---|

| Recurrent laryngeal nerve injury | Loss of all laryngeal muscles except cricothyroid. Hoarseness. |
|---|---|

**Aphasia**

Aphasia = higher-order inability to speak. Dysarthria = motor inability to speak.

Broca's

Nonfluent aphasia with intact comprehension. Broca's area—inferior frontal gyrus.

**Broca's Broken Boca.**

Wernicke's

Fluent aphasia with impaired comprehension. Wernicke's area—superior temporal gyrus.

Wernicke's is **W**ordy but makes no sense.

Global

Nonfluent aphasia with impaired comprehension. Both Broca's and Wernicke's areas affected.

Wernicke's = "**W**hat?"

Conduction

Poor repetition but fluent speech, intact comprehension. Arcuate fasciculus—connects Broca's, Wernicke's areas.

## Cerebral arteries—cortical distribution

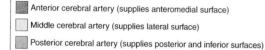

- Anterior cerebral artery (supplies anteromedial surface)
- Middle cerebral artery (supplies lateral surface)
- Posterior cerebral artery (supplies posterior and inferior surfaces)

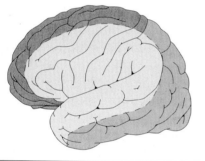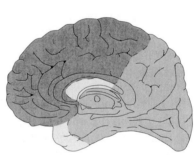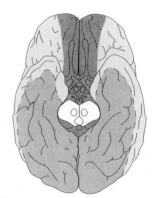

## Circle of Willis

Right anterior cerebral artery
Middle cerebral artery
Posterior communicating artery
Basilar artery
Vertebral artery

Anterior communicating artery
Optic chiasm
Internal carotid artery (ICA)
Lateral striate
CN III
Posterior cerebral artery
Anterior inferior cerebellar artery (AICA)
Posterior inferior cerebellar artery (PICA)

Anterior spinal artery

| Region | Associated area/deficit |
| --- | --- |
| Anterior spinal artery (medial medullary syndrome) | Contralateral hemiparesis (lower extremities), medial lemniscus ($\downarrow$ contralateral proprioception), ipsilateral paralysis of hypoglossal nerve. |
| PICA (lateral medullary syndrome, aka Wallenberg's) | Contralateral loss of pain and temperature, ipsilateral dysphagia, hoarseness, $\downarrow$ gag reflex, vertigo, diplopia, nystagmus, vomiting, ipsilateral Horner's, ipsilateral facial pain and temperature, trigeminal nucleus (spinal tract and nucleus), ipsilateral ataxia. |
| AICA (lateral inferior pontine syndrome) | Ipsilateral facial paralysis, ipsilateral cochlear nucleus, vestibular (nystagmus), ipsilateral facial pain and temperature, ipsilateral dystaxia (MCP, ICP). |
| Posterior cerebral artery | Contralateral homonymous hemianopia with macular sparing; supplies occipital cortex. |
| Middle cerebral artery | Contralateral face and arm paralysis and sensory loss, aphasia (dominant sphere), left-sided neglect. |
| Anterior cerebral artery | Supplies medial surface of the brain, leg-foot area of motor and sensory cortices. |
| Anterior communicating artery | Most common site of circle of Willis aneurysm; lesions may cause visual field defects. |
| Posterior communicating artery | Common area of aneurysm; causes CN III palsy. |
| Lateral striate | Divisions of middle cerebral artery; supply internal capsule, caudate, putamen, globus pallidus. "Arteries of stroke"; infarct of the posterior limb of the internal capsule causes pure motor hemiparesis. |
| Watershed zones | Between anterior cerebral/middle cerebral, posterior cerebral/middle cerebral arteries. Damage in severe hypotension $\rightarrow$ upper leg/upper arm weakness, defects in higher-order visual processing. |
| Basilar artery | Infarct causes "locked-in syndrome" (CN III is typically intact). |
| In general, stroke of anterior circle | General sensory and motor dysfunction, aphasia. |
| In general, stroke of posterior circle | Cranial nerve deficits (vertigo, visual deficits), coma, cerebellar deficits (ataxia). Dominant hemisphere (ataxia), nondominant (neglect). |

---

**Aneurysms**

Berry aneurysms—occur at the bifurcations in the circle of Willis. Most common site is bifurcation of the anterior communicating artery. Rupture (most common complication) leads to hemorrhagic stroke/subarachnoid hemorrhage. Associated with adult polycystic kidney disease, Ehlers-Danlos syndrome, and Marfan's syndrome. Other risk factors: advanced age, hypertension, smoking, race (higher risk in blacks) (see Image 46).

Charcot-Bouchard microaneurysms—associated with chronic hypertension; affects small vessels (e.g., in basal ganglia, thalamus).

## Intracranial hemorrhage

### Epidural hematoma

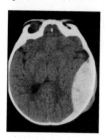

(Reproduced, with permission, from the PEIR Digital Library.)

Rupture of middle meningeal artery (branch of maxillary artery), often 2° to fracture of temporal bone (see Image 44). Lucid interval. Rapid expansion under systemic arterial pressure → transtentorial herniation, CN III palsy.

CT shows "biconvex disk" not crossing suture lines. Can cross falx, tentorium.

### Subdural hematoma

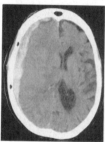

(Reproduced, with permission, from Chen MY et al. *Basic Radiology*, 1st ed. New York: McGraw-Hill, 2005, Fig. 12-32.)

Rupture of bridging veins. Slow venous bleeding (less pressure = hematoma develops over time) with delayed onset of symptoms. Seen in elderly individuals, alcoholics, blunt trauma, shaken baby (predisposing factors—brain atrophy, shaking, whiplash) (see Image 43).

Crescent-shaped hemorrhage that crosses suture lines. Gyri are preserved, since pressure is distributed equally. Cannot cross falx, tentorium.

### Subarachnoid hemorrhage

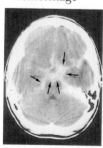

Rupture of an aneurysm (usually berry aneurysm in Marfan's, Ehlers-Danlos, APCKD) or an AVM. Patients complain of "worst headache of my life." Bloody or yellow (xanthochromic) spinal tap. 2–3 days afterward, there is a risk of vasospasm due to blood breakdown products, which irritate vessels (treat with calcium channel blockers).

### Parenchymal hematoma

Caused by hypertension, amyloid angiopathy—lobar strokes all over brain (see Image 96), diabetes mellitus, and tumor. Typically occurs in basal ganglia and internal capsule.

**Ischemic brain disease**

Irreversible damage after 5 minutes. Most vulnerable—hippocampus, neocortex, cerebellum, watershed areas. Irreversible neuronal injury—red neurons (12–48 hours), necrosis + neutrophils (24–72 hours), macrophages (3–5 days), reactive gliosis + vascular proliferation (1–2 weeks), glial scar (> 2 weeks).

Atherosclerosis—thrombi lead to ischemic stroke with subsequent necrosis (red neurons). Form cystic cavity with reactive gliosis.

Hemorrhagic stroke—intracerebral bleeding, often due to aneurysm rupture. May be 2° to ischemic stroke following reperfusion (↑ vessel fragility).

Ischemic stroke—emboli block large vessels; etiologies include atrial fibrillation, carotid dissection, patent foramen ovale, endocarditis. Lacunar strokes block small vessels, are 2° to hypertension. Treatment: tPA within 3 hours.

Transient ischemic attack (TIA)—brief, reversible episode of neurologic dysfunction due to focal ischemia. Typically, symptoms last for < 24 hours.

Stroke imaging: bright on diffusion-weighted MRI in 3–30 minutes and remains bright for 10 days, dark on CT in ~ 24 hours.

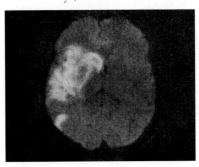

**Right MCA stroke: diffusion MRI**
(Reproduced, with permission, from USMLERx.com.)

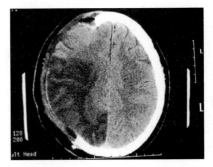

**Right MCA stroke: CT**
(Reproduced, with permission, from Brunicardi FC et al. *Schwartz's Principles of Surgery*, 8th ed. New York: McGraw-Hill, 2004, Fig. 41-6B.)

**Dural venous sinuses**

Venous sinuses run in the dura mater where its meningeal and periosteal layers separate. Cerebral veins → venous sinuses → internal jugular vein.

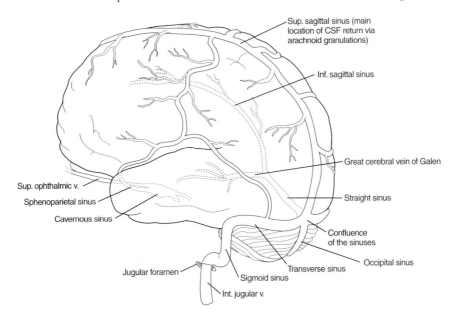

(Adapted, with permission, from White JS. *USMLE Road Map: Gross Anatomy*, 1st ed. New York: McGraw-Hill, 2003.)

**Ventricular system**

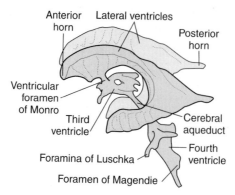

CSF is made by the choroid plexus; it is reabsorbed by venous sinus arachnoid granulations.

Lateral ventricle → 3rd ventricle via foramen of Monro.
3rd ventricle → 4th ventricle via cerebral aqueduct.
4th ventricle → subarachnoid space via:
    Foramina of **L**uschka = **L**ateral.
    Foramen of **M**agendie = **M**edial.

**Hydrocephalus**

| | |
|---|---|
| Normal pressure hydrocephalus | "Wet, wobbly, and wacky." Does **not** result in ↑ subarachnoid space volume. Expansion of ventricles distorts the fibers of the corona radiata and leads to the clinical triad of dementia, ataxia, and urinary incontinence (a reversible cause of dementia in the elderly). |
| Communicating hydrocephalus | ↓ CSF absorption by arachnoid villi, which can lead to ↑ intracranial pressure, papilledema, and herniation (e.g., arachnoid scarring post-meningitis). |
| Obstructive (noncommunicating) hydrocephalus | Caused by a structural blockage of CSF circulation within the ventricular system (e.g., stenosis of the aqueduct of Sylvius). |
| Hydrocephalus ex vacuo | Appearance of ↑ CSF in atrophy (e.g., Alzheimer's disease, advanced HIV, Pick's disease). Intracranial pressure is normal; triad is not seen. |

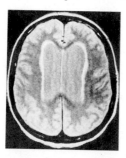

(Reproduced, with permission, from Ropper AH et al. *Adams and Victor's Principles of Neurology,* 8th ed. New York: McGraw-Hill, 2005, Fig. 30-2.)

**Spinal nerves**

There are 31 spinal nerves altogether: 8 cervical, 12 thoracic, 5 lumbar, 5 sacral, 1 coccygeal.
Nerves C1–C7 exit via intervertebral foramina above the corresponding vertebra. All other nerves exit below.

31, just like 31 flavors!
Vertebral disk herniation (nucleus pulposus herniates through annulus fibrosus) usually occurs between L5 and S1.

HIGH-YIELD SYSTEMS

NEUROLOGY

| | | |
|---|---|---|
| **Spinal cord—lower extent** | In adults, spinal cord extends to lower border of L1–L2; subarachnoid space extends to lower border of S2. Lumbar puncture is usually performed in L3–L4 or L4–L5 interspaces, at level of cauda equina. | To keep the cord **alive**, keep the spinal needle between **L3** and **L5.** |
| **Lumbar puncture** 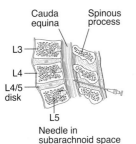 Cauda equina   Spinous process<br>L3<br>L4<br>L4/5 disk<br>L5<br>Needle in subarachnoid space | CSF obtained from lumbar subarachnoid space between L4 and L5 (at the level of iliac crests). Structures pierced as follows:<br>1. Skin/superficial fascia<br>2. Ligaments (supraspinous, interspinous, ligamentum flavum)<br>3. Epidural space<br>4. Dura mater<br>5. Subdural space<br>6. Arachnoid<br>7. Subarachnoid space—CSF | **Pia** is not **pier**ced. |

### Spinal cord and associated tracts

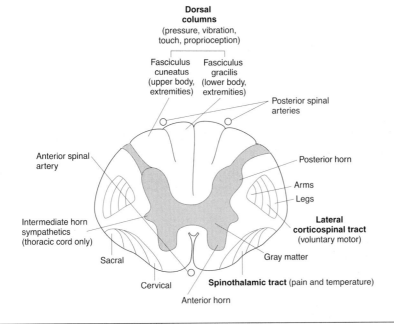

Dorsal columns (pressure, vibration, touch, proprioception)

Fasciculus cuneatus (upper body, extremities)   Fasciculus gracilis (lower body, extremities)

Posterior spinal arteries

Anterior spinal artery

Posterior horn

Arms

Legs

Intermediate horn sympathetics (thoracic cord only)

Lateral corticospinal tract (voluntary motor)

Sacral

Gray matter

Cervical

Spinothalamic tract (pain and temperature)

Anterior horn

Legs are Lateral in Lateral corticospinal, spinothalamic tracts.

Dorsal column is organized as you are, with hands at sides. Arms outside, legs inside.

**Spinal tract anatomy and functions**  Remember, ascending tracts synapse and **then** cross.

| Tract and Function | 1st-Order Neuron | Synapse 1 | 2nd-Order Neuron | Synapse 2 | 3rd-Order Neuron |
|---|---|---|---|---|---|
| Dorsal column—medial lemniscal pathway (ascending pressure, vibration, touch, and proprioceptive sensation) | Sensory nerve ending → cell body in dorsal root ganglion → enters spinal cord, ascends ipsilaterally in dorsal column | Ipsilateral nucleus cuneatus or gracilis (medulla) | **Decussates** in medulla → ascends contralaterally in medial lemniscus | VPL of thalamus | Sensory cortex |
| Spinothalamic tract (ascending pain and temperature sensation) | Sensory nerve ending (A-delta and C fibers) (cell body in dorsal root ganglion) → enters spinal cord | Ipsilateral gray matter (spinal cord) | **Decussates** at anterior white commissure → ascends contralaterally | VPL of thalamus | Sensory cortex |
| Lateral corticospinal tract (descending voluntary movement of contralateral limbs) | **Upper motor neuron:** cell body in 1° motor cortex → descends ipsilaterally (through internal capsule) until **decussating** at caudal medulla (pyramidal decussation) → descends contralaterally | Cell body of anterior horn (spinal cord) | **Lower motor neuron:** Leaves spinal cord | Neuromuscular junction | |

**Motor neuron signs**

| Sign | UMN lesion | LMN lesion |
|---|---|---|
| Weakness | + | + |
| Atrophy | − | + |
| Fasciculation | − | + |
| Reflexes | ↑ | ↓ |
| Tone | ↑ | ↓ |
| Babinski | + | − |
| Spastic paralysis | + | − |
| Clasp knife spasticity | + | − |

Lower MN = everything **lowered** (less muscle mass, ↓ muscle tone, ↓ reflexes, downgoing toes).

Upper MN = everything **up** (tone, DTRs, toes).

Upgoing Babinski is normal in infants.

Fasciculation = muscle twitching.

## Spinal cord lessons

Poliomyelitis and Werdnig-Hoffmann disease: lower motor neuron lesions only, due to destruction of anterior horns; flaccid paralysis

Multiple sclerosis: mostly white matter of cervical region; random and asymmetric lesions, due to demyelination; scanning speech, intention tremor, nystagmus

ALS: combined upper and lower motor neuron deficits with no sensory deficit; both upper and lower motor neuron signs

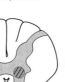 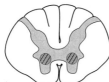 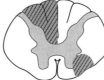 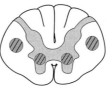

Complete occlusion of anterior spinal artery; spares dorsal columns and tract of Lissauer; upper thoracic ASA territory is a watershed area, as artery of Adamkiewicz supplies ASA below ~ T8

Tabes dorsalis (3° syphilis): degeneration of dorsal roots and dorsal columns; impaired proprioception, locomotor ataxia

Syringomyelia: damages anterior white commissure of spinothalamic tract (2nd-order neurons), resulting in bilateral loss of pain and temperature sensation (usually C8–T1); seen with Arnold-Chiari II; can expand and affect other tracts

Vitamin $B_{12}$ neuropathy, vitamin E deficiency, and Friedreich's ataxia: demyelination of dorsal columns, lateral corticospinal tracts, and spinocerebellar tracts; ataxic gait, hyperreflexia, impaired position and vibration sense

Posterior spinal arteries

 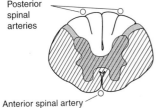 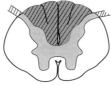 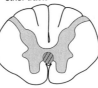 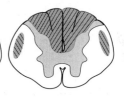

Anterior spinal artery

| | |
|---|---|
| **Poliomyelitis** | Caused by poliovirus, which is transmitted by the fecal-oral route. Replicates in the oropharynx and small intestine before spreading through the bloodstream to the CNS, where it leads to the destruction of cells in the anterior horn of the spinal cord, leading in turn to LMN destruction. |
| Symptoms | Malaise, headache, fever, nausea, abdominal pain, sore throat. Signs of LMN lesions—muscle weakness and atrophy, fasciculations, fibrillation, and hyporeflexia. |
| Findings | CSF with lymphocytic pleocytosis with slight elevation of protein (with no change in CSF glucose). Virus recovered from stool or throat. |
| **Werdnig-Hoffman disease** | Also known as infantile spinal muscular atrophy. Autosomal-recessive inheritance; presents at birth as a "floppy baby," tongue fasciculations; median age of death 7 months. Associated with degeneration of anterior horns. LMN involvement only. |
| **Amyotrophic lateral sclerosis** | Associated with **both** LMN and UMN signs; no sensory, cognitive, or oculomotor deficits. Can be caused by defect in superoxide dismutase 1 (SOD1), betel nut ingestion. Commonly presents as fasciculations. Commonly known as Lou Gehrig's disease. |

**Tabes dorsalis**

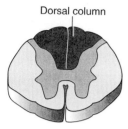

Dorsal column

Degeneration of dorsal columns and dorsal roots due to 3° syphilis, resulting in impaired proprioception and locomotor ataxia. Associated with Charcot's joints, shooting (lightning) pain (see Image 12), Argyll Robertson pupils (reactive to accommodation but not to light), absence of DTRs, positive Romberg, and sensory ataxia at night.

Argyll Robertson pupils are also known as "prostitute's pupils" because they accommodate but do not react.

---

**Friedreich's ataxia**

Autosomal-recessive trinucleotide repeat disorder (GAA; frataxin gene). Leads to impairment in mitochondrial functioning. Staggering gait, frequent falling, nystagmus, dysarthria, pes cavus, hammer toes, hypertrophic cardiomyopathy (cause of death). Presents in childhood with kyphoscoliosis.

Friedreich is Fratastic **(frataxin):** he's your favorite frat brother, always stumbling, staggering, and falling.

---

**Brown-Séquard syndrome**

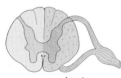

Lesion

Hemisection of spinal cord. Findings:
1. Ipsilateral UMN signs (corticospinal tract) below lesion
2. Ipsilateral loss of tactile, vibration, proprioception sense (dorsal column) below lesion
3. Contralateral pain and temperature loss (spinothalamic tract) below lesion
4. Ipsilateral loss of all sensation at level of lesion
5. LMN signs (e.g., flaccid paralysis) at level of lesion

If lesion occurs above T1, presents with Horner's syndrome.

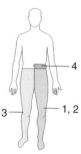

| **Horner's syndrome** | Sympathectomy of face: | **PAM** is **horny** (Horner's). |

**Horner's syndrome** | Sympathectomy of face:
1. **P**tosis (slight drooping of eyelid: superior tarsal muscle)
2. **A**nhidrosis (absence of sweating) and flushing (rubor) of affected side of face
3. **M**iosis (pupil constriction)

Associated with lesion of spinal cord above T1 (e.g., Pancoast's tumor, Brown-Séquard syndrome [cord hemisection], late-stage syringomyelia).

**PAM** is **horny** (Horner's).

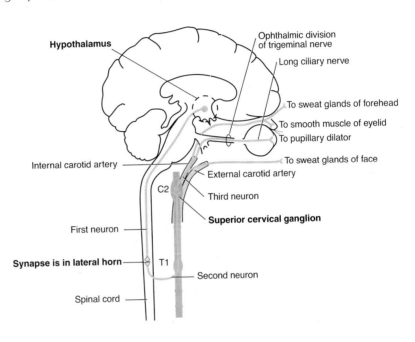

The 3-neuron oculosympathetic pathway projects from the hypothalamus to the intermediolateral column of the spinal cord, then to the superior cervical (sympathetic) ganglion, and finally to the pupil, the smooth muscle of the eyelids, and the sweat glands of the forehead and face. Interruption of any of these pathways results in Horner's syndrome.

| **Landmark dermatomes** | | |

**Landmark dermatomes**

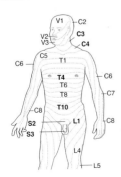

C2—posterior half of a skull "cap."
C3—high turtleneck shirt.
C4—low-collar shirt.

T4—at the nipple.
T7—at the xiphoid process.
T10—at the umbilicus (important for early appendicitis pain referral).
L1—at the inguinal ligament.
L4—includes the kneecaps.
S2, S3, S4—erection and sensation of penile and anal zones.

Diaphragm and gallbladder pain referred to the right shoulder via the phrenic nerve.
**T4** at the **teat pore.**

**T10** at the belly but**TEN.**

L1 is **IL** (Inguinal Ligament).
Down on **L4s (all fours).**
"**S2, 3, 4** keep the penis off the floor."

### Spindle muscle control

| | | |
|---|---|---|
| Muscle spindle | In parallel with extrafusal muscle fibers. Muscle stretch → intrafusal stretch → stimulates Ia afferent → dorsal horn → stimulates α motor neuron → reflex muscle (extrafusal) contraction (monosynaptic reflex). In contrast, Golgi tendons are perpendicular to intrafusal muscle → Ib afferent —\| α motor neuron. | Muscle spindles monitor muscle length (help you pick up a heavy suitcase when you didn't know how heavy it was). Golgi Tendon organs monitor muscle Tension and prevent tendon tear (make you drop a heavy suitcase you've been holding too long). |
| Gamma loop | CNS stimulates γ motor neuron → contracts intrafusal fiber at central part of muscle spindle → ↑ sensitivity of reflex arc. Can be influenced by the brain. | |

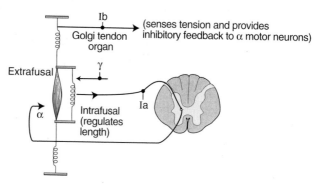

### Clinical reflexes

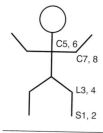

Biceps = C5 nerve root.
Triceps = C7 nerve root.
Patella = L4 nerve root.
Achilles = S1 nerve root.
Babinski—dorsiflexion of the big toe and fanning of other toes; sign of UMN lesion, but normal reflex in 1st year of life.

Reflexes count up in order:
S1, 2
L3, 4
C5, 6
C7, 8

### Primitive reflexes

1. Moro reflex—"hang on for life" reflex—abduct/extend limbs when startled, and then draw together
2. Rooting reflex—movement of head toward one side if cheek or mouth is stroked (nipple seeking)
3. Sucking reflex—sucking response when roof of mouth is touched
4. Palmar and plantar reflexes—curling of fingers/toes if palms of hands/feet are stroked
5. Babinski reflex—dorsiflexion of large toe and fanning of other toes with plantar stimulation

Normally disappear within 1st year of life. May reemerge following frontal lobe lesion.

## Brain stem—ventral view

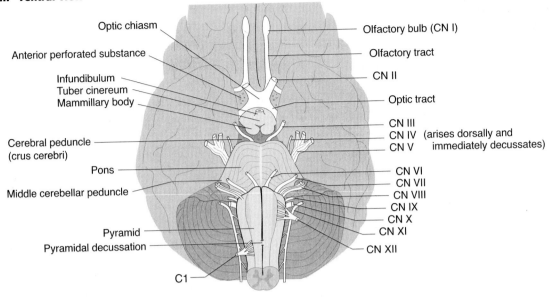

Optic chiasm

Anterior perforated substance

Infundibulum
Tuber cinereum
Mammillary body

Cerebral peduncle
(crus cerebri)

Pons

Middle cerebellar peduncle

Pyramid

Pyramidal decussation

C1

Olfactory bulb (CN I)

Olfactory tract

CN II

Optic tract

CN III
CN IV  (arises dorsally and
CN V        immediately decussates)

CN VI
CN VII
CN VIII
CN IX
CN X
CN XI
CN XII

CNs that lie medially at brain stem: III, VI, XII. 3(×2) = 6(×2) = 12 (**M**otor = **M**edial).

## Brain stem—dorsal view (cerebellum removed)

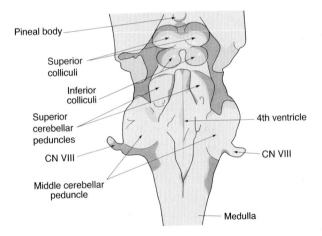

Pineal body

Superior
colliculi

Inferior
colliculi

Superior
cerebellar
peduncles

CN VIII

Middle cerebellar
peduncle

4th ventricle

CN VIII

Medulla

Pineal gland—melatonin secretion, circadian rhythms.

Superior colliculi—conjugate vertical gaze center.

Inferior colliculi—auditory.

**Parinaud syndrome**—paralysis of conjugate vertical gaze due to lesion in superior colliculi (e.g., pinealoma).

Your eyes are **above** your ears, and the superior colliculus (visual) is **above** the inferior colliculus (auditory).

**Cranial nerves**

| Nerve | CN | Function | Type | Mnemonic |
|---|---|---|---|---|
| Olfactory | I | Smell (only CN without thalamic relay to cortex) | Sensory | Some |
| Optic | II | Sight | Sensory | Say |
| Oculomotor | III | Eye movement (SR, IR, MR, IO), pupillary constriction (PS: E-W nucleus, muscarinic-R), accommodation, eyelid opening (levator palpebrae) | Motor | Marry |
| Trochlear | IV | Eye movement (SO) | Motor | Money |
| Trigeminal | V | Mastication, facial sensation (ophthalmic, maxillary, mandibular divisions) | Both | But |
| Abducens | VI | Eye movement (LR) | Motor | My |
| Facial | VII | Facial movement, taste from anterior $2/3$ of tongue, lacrimation, salivation (submandibular and sublingual glands), eyelid closing (orbicularis oculi), stapedius muscle in ear | Both | Brother |
| Vestibulocochlear | VIII | Hearing, balance | Sensory | Says |
| Glossopharyngeal | IX | Taste from posterior $1/3$ of tongue, swallowing, salivation (parotid gland), monitoring carotid body and sinus chemo- and baroreceptors, and stylopharyngeus (elevates pharynx, larynx) | Both | Big |
| Vagus | X | Taste from epiglottic region, swallowing, palate elevation, midline uvula, talking, coughing, thoracoabdominal viscera, monitoring aortic arch chemo- and baroreceptors | Both | Brains |
| Accessory | XI | Head turning, shoulder shrugging (SCM, trapezius) | Motor | Matter |
| Hypoglossal | XII | Tongue movement | Motor | Most |

**Cranial nerve nuclei**

Located in tegmentum portion of brain stem (between dorsal and ventral portions).
1. Midbrain—nuclei of CN III, IV
2. Pons—nuclei of CN V, VI, VII, VIII
3. Medulla—nuclei of CN IX, X, XI, XII

Lateral nuclei = sensory (alar plate).
— Sulcus limitans —
Medial nuclei = **M**otor (basal plate).

**Cranial nerve reflexes**

| Reflex | Afferent | Efferent |
|---|---|---|
| Corneal | $V_1$ ophthalmic (nasociliary branch: levator palpebrae) | VII (temporal branch: orbicularis oculi) |
| Lacrimation | $V_1$ (loss of reflex does not preclude emotional tears) | VII |
| Jaw jerk | $V_3$ (sensory—muscle spindle from masseter) | $V_3$ (motor—masseter) |
| Pupillary | II | III |
| Gag | IX | IX, X |

| | | |
|---|---|---|
| **Vagal nuclei** | | |
| Nucleus Solitarius | Visceral **S**ensory information (e.g., taste, baroreceptors, gut distention). | VII, IX, X. |
| Nucleus a**M**biguus | **M**otor innervation of pharynx, larynx, and upper esophagus (e.g., swallowing, palate elevation). | IX, X, XI. |
| Dorsal motor nucleus | Sends autonomic (parasympathetic) fibers to heart, lungs, and upper GI. | |

| | | |
|---|---|---|
| **Cranial nerve and vessel pathways** | Cribriform plate (CN I). | Divisions of CN V exit owing to **S**tanding **R**oom **O**nly. |
| | Middle cranial fossa (CN II–VI)—through sphenoid bone: | |

Middle cranial fossa (CN II–VI)—through sphenoid bone:
1. Optic canal (CN II, ophthalmic artery, central retinal vein)
2. **S**uperior orbital fissure (CN III, IV, V$_1$, VI, ophthalmic vein, sympathetic fibers)
3. Foramen **R**otundum (CN V$_2$)
4. Foramen **O**vale (CN V$_3$)
5. Foramen spinosum (middle meningeal artery)

Posterior cranial fossa (CN VII–XII)—through temporal or occipital bone:
1. Internal auditory meatus (CN VII, VIII)
2. Jugular foramen (CN IX, X, XI, jugular vein)
3. Hypoglossal canal (CN XII)
4. Foramen magnum (spinal roots of CN XI, brain stem, vertebral arteries)

**Cavernous sinus**

A collection of venous sinuses on either side of the pituitary. Blood from eye and superficial cortex → cavernous sinus → internal jugular vein.

CN III, IV, $V_1$, $V_2$, and VI and postganglionic sympathetic fibers en route to the orbit all pass through the cavernous sinus. Only CN VI is "free-floating." Cavernous portion of internal carotid artery is also here.

The nerves that control extraocular muscles (plus $V_1$ and $V_2$) pass through the cavernous sinus.

Cavernous sinus syndrome (e.g., due to mass effect)—ophthalmoplegia, ophthalmic and maxillary sensory loss.

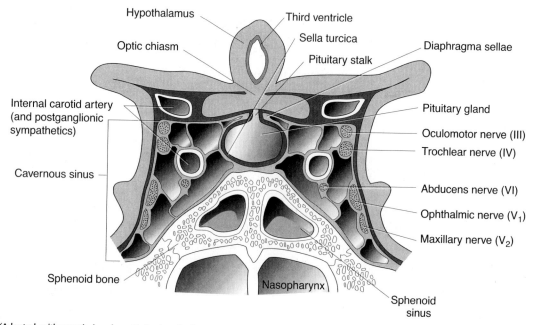

(Adapted, with permission, from Stobo J et al. *The Principles and Practice of Medicine,* 23rd ed. Stamford, CT: Appleton & Lange, 1996: 277.)

**Cranial nerve lesions**

CN XII lesion (LMN)—tongue deviates **toward** side of lesion (lick your wounds). Decussates before medulla and synapse on contralateral hypoglossal nucleus.

CN V motor lesion—jaw deviates **toward** side of lesion. Bilateral cortical input to lateral pterygoid muscle.

CN X lesion—uvula deviates **away** from side of lesion. Weak side collapses and uvula points away.

CN XI lesion—weakness turning head to contralateral side of lesion (SCM). Shoulder droop on side of lesion (trapezius).

**Facial lesions**

UMN lesion

Lesion of motor cortex or connection between cortex and facial nucleus.
Contralateral paralysis of lower face only, since upper face receives bilateral UMN innervation.

LMN lesion

Ipsilateral paralysis of upper **and** lower face.

Bell's palsy

Complete destruction of the facial nucleus itself or its branchial efferent fibers (facial nerve proper).
Peripheral ipsilateral facial paralysis with inability to close eye on involved side.
Can occur idiopathically; gradual recovery in most cases.
Seen as a complication in AIDS, Lyme disease, Herpes zoster, Sarcoidosis, Tumors, Diabetes (**AL**exander gra**H**am **Bell** with **STD**).

Face area of motor cortex

Cortico-bulbar tract (UMN lesion = **central facial**)

Facial nucleus

Upper division
Lower division

LMN lesion
*Cannot wrinkle forehead.

CN VII (LMN lesion = **Bell's palsy**)

---

**KLM sounds: kuh, la, mi**

Kuh-kuh-kuh tests palate elevation (CN X—vagus).
La-la-la tests tongue (CN XII—hypoglossal).
Mi-mi-mi tests lips (CN VII—facial).

Say it aloud.
It would be a **K**a**L**a**M**ity to lose CN X, XII, and VII.

---

**Mastication muscles**

3 muscles close jaw: **M**asseter, te**M**poralis, **M**edial pterygoid. 1 opens: lateral pterygoid. All are innervated by the trigeminal nerve (V₃).

**M**'s Munch.
**L**ateral **L**owers (when speaking of pterygoids with respect to jaw motion).
"It takes more muscle to keep your mouth shut."

---

**Muscles with glossus**

All muscles with root *glossus* in their names (**except palatoglossus**, innervated by vagus nerve) are innervated by hypo*glossal* nerve.

*Palat*: vagus nerve.
*Glossus*: hypo*glossal* nerve.

---

**Muscles with palat**

All muscles with root *palat* in their names (**except tensor veli palatini**, innervated by mandibular branch of CN V) are innervated by vagus nerve.

*Palat*: vagus nerve (except **TENS**or, who was too **TENSE**).

**Inner ear**

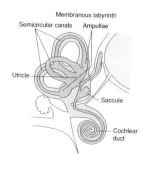

Membranous labyrinth
Semicircular canals  Ampullae
Utricle
Saccule
Cochlear duct

Consists of a series of tubes in the temporal bone (bony labyrinth) filled with perilymph ($Na^+$ rich, similar to ECF) that includes cochlea, vestibule, and semicircular canals.

Within the bony labyrinth is a 2nd series of tubes (membranous labyrinth) filled with endolymph ($K^+$ rich, similar to ICF) that includes cochlear duct (within the cochlea), utricle and saccule (within the vestibule), and semicircular canals. Hair cells (located within the organ of Corti) are the sensory elements in both vestibular apparatus (spatial orientation) and cochlea (hearing).

Sound enters (middle ear):
1. Vibration of tympanic membrane → ossicles →
2. Oval window →
3. Vibration of basilar membrane → bending of hair cell cilia against tectorial membrane →
4. Hair cell bending = hyper- or depolarization of CN VIII

Hearing loss:
1. Normal: air (AC) > bone conduction (BC) (Rinne)
2. If BC > AC: conduction deafness in that ear (Weber lateralizes to that ear)
3. If AC > BC (normal) but there is sensorineural loss, Weber lateralizes to opposite ear

*Peri*—think outside of cell ($Na^+$).
*Endo*—think inside of cell ($K^+$).
Endolymph is made by the stria vascularis.
Utricle (horizontal) and saccule (vertical) contain maculae—detect linear acceleration.
Semicircular canals contain Ampullae—detect Angular acceleration.
Cochlear membrane = scuba flipper.

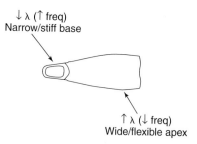

↓ λ (↑ freq)
Narrow/stiff base

↑ λ (↓ freq)
Wide/flexible apex

Hearing loss in the elderly—high frequency → low frequency.

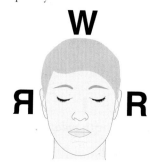

## Eye and retina

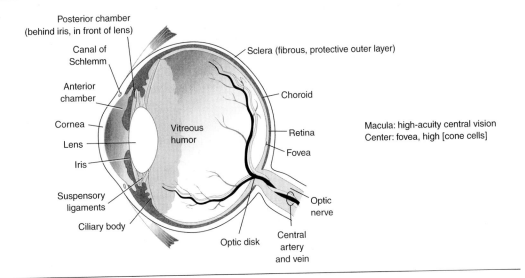

Posterior chamber (behind iris, in front of lens)

Canal of Schlemm

Anterior chamber

Cornea

Lens

Iris

Suspensory ligaments

Ciliary body

Optic disk

Sclera (fibrous, protective outer layer)

Choroid

Retina

Fovea

Vitreous humor

Optic nerve

Central artery and vein

Macula: high-acuity central vision
Center: fovea, high [cone cells]

## Eye pathology

| | |
|---|---|
| Retinitis | Retinal necrosis + edema → atrophic scar. |
| Iritis | Systemic inflammation (e.g., Reiter's). |
| Near vision | Ciliary muscle contracts (zonular fibers relax → lens relaxes → more convex). |
| Distant vision | Ciliary muscle relaxes (lens flattens). |
| Aging | Sclerosis and ↓ elasticity cause lens shape to change. |
| Retinal artery occlusion | Acute, painless monocular loss of vision; pale retina and cherry-red macula (has its own blood supply—choroid artery). |

## Aqueous humor pathway

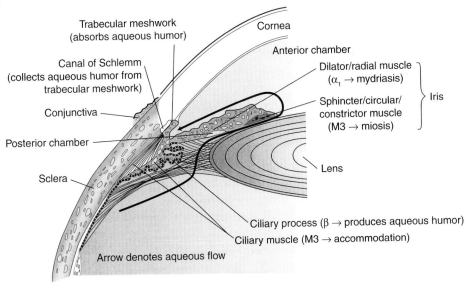

Trabecular meshwork (absorbs aqueous humor)

Canal of Schlemm (collects aqueous humor from trabecular meshwork)

Conjunctiva

Posterior chamber

Sclera

Cornea

Anterior chamber

Dilator/radial muscle ($\alpha_1$ → mydriasis)

Sphincter/circular/ constrictor muscle (M3 → miosis)

Iris

Lens

Ciliary process ($\beta$ → produces aqueous humor)

Ciliary muscle (M3 → accommodation)

Arrow denotes aqueous flow

**Glaucoma**

Impaired flow of aqueous humor → ↑ intraocular pressure → optic disk atrophy with cupping.

Open/wide angle—obstructed outflow (e.g., canal of Schlemm); associated with myopia, ↑ age, African-American race. More common, "silent," painless.

Closed/narrow angle—obstruction of flow between iris and cornea → pressure buildup behind iris. Very painful, ↓ vision, rock-hard eye, frontal headache. An ophthalmologic emergency. Do not give epinephrine.

Closed/narrow-angle glaucoma

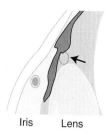

1. Iris and lens stick together
2. Pressure buildup behind iris

Iris    Lens

Open/wide-angle glaucoma

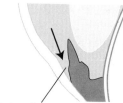

Obstruction of drainage

Trabecular meshwork

---

**Cataract**

Painless, bilateral opacification of lens → ↓ in vision. Risk factors: age, smoking, EtOH, sunlight, classic galactosemia, galactokinase deficiency, diabetes (sorbitol), trauma, infection.

---

**Papilledema**

↑ in intracranial pressure → elevated optic disk with blurred margins, bigger blind spot (can be seen in hydrocephalus).

---

**Extraocular muscles and nerves**

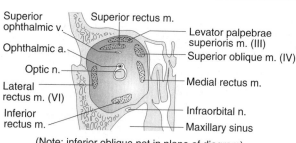

Superior ophthalmic v.
Superior rectus m.
Levator palpebrae superioris m. (III)
Superior oblique m. (IV)
Ophthalmic a.
Optic n.
Medial rectus m.
Lateral rectus m. (VI)
Inferior rectus m.
Infraorbital n.
Maxillary sinus

(Note: inferior oblique not in plane of diagram)

CN III damage—eye looks down and out; ptosis, pupillary dilation, loss of accommodation.
CN IV damage—diplopia with a defective downward gaze (adjust by tilting head toward lesion).
CN VI damage—medially directed eye.

CN VI innervates the Lateral Rectus.
CN IV innervates the Superior Oblique.
CN III innervates the Rest.
The "chemical formula" $LR_6SO_4R_3$.
The superior oblique abducts, intorts, and depresses while adducted.

| Testing extraocular muscles | To test the function of each muscle, have the patient look in the following directions (e.g., to test SO, have patient depress eye from adducted position): | IOU: to test Inferior Oblique, have patient look Up. |
|---|---|---|

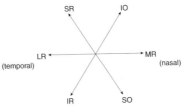

## Strabismus vs. amblyopia

| Strabismus | Misalignment of eyes. Multiple etiologies. |
|---|---|
| Amblyopia | Reduction of vision from disuse in critical period. May be 2° to strabismus, deprivation, unequal refractive errors. |

| Pupillary control | 1. Constriction (miosis)—Pupillary sphincter muscle (aka circular muscle). Parasympathetic. Innervation—CN III from Edinger-Westphal nucleus → ciliary ganglion.<br>2. Dilation (myDriasis)—radial muscle (aka pupillary dilator muscle), sympathetic. Innervation—T1 preganglionic sympathetic → superior cervical ganglion → postganglionic sympathetic → long ciliary nerve. |
|---|---|

| Pupillary light reflex | Light in either retina sends a signal via CN II to pretectal nuclei (dashed lines) in midbrain that activate bilateral Edinger-Westphal nuclei; pupils contract bilaterally (consensual reflex).<br>Result: illumination of 1 eye results in bilateral pupillary constriction.<br>Marcus Gunn pupil—afferent pupillary defect (e.g., due to optic nerve damage or retinal detachment). ↓ bilateral pupillary constriction when light is shone in affected eye. |
|---|---|

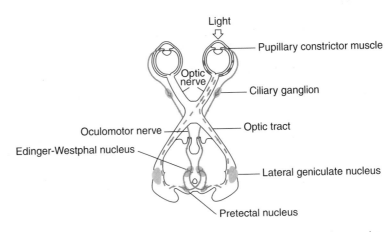

(Adapted, with permission, from Simon RP et al. *Clinical Neurology*, 3rd ed. Stamford, CT: Appleton & Lange, 1996.)

### Cranial nerve III in cross section

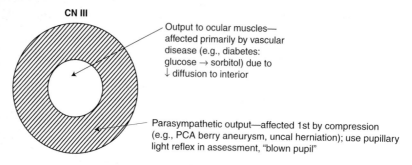

**CN III**

Output to ocular muscles—affected primarily by vascular disease (e.g., diabetes: glucose → sorbitol) due to ↓ diffusion to interior

Parasympathetic output—affected 1st by compression (e.g., PCA berry aneurysm, uncal herniation); use pupillary light reflex in assessment, "blown pupil"

| | |
|---|---|
| **Retinal detachment** | Separation of neurosensory layer of retina from pigment epithelium → degeneration of photoreceptors → vision loss. May be 2° to trauma, diabetes. |
| **Age-related macular degeneration (ARMD)** | Degeneration of macula (central area of retina). Causes loss of central vision (scotomas). "Dry"/atrophic ARMD is slow, due to fat deposits and causes gradual ↓ in vision. "Wet" ARMD is rapid, due to neovascularization. |

### Visual field defects

1. Right anopia
2. Bitemporal hemianopia
3. Left homonymous hemianopia
4. Left upper quadrantic anopia (right temporal lesion, MCA)
5. Left lower quadrantic anopia (right parietal lesion, MCA)
6. Left hemianopia with macular sparing (PCA), macula → bilateral projection to occiput
7. Central scotoma (macular degeneration)

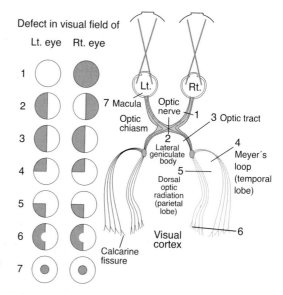

Defect in visual field of

Lt. eye   Rt. eye

7 Macula    Optic nerve
Optic chiasm    1
Optic    3 Optic tract
2
Lateral geniculate body    4 Meyer's loop (temporal lobe)
5
Dorsal optic radiation (parietal lobe)
Visual cortex
Calcarine fissure    6

Note: When an image hits 1° visual cortex, it is upside down and left-right reversed.

Meyer's loop—inferior retina; loops around inferior horn of lateral ventricle. Dorsal optic radiation—superior retina; takes shortest path via internal capsule.

| **Internuclear ophthalmoplegia (MLF syndrome)** | Lesion in the medial longitudinal fasciculus (MLF) → medial rectus palsy on attempted lateral gaze. Nystagmus in abducting eye. Convergence is normal. Syndrome is seen in many patients with multiple sclerosis. | **MLF = MS.** When looking left, the left nucleus of CN VI fires, which contracts the left lateral rectus and stimulates the contralateral (right) nucleus of CN III via the right MLF to contract the right medial rectus. |

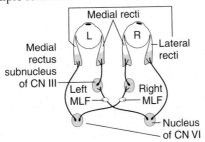

Looking to the left with right MLF damage

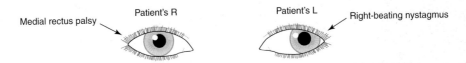

Medial rectus palsy — Patient's R     Patient's L — Right-beating nystagmus

| **Vestibular apparatus** | Nystagmus with quick-phase correction:<br>—Cold water: nystagmus toward lesion with quick phase to Opposite side.<br>—Warm water: nystagmus to opposite side with quick phase to Same side. | COWS. |

**Dementia**  A ↓ in cognitive ability, memory, or function with intact consciousness.

| Disease | Description | Histologic/Gross Findings |
|---|---|---|
| Alzheimer's disease | Most common cause in elderly. Down syndrome patients have an ↑ risk of developing Alzheimer's.<br>Familial form (10%) associated with the following genes (see Image 41):<br>  ▪ **Early onset:** APP (21), presenilin-1 (14), presenilin-2 (1)<br>  ▪ **Late onset:** ApoE4 (19)<br>ApoE2 (19) is protective. | ▪ Widespread cortical atrophy<br>▪ ↓ ACh<br>▪ Senile plaques (extracellular β-amyloid core): may cause amyloid angiopathy → intracranial hemorrhage (Aβ-amyloid synthesized by cleaving amyloid protein)<br>▪ Neurofibrillary tangles (intracellular, abnormally phosphorylated tau protein = insoluble cytoskeletal elements; tangles correlate with degree of dementia) |
| Pick's disease (frontotemporal dementia) | Dementia, aphasia, parkinsonian aspects; change in personality.<br>Spares parietal lobe and posterior ⅔ of superior temporal gyrus. | ▪ Pick bodies (intracellular, aggregated tau protein)<br>▪ Frontotemporal atrophy |
| Lewy body dementia | Parkinsonism with dementia and hallucinations. | ▪ α-synuclein defect |
| Creutzfeldt-Jakob disease (CJD) | Rapidly progressive (weeks to months) dementia with myoclonus. | ▪ Spongiform cortex<br>▪ Prions (α helix → β sheet [resistant to proteases]) |
| Other causes | **Multi-infarct** (2nd most common in elderly), **syphilis, HIV, vitamin B$_{12}$ deficiency, Wilson's disease.** | |

**Multiple sclerosis**  Autoimmune inflammation and demyelination of CNS (brain and spinal cord). Patients can present with optic neuritis (sudden loss of vision), MLF syndrome (internuclear ophthalmoplegia), hemiparesis, hemisensory symptoms, or bladder/bowel incontinence. Relapsing and remitting course. Most often affects women in their 20s and 30s; more common in whites.

Findings: ↑ protein (IgG) in CSF. Oligoclonal bands are diagnostic. MRI is gold standard. Periventricular plaques (areas of oligodendrocyte loss and reactive gliosis) with preservation of axons (see Image 47).

Charcot's classic triad of **MS** is a **SIN:**

Scanning speech
Intention tremor,
  Incontinence,
  Internuclear ophthalmoplegia
Nystagmus
Treatment: β-interferon or immunosuppressant therapy. Symptomatic treatment for neurogenic bladder, spasticity, pain.

| | | |
|---|---|---|
| **Guillain-Barré syndrome (acute inflammatory demyelinating polyradiculopathy)** | Inflammation and demyelination of peripheral nerves and motor fibers of ventral roots (sensory effect less severe than motor), causing symmetric ascending muscle weakness beginning in distal lower extremities. Facial paralysis in 50% of cases. Autonomic function may be severely affected (e.g., cardiac irregularities, hypertension, or hypotension). Almost all patients survive; the majority recover completely after weeks to months.<br><br>Findings: ↑ CSF protein with normal cell count (albuminocytologic dissociation). ↑ protein → papilledema. | Associated with infections → autoimmune attack of peripheral myelin due to molecular mimicry (e.g., *Campylobacter jejuni* or herpesvirus infection), inoculations, and stress, but no definitive link to pathogens.<br>Respiratory support is critical until recovery. Additional treatment: plasmapheresis, IV immune globulins. |
| **Other demyelinating and dysmyelinating diseases** | **Progressive multifocal leukoencephalopathy (PML)**—demyelination of CNS due to destruction of oligodendrocytes. Associated with JC virus and seen in 2–4% of AIDS patients (reactivation of latent viral infection). Rapidly progressive, usually fatal.<br>**Acute disseminated (postinfectious) encephalomyelitis**—multifocal perivenular inflammation and demyelination after infection (e.g., chickenpox, measles) or certain vaccinations (e.g., rabies, smallpox).<br>**Metachromatic leukodystrophy**—autosomal-recessive lysosomal storage disease, most commonly due to arylsulfatase A deficiency. Buildup of sulfatides leads to impaired production of myelin sheath.<br>**Charcot-Marie-Tooth disease**—also known as hereditary motor and sensory neuropathy (HMSN). Group of progressive hereditary nerve disorders related to the defective production of proteins involved in the structure and function of peripheral nerves or the myelin sheath. | |
| **Seizures** | Seizure—characterized by synchronized, high-frequency neuronal firing. Variety of forms.<br>Partial seizures—1 area of the brain. Most commonly originates in mesial temporal lobe. Often preceded by seizure aura; can secondarily generalize.<br>  1. Simple partial (consciousness intact)—motor, sensory, autonomic, psychic<br>  2. Complex partial (impaired consciousness)<br>Generalized seizures—diffuse.<br>  1. Absence (petit mal, 3 Hz, no postictal confusion)—blank stare<br>  2. Myoclonic—quick, repetitive jerks<br>  3. Tonic-clonic (grand mal)—alternating stiffening and movement<br>  4. Tonic—stiffening<br>  5. Atonic—"drop" seizures (falls to floor); commonly mistaken for fainting | Epilepsy—a disorder of recurrent seizures (febrile seizures are not epilepsy).<br>Causes of seizures by age:<br>  Children—genetic, infection (febrile), trauma, congenital, metabolic.<br>  Adults—tumors, trauma, stroke, infection.<br>  Elderly—stroke, tumor, trauma, metabolic, infection. |

**Headache**

Pain due to irritation of structures such as dura, cranial nerves, or extracranial structures, not brain parenchyma itself.

Migraine—unilateral; 4–72 hours of pulsating pain with nausea, photophobia, or phonophobia. +/– "aura" of neurologic symptoms before headache, including visual, sensory, speech disturbances. Due to irritation of CN V and release of substance P, CGRP, vasoactive peptides. Treatment: propranolol; NSAIDs; sumatriptan for acute migraines.

Tension headache—bilateral; > 30 minutes of steady pain. Not aggravated by light or noise; no aura.

Cluster headache—unilateral; repetitive brief headaches characterized by periorbital pain associated with ipsilateral lacrimation, rhinorrhea, Horner's syndrome. Much more common in males. Treatment: sumatriptan.

Other causes of headache include subarachnoid hemorrhage ("worst headache of life"), meningitis, hydrocephalus, neoplasia, arteritis.

**Vertigo**

Illusion of movement, not to be confused with dizziness or lightheadedness.

Peripheral vertigo—more common. Inner ear etiology (e.g., semicircular canal debris, vestibular nerve infection, Ménière's disease). Positional testing → delayed horizontal nystagmus.

Central vertigo—brain stem or cerebellar lesion (e.g., vestibular nuclei, posterior fossa tumor). Positional testing → immediate nystagmus in any direction; may change directions.

**Neurocutaneous disorders**

Sturge-Weber syndrome

Congenital disorder with port-wine stains (aka nevus flammeus), typically in $V_1$ ophthalmic distribution; ipsilateral leptomeningeal angiomas, pheochromocytomas.

Can cause glaucoma, seizures, hemiparesis, and mental retardation. Occurs sporadically.

Tuberous sclerosis

Hamartomas in CNS, skin, organs; cardiac rhabdomyoma, renal angiomyolipoma, subependymal giant cell astrocytoma, mitral regurgitation, seizures, hypopigmented "ash leaf spots," sebaceous adenoma, shagreen patch. Autosomal dominant.

Neurofibromatosis type I (von Recklinghausen's disease)

Café-au-lait spots, Lisch nodules (pigmented iris hamartomas), neurofibromas in skin, optic gliomas, pheochromocytomas. Autosomal dominant. Mutated NF-1 gene on chromosome 17.

von Hippel–Lindau disease

Cavernous hemangiomas in skin, mucosa, organs; bilateral renal cell carcinoma, hemangioblastoma in retina, brain stem, cerebellum; pheochromocytomas. Autosomal dominant; mutated tumor suppressor VHL on chromosome 3.

HIGH-YIELD SYSTEMS

NEUROLOGY

**Primary brain tumors**

Clinical presentation due to mass effects (e.g., seizures, dementia, focal lesions); 1° brain tumors rarely undergo metastasis. The majority of adult 1° tumors are supratentorial, while the majority of childhood 1° tumors are infratentorial. Note: half of adult brain tumors are metastases (well circumscribed; usually present at the gray-white junction).

**Adult peak incidence**

Glioblastoma multiforme (grade IV astrocytoma)
Most common 1° brain tumor. Prognosis grave; < 1-year life expectancy. Found in cerebral hemispheres. Can cross corpus callosum ("butterfly glioma") (see Image 48). Stain astrocytes for GFAP.
"Pseudopalisading" pleomorphic tumor cells—border central areas of necrosis and hemorrhage.

Meningioma
2nd most common 1° brain tumor. Most often occurs in convexities of hemispheres and parasagittal region. Arises from arachnoid cells external to brain. Resectable.
Spindle cells concentrically arranged in a whorled pattern; **psammoma bodies** (laminated calcifications).

Schwannoma
3rd most common 1° brain tumor. Schwann cell origin; often localized to CN VIII → acoustic schwannoma. Resectable. Usually found at cerebellopontine angle; S-100 positive.
Bilateral schwannoma found in neurofibromatosis type 2.

Oligodendroglioma
Relatively rare, slow growing. Most often in frontal lobes. Chicken-wire capillary pattern (see Image 49).
Oligodendrocytes = "fried egg" cells—round nuclei with clear cytoplasm. Often calcified in oligodendroglioma.

Pituitary adenoma
Most commonly prolactinoma. Bitemporal hemianopia (due to pressure on optic chiasm) and hyper- or hypopituitarism are sequelae.
Rathke's pouch.

**Childhood peak incidence**

Pilocytic (low-grade) astrocytoma
Usually well circumscribed. In children, most often found in posterior fossa. May be supratentorial. GFAP positive. Benign; good prognosis.
Rosenthal fibers—eosinophilic, corkscrew fibers. Cystic + solid (gross).

Medulloblastoma
Highly malignant cerebellar tumor. A form of primitive neuroectodermal tumor (PNET). Can compress 4th ventricle, causing hydrocephalus.
Rosettes or perivascular pseudorosette pattern of cells. Solid (gross), small blue cells (histology). Radiosensitive.

Ependymoma
Ependymal cell tumors most commonly found in 4th ventricle. Can cause hydrocephalus. Poor prognosis.
Characteristic perivascular pseudorosettes. Rod-shaped blepharoplasts (basal ciliary bodies) found near nucleus.

Hemangioblastoma
Most often cerebellar; associated with von Hippel–Lindau syndrome when found with retinal angiomas. Can produce EPO → 2° polycythemia.
Foamy cells and high vascularity are characteristic.

Craniopharyngioma
Benign childhood tumor, confused with pituitary adenoma (can also cause bitemporal hemianopia). Most common childhood supratentorial tumor.
Derived from remnants of Rathke's pouch. Calcification is common (tooth enamel–like).

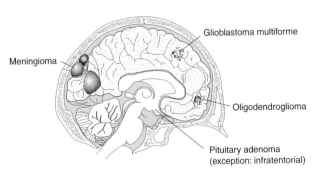

Supratentorial/adult tumors

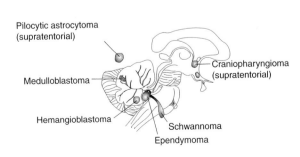

Infratentorial/childhood tumors

### Herniation syndromes

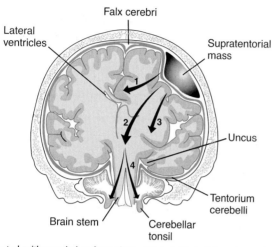

1. Cingulate (subfalcine) herniation under falx cerebri
2. Downward transtentorial (central) herniation
3. Uncal herniation
4. Cerebellar tonsillar herniation into the foramen magnum

Can compress anterior cerebral artery.
Coma and death result when these herniations compress the brain stem.
Uncus = medial temporal lobe.

(Adapted, with permission, from Simon RP et al. *Clinical Neurology*, 4th ed. Stamford, CT: Appleton & Lange, 1999: 314.)

### Uncal herniation

| Clinical signs | Cause |
|---|---|
| Ipsilateral dilated pupil/ptosis | Stretching of CN III (innervates levator palpebrae) |
| Contralateral homonymous hemianopia | Compression of ipsilateral posterior cerebral artery |
| Ipsilateral paresis | Compression of contralateral crus cerebri (Kernohan's notch) |
| Duret hemorrhages— paramedian artery rupture | Caudal displacement of brain stem |

### Differential diagnosis of brain lesions

| | |
|---|---|
| Ring-enhancing lesion | Metastases, abscesses, toxoplasmosis, AIDS lymphoma. |
| Uniformly enhancing lesion | Lymphoma, meningioma, metastases (usually ring enhancing). |
| Heterogeneously enhancing lesion | Glioblastoma multiforme. |

### Glaucoma drugs

| Drug | Mechanism | Side effects |
|---|---|---|
| **α-agonists** | | |
| Epinephrine | ↓ aqueous humor synthesis due to vasoconstriction | Mydriasis, stinging; do not use in closed-angle glaucoma |
| Brimonidine | ↓ aqueous humor synthesis | No pupillary or vision changes |
| **β-blockers** | | |
| Timolol, betaxolol, carteolol | ↓ aqueous humor secretion | No pupillary or vision changes |
| **Diuretics** | | |
| Acetazolamide | ↓ aqueous humor secretion due to ↓ $HCO_3^-$ (via inhibition of carbonic anhydrase) | No pupillary or vision changes |
| **Cholinomimetics** | | |
| Direct (pilocarpine, carbachol), indirect (physostigmine, echothiophate) | ↑ outflow of aqueous humor; contract ciliary muscle and open trabecular meshwork; use pilocarpine in emergencies; very effective at opening meshwork into canal of Schlemm | Miosis, cyclospasm |
| **Prostaglandin** | | |
| Latanoprost ($PGF_{2\alpha}$) | ↑ outflow of aqueous humor | Darkens color of iris (browning) |

### Opioid analgesics

| | |
|---|---|
| Mechanism | Morphine, fentanyl, codeine, heroin, methadone, meperidine, dextromethorphan. Act as agonists at opioid receptors (mu = morphine, delta = enkephalin, kappa = dynorphin) to modulate synaptic transmission—open $K^+$ channels, close $Ca^{2+}$ channels → ↓ synaptic transmission. Inhibit release of ACh, NE, 5-HT, glutamate, substance P. |
| Clinical use | Pain, cough suppression (dextromethorphan), diarrhea (loperamide and diphenoxylate), acute pulmonary edema, maintenance programs for addicts (methadone). |
| Toxicity | Addiction, **respiratory depression**, constipation, miosis (**pinpoint pupils**), additive **CNS depression** with other drugs. Tolerance does not develop to miosis and constipation. Toxicity treated with naloxone or naltrexone (opioid receptor antagonist). |

### Butorphanol

| | |
|---|---|
| Mechanism | Partial agonist at opioid mu receptors, agonist at kappa receptors. |
| Clinical use | Pain; causes less respiratory depression than full agonists. |
| Toxicity | Causes withdrawal if on full opioid agonist. |

### Tramadol

| | |
|---|---|
| Mechanism | Very weak opioid agonist; also inhibits serotonin and NE reuptake (works on multiple neurotransmitters—"**tram it all**" in). |
| Clinical use | Chronic pain. |
| Toxicity | Similar to opioids. Decreases seizure threshold. |

## Epilepsy drugs

| | PARTIAL | | GENERALIZED | | | Mechanism | Notes |
|---|---|---|---|---|---|---|---|
| | Simple | Complex | Tonic-Clonic | Absence | Status | | |
| Phenytoin | ✓ | ✓ | 1st line | | 1st line for prophylaxis | ↑ Na⁺ channel inactivation | Fosphenytoin for parenteral use |
| Carbamazepine | ✓ | ✓ | 1st line | | | ↑ Na⁺ channel inactivation | 1st line for trigeminal neuralgia |
| Lamotrigine | ✓ | ✓ | ✓ | | | Blocks voltage-gated Na⁺ channels | |
| Gabapentin | ✓ | ✓ | ✓ | | | Designed as GABA analog, but primarily inhibits HVA calcium channels | Also used for peripheral neuropathy, bipolar disorder |
| Topiramate | ✓ | ✓ | ✓ | | | Blocks Na⁺ channels, ↑ GABA action | |
| Phenobarbital | ✓ | ✓ | ✓ | | | ↑ GABA_A action | 1st line in pregnant women, children |
| Valproic acid | ✓ | ✓ | 1st line | ✓ | | ↑ Na⁺ channel inactivation, ↑ GABA concentration | Also used for myoclonic seizures |
| Ethosuximide | | | | 1st line | | Blocks thalamic T-type Ca²⁺ channels | |
| Benzodiazepines (diazepam or lorazepam) | | | | | 1st line for acute | ↑ GABA_A action | Also used for seizures of eclampsia (1st line to prevent seizures of eclampsia is MgSO₄) |
| Tiagabine | ✓ | ✓ | | | | Inhibits GABA reuptake | |
| Vigabatrin | ✓ | ✓ | | | | Irreversibly inhibits GABA transaminase → ↑ GABA | |
| Levetiracetam | ✓ | ✓ | ✓ | | | Mechanism unknown; may modulate GABA and glutamate release | |

## Epilepsy drug toxicities

| | |
|---|---|
| Benzodiazepines | Sedation, tolerance, dependence. |
| Carbamazepine | Diplopia, ataxia, blood dyscrasias (agranulocytosis, aplastic anemia), liver toxicity, teratogenesis, induction of cytochrome P-450, SIADH, Stevens-Johnson syndrome. |
| Ethosuximide | GI distress, fatigue, headache, urticaria, Stevens-Johnson syndrome. |
| Phenobarbital | Sedation, tolerance, dependence, induction of cytochrome P-450. |
| Phenytoin | Nystagmus, diplopia, ataxia, sedation, gingival hyperplasia, hirsutism, megaloblastic anemia, teratogenesis (fetal hydantoin syndrome), SLE-like syndrome, induction of cytochrome P-450. |
| Valproic acid | GI distress, rare but fatal hepatotoxicity (measure LFTs), neural tube defects in fetus (spina bifida), tremor, weight gain. Contraindicated in pregnancy. |
| Lamotrigine | Stevens-Johnson syndrome. |
| Gabapentin | Sedation, ataxia. |
| Topiramate | Sedation, mental dulling, kidney stones, weight loss. |

EFGH—Ethosuximide, Fatigue, GI, Headache.

Stevens-Johnson syndrome—prodrome of malaise and fever followed by rapid onset of erythematous/purpuric macules (oral, ocular, genital). Skin lesions progress to epidermal necrosis and sloughing.

## Phenytoin

| | |
|---|---|
| Mechanism | Use-dependent blockade of $Na^+$ channels; ↑ refractory period; inhibition of glutamate release from excitatory presynaptic neuron. |
| Clinical use | Tonic-clonic seizures. Also a class IB antiarrhythmic. |
| Toxicity | Nystagmus, ataxia, diplopia, sedation, SLE-like syndrome, induction of cytochrome P-450. Chronic use produces gingival hyperplasia in children, peripheral neuropathy, hirsutism, megaloblastic anemia (↓ folate absorption). Teratogenic (fetal hydantoin syndrome). |

## Barbiturates

| | |
|---|---|
| | Phenobarbital, pentobarbital, thiopental, secobarbital. |
| Mechanism | Facilitate $GABA_A$ action by ↑ **duration** of $Cl^-$ channel opening, thus ↓ neuron firing. |
| Clinical use | Sedative for anxiety, seizures, insomnia, induction of anesthesia (thiopental). |
| Toxicity | Dependence, additive CNS depression effects with alcohol, respiratory or cardiovascular depression (can lead to death), drug interactions owing to induction of liver microsomal enzymes (cytochrome P-450). Treat overdose with symptom management (assist respiration, ↑ BP). |

BarbiDURATe (↑ DURATion). Contraindicated in porphyria.

**Benzodiazepines**

Diazepam, lorazepam, triazolam, temazepam, oxazepam, midazolam, chlordiazepoxide, alprazolam.

Mechanism

Facilitate GABA$_A$ action by ↑ **frequency** of Cl$^-$ channel opening. ↓ REM sleep. Most have long half-lives and active metabolites.

Clinical use

Anxiety, spasticity, status epilepticus (lorazepam and diazepam), detoxification (especially alcohol withdrawal–DTs), night terrors, sleepwalking, general anesthetic (amnesia, muscle relaxation), hypnotic (insomnia).

Toxicity

Dependence, additive CNS depression effects with alcohol. Less risk of respiratory depression and coma than with barbiturates.

Treat overdose with flumazenil (competitive antagonist at GABA benzodiazepine receptor).

**FRE**nzodiazepines (↑ **FRE**quency).
Short acting = **TOM** Thumb = **T**riazolam, **O**xazepam, **M**idazolam. Highest addictive potential.
Benzos, barbs, and EtOH all bind GABA(A)-R, which is a ligand-gated chloride channel.

**Anesthetics— general principles**

CNS drugs must be lipid soluble (cross the blood-brain barrier) or be actively transported.

Drugs with ↓ solubility in blood = rapid induction and recovery times.

Drugs with ↑ solubility in lipids = ↑ potency = $\dfrac{1}{MAC}$

where MAC = minimal alveolar concentration at which 50% of the population is anesthetized. Varies with age.

Examples: N$_2$O has low blood and lipid solubility, and thus fast induction and low potency. Halothane, in contrast, has ↑ lipid and blood solubility, and thus high potency and slow induction.

| Organ | Mechanism of Action |
|---|---|
| Lungs | ↑ rate + depth of ventilation = ↑ gas tension |
| Blood | ↑ blood solubility = ↑ blood/gas partition coefficient = ↑ solubility = ↑ gas required to saturate blood = **slower** onset of action |
| Tissue (e.g., brain) | AV concentration gradient ↑ = ↑ solubility = ↑ gas required to saturate tissue = **slower** onset of action |

**Inhaled anesthetics**

Halothane, enflurane, isoflurane, sevoflurane, methoxyflurane, nitrous oxide.

Mechanism

Mechanism unknown.

Effects

Myocardial depression, respiratory depression, nausea/emesis, ↑ cerebral blood flow (↓ cerebral metabolic demand).

Toxicity

Hepatotoxicity (halothane), nephrotoxicity (methoxyflurane), proconvulsant (enflurane), malignant hyperthermia (rare), expansion of trapped gas (nitrous oxide).

## Intravenous anesthetics

**Barbiturates** — Thiopental—high potency, high lipid solubility, rapid entry into brain. Used for induction of anesthesia and short surgical procedures. Effect terminated by rapid redistribution into tissue and fat. ↓ cerebral blood flow.

**B. B. King on OPIATES PROPOses FOOLishly.**

**Benzodiazepines** — Midazolam most common drug used for endoscopy; used adjunctively with gaseous anesthetics and narcotics. May cause severe postoperative respiratory depression, ↓ BP (treat overdose with flumazenil), and amnesia.

**Arylcyclohexylamines (Ketamine)** — PCP analogs that act as dissociative anesthetics. Block NMDA receptors. Cardiovascular stimulants. Cause disorientation, hallucination, and bad dreams. ↑ cerebral blood flow.

**Opiates** — Morphine, fentanyl used with other CNS depressants during general anesthesia.

**Propofol** — Used for rapid anesthesia induction and short procedures. Less postoperative nausea than thiopental. Potentiates $GABA_A$.

## Local anesthetics

Esters—procaine, cocaine, tetracaine; amides—lIdocaIne, mepIvacaIne, bupIvacaIne (amIdes have 2 I's in name).

**Mechanism** — Block $Na^+$ channels by binding to specific receptors on inner portion of channel. Preferentially bind to activated $Na^+$ channels, so most effective in rapidly firing neurons. 3° amine local anesthetics penetrate membrane in uncharged form, then bind to ion channels as charged form.

**Principle**
1. In infected (acidic) tissue, alkaline anesthetics are charged and cannot penetrate membrane effectively. More anesthetic is needed in these cases.
2. Order of nerve blockade—small-diameter fibers > large diameter. Myelinated fibers > unmyelinated fibers. Overall, size factor predominates over myelination such that small myelinated fibers > small unmyelinated fibers > large myelinated fibers > large unmyelinated fibers. Order of loss—pain (lose first) > temperature > touch > pressure (lose last).
3. Except for cocaine, given with vasoconstrictors (usually epinephrine) to enhance local action—↓ bleeding, ↑ anesthesia by ↓ systemic concentration.

**Clinical use** — Minor surgical procedures, spinal anesthesia. If allergic to esters, give amides.

**Toxicity** — CNS excitation, severe cardiovascular toxicity (bupivacaine), hypertension, hypotension, and arrhythmias (cocaine).

## Neuromuscular blocking drugs

Used for muscle paralysis in surgery or mechanical ventilation. Selective for motor (vs. autonomic) nicotinic receptor.

**Depolarizing** — Succinylcholine (complications include hypercalcemia and hyperkalemia).
Reversal of blockade:
  Phase I (prolonged depolarization)—no antidote. Block potentiated by cholinesterase inhibitors.
  Phase II (repolarized but blocked)—antidote consists of cholinesterase inhibitors (e.g., neostigmine).

**Nondepolarizing** — Tubocurarine, atracurium, mivacurium, pancuronium, vecuronium, rocuronium. Competitive—compete with ACh for receptors.
Reversal of blockade—neostigmine, edrophonium, and other cholinesterase inhibitors.

**Dantrolene**

Used in the treatment of **malignant hyperthermia**, which is caused by the concomitant use of inhalation anesthetics (except $N_2O$) and succinylcholine. Also used to treat **neuroleptic malignant syndrome** (a toxicity of antipsychotic drugs).

Mechanism: prevents the release of $Ca^{2+}$ from the sarcoplasmic reticulum of skeletal muscle.

---

**Parkinson's disease drugs**

Parkinsonism is due to loss of dopaminergic neurons and excess cholinergic activity.

| Strategy | Agents | |
|---|---|---|
| Agonize dopamine receptors | Bromocriptine, pergolide (ergot alkaloid and partial dopamine agonist), pramipexole, ropinirole (non-ergot); non-ergots are preferred | **BALSA:** Bromocriptine |
| ↑ dopamine | Amantadine (may ↑ dopamine release); also used as an antiviral against influenza A and rubella; toxicity = ataxia | Amantadine Levodopa (with carbidopa) |
| | L-dopa/carbidopa (converted to dopamine in CNS) | Selegiline (and COMT inhibitors) Antimuscarinics |
| Prevent dopamine breakdown | Selegiline (selective MAO type B inhibitor); entacapone, tolcapone (COMT inhibitors—prevent L-dopa degradation, thereby increasing dopamine availability) | |
| Curb excess cholinergic activity | **Benz**tropine (Antimuscarinic; improves tremor and rigidity but has little effect on bradykinesia) | **Park** your Mercedes-**Benz**. |

For essential or familial tremors, use a β-blocker (e.g., propranolol).

---

**L-dopa (levodopa)/carbidopa**

| | |
|---|---|
| Mechanism | ↑ level of dopamine in brain. Unlike dopamine, L-dopa can cross blood-brain barrier and is converted by dopa decarboxylase in the CNS to dopamine. |
| Clinical use | Parkinsonism. |
| Toxicity | Arrhythmias from peripheral conversion to dopamine. Long-term use can → dyskinesia following administration, akinesia between doses. Carbidopa, a peripheral decarboxylase inhibitor, is given with L-dopa in order to ↑ the bioavailability of L-dopa in the brain and to limit peripheral side effects. |

---

**Selegiline**

| | |
|---|---|
| Mechanism | Selectively inhibits MAO-B, which preferentially metabolizes dopamine over NE and 5-HT, thereby increasing the availability of dopamine. |
| Clinical use | Adjunctive agent to L-dopa in treatment of Parkinson's disease. |
| Toxicity | May enhance adverse effects of L-dopa. |

## Alzheimer's drugs

### Memantine

| | |
|---|---|
| Mechanism | NMDA receptor antagonist; helps prevent excitotoxicity (mediated by $Ca^{2+}$). |
| Toxicity | Dizziness, confusion, hallucinations. |

### Donepezil, galantamine, rivastigmine

| | |
|---|---|
| Mechanism | Acetylcholinesterase inhibitors. |
| Toxicity | Nausea, dizziness, insomnia. |

## Huntington's drugs

Disease — ↑ dopamine, ↓ GABA + ACh.
Reserpine + tetrabenazine — amine depleting.
Haloperidol — dopamine receptor antagonist.

## Sumatriptan

| | | |
|---|---|---|
| Mechanism | $5\text{-}HT_{1B/1D}$ agonist. Causes vasoconstriction, inhibition of trigeminal activation and vasoactive peptide release. Half-life < 2 hours. | A **SUM**o wrestler **TRIP**s **AN**d falls on your **head.** |
| Clinical use | Acute migraine, cluster headache attacks. | |
| Toxicity | Coronary vasospasm (contraindicated in patients with CAD or Prinzmetal's angina), mild tingling. | |

# Psychiatry

*"A Freudian slip is when you say one thing but mean your mother."*
— Anonymous

*"Men will always be mad, and those who think they can cure them are the maddest of all."*
— Voltaire

*"Anyone who goes to a psychiatrist ought to have his head examined."*
— Samuel Goldwyn

▸ Psychology

▸ Pathology

▸ Pharmacology

| | | |
|---|---|---|
| **Intelligence quotient** | Stanford-Binet—calculates IQ as mental age/ chronological age × 100. | Standard-Binet IQ test. |
| | Wechsler Adult Intelligence Scale (WAIS III)— uses 14 subtests (7 verbal, 7 performance). Can quantify intellectual decline. | |
| | Wechsler Intelligence Scale for Children (**WISC**)— used for children between ages 6 and 16. | Kids **WISC** cookie crumbs off the table. |
| | Mean is defined at 100, with standard deviation of 15. | |
| | IQ < 70 is one of the criteria for diagnosis of mental retardation (MR). | |
| | IQ < 40—severe MR. IQ < 20—profound MR. | |
| **Simple learning** | Habituation—repeated stimulation leads to ↓ response. | |
| | Sensitization—repeated stimulation leads to ↑ response. | |
| **Classical conditioning** | Learning in which a natural response (salivation) is elicited by a conditioned, or learned, stimulus (bell) that previously was presented in conjunction with an unconditioned stimulus (food). | Pavlov's classical experiments with dogs—ringing the bell provoked salivation. |
| **Operant conditioning** | Learning in which a particular action is elicited because it produces a reward. | |
| | Positive reinforcement—desired reward produces action (mouse presses button to get food). | |
| | Negative reinforcement—removal of aversive stimulus elicits behavior (mouse presses button to avoid shock). | |
| | Punishment—application of aversive stimulus extinguishes unwanted behavior. | |
| | Extinction—discontinuation of reinforcement eliminates behavior. | |
| **Reinforcement schedules** | Pattern of reinforcement determines how quickly a behavior is learned or extinguished. | |
| Continuous | Reward received after every response. Rapidly extinguished. | Think vending machine—stop using it if it does not deliver. |
| Variable ratio | Reward received after random number of responses. Slowly extinguished. | Think slot machine—continue to play even if it rarely rewards. |

## Transference and countertransference

| | |
|---|---|
| Transference | Patient projects feelings about formative or other important persons onto physician (e.g., psychiatrist = parent). |
| Countertransference | Doctor projects feelings about formative or other important persons onto patient. |

| | | |
|---|---|---|
| **Freud's structural theory of the mind** | The central goal of Freudian psychoanalysis is to make the patient aware of what is hidden in his/her unconscious. | |
| Id | Primal urges, food, sex, and aggression. The id "drives"; Instinct. Entirely subconscious. | "I want it." |
| Ego | Mediator between primal urges and behavior accepted in reality. | "Take it and you will get in trouble." |
| Superego | Moral values, conscience; can lead to self-blame and attacks on ego. | "You know you can't have it. Taking it is wrong." |

| | |
|---|---|
| **Oedipus complex** | Repressed sexual feelings of a child for the opposite-sex parent, accompanied by rivalry with same-sex parent. First described by Freud. |

| | |
|---|---|
| **Social learning** | Shaping—behavior achieved following reward of closer and closer approximations of desired behavior. Modeling—behavior acquired by watching others and assimilating actions into one's own repertoire. |

| | |
|---|---|
| **Erikson's stages of psychosocial development** | 8 stages of normal development, each posing a new crisis. Unsuccessful completion of a stage may manifest as psychosocial maladaption later in life. Examples include the Oral Sensory Stage at 0 to 12–18 months, where trust vs. mistrust is crisis, and the Adolescence Stage at 12–20 years, where identity vs. role confusion is crisis. |

**Ego defenses**
Unconscious mental processes of the ego used to resolve conflict and prevent feelings of anxiety and depression.

**Immature—more primitive**

| | | |
|---|---|---|
| Acting out | Unacceptable feelings and thoughts are expressed through actions. | Tantrums. |
| Dissociation | Temporary, drastic change in personality, memory, consciousness, or motor behavior to avoid emotional stress. | Extreme forms can result in dissociative identity disorder (multiple personality disorder). |
| Denial | Avoidance of awareness of some painful reality. | A common reaction in newly diagnosed AIDS and cancer patients. |
| Displacement | Process whereby avoided ideas and feelings are transferred to some neutral person or object (vs. projection). | Mother places blame on child because she is angry at her husband. |
| Fixation | Partially remaining at a more childish level of development (vs. regression). | Men fixating on sports games. |
| Identification | Modeling behavior after another person who is more powerful (though not necessarily admired). | Abused child identifies himself/herself as an abuser. |
| Isolation of affect | Separation of feelings from ideas and events. | Describing murder in graphic detail with no emotional response. |
| Projection | An unacceptable internal impulse is attributed to an external source. | A man who wants another woman thinks his wife is cheating on him. |
| Rationalization | Proclaiming logical reasons for actions actually performed for other reasons, usually to avoid self-blame. | After getting fired, claiming that the job was not important anyway. |
| Reaction formation | Process whereby a warded-off idea or feeling is replaced by an (unconsciously derived) emphasis on its opposite. | A patient with libidinous thoughts enters a monastery. |
| Regression | Turning back the maturational clock and going back to earlier modes of dealing with the world. | Seen in children under stress (e.g., bedwetting) and in patients on dialysis (e.g., crying). |
| Repression | Involuntary withholding of an idea or feeling from conscious awareness. | Not remembering a conflictual or traumatic experience; pressing bad thoughts into the unconscious. |
| Splitting | Belief that people are either all good or all bad at different times due to intolerance of ambiguity. Seen in borderline personality disorder. | A patient says that all the nurses are cold and insensitive but that the doctors are warm and friendly. |

**Mature—less primitive**

| | | |
|---|---|---|
| Altruism | Guilty feelings alleviated by unsolicited generosity toward others. | Mafia boss makes large donation to charity. |
| Humor | Appreciating the amusing nature of an anxiety-provoking or adverse situation. | Nervous medical student jokes about the boards. |
| Sublimation | Process whereby one replaces an unacceptable wish with a course of action that is similar to the wish but does not conflict with one's value system. | Actress uses experience of abuse to enhance her acting. Think of sublimation as it is used in chemistry: a substance changing from a solid to a gas. |
| Suppression | Voluntary withholding of an idea or feeling from conscious awareness (vs. repression). | Choosing not to think about the USMLE until the week of the exam. |

**Mature** women wear a **SASH: S**ublimation, **A**ltruism, **S**uppression, **H**umor.

| | | |
|---|---|---|
| **Infant deprivation effects** | Long-term deprivation of affection results in: <br> 1. ↓ muscle tone <br> 2. Poor language skills <br> 3. Poor socialization skills <br> 4. Lack of basic trust <br> 5. Anaclitic depression <br> 6. Weight loss <br> 7. Physical illness <br> Severe deprivation can result in infant death. | The **4 W's: W**eak, **W**ordless, **W**anting (socially), **W**ary. <br> Deprived babies say **W**ah, Wah, Wah, Wah. <br> Deprivation for > 6 months can lead to irreversible changes. |

**Child abuse**

| | Physical abuse | Sexual abuse |
|---|---|---|
| Evidence | Healed fractures on x-ray, cigarette burns, subdural hematomas, multiple bruises, retinal hemorrhage or detachment | Genital/anal trauma, STDs, UTIs |
| Abuser Epidemiology | Usually female and the 1° caregiver <br> ~3000 deaths/year in the United States | Known to victim, usually male <br> Peak incidence 9–12 years of age |

| | |
|---|---|
| **Child neglect** | Failure to provide a child with adequate food, shelter, supervision, education, and/or affection. Most common form of child maltreatment. Evidence: poor hygiene, malnutrition, withdrawal, impaired social/emotional development, failure to thrive. As with child abuse, child neglect must be reported to local child protective services. |
| **Anaclitic depression (hospitalism)** | Depression in an infant attributable to continued separation from caregiver. Infant becomes withdrawn and unresponsive. Reversible, but prolonged separation can result in failure to thrive or other developmental disturbances (e.g., delayed speech). |
| **Regression in children** | Children regress to younger patterns of behavior under conditions of stress such as physical illness, punishment, birth of a new sibling, or fatigue (e.g., bedwetting in a previously toilet-trained child when hospitalized). |

| | |
|---|---|
| **Childhood and early-onset disorders** | Attention-deficit hyperactivity disorder (ADHD)—limited attention span and poor impulse control. Onset before age 7. Characterized by hyperactivity, motor impairment, and emotional lability. Normal intelligence, but commonly coexists with difficulties in school. May continue into adulthood in as many as 50% of individuals. Associated with ↓ frontal lobe volumes. Treatment: methylphenidate (Ritalin), amphetamines (Dexedrine), atomoxetine (nonstimulant SNRI). |
| | Conduct disorder—repetitive and pervasive behavior violating social norms (physical aggression, destruction of property, theft). After 18 years of age, diagnosed as antisocial personality disorder. |
| | Oppositional defiant disorder—enduring pattern of hostile, defiant behavior toward authority figures in the absence of serious violations of social norms. |
| | Tourette's syndrome—characterized by sudden, rapid, recurrent, nonrhythmic, stereotyped motor movements or vocalizations (tics) that persist for > 1 year. Lifetime prevalence of 0.1–1.0% in the general population. Coprolalia (obscene speech) found in only 20% of patients. Associated with OCD. Onset at < 18 years of age. Treatment: antipsychotics (e.g., haloperidol). |
| | Separation anxiety disorder—overwhelming fear of separation from home or loss of attachment figure. May lead to factitious physical complaints to avoid going to school. Common onset at 7–9 years of age. |
| **Pervasive developmental disorders** | Autistic disorder—severe language impairment and poor social interactions. Greater focus on objects than on people. Characterized by repetitive behavior and usually below-normal intelligence. Rarely, may have unusual abilities (savants). More common in boys. Treatment: behavioral and supportive therapy to improve communication and social skills. |
| | Asperger's disorder—a milder form of autism. Characterized by all-absorbing interests, repetitive behavior, and problems with social relationships. Children are of normal intelligence and lack verbal or cognitive deficits. No language impairment. |
| | Rett's disorder—X-linked disorder seen almost exclusively in girls (affected males die in utero or shortly after birth). Normal to age 4, followed by regression characterized by loss of development, mental retardation, loss of verbal abilities, ataxia, and stereotyped hand-wringing. |
| | Childhood disintegrative disorder—marked regression in multiple areas of functioning after at least 2 years of apparently normal development. Significant loss of expressive or receptive language skills, social skills or adaptive behavior, bowel or bladder control, play, or motor skills. Common onset between 3 and 4 years of age. More common in boys. |
| **Neurotransmitter changes with disease** | Anxiety—↑ NE, ↓ GABA, ↓ serotonin (5-HT). |
| | Depression—↓ NE, ↓ serotonin (5-HT), ↓ dopamine. |
| | Alzheimer's dementia—↓ ACh. |
| | Huntington's disease—↓ GABA, ↓ ACh. |
| | Schizophrenia—↑ dopamine. |
| | Parkinson's disease—↓ dopamine, ↑ ACh. |

HIGH-YIELD PRINCIPLES

PSYCHIATRY

| | | |
|---|---|---|
| **Orientation** | Patient's ability to know who he or she is, what date and time it is, and what his or her present circumstances are.<br><br>Common causes of loss of orientation: alcohol, drugs, fluid/electrolyte imbalance, head trauma, hypoglycemia, nutritional deficiencies. | Order of loss: 1st—time; 2nd—place; last—person. |
| **Amnesia types** | *Retro*grade amnesia—inability to remember things that occurred before a CNS insult.<br>*Antero*grade amnesia—inability to remember things that occurred after a CNS insult (no new memory).<br>Korsakoff's amnesia—classic anterograde amnesia caused by thiamine deficiency. Leads to bilateral destruction of mammillary bodies. May also lead to some retrograde amnesia. Seen in alcoholics, and associated with confabulations.<br>Dissociative amnesia—inability to recall important personal information, usually subsequent to severe trauma or stress. | |
| **Delirium** | **Waxing and waning level of consciousness with acute onset;** rapid ↓ in attention span and level of arousal. Characterized by acute changes in mental status, disorganized thinking, hallucinations (often visual), illusions, misperceptions, disturbance in sleep-wake cycle, cognitive dysfunction. Most common psychiatric illness on medical and surgical floors. Abnormal EEG. | Deli**RIUM** = changes in senso**RIUM.**<br>Check for drugs with anticholinergic effects.<br>Often reversible. |
| **Dementia** | **Gradual ↓ in cognition with no change in level of consciousness.** Characterized by memory deficits, aphasia, apraxia, agnosia, loss of abstract thought, behavioral/personality changes, impaired judgment. Patient is alert.<br>↑ incidence with age. More often gradual onset. Normal EEG.<br>Caused by Alzheimer's disease, vascular thrombosis/hemorrhage (may have acute/subacute onset), HIV, Pick's disease, substance abuse, CJD. | De**MEM**tia is characterized by **MEM**ory loss. Usually irreversible.<br>In elderly patients, depression may present like dementia (pseudodementia). |
| **Hallucination vs. illusion vs. delusion vs. loose association** | Hallucinations—perceptions in the absence of external stimuli (e.g., seeing a light that is not actually present).<br>Illusions—misinterpretations of actual external stimuli (e.g., seeing a light and thinking that it is the sun).<br>Delusions—false beliefs not shared with other members of culture/subculture that are firmly maintained in spite of obvious proof to the contrary (e.g., thinking the CIA is spying on you).<br>Loose associations—disorders in the form of thought (the way ideas are tied together). | |

**Hallucination types**

Visual hallucinations—common in delirium.

Auditory hallucinations—common in schizophrenia.

Olfactory hallucination—often occurs as an aura of psychomotor epilepsy.

Gustatory hallucination—rare.

Tactile hallucinations—common in alcohol withdrawal (e.g., formication—the sensation of ants crawling on one's skin). Also seen in cocaine abusers ("cocaine bugs").

HypnaGOgic hallucination—occurs while GOing to sleep.

HypnoPOMPic hallucination—occurs while waking from sleep (POMPous upon awakening).

**Schizophrenia**

Periods of psychosis and disturbed behavior with a decline in functioning lasting > 6 months. Associated with ↑ dopaminergic activity, ↓ dendritic branching. Marijuana use is a risk factor for schizophrenia in teens.

Diagnosis requires 2 or more of the following (1–4 are "positive symptoms"):

1. Delusions
2. Hallucinations—often auditory
3. Disorganized speech (loose associations)
4. Disorganized or catatonic behavior
5. "Negative symptoms"—flat affect, social withdrawal, lack of motivation, lack of speech or thought

**Brief psychotic disorder**—< 1 month, usually stress related.

**Schizophreniform disorder**—1–6 months.

**Schizoaffective disorder**—at least 2 weeks of stable mood with psychotic symptoms, plus a major depressive, manic, or mixed (both) episode. 2 subtypes: bipolar or depressive.

5 subtypes:

1. Paranoid (delusions)
2. Disorganized (with regard to speech, behavior, and affect)
3. Catatonic (automatisms)
4. Undifferentiated (elements of all types)
5. Residual

Genetic factors outweigh environmental factors in the etiology of schizophrenia.

Lifetime prevalence—1.5% (males = females, blacks = whites). Presents earlier in men (late teens to early 20s vs. late 20s to early 30s in women). Patients are at ↑ risk for suicide.

**Delusional disorder**

Fixed, persistent, nonbizarre belief system lasting > 1 month. Functioning otherwise not impaired. Often self-limited.

Shared psychotic disorder (folie à deux)—development of delusions in a person in a close relationship with someone with delusional disorder. Often resolves upon separation.

**Dissociative disorders**

Dissociative identity disorder—formerly known as multiple personality disorder. Presence of 2 or more distinct identities or personality states. More common in women. Associated with history of sexual abuse.

Depersonalization disorder—persistent feelings of detachment or estrangement from oneself.

Dissociative fugue—abrupt change in geographic location with inability to recall past, confusion about personal identity, or assumption of a new identity. Associated with traumatic circumstances (e.g., natural disasters, wartime, trauma). Leads to significant distress or impairment. Not the result of substance abuse or general medical condition.

| | | |
|---|---|---|
| **Manic episode** | Distinct period of abnormally and persistently elevated, expansive, or irritable mood lasting at least 1 week. Often disturbing to patient. | |
| | Diagnosis requires 3 or more of the following are present during mood disturbance: | Maniacs **DIG FAST.** |
| | 1. **D**istractibility | |
| | 2. **I**rresponsibility—seeks pleasure without regard to consequences (hedonistic) | |
| | 3. **G**randiosity—inflated self-esteem | |
| | 4. **F**light of ideas—racing thoughts | |
| | 5. ↑ in goal-directed **A**ctivity/psychomotor **A**gitation | |
| | 6. ↓ need for **S**leep | |
| | 7. **T**alkativeness or pressured speech | |
| **Hypomanic episode** | Like manic episode except mood disturbance is not severe enough to cause marked impairment in social and/or occupational functioning or to necessitate hospitalization. No psychotic features. | |
| **Bipolar disorder** | Defined by the presence of at least 1 manic (bipolar I) or hypomanic (bipolar II) episode. Depressive symptoms always occur eventually. Patient's mood and functioning usually return to normal between episodes. Use of antidepressants can lead to ↑ mania. Engagement in pleasurable activities with potentially painful consequences can be seen. High suicide risk. Treatment: mood stabilizers (e.g., lithium, valproic acid, carbamazepine), atypical antipsychotics. | |
| | Cyclothymic disorder—milder form of bipolar disorder lasting at least 2 years. | |
| **Major depressive episode** | Characterized by at least 5 of the following 9 symptoms for 2 weeks (symptoms must include patient-reported depressed mood or anhedonia): | **SIG E CAPS.** |
| | 1. **S**leep disturbance | Commonly used mnemonic for depression screening. Historically used by physicians in prescription writing. **SIG** is short for *signatura* (Latin for "directions"). Depressed patients were **directed** to take **E**nergy **CAPS**ules. |
| | 2. Loss of **I**nterest (anhedonia) | |
| | 3. **G**uilt or feelings of worthlessness | |
| | 4. Loss of **E**nergy | |
| | 5. Loss of **C**oncentration | |
| | 6. **A**ppetite/weight changes | |
| | 7. **P**sychomotor retardation or agitation | |
| | 8. **S**uicidal ideations | |
| | 9. Depressed mood | Lifetime prevalence of major depressive episode—5–12% male, 10–25% female. |
| | Major depressive disorder, recurrent—requires 2 or more major depressive episodes with a symptom-free interval of 2 months. | |
| | Dysthymia—milder form of depression lasting at least 2 years. | |
| | Seasonal affective disorder—associated with winter season; improves in response to full-spectrum light exposure. | |

| | |
|---|---|
| **Sleep patterns of depressed patients** | Patients with depression typically have the following changes in their sleep stages:<br>1. ↓ slow-wave sleep<br>2. ↓ REM latency<br>3. ↑ REM early in sleep cycle<br>4. ↑ total REM sleep<br>5. Repeated nighttime awakenings<br>6. Early-morning awakening (important screening question) |
| **Atypical depression** | Differs from classical forms of depression. Characterized by hypersomnia, overeating, and mood reactivity (the ability to experience improved mood in response to positive events vs. persistent sadness). Associated with weight gain and sensitivity to rejection. Most common subtype of depression. Treatment: MAO inhibitors, SSRIs. |
| **Electroconvulsive therapy (ECT)** | Treatment option for major depressive disorder refractory to other treatment. Produces a painless seizure in an anesthetized patient. Major adverse effects are disorientation and anterograde/retrograde amnesia (can be minimized when ECT is performed unilaterally). |
| **Risk factors for suicide completion** | **S**ex (male), **A**ge (teenager or elderly), **D**epression, **P**revious attempt, **E**thanol or drug use, loss of **R**ational thinking, **S**ickness (medical illness, 3 or more prescription medications), **O**rganized plan, **N**o spouse (divorced, widowed, or single, especially if childless), **S**ocial support lacking. Women try more often; men succeed more often. | **SAD PERSONS.** |
| **Panic disorder** | Defined by the presence of recurrent periods of intense fear and discomfort peaking in 10 minutes with at least 4 of the following: **P**alpitations, **P**aresthesias, **A**bdominal distress, **N**ausea, **I**ntense fear of dying or losing control, l**I**ght-headedness, **C**hest pain, **C**hills, **C**hoking, dis**C**onnectedness, **S**weating, **S**haking, **S**hortness of breath. Treatment: cognitive behavioral therapy (CBT), SSRIs, TCAs, benzodiazepines. | **PANICS.** Described in context of occurrence (e.g., panic disorder with agoraphobia). Associated with persistent fear of having another attack. |
| **Specific phobia** | Fear that is excessive or unreasonable and interferes with normal function. **Cued** by presence or anticipation of a specific object or situation. Person recognizes fear is excessive. Can treat with systematic desensitization.<br>**Social phobia** (social anxiety disorder)—exaggerated fear of embarrassment in social situations (e.g., public speaking, using public restrooms). Treatment: SSRIs. |
| **Obsessive-compulsive disorder (OCD)** | Recurring, intrusive thoughts, feelings, or sensations (obsessions) that cause severe distress; relieved in part by the performance of repetitive actions (compulsions). Ego dystonic: behavior inconsistent with one's own beliefs and attitudes (vs. obsessive-compulsive personality disorder). Associated with Tourette's disorder. Treatment: SSRIs, clomipramine. |

| | |
|---|---|
| **Post-traumatic stress disorder** | Persistent reexperiencing of a previous traumatic event. May involve nightmares or flashbacks, intense fear, helplessness, or horror. Leads to avoidance of stimuli associated with the trauma and persistently ↑ arousal. **Disturbance lasts > 1 month,** with onset > 1 month after event, and causes significant distress and/or impaired functioning. Treatment: psychotherapy, SSRIs.<br>Acute stress disorder—lasts between 2 days and 1 month. |
| **Generalized anxiety disorder** | Pattern of uncontrollable anxiety for at least 6 months that is unrelated to a specific person, situation, or event. Associated with sleep disturbance, fatigue, and difficulty concentrating. Treatment: benzodiazepines, buspirone, SSRIs.<br>Adjustment disorder—emotional symptoms (anxiety, depression) causing impairment following an identifiable psychosocial stressor (e.g., divorce, illness) and lasting < 6 months (> 6 months in presence of chronic stressor). |
| **Malingering** | Patient consciously fakes or claims to have a disorder in order to attain a specific 2° gain (e.g., avoiding work, obtaining drugs). Avoids treatment by medical personnel; complaints cease after gain (vs. factitious disorder). |
| **Factitious disorder** | Patient consciously creates physical and/or psychological symptoms in order to assume "sick role" and to get medical attention (1° gain).<br>Munchausen's syndrome—**chronic** factitious disorder with predominantly physical signs and symptoms. Characterized by a history of multiple hospital admissions and willingness to receive invasive procedures.<br>Munchausen's syndrome by proxy—when illness in a child is caused by the caregiver. Motivation is to assume a sick role by proxy. Form of child abuse. |
| **Somatoform disorders** | Category of disorders characterized by physical symptoms with no identifiable physical cause. Both illness production and motivation are unconscious drives. Symptoms not intentionally produced or feigned. More common in women. Several types:<br>1. Somatization disorder—variety of complaints in multiple organ systems (at least 4 pain, 2 GI, 1 sexual, 1 pseudoneurologic) over a period of years<br>2. Conversion—motor or sensory symptoms (e.g., paralysis, blindness, mutism), often following an acute stressor; patient is aware of but indifferent toward symptoms ("la belle indifférence")<br>3. Hypochondriasis—preoccupation with and fear of having a serious illness despite medical evaluation and reassurance<br>4. Body dysmorphic disorder—preoccupation with minor or imagined defect in appearance, leading to significant emotional distress or impaired functioning; patients often repeatedly seek cosmetic surgery<br>5. Pain disorder—prolonged pain with no physical findings |
| **Personality** | Personality trait—an enduring, repetitive pattern of perceiving, relating to, and thinking about the environment and oneself that is exhibited in a wide range of important social and personal contexts.<br>Personality disorder—inflexible, maladaptive, and rigidly pervasive pattern of behavior causing subjective distress and/or impaired functioning; person is usually not aware of problem. Stable by early adulthood; not usually diagnosed in children. |

| | | |
|---|---|---|
| **Cluster A personality disorders** | Odd or eccentric; inability to develop meaningful social relationships. No psychosis; genetic association with schizophrenia. Types: | "**Weird**" (Accusatory, Aloof, Awkward). |
| | 1. Paranoid—pervasive distrust and suspiciousness; projection is major defense mechanism | |
| | 2. Schizoid—voluntary social withdrawal, limited emotional expression, content with social isolation (vs. avoidant) | SchizoiD = Distant. |
| | 3. Schizotypal—eccentric appearance, odd beliefs or magical thinking, interpersonal awkwardness | SchizoTypal = magical Thinking. |
| **Cluster B personality disorders** | Dramatic, emotional, or erratic; genetic association with mood disorders and substance abuse. Types: | "**Wild**" (Bad to the Bone). |
| | 1. Antisocial—disregard for and violation of rights of others, criminality; males > females; conduct disorder if < 18 years | AntiSOCial = SOCiopath. |
| | 2. Borderline—unstable mood and interpersonal relationships, impulsiveness, self-mutilation, sense of emptiness; females > males; splitting is a major defense mechanism | |
| | 3. Histrionic—excessive emotionality and excitability, attention seeking, sexually provocative, overly concerned with appearance | |
| | 4. Narcissistic—grandiosity, sense of entitlement; lacks empathy and requires excessive admiration; often demands the "best" and reacts to criticism with rage | |
| **Cluster C personality disorders** | Anxious or fearful; genetic association with anxiety disorders. Types: | "**Worried**" (Cowardly, Compulsive, Clingy). |
| | 1. Avoidant—hypersensitive to rejection, socially inhibited, timid, feelings of inadequacy, desires relationships with others (vs. schizoid) | |
| | 2. Obsessive-compulsive—preoccupation with order, perfectionism, and control; ego syntonic: behavior consistent with one's own beliefs and attitudes (vs. OCD) | |
| | 3. Dependent—submissive and clinging, excessive need to be taken care of, low self-confidence | |

| Keeping "schizo-" straight | Schizoid | < | Schizotypal (schizoid + odd thinking) | < | Schizophrenic (greater odd thinking than schizotypal) | < | Schizoaffective (schizophrenic psychotic symptoms + bipolar or depressive mood disorder) |
|---|---|---|---|---|---|---|---|

Schizophrenia time course:
    < 1 mo—brief psychotic disorder, usually stress related.
    1–6 mo—schizophreniform disorder.
    > 6 mo—schizophrenia.

**Eating disorders**

**Anorexia nervosa**—excessive dieting +/– purging; intense fear of gaining weight, body image distortion, and ↑ exercise, leading to body weight < 85% below ideal body weight. Associated with ↓ bone density. Severe weight loss, metatarsal stress fractures, amenorrhea, anemia, and electrolyte disturbances. Seen primarily in adolescent girls. Commonly coexists with depression.

**Bulimia nervosa**—binge eating +/– purging; followed by self-induced vomiting or use of laxatives, diuretics, or emetics. Body weight often maintained within normal range. Associated with parotitis, enamel erosion, electrolyte disturbances, alkalosis, dorsal hand calluses from inducing vomiting (Russell's sign).

**Gender identity disorder**

Strong, persistent cross-gender identification. Characterized by persistent discomfort with one's sex, causing significant distress and/or impaired functioning.

**Substance dependence**

Maladaptive pattern of substance use defined as 3 or more of the following signs in 1 year:
1. Tolerance—need more to achieve same effect
2. Withdrawal
3. Substance taken in larger amounts or over longer time than desired
4. Persistent desire or unsuccessful attempts to cut down
5. Significant energy spent obtaining, using, or recovering from substance
6. Important social, occupational, or recreational activities reduced because of substance use
7. Continued use in spite of knowing the problems that it causes

**Substance abuse**

Maladaptive pattern leading to clinically significant impairment or distress. Symptoms have NEVER met criteria for substance dependence.
1. Recurrent use resulting in failure to fulfill major obligations at work, school, or home
2. Recurrent use in physically hazardous situations
3. Recurrent substance-related legal problems
4. Continued use in spite of persistent problems caused by use

**Substance withdrawal**

Behavioral, physiologic, and cognitive state caused by cessation or reduction of heavy and prolonged substance use. Signs and symptoms often opposite to those seen in intoxication.

## Signs and symptoms of substance abuse

| Drug | Intoxication | Withdrawal |
|---|---|---|
| **Depressants** | | |
| Alcohol | Disinhibition, emotional lability, slurred speech, ataxia, coma, blackouts. Serum γ-glutamyltransferase (**GGT**)—sensitive indicator of alcohol use. Treatment: naltrexone, disulfiram. | Tremor, tachycardia, hypertension, malaise, nausea, seizures, delirium tremens (DTs), tremulousness, agitation, hallucinations (including tactile). Treatment for DTs: benzodiazepines. |
| Opioids (e.g., morphine, heroin, methadone) | CNS depression, nausea and vomiting, constipation, pupillary constriction (**pinpoint pupils**), seizures (overdose is life-threatening). Treatment: naloxone, naltrexone. | Anxiety, insomnia, anorexia, sweating, dilated pupils, piloerection ("cold turkey"), fever, rhinorrhea, nausea, stomach cramps, diarrhea ("flulike" symptoms), yawning. Treatment: symptomatic, naloxone + buprenorphine (Suboxone), methadone. |
| Barbiturates | Low safety margin, **respiratory depression.** Treatment: symptom management (assist respiration, ↑ BP). | Anxiety, seizures, delirium, life-threatening cardiovascular collapse. |
| Benzodiazepines | Greater safety margin. Amnesia, ataxia, somnolence, minor respiratory depression. Additive effects with alcohol. Treatment: flumazenil (competitive GABA antagonist). | Rebound anxiety, seizures, tremor, insomnia. |
| **Stimulants** | | |
| Amphetamines | Psychomotor agitation, impaired judgment, pupillary dilation, hypertension, tachycardia, euphoria, prolonged wakefulness and attention, cardiac arrhythmias, delusions, hallucinations, fever. | Post-use "crash," including depression, lethargy, headache, stomach cramps, hunger, hypersomnolence. |
| Cocaine | Euphoria, psychomotor agitation, impaired judgment, tachycardia, pupillary dilation, hypertension, hallucinations (including tactile), paranoid ideations, angina, sudden cardiac death. Treatment: benzodiazepines. | Post-use "crash," including severe depression and suicidality, hypersomnolence, fatigue, malaise, severe psychological craving. |
| Caffeine | Restlessness, insomnia, ↑ diuresis, muscle twitching, cardiac arrhythmias. | Headache, lethargy, depression, weight gain. |
| Nicotine | Restlessness, insomnia, anxiety, arrhythmias. | Irritability, headache, anxiety, weight gain, craving. Treatment: bupropion/varenicline. |
| **Hallucinogens** | | |
| PCP | **Belligerence,** impulsiveness, fever, psychomotor agitation, vertical and horizontal nystagmus, tachycardia, ataxia, homicidality, psychosis, delirium. | Depression, anxiety, irritability, restlessness, anergia, disturbances of thought and sleep. |
| LSD | Marked anxiety or depression, delusions, visual hallucinations, **flashbacks,** pupillary dilation. | |
| Marijuana | Euphoria, anxiety, paranoid delusions, perception of slowed time, impaired judgment, social withdrawal, ↑ appetite, dry mouth, hallucinations. | Irritability, depression, insomnia, nausea, anorexia. Most symptoms peak in 48 hours and last for 5–7 days. Can be detected in urine up to 1 month after last use. |

| | |
|---|---|
| **Heroin addiction** | Users at ↑ risk for hepatitis, abscesses, overdose, hemorrhoids, AIDS, and right-sided endocarditis. Look for track marks (needle sticks in veins). Symptoms of opioid intoxication (pinpoint pupils, respiratory depression, coma).<br><br>Treatment: naloxone and naltrexone—competitively inhibit opioids; used in cases of overdose.<br><br>Methadone—long-acting oral opiate; used for heroin detoxification or long-term maintenance.<br><br>Suboxone—naloxone + buprenorphine (partial agonist); long acting with fewer withdrawal symptoms than methadone. Naloxone is not active when taken orally, so withdrawal symptoms occur only if injected (lower abuse potential). |
| **Alcoholism** | Physiologic tolerance and dependence with symptoms of withdrawal (tremor, tachycardia, hypertension, malaise, nausea, DTs) when intake is interrupted.<br><br>Complications: alcoholic cirrhosis, hepatitis, pancreatitis, peripheral neuropathy, testicular atrophy.<br><br>Wernicke-Korsakoff syndrome—caused by thiamine deficiency. Triad of confusion, ophthalmoplegia, and ataxia (Wernicke's encephalopathy). May progress to irreversible memory loss, confabulation, personality change (Korsakoff's psychosis). Associated with periventricular hemorrhage/necrosis of mammillary bodies. Treatment: IV vitamin $B_1$ (thiamine).<br><br>Mallory-Weiss syndrome—longitudinal lacerations at the gastroesophageal junction caused by excessive vomiting. Often presents with hematemesis. Associated with pain (vs. esophageal varices).<br><br>Treatment: disulfiram (to condition the patient to abstain from alcohol use), supportive care. Alcoholics Anonymous and other peer support groups are helpful in sustaining abstinence. |
| **Delirium tremens (DTs)** | Life-threatening alcohol withdrawal syndrome that peaks 2–5 days after last drink.<br><br>Symptoms in order of appearance: autonomic system hyperactivity (tachycardia, tremors, anxiety, seizures), psychotic symptoms (hallucinations, delusions), confusion.<br><br>Treatment: benzodiazepines. |

## Treatment for selected psychiatric conditions

| Psychiatric condition | Drug |
|---|---|
| Alcohol withdrawal | Benzodiazepines |
| Anorexia/bulimia | SSRIs |
| Anxiety | Benzodiazepines |
| | Buspirone |
| | SSRIs |
| ADHD | Methylphenidate (Ritalin) |
| | Amphetamines (Dexedrine) |
| Atypical depression | MAO inhibitors |
| | SSRIs |
| Bipolar disorder | "Mood stabilizers": |
| |    Lithium |
| |     Valproic acid |
| |     Carbamazepine |
| | Atypical antipsychotics |
| Depression | SSRIs, SNRIs |
| | TCAs |
| Depression with insomnia | Mirtazapine |
| Obsessive-compulsive disorder | SSRIs |
| | Clomipramine |
| Panic disorder | SSRIs |
| | TCAs |
| | Benzodiazepines |
| PTSD | SSRIs |
| Schizophrenia | Antipsychotics |
| Tourette's syndrome | Antipsychotics (haloperidol) |
| Social phobias | SSRIs |

## Methylphenidate (Ritalin)

| | |
|---|---|
| Mechanism | ↑ presynaptic NE vesicular release (like amphetamines). However, the mechanism for relieving ADHD symptoms is not known. |
| Clinical use | ADHD. |

| **Antipsychotics (neuroleptics)** | Haloperidol, trifluoperazine, fluphenazine, thioridazine, chlorpromazine (haloperidol + "-azine"s). | |
|---|---|---|
| Mechanism | All typical antipsychotics block dopamine $D_2$ receptors ($\uparrow [cAMP]_1$). | High potency: haloperidol, trifluoperazine, fluphenazine—neurologic side effects. |
| Clinical use | Schizophrenia (primarily positive symptoms), psychosis, acute mania, Tourette's syndrome. | Low potency: thioridazine, chlorpromazine—non-neurologic side effects. |
| Toxicity | 1. Highly lipid soluble and stored in body fat; thus, very slow to be removed from body | Chlorpromazine—Corneal deposits; Thioridazine—reTinal deposits. |
| | 2. Extrapyramidal system (EPS) side effects | Evolution of EPS side effects: |
| | 3. Endocrine side effects (e.g., dopamine receptor antagonism → hyperprolactinemia → galactorrhea) | 4 h acute dystonia (muscle spasm, stiffness, oculogyric crisis) |
| | 4. Side effects arising from blocking muscarinic (dry mouth, constipation), α (hypotension), and histamine (sedation) receptors | 4 d akinesia (parkinsonian symptoms) |
| | **Other toxicities: Neuroleptic malignant syndrome (NMS)**—rigidity, myoglobinuria, autonomic instability, hyperpyrexia. Treatment: dantrolene, agonists (e.g., bromocriptine). | 4 wk akathisia (restlessness) |
| | | 4 mo tardive dyskinesia |
| | **Tardive dyskinesia**—stereotypic oral-facial movements due to long-term antipsychotic use. Often irreversible. | For NMS, think **FEVER**: **F**ever **E**ncephalopathy **V**itals unstable **E**levated enzymes **R**igidity of muscles |

| **Atypical antipsychotics** | Olanzapine, **clozapine, quetiapine, risperidone, aripiprazole, ziprasidone.** | It's **atypical** for **old clos**ets to **quietly risper** from **A to Z.** |
|---|---|---|
| Mechanism | Block $5\text{-}HT_2$, α, H1, and dopamine receptors. | |
| Clinical use | Schizophrenia (useful for both positive and negative symptoms). **Olanzapine** is also used for OCD, anxiety disorder, depression, mania, Tourette's syndrome. | |
| Toxicity | Fewer extrapyramidal and anticholinergic side effects than traditional antipsychotics. Olanzapine/clozapine may cause significant weight gain. **Clozapine** may cause agranulocytosis (requires weekly WBC monitoring). | |

| **Lithium** | | |
|---|---|---|
| Mechanism | Not established; possibly related to inhibition of phosphoinositol cascade. | **LMNOP:** |
| Clinical use | Mood stabilizer for bipolar disorder; blocks relapse and acute manic events. Also SIADH. | Lithium side effects— **M**ovement (tremor) **N**ephrogenic diabetes insipidus |
| Toxicity | Tremor, sedation, edema, heart block, hypothyroidism, polyuria (ADH antagonist causing nephrogenic diabetes insipidus), teratogenesis. Narrow therapeutic window requires close monitoring of serum levels. | Hyp**O**thyroidism **P**regnancy problems |

### Buspirone

| | |
|---|---|
| Mechanism | Stimulates 5-HT$_{1A}$ receptors |
| Clinical use | Generalized anxiety disorder. Does not cause sedation, addiction, or tolerance. Does not interact with alcohol (vs. barbiturates, benzodiazepines). |

### Antidepressants

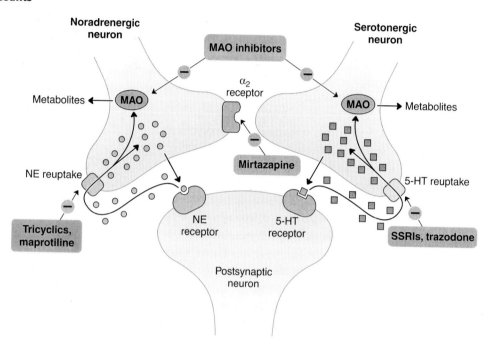

(Adapted, with permission, from Katzung BG, Trevor AJ. *USMLE Road Map: Pharmacology,* 1st ed. New York: McGraw-Hill, 2003: 80.)

| | | |
|---|---|---|
| **Tricyclic antidepressants** | Imipramine, amitriptyline, desipramine, nortriptyline, clomipramine, doxepin, amoxapine. | |
| Mechanism | Block reuptake of NE and serotonin. | |
| Clinical use | Major depression, bedwetting (imipramine), OCD (clomipramine), fibromyalgia. | |
| Side effects | Sedation, α-blocking effects, atropine-like (anticholinergic) side effects (tachycardia, urinary retention). 3° TCAs (amitriptyline) have more anticholinergic effects than do 2° TCAs (nortriptyline). Desipramine is the least sedating and has lower seizure threshold. | |
| Toxicity | **Tri-C's:** Convulsions, Coma, Cardiotoxicity (arrhythmias); also respiratory depression, hyperpyrexia. Confusion and hallucinations in elderly due to anticholinergic side effects (use nortriptyline). Treatment: NaHCO$_3$ for CV toxicity. | |
| **SSRIs** | Fluoxetine, paroxetine, sertraline, citalopram. | |
| Mechanism | Serotonin-specific reuptake inhibitors. | It normally takes 2–3 weeks for antidepressants to have an effect. |
| Clinical use | Depression, OCD, bulimia, social phobias. | |
| Toxicity | Fewer than TCAs. GI distress, sexual dysfunction (anorgasmia). **"Serotonin syndrome"** with any drug that ↑ serotonin (e.g., MAO inhibitors) —hyperthermia, muscle rigidity, cardiovascular collapse, flushing, diarrhea, seizures. Treatment: cyproheptadine (5-HT$_2$ receptor antagonist). | |

| **SNRIs** | Venlafaxine, duloxetine. |
|---|---|
| Mechanism | Inhibit serotonin and NE reuptake. |
| Clinical use | Depression. Venlafaxine is also used in generalized anxiety disorder; duloxetine is also indicated for diabetic peripheral neuropathy. Duloxetine has greater effect on NE. |
| Toxicity | ↑ BP most common; also stimulant effects, sedation, nausea. |

| **Monoamine oxidase (MAO) inhibitors** | Phenelzine, tranylcypromine, isocarboxazid, selegiline (selective MAO-B inhibitor). |
|---|---|
| Mechanism | Nonselective MAO inhibition → ↑ levels of amine neurotransmitters. |
| Clinical use | Atypical depression, anxiety, hypochondriasis. |
| Toxicity | Hypertensive crisis with tyramine ingestion (in many foods, such as wine and cheese) and β-agonists; CNS stimulation. Contraindicated with SSRIs or meperidine (to prevent serotonin syndrome). |

| **Atypical antidepressants** | | |
|---|---|---|
| Bupropion (Wellbutrin) | Also used for smoking cessation. ↑ NE and dopamine via unknown mechanism. Toxicity: stimulant effects (tachycardia, insomnia), headache, seizure in bulimic patients. No sexual side effects. | |
| Mirtazapine | $\alpha_2$ antagonist (↑ release of NE and serotonin) and potent 5-HT$_2$ and 5-HT$_3$ receptor antagonist. Toxicity: sedation, ↑ appetite, weight gain, dry mouth. | |
| Maprotiline | Blocks NE reuptake. Toxicity: sedation, orthostatic hypotension. | |
| Trazodone | Primarily inhibits serotonin reuptake. Used for insomnia, as high doses are needed for antidepressant effects. Toxicity: sedation, nausea, priapism, postural hypotension. | Called Trazo**BONE** due to male-specific side effects. |

# Renal

*"But I know all about love already. I know precious little about kidneys."*
—Aldous Huxley, *Antic Hay*

*"This too shall pass. Just like a kidney stone."*

—Hunter Madsen

### Kidney anatomy and glomerular structure

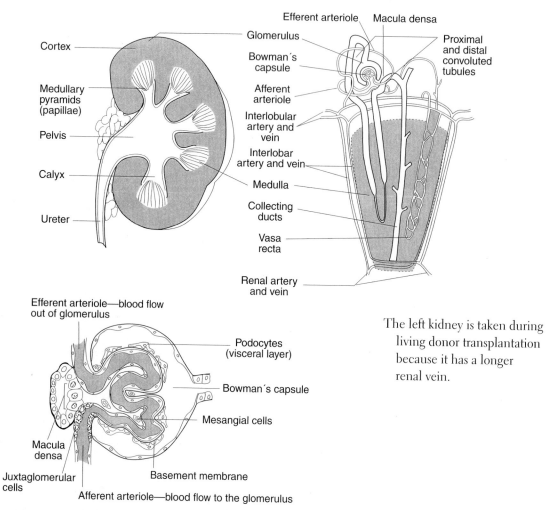

The left kidney is taken during living donor transplantation because it has a longer renal vein.

(Adapted, with permission, from McPhee S et al. *Pathophysiology of Disease: An Introduction to Clinical Medicine*, 3rd ed. New York: McGraw-Hill, 2000: 284.)

| Ureters: course | Ureters pass **under** uterine artery and **under** ductus deferens (retroperitoneal). | Water (ureters) **under** the bridge (artery, ductus deferens). |
| --- | --- | --- |

## Fluid compartments

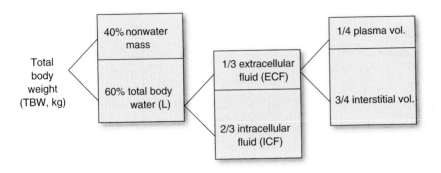

ECF: ↑ NaCl, ↓ $K^+$.
ICF: ↑ $K^+$, ↓ NaCl
   (**HIKIN'**: **HI**gh **K**
   **IN**tracellular).
TBW – ECF = ICF.
ECF – PV = interstitial volume.
60–40–20 rule (% of body weight):
   60% total body water
   40% ICF
   20% ECF
Plasma volume measured by
   radiolabeled albumin.
Extracellular volume measured
   by inulin.
Osmolarity = 290 mOsm.

| | | |
|---|---|---|
| **Glomerular filtration barrier** | Responsible for filtration of plasma according to size and net charge. Composed of: 1. Fenestrated capillary endothelium (size barrier) 2. Fused basement membrane with heparan sulfate (negative charge barrier) 3. Epithelial layer consisting of podocyte foot processes | The charge barrier is lost in **nephrotic syndrome,** resulting in albuminuria, hypoproteinemia, generalized edema, and hyperlipidemia. |
| **Renal clearance** | $C_x = U_x V/P_x$ = volume of plasma from which the substance is completely cleared per unit time. $C_x <$ GFR: net tubular reabsorption of X. $C_x >$ GFR: net tubular secretion of X. $C_x =$ GFR: no net secretion or reabsorption. | Be familiar with calculations. $C_x$ = clearance of X. Units are mL/min. $U_x$ = urine concentration of X. $P_x$ = plasma concentration of X. V = urine flow rate. |
| **Glomerular filtration rate (GFR)** | Inulin can be used to calculate GFR because it is freely filtered and is neither reabsorbed nor secreted. $GFR = U_{inulin} \times V/P_{inulin} = C_{inulin}$ $= K_f [(P_{GC} - P_{BS}) - (\pi_{GC} - \pi_{BS})].$ (GC = glomerular capillary; BS = Bowman's space.) $\pi_{BS}$ normally equals zero. | Normal GFR ≈ 100 mL/min. Creatinine clearance is an approximate measure of GFR. Slightly overestimates GFR because creatinine is moderately secreted by the renal tubules. |
| **Effective renal plasma flow (ERPF)** | ERPF can be estimated using PAH clearance because it is both filtered and actively secreted in the proximal tubule. All PAH entering the kidney is excreted. $ERPF = U_{PAH} \times V/P_{PAH} = C_{PAH}.$ RBF = RPF/(1 – Hct). ERPF underestimates true RPF by ~10%. | |

**Filtration**

Filtration fraction (FF) = GFR/RPF.
Normal FF = 20%.
Filtered load = GFR × plasma concentration.

GFR can be estimated with creatinine.
RPF is best estimated with PAH.

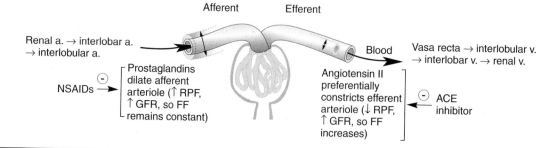

Renal a. → interlobar a. → interlobular a.

NSAIDs → $\ominus$ → Prostaglandins dilate afferent arteriole (↑ RPF, ↑ GFR, so FF remains constant)

Afferent     Efferent

Blood

Angiotensin II preferentially constricts efferent arteriole (↓ RPF, ↑ GFR, so FF increases)

$\ominus$ ACE inhibitor

Vasa recta → interlobular v. → interlobar v. → renal v.

**Changes in glomerular dynamics**

| Effect | RPF | GFR | FF (GFR/RPF) |
|---|---|---|---|
| Afferent arteriole constriction | ↓ | ↓ | NC |
| Efferent arteriole constriction | ↓ | ↑ | ↑ |
| ↑ plasma protein concentration | NC | ↓ | ↓ |
| ↓ plasma protein concentration | NC | ↑ | ↑ |
| Constriction of ureter | NC | ↓ | ↓ |

**Free water clearance**

Ability to dilute urine. Given urine flow rate, urine osmolarity, and plasma osmolarity, be able to calculate free water clearance:
Free water $(C_{H_2O})$ = total urine (V) – water occupied with solute $(C_{osm})$.
$C_{H_2O} = V - C_{osm}$.
V = urine flow rate; $C_{osm} = U_{osm}V/P_{osm}$.
With ADH: $C_{H_2O} < 0$ (retention of free water).
Without ADH: $C_{H_2O} > 0$ (excretion of free water).
Isotonic urine: $C_{H_2O} = 0$ (seen with loop diuretics).

**Calculation of reabsorption and secretion rate**

Filtered load = GFR × $P_x$.
Excretion rate = V × $U_x$.
Reabsorption = filtered – excreted.
Secretion = excreted – filtered.

**Glucose clearance**

Glucose at a normal plasma level is completely reabsorbed in proximal tubule by $Na^+$/glucose cotransport.
At plasma glucose of 160–200 mg/dL, glucosuria begins (threshold). At 350 mg/dL, all transporters are fully saturated $(T_m)$.

Glucosuria is an important clinical clue to diabetes mellitus.

**Amino acid clearance**

Sodium-dependent transporters in proximal tubule reabsorb amino acids by at least 3 distinct carrier systems, with competitive inhibition within each group.
Deficiency of neutral amino acid (tryptophan) transporter is called Hartnup's disease; results in pellagra.

## Nephron physiology

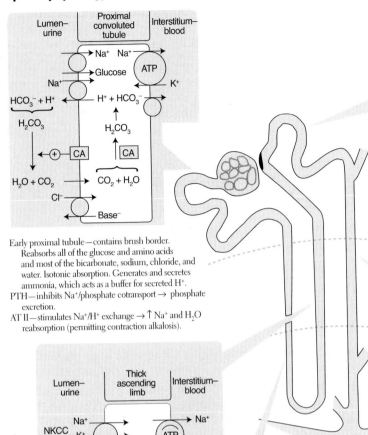

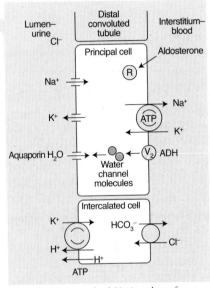

Early proximal tubule—contains brush border. Reabsorbs all of the glucose and amino acids and most of the bicarbonate, sodium, chloride, and water. Isotonic absorption. Generates and secretes ammonia, which acts as a buffer for secreted $H^+$.
PTH—inhibits $Na^+$/phosphate cotransport → phosphate excretion.
AT II—stimulates $Na^+$/$H^+$ exchange → ↑ $Na^+$ and $H_2O$ reabsorption (permitting contraction alkalosis).

Early distal convoluted tubule—actively reabsorbs $Na^+$, $Cl^-$. Diluting segment. Makes urine hypotonic.
PTH—↑ $Ca^{2+}$/$Na^+$ exchange → $Ca^{2+}$ reabsorption.

Thin descending loop of Henle—passively reabsorbs water via medullary hypertonicity (impermeable to sodium). Concentrating segment. Makes urine hypertonic.

Thick ascending loop of Henle—actively reabsorbs $Na^+$, $K^+$, and $Cl^-$ and indirectly induces the paracellular reabsorption of $Mg^{2+}$ and $Ca^{2+}$. Impermeable to $H_2O$. Makes urine less concentrated as it ascends.

Collecting tubules—reabsorb $Na^+$ in exchange for secreting $K^+$ and $H^+$ (regulated by aldosterone).
Aldosterone—leads to insertion of $Na^+$ channel on luminal side.
ADH—acts at $V_2$ receptors → insertion of aquaporin $H_2O$ channels on luminal side.

## Relative concentrations along proximal tubule

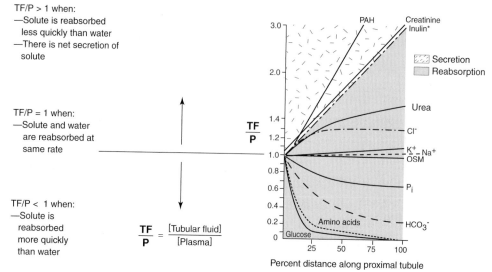

TF/P > 1 when:
—Solute is reabsorbed less quickly than water
—There is net secretion of solute

TF/P = 1 when:
—Solute and water are reabsorbed at same rate

$$\frac{TF}{P} = \frac{[\text{Tubular fluid}]}{[\text{Plasma}]}$$

TF/P < 1 when:
—Solute is reabsorbed more quickly than water

PAH
Creatinine
Inulin*

Secretion
Reabsorption

Urea
Cl⁻
K⁺ Na⁺
OSM
P$_i$
Amino acids
HCO$_3$⁻
Glucose

Percent distance along proximal tubule

\* Neither secreted nor reabsorbed; concentration increases as water is reabsorbed.

(Adapted, with permission, from Ganong WF. *Review of Medical Physiology*, 22nd ed. New York: McGraw-Hill, 2005.)

Tubular creatinine and inulin ↑ in concentration (but not amount) along the proximal tubule due to water reabsorption.

Cl⁻ reabsorption occurs at a slower rate than Na⁺ in the proximal ⅓ of the proximal tubule and then matches the rate of Na⁺ reabsorption more distally. Thus, its relative concentration ↑ before it plateaus.

Na⁺ reabsorption drives H₂O reabsorption, so it nearly matches osm.

## Renin-angiotensin-aldosterone system

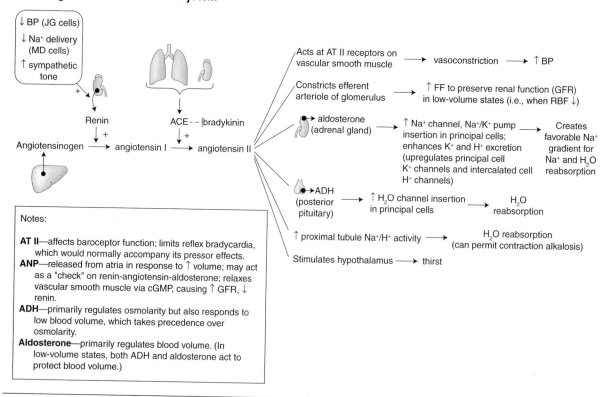

↓ BP (JG cells)
↓ Na⁺ delivery (MD cells)
↑ sympathetic tone

Renin
Angiotensinogen → angiotensin I → angiotensin II
ACE– –|bradykinin

Acts at AT II receptors on vascular smooth muscle → vasoconstriction → ↑ BP

Constricts efferent arteriole of glomerulus → ↑ FF to preserve renal function (GFR) in low-volume states (i.e., when RBF ↓)

aldosterone (adrenal gland) → ↑ Na⁺ channel, Na⁺/K⁺ pump insertion in principal cells; enhances K⁺ and H⁺ excretion (upregulates principal cell K⁺ channels and intercalated cell H⁺ channels) → Creates favorable Na⁺ gradient for Na⁺ and H₂O reabsorption

ADH (posterior pituitary) → ↑ H₂O channel insertion in principal cells → H₂O reabsorption

↑ proximal tubule Na⁺/H⁺ activity → H₂O reabsorption (can permit contraction alkalosis)

Stimulates hypothalamus → thirst

Notes:

**AT II**—affects baroceptor function; limits reflex bradycardia, which would normally accompany its pressor effects.
**ANP**—released from atria in response to ↑ volume; may act as a "check" on renin-angiotensin-aldosterone; relaxes vascular smooth muscle via cGMP, causing ↑ GFR, ↓ renin.
**ADH**—primarily regulates osmolarity but also responds to low blood volume, which takes precedence over osmolarity.
**Aldosterone**—primarily regulates blood volume. (In low-volume states, both ADH and aldosterone act to protect blood volume.)

| | | |
|---|---|---|
| **Juxtaglomerular apparatus (JGA)** | JGA—JG cells (modified smooth muscle of afferent arteriole) and macula densa ($Na^+$ sensor, part of the distal convoluted tubule). JG cells secrete renin (leading to ↑ angiotensin II and aldosterone levels) in response to ↓ renal blood pressure, ↓ $Na^+$ delivery to distal tubule, and ↑ sympathetic tone ($\beta_1$). | JGA defends glomerular filtration rate via renin-angiotensin-aldosterone system. *Juxta* = close by. |
| **Kidney endocrine functions** | 1. **Erythropoietin**—released in response to hypoxia from endothelial cells of peritubular capillaries. <br> 2. **1,25-(OH)$_2$ vitamin D**—proximal tubule cells convert 25-OH vitamin D to 1,25-(OH)$_2$ vitamin D, which ↑ intestinal reabsorption of both calcium and phosphate. Parathyroid hormone (PTH) acts directly on the kidney and ↑ renal calcium reabsorption and ↓ renal phosphate reabsorption. However, PTH also acts indirectly, stimulating proximal tubule cells to make 1,25-(OH)$_2$ vitamin D, which ↑ intestinal absorption of both **calcium** and **phosphate**. <br> 3. **Renin**—secreted by JG cells in response to ↓ renal arterial pressure and ↑ renal sympathetic discharge ($\beta_1$ effect). <br> 4. **Prostaglandins**—paracrine secretion vasodilates the afferent arterioles to ↑ GFR. | NSAIDs can cause acute renal failure by inhibiting the renal production of prostaglandins, which keep the afferent arterioles vasodilated to maintain GFR. |

25-OH vitamin D ——————→ 1,25-(OH)$_2$ vitamin D
1α-hydroxylase

⊕

PTH

## Hormones acting on kidney

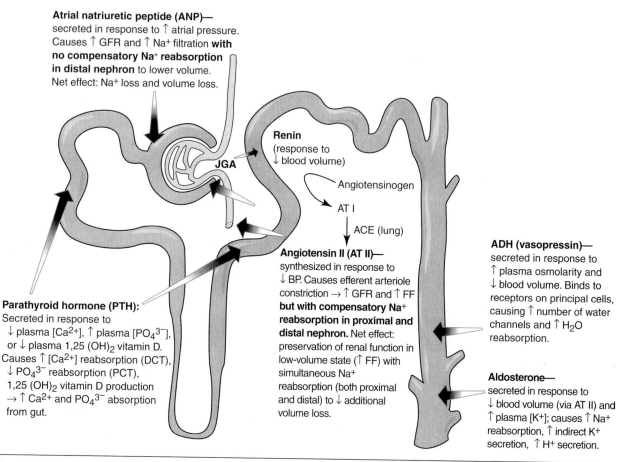

**Atrial natriuretic peptide (ANP)—** secreted in response to ↑ atrial pressure. Causes ↑ GFR and ↑ $Na^+$ filtration **with no compensatory $Na^+$ reabsorption in distal nephron** to lower volume. Net effect: $Na^+$ loss and volume loss.

**Renin** (response to ↓ blood volume)

Angiotensinogen

AT I

↓ ACE (lung)

**Angiotensin II (AT II)—** synthesized in response to ↓ BP. Causes efferent arteriole constriction → ↑ GFR and ↑ FF **but with compensatory $Na^+$ reabsorption in proximal and distal nephron.** Net effect: preservation of renal function in low-volume state (↑ FF) with simultaneous $Na^+$ reabsorption (both proximal and distal) to ↓ additional volume loss.

JGA

**Parathyroid hormone (PTH):** Secreted in response to ↓ plasma $[Ca^{2+}]$, ↑ plasma $[PO_4^{3-}]$, or ↓ plasma 1,25 $(OH)_2$ vitamin D. Causes ↑ $[Ca^{2+}]$ reabsorption (DCT), ↓ $PO_4^{3-}$ reabsorption (PCT), 1,25 $(OH)_2$ vitamin D production → ↑ $Ca^{2+}$ and $PO_4^{3-}$ absorption from gut.

**ADH (vasopressin)—** secreted in response to ↑ plasma osmolarity and ↓ blood volume. Binds to receptors on principal cells, causing ↑ number of water channels and ↑ $H_2O$ reabsorption.

**Aldosterone—** secreted in response to ↓ blood volume (via AT II) and ↑ plasma $[K^+]$; causes ↑ $Na^+$ reabsorption, ↑ indirect $K^+$ secretion, ↑ $H^+$ secretion.

## Potassium shifts

Shift out of cell (causing hyperkalemia):
1. Insulin deficiency (↓ $Na^+/K^+$ ATPase)
2. β-adrenergic antagonists (↓ $Na^+/K^+$ ATPase)
3. Acidosis, severe exercise ($K^+/H^+$ exchanger)
4. Hyperosmolarity
5. Digitalis (blocks $Na^+/K^+$ ATPase)
6. Cell lysis

Shift into cell (causing hypokalemia):
1. Insulin (↑ $Na^+/K^+$ ATPase)
2. β-adrenergic agonists (↑ $Na^+/K^+$ ATPase)
3. Alkalosis ($K^+/H^+$ exchanger)
4. Hypo-osmolarity

## Acid-base physiology

|                       | pH | $P_{CO_2}$ | $[HCO_3^-]$ |
| --------------------- | -- | ---------- | ----------- |
| Metabolic acidosis    | ↓  | ↓          | ↓           |
| Metabolic alkalosis   | ↑  | ↑          | ↑           |
| Respiratory acidosis  | ↓  | ↑          | ↑           |
| Respiratory alkalosis | ↑  | ↓          | ↓           |

**Compensatory response**
Hyperventilation
Hypoventilation
↑ renal $[HCO_3^-]$ reabsorption
↓ renal $[HCO_3^-]$ reabsorption

Henderson-Hasselbalch equation: $pH = pKa + \log \dfrac{[HCO_3^-]}{0.03\ P_{CO_2}}$

Key: ↑ ↓ = 1° disturbance; ↓ ↑ = compensatory response.

Respiratory compensation in response to metabolic acidosis can be quantified with Winter's formula:

$$P_{CO_2} = 1.5\ (HCO_3^-) + 8 +/- 2$$

$P_{CO_2}$ ↑ 0.7 mmHg for every ↑ 1 mEq/L $HCO_3^-$

## Acidosis/alkalosis

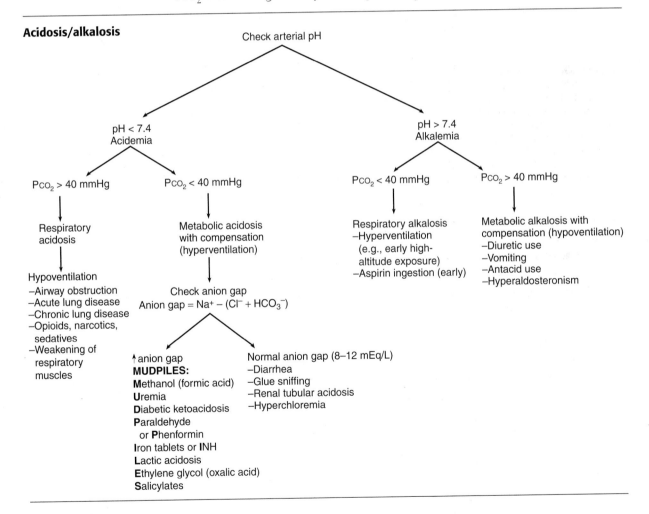

Check arterial pH

**pH < 7.4 Acidemia**

$P_{CO_2}$ > 40 mmHg

Respiratory acidosis

Hypoventilation
–Airway obstruction
–Acute lung disease
–Chronic lung disease
–Opioids, narcotics, sedatives
–Weakening of respiratory muscles

$P_{CO_2}$ < 40 mmHg

Metabolic acidosis with compensation (hyperventilation)

Check anion gap
Anion gap = $Na^+ - (Cl^- + HCO_3^-)$

↑anion gap
**MUDPILES:**
**M**ethanol (formic acid)
**U**remia
**D**iabetic ketoacidosis
**P**araldehyde or **P**henformin
**I**ron tablets or **INH**
**L**actic acidosis
**E**thylene glycol (oxalic acid)
**S**alicylates

Normal anion gap (8–12 mEq/L)
–Diarrhea
–Glue sniffing
–Renal tubular acidosis
–Hyperchloremia

**pH > 7.4 Alkalemia**

$P_{CO_2}$ < 40 mmHg

Respiratory alkalosis
–Hyperventilation (e.g., early high-altitude exposure)
–Aspirin ingestion (early)

$P_{CO_2}$ > 40 mmHg

Metabolic alkalosis with compensation (hypoventilation)
–Diuretic use
–Vomiting
–Antacid use
–Hyperaldosteronism

## Renal tubular acidosis (RTA)

| | |
|---|---|
| Type 1 ("distal") | Defect in collecting tubule's ability to excrete $H^+$. Associated with hypokalemia and risk for calcium-containing kidney stones. |
| Type 2 ("proximal") | Defect in proximal tubule $HCO_3^-$ reabsorption. Associated with hypokalemia and hypophosphatemic rickets. |
| Type 4 ("hyperkalemic") | Hypoaldosteronism or lack of collecting tubule response to aldosterone → hyperkalemia → inhibition of ammonia excretion in proximal tubule. Leads to ↓ urine pH due to ↓ buffering capacity. |

## Acid-base nomogram

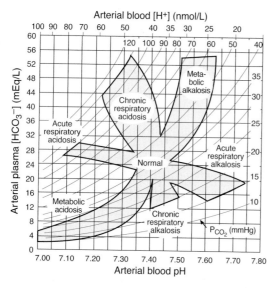

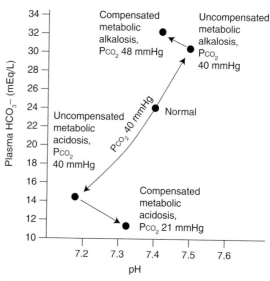

(Reproduced, with permission, from DuBose TD Jr, Cogan MG, Rector FC Jr. Acid-base disorders. In Brenner BM, Rector FC Jr (eds). *The Kidney*, 4th ed. Philadelphia: Saunders, 1991.)

(Reproduced, with permission, from Ganong WF. *Review of Medical Physiology*, 22nd ed. New York: McGraw-Hill, 2005: 735.)

## Casts in urine

RBC casts—glomerulonephritis, ischemia, or malignant hypertension.

WBC casts—tubulointerstitial inflammation, acute pyelonephritis, transplant rejection.

Granular ("muddy brown") casts—acute tubular necrosis.

Waxy casts—advanced renal disease/CRF.

Hyaline casts—nonspecific.

Presence of casts indicates that hematuria/pyuria is of renal origin.

Bladder cancer, kidney stones → RBCs, no casts.

Acute cystitis → WBCs, no casts.

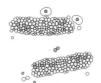   

Red blood cell casts    White blood cell casts    Hyaline casts    Granular casts

## Glomerular disorders

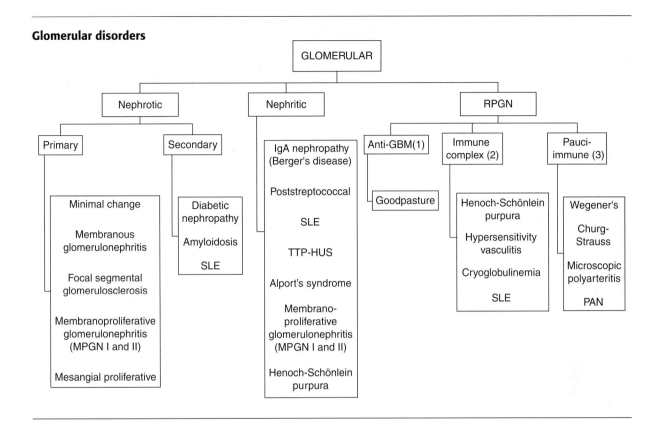

| | | |
|---|---|---|
| **Nephritic syndrome** | NephrItic syndrome = an **I**nflammatory process. When it involves glomeruli, it leads to hematuria and RBC casts in urine. Associated with azotemia, oliguria, hypertension, and proteinuria (< 3.5 g/day). | |
| Acute poststreptococcal glomerulonephritis | LM—glomeruli enlarged and hypercellular, neutrophils, "lumpy-bumpy" appearance. EM—subepithelial immune complex (IC) humps. IF—granular. | Most frequently seen in children. Peripheral and periorbital edema. Resolves spontaneously. |
| Rapidly progressive (crescentic) glomerulonephritis (RPGN) | LM and IF—crescent-moon shape. Crescent consists of fibrin and plasma proteins with glomerular parietal cells, monocytes, and macrophages. Several disease processes may result in this pattern, including:<br>  1. **Goodpasture syndrome**—type II hypersensitivity; antibodies to GBM → linear IF<br>  2. **Wegener's granulomatosis**<br>  3. **Microscopic polyarteritis** | Poor prognosis.<br><br><br><br>Male-dominant disease. Hematuria/hemoptysis (lung involvement).<br>c-ANCA.<br>p-ANCA. |
| Diffuse proliferative glomerulonephritis (due to SLE or MPGN) | Subendothelial DNA-anti-DNA ICs → "wire looping" of capillaries. Granular IF. | Most common cause of death in SLE. SLE and MPGN can present as nephrotic syndrome (see below). |
| Berger's disease (IgA glomerulopathy) | ↑ synthesis of IgA. LM and IF—ICs deposit in mesangium. | Often presents/flares with a URI or acute gastroenteritis. |
| Alport's syndrome | Mutation in type IV collagen → split basement membrane. | Nerve disorders, ocular disorders, deafness. |

(LM = light microscopy; EM = electron microscopy; IF = immunofluorescence.)

| **Nephrotic syndrome** | NephrOtic syndrome presents with massive prOteinuria (> 3.5g/day, frothy urine), hyperlipidemia, fatty casts, edema. Associated with thromboembolism and ↑ risk of infection (loss of immunoglobulins). | |
|---|---|---|
| Membranous glomerulonephritis (diffuse membranous glomerulopathy) | LM—diffuse capillary and GBM thickening. EM— "spike and dome" appearance with subepithelial deposits. IF—granular. SLE's nephrotic presentation (see Image 86). | Caused by drugs, infections, SLE, solid tumors. Most common cause of adult nephrotic syndrome. |
| Minimal change disease (lipoid nephrosis) | LM—normal glomeruli. EM—foot process effacement (see Image 85). Selective loss of albumin, not globulins, due to GBM polyanion loss. | May be triggered by a recent infection or an immune stimulus. Most common in children. Responds to corticosteroids. |
| Amyloidosis | LM—Congo red stain, apple-green birefringence. | Associated with multiple myeloma, chronic conditions, TB, rheumatoid arthritis. |
| Diabetic glomerulo-nephropathy | Nonenzymatic glycosylation (NEG) of GBM → ↑ permeability, thickening. NEG of efferent arterioles → ↑ GFR → mesangial expansion. LM—mesangial expansion, GBM thickening, nodular glomerulosclerosis (Kimmelstiel-Wilson lesion) (see Image 87). | |
| Focal segmental glomerulosclerosis | LM—segmental sclerosis and hyalinosis. | Most common glomerular disease in HIV patients. More severe in HIV patients. |
| Membrano-proliferative glomerulonephritis | Subendothelial ICs with granular IF. Type I EM— "tram-track" appearance due to GBM splitting caused by mesangial ingrowth. Type II EM— "dense deposits." | Can present as nephritic syndrome. Usually progresses slowly to CRF. Type I is associated with HBV > HCV; type II is associated with C3 nephritic factor. |

## Glomerular histopathology

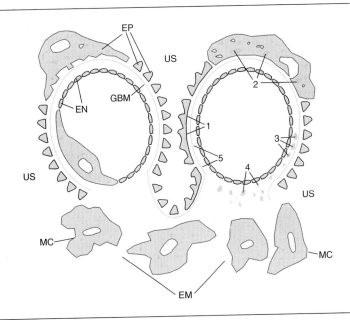

EP = epithelium with foot processes
US = urinary space
GBM = glomerular basement membrane
EN = fenestrated endothelium
MC = mesangial cells
EM = extracellular matrix

1 = effacement of epithelial foot processes (common in all forms of glomerular injury with proteinuria)
2 = large irregular subepithelial deposits or "humps" (acute glomerulonephritis)
3 = subendothelial deposits in lupus glomerulonephritis
4 = mesangial deposits (IgA nephropathy)
5 = antibody binding to GBM—smooth linear pattern on immunofluorescence (Goodpasture's)

| | | |
|---|---|---|
| **Kidney stones** | Can lead to severe complications, such as hydronephrosis and pyelonephritis. Treat and prevent by encouraging fluid intake. | |
| Calcium | Most common kidney stones (75–85%). Calcium oxalate (see Image 88), calcium phosphate, or both. Conditions that cause hypercalcemia (cancer, ↑ PTH, ↑ vitamin D, milk-alkali syndrome) can lead to hypercalciuria and stones. Tend to recur. | Radiopaque. Oxalate crystals can result from ethylene glycol (antifreeze) or vitamin C abuse. |
| Ammonium magnesium phosphate (**struvite**) | 2nd most common kidney stone. Caused by infection with urease-positive bugs (*Proteus vulgaris, Staphylococcus, Klebsiella*). Can form **staghorn calculi** that can be a nidus for UTIs. | Radiopaque or radiolucent. Worsened by alkaluria. |
| Uric acid | Strong association with hyperuricemia (e.g., gout). Often seen as a result of diseases with ↑ cell turnover, such as leukemia and myeloproliferative disorders. | RadiolUcent. |
| Cystine | Most often 2° to cystinuria. Hexagonal shape. Rarely, may form cystine staghorn calculi. | Faintly radiopaque. Treat with alkalinization of urine. |

**Renal cell carcinoma**

Most common renal malignancy. Invades IVC and spreads hematogenously; metastasizes to lung, bone. Most common in men ages 50–70. ↑ incidence with smoking and obesity. Associated with von Hippel–Lindau and gene deletion in chromosome 3. Originates in renal tubule cells → polygonal clear cells. Manifests clinically with hematuria, palpable mass, 2° polycythemia, flank pain, fever, and weight loss. Associated with paraneoplastic syndromes (ectopic EPO, ACTH, PTHrP, and prolactin) (see Image 89).

**Wilms' tumor (nephroblastoma)**

Most common renal malignancy of early childhood (ages 2–4). Presents with huge, palpable flank mass and/or hematuria. May be associated with hemihypertrophy syndromes. Contains embryonic glomerular structures. Deletion of tumor suppressor gene *WT1* on chromosome 11. Can be part of **WAGR** complex: **W**ilms' tumor, **A**niridia, **G**enitourinary malformation, and mental-motor **R**etardation.

**Transitional cell carcinoma**

Most common tumor of urinary tract system (can occur in renal calyces, renal pelvis, ureters, and bladder). Painless hematuria is suggestive of bladder cancer. Associated with problems in your **P**ee **SAC**: **P**henacetin, **S**moking, **A**niline dyes, and **C**yclophosphamide (see Image 82).

**Pyelonephritis**

| | |
|---|---|
| Acute | Affects cortex with relative sparing of glomeruli/vessels. White cell casts in urine are classic (see Image 81A). Presents with fever, CVA tenderness, nausea, and vomiting. |
| Chronic | Coarse, asymmetric corticomedullary scarring, blunted calyx. Tubules can contain eosinophilic casts (thyroidization of kidney) (see Image 81B). |

**Drug-induced interstitial nephritis**

Acute interstitial renal inflammation. Pyuria (typically eosinophils) and azotemia occurring 1–2 weeks after administration. Associated with fever, rash, hematuria, and CVA tenderness. Drugs (e.g., diuretics, NSAIDs, penicillin derivatives, sulfonamides, rifampin) act as haptens, inducing hypersensitivity.

| Diffuse cortical necrosis | Acute generalized infarction of cortices of both kidneys. Likely due to a combination of vasospasm and DIC. Associated with obstetric catastrophes (e.g., abruptio placentae) and septic shock. |
|---|---|
| Acute tubular necrosis | Most common cause of acute renal failure in hospital. Self-reversible, but fatal if left untreated (provide supportive dialysis). Associated with renal ischemia (e.g., shock, sepsis), crush injury (myoglobulinuria), toxins. Death most often occurs during initial oliguric phase.<br>Loss of cell polarity, epithelial cell detachment, necrosis, granular ("muddy brown") casts. 3 stages: inciting event → maintenance (low urine) → recovery (2–3 weeks). |
| Renal papillary necrosis | Sloughing of renal papillae → gross hematuria, proteinuria. May be triggered by a recent infection or immune stimulus. Associated with:<br>1. Diabetes mellitus<br>2. Acute pyelonephritis<br>3. Chronic phenacetin use (acetaminophen is phenacetin derivative)<br>4. Sickle cell anemia |
| Acute renal failure (acute kidney injury) | In normal nephron, BUN is reabsorbed (for countercurrent multiplication), but creatinine is not.<br>Acute renal failure is defined as an abrupt decline in renal function with ↑ creatinine and ↑ BUN over a period of several days.<br>1. Prerenal azotemia—↓ RBF (e.g., hypotension) → ↓ GFR. $Na^+/H_2O$ and urea retained by kidney, so BUN/creatinine ratio ↑ in attempt to conserve volume.<br>2. Intrinsic renal—generally due to acute tubular necrosis or ischemia/toxins; less commonly due to acute glomerulonephritis (e.g., RPGN). Patchy necrosis leads to debris obstructing tubule and fluid backflow across necrotic tubule → ↓ GFR. Urine has epithelial/granular casts. BUN reabsorption is impaired → ↓ BUN/creatinine ratio.<br>3. Postrenal—outflow obstruction (stones, BPH, neoplasia, congenital anomalies). Develops only with bilateral obstruction. |

| Variable | Prerenal | Renal | Postrenal |
|---|---|---|---|
| Urine osmolality | > 500 | < 350 | < 350 |
| Urine Na | < 10 | > 20 | > 40 |
| $Fe_{Na}$ | < 1% | > 2% | > 4% |
| Serum BUN/Cr | > 20 | < 15 | > 15 |

| | | |
|---|---|---|
| **Consequences of renal failure** | Inability to make urine and excrete nitrogenous wastes. | 2 forms of renal failure—acute (e.g., ATN) and chronic (e.g., hypertension and diabetes). |

Consequences:

1. $Na^+/H_2O$ retention (CHF, pulmonary edema, hypertension)
2. Hyperkalemia
3. Metabolic acidosis
4. Uremia—clinical syndrome marked by ↑ BUN and ↑ creatinine
   a. Nausea and anorexia
   b. Pericarditis
   c. Asterixis
   d. Encephalopathy
   e. Platelet dysfunction
5. Anemia (failure of erythropoietin production)
6. Renal osteodystrophy (failure of vitamin D hydroxylation)
7. Dyslipidemia (especially ↑ triglycerides)
8. Growth retardation and developmental delay (in children)

---

**Fanconi's syndrome** 

↓ proximal tubule transport of amino acids, glucose, phosphate, uric acid, protein, and electrolytes. Can be congenital or acquired. Causes include Wilson's disease, glycogen storage diseases, and drugs (e.g., cisplatin, expired tetracycline).

| Defect | Complications |
|---|---|
| ↓ phosphate reabsorption | Rickets |
| ↓ $HCO_3^-$ reabsorption | Metabolic acidosis (type 2 RTA) |
| ↓ early $Na^+$ reabsorption | ↑ distal $Na^+$ reabsorption → hypokalemia |

## Cysts

| | |
|---|---|
| ADPKD (formerly adult polycystic kidney disease) | Multiple, large, bilateral cysts that ultimately destroy the parenchyma. Enlarged kidneys. Presents with flank pain, hematuria, hypertension, urinary infection, progressive renal failure. Autosomal-dominant mutation in *APKD1* or *APKD2*. Death from complications of chronic kidney disease or hypertension (due to ↑ renin production). Associated with polycystic liver disease, berry aneurysms, mitral valve prolapse. |

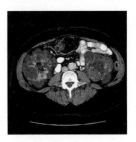

(Reproduced, with permission, from the PEIR Digital Library.)

| | |
|---|---|
| ARPKD (formerly infantile polycystic kidney disease) | Infantile presentation in parenchyma. Autosomal recessive. Associated with congenital hepatic fibrosis. Significant renal failure in utero can lead to Potter's; concerns beyond neonatal period are hypertension, portal hypertension, and progressive renal insufficiency. |
| Dialysis cysts | Cortical and medullary cysts resulting from long-standing dialysis. |
| Simple cysts | Benign, incidental finding. Cortex only. |
| Medullary cystic disease | Medullary cysts sometimes lead to fibrosis and progressive renal insufficiency with urinary concentrating defects. Ultrasound shows small kidney. Poor prognosis. |

## Electrolyte disturbances

| Electrolyte | Low serum concentration | High serum concentration |
|---|---|---|
| $Na^+$ | Disorientation, stupor, coma | Neurologic: irritability, delirium, coma |
| $Cl^-$ | 2° to metabolic alkalosis, hypokalemia, hypovolemia, ↑ aldosterone | 2° to non–anion gap acidosis |
| $K^+$ | U waves on ECG, flattened T waves, arrhythmias, paralysis | Peaked T waves, wide QRS, arrhythmias |
| $Ca^{2+}$ | Tetany, neuromuscular irritability | Delirium, renal stones, abdominal pain, not necessarily calciuria |
| $Mg^{2+}$ | Neuromuscular irritability, arrhythmias | Delirium, ↓ DTRs, cardiopulmonary arrest |
| $PO_4^{3-}$ | Low-mineral ion product causes bone loss, osteomalacia | High-mineral ion product causes renal stones, metastatic calcifications |

## Diuretics: site of action

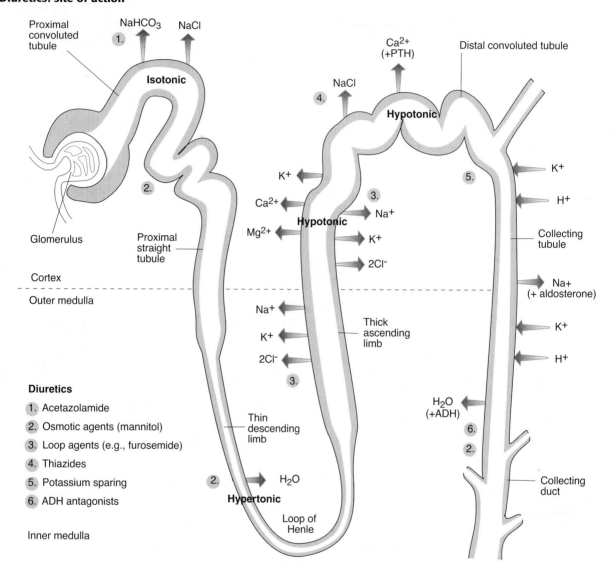

Proximal convoluted tubule

NaHCO₃   NaCl

1.

Isotonic

2.

Glomerulus

Proximal straight tubule

Cortex

Outer medulla

Ca²⁺ (+PTH)

Distal convoluted tubule

NaCl

4.

Hypotonic

K⁺

Ca²⁺

3.

Na⁺

Hypotonic

Mg²⁺

K⁺

2Cl⁻

Na⁺

K⁺

2Cl⁻

Thick ascending limb

3.

5.

K⁺

H⁺

Collecting tubule

Na⁺ (+ aldosterone)

K⁺

H⁺

H₂O (+ADH)

6.

2.

Collecting duct

Thin descending limb

### Diuretics

1. Acetazolamide
2. Osmotic agents (mannitol)
3. Loop agents (e.g., furosemide)
4. Thiazides
5. Potassium sparing
6. ADH antagonists

Inner medulla

2.

H₂O

Hypertonic

Loop of Henle

(Adapted, with permission, from Katzung BG. *Basic and Clinical Pharmacology,* 7th ed. Stamford, CT: Appleton & Lange, 1997: 243.)

## Mannitol

**Mechanism**
Osmotic diuretic, ↑ tubular fluid osmolarity, producing ↑ urine flow.

**Clinical use**
Shock, drug overdose, ↓ intracranial/intraocular pressure.

**Toxicity**
Pulmonary edema, dehydration. Contraindicated in anuria, CHF.

## Acetazolamide

**Mechanism**
Carbonic anhydrase inhibitor. Causes self-limited $NaHCO_3$ diuresis and reduction in total-body $HCO_3^-$ stores.

**Clinical use**
Glaucoma, urinary alkalinization, metabolic alkalosis, altitude sickness.

**Toxicity**
Hyperchloremic metabolic acidosis, neuropathy, $NH_3$ toxicity, sulfa allergy.

**ACID**azolamide causes **ACID**osis.

## Furosemide

**Mechanism**
Sulfonamide loop diuretic. Inhibits cotransport system ($Na^+$, $K^+$, $2 Cl^-$) of thick ascending limb of loop of Henle. Abolishes hypertonicity of medulla, preventing concentration of urine. ↑ $Ca^{2+}$ excretion. Loops Lose calcium.

**Clinical use**
Edematous states (CHF, cirrhosis, nephrotic syndrome, pulmonary edema), hypertension, hypercalcemia.

**Toxicity**
**O**totoxicity, **H**ypokalemia, **D**ehydration, **A**llergy (sulfa), **N**ephritis (interstitial), **G**out.

**OH DANG!**

## Ethacrynic acid

**Mechanism**
Phenoxyacetic acid derivative (NOT a sulfonamide). Essentially same action as furosemide.

**Clinical use**
Diuresis in patients allergic to sulfa drugs.

**Toxicity**
Similar to furosemide; can be used in hyperuricemia, acute gout (never used to treat gout).

## Hydrochlorothiazide

**Mechanism**
Thiazide diuretic. Inhibits NaCl reabsorption in early distal tubule, reducing diluting capacity of the nephron. ↓ $Ca^{2+}$ excretion.

**Clinical use**
Hypertension, CHF, idiopathic hypercalciuria, nephrogenic diabetes insipidus.

**Toxicity**
Hypokalemic metabolic alkalosis, hyponatremia, hyper**G**lycemia, hyper**L**ipidemia, hyper**U**ricemia, and hyper**C**alcemia. Sulfa allergy.

**HyperGLUC.**

| | | |
|---|---|---|
| **$K^+$-sparing diuretics** | Spironolactone, Triamterene, Amiloride, eplerenone. | The $K^+$ **STA**ys. |
| Mechanism | Spironolactone is a competitive aldosterone receptor antagonist in the cortical collecting tubule. Triamterene and amiloride act at the same part of the tubule by blocking $Na^+$ channels in the CCT. | |
| Clinical use | Hyperaldosteronism, $K^+$ depletion, CHF. | |
| Toxicity | Hyperkalemia (can lead to arrhythmias), endocrine effects with aldosterone antagonists (e.g., spironolactone causes gynecomastia, antiandrogen effects). | |

### Diuretics: electrolyte changes

| | |
|---|---|
| Urine NaCl | ↑ (all diuretics—carbonic anhydrase inhibitors, loop diuretics, thiazides, $K^+$-sparing diuretics). Serum NaCl may ↓ as a result. |
| Urine $K^+$ | ↑ (all except $K^+$-sparing diuretics). Serum $K^+$ may ↓ as a result. |
| Blood pH | ↓ (acidemia): Carbonic anhydrase inhibitors— ↓ $HCO_3^-$ reabsorption. $K^+$ sparing—aldosterone blockade prevents $K^+$ secretion and $H^+$ secretion. Additionally, hyperkalemia leads to $K^+$ entering all cells (via $H^+/K^+$ exchanger) in exchange for $H^+$ exiting cells. |
| | ↑ (alkalemia): Loop diuretics and thiazides cause alkalemia through several mechanisms: |
| | 1. Volume contraction → ↑ AT II → ↑ $Na^+/H^+$ exchange in proximal tubule → ↑ $HCO_3^-$ ("contraction alkalosis") |
| | 2. $K^+$ loss leads to $K^+$ exiting all cells (via $H^+/K^+$ exchanger) in exchange for $H^+$ entering cells |
| | 3. In low $K^+$ state, $H^+$ (rather than $K^+$) is exchanged for $Na^+$ in cortical collecting tubule, leading to alkalosis and "paradoxical aciduria" |
| Urine $Ca^{2+}$ | ↑ loop diuretics: Abolish lumen-positive potential in thick ascending limb of loop of Henle → ↓ paracellular $Ca^+$ reabsorption → hypocalcemia, ↑ urinary $Ca^{2+}$. |
| | ↓ thiazides: Volume depletion → upregulation of sodium reabsorption → enhanced paracellular $Ca^{2+}$ reabsorption in proximal tubule and loop of Henle. Thiazides also block luminal $Na^+/Cl^-$ cotransport in distal convoluted tubule → ↑ $Na^+$ gradient → ↑ interstitial $Na^+/Ca^{2+}$ exchange → hypercalcemia. |

| | | |
|---|---|---|
| **ACE inhibitors** | Captopril, enalapril, lisinopril. | |
| Mechanism | Inhibit angiotensin-converting enzyme, reducing levels of angiotensin II and preventing inactivation of bradykinin, a potent vasodilator. **Renin release is** ↑ due to loss of feedback inhibition. | **Losartan** is an angiotensin II receptor antagonist. It is **not** an ACE inhibitor and does not cause cough. |
| Clinical use | Hypertension, CHF, diabetic renal disease. | |
| Toxicity | **C**ough, **A**ngioedema, **P**roteinuria, **T**aste changes, hyp**O**tension, **P**regnancy problems (fetal renal damage), **R**ash, **I**ncreased renin, **L**ower angiotensin II. Also **hyperkalemia.** Avoid with bilateral renal artery stenosis because ACE inhibitors significantly ↓ GFR by preventing constriction of efferent arterioles. | **CAPTOPRIL.** |

# Reproductive

*"Artificial insemination is when the farmer does it to the cow instead of the bull."*

—Student essay

*"Whoever called it necking was a poor judge of anatomy."*

—Groucho Marx

*"See, the problem is that God gives men a brain and a penis, and only enough blood to run one at a time."*

—Robin Williams

▸ Anatomy

▸ Physiology

▸ Pathology

▸ Pharmacology

**Gonadal drainage**

Venous drainage

Left ovary/testis → left gonadal vein → left renal vein → IVC.

Right ovary/testis → right gonadal vein → IVC.

Lymphatic drainage

Ovaries/testes → para-aortic lymph nodes.

Distal ⅓ of vagina/vulva/scrotum → superficial inguinal nodes.

Proximal ⅔ of vagina/uterus → obturator, external iliac and hypogastric nodes.

Just as the left adrenal vein drains to the left renal vein before the IVC.

As a result, varicocele is more common on left.

**Female reproductive anatomy**

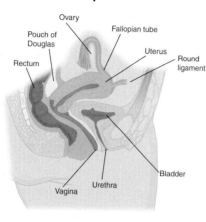
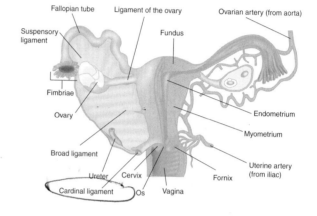

| Ligament | Connects | Structures contained | Notes |
|---|---|---|---|
| Suspensory ligament of the ovaries | Ovaries to lateral pelvic wall | Ovarian vessels | |
| Cardinal ligament | Cervix to side wall of pelvis | Uterine vessels | |
| **Round** ligament of the uterus | Uterine fundus to labia majora | | **Round** like the number of structures it carries: 0. Derivative of gubernaculum. Travels through **round** inguinal canal. |
| Broad ligament | Uterus, fallopian tubes, and ovaries to pelvic side wall | Ovaries, fallopian tubes, and round ligaments of uterus | |
| Ligament of the ovary | Ovary to uterus | | |

## Male reproductive anatomy

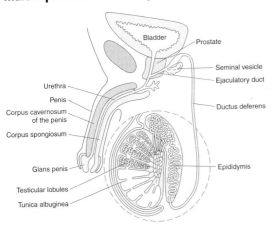

(Reproduced, with permission, from Junqueira LC et al. *Basic Histology*, 9th ed. New York: McGraw-Hill, 1998.)

Pathway of sperm during ejaculation—**SEVEN UP**:

Seminiferous tubules
Epididymis
Vas deferens
Ejaculatory ducts
(Nothing)
Urethra
Penis

| Autonomic innervation of the male sexual response | Erection—**P**arasympathetic nervous system (pelvic nerve): 1. NO → ↑ cGMP → smooth muscle relaxation → vasodilation → proerectile. 2. NE → ↑ $[Ca^2]_{in}$ → smooth muscle contraction → vasoconstriction → antierectile. Emission—**S**ympathetic nervous system (hypogastric nerve). Ejaculation—visceral and somatic nerves (pudendal nerve). | **P**oint and **S**hoot. Sildenafil and vardenafil inhibit cGMP breakdown. |
|---|---|---|
| **Derivation of sperm parts** | Occurs during final phase of spermatogenesis (spermiogenesis): spermatid → spermatozoa. Acrosome is derived from the Golgi apparatus and flagellum (tail) from one of the centrioles. Middle piece (neck) has **M**itochondria. Feeds on **F**ructose. Tail forms from centrioles. | 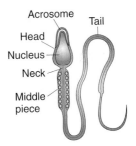 |

## Seminiferous tubules

| Cell | Function | Location/notes |
|---|---|---|
| Spermatogonia (germ cells) | Maintain germ pool and produce 1° spermatocytes | Line seminiferous tubules |
| Sertoli cells (non–germ cells) | Secrete inhibin → inhibit FSH<br>Secrete androgen-binding protein (ABP) → maintain levels of testosterone<br>Tight junctions between adjacent Sertoli cells form blood-testis barrier → isolate gametes from autoimmune attack<br>Support and nourish developing spermatozoa<br>Regulate spermatogenesis<br>Produce anti-müllerian hormone | Line seminiferous tubules<br>Sertoli cells Support Sperm Synthesis |
| Leydig cells (endocrine cells) | Secrete testosterone | Interstitium |

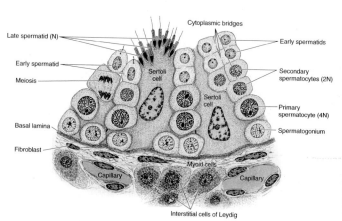
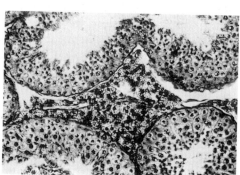

(Reproduced, with permission, from Junqueira LC, Cameiro J. *Basic Histology*, 11th ed. New York: McGraw-Hill, 2005: 420.)

## Composition of semen

| | |
|---|---|
| Seminal vesicle products (60% of total volume) | Fructose, ascorbic acid, prostaglandins, phosphorylcholine, flavins. |
| Prostate products (20% of total volume) | Zinc, citric acid, phospholipids, acid phosphatase, fibrinolysin. |
| Sperm | |

**Spermatogenesis**

Spermatogenesis begins at puberty with spermatogonia. Full development takes 2 months. Occurs in seminiferous tubules. Produces spermatids that undergo spermiogenesis (loss of cytoplasmic contents, gain of acrosomal cap) to form mature spermatozoan.

"**Gonium**" is **going** to be a sperm; "**Zoan**" is "**Zooming**" out of cell.

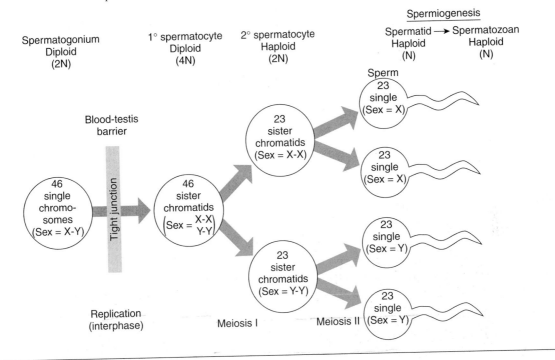

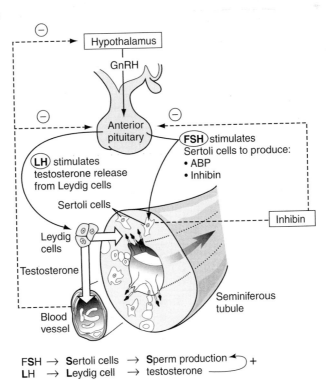

## Regulation of spermatogenesis

FSH → **S**ertoli cells → **S**perm production ⤹ +
LH → **L**eydig cell → testosterone

**Androgens**

Testosterone, dihydrotestosterone (DHT), androstenedione.

Source

DHT and testosterone (testis), androstenedione (adrenal).

Potency—DHT > testosterone > androstenedione.

Function

**Testosterone:**
1. Differentiation of epididymis, vas deferens, seminal vesicles
2. Growth spurt
   —Penis
   —Seminal vesicles
   —Sperm
   —Muscle
   —RBCs
3. Deepening of voice
4. Closing of epiphyseal plates (via estrogen converted from testosterone)
5. Libido

**DHT:**

Early—differentiation of penis, scrotum, prostate.
Late—prostate growth, balding, sebaceous gland activity.

Testosterone is converted to DHT by the enzyme 5α-reductase, which is inhibited by finasteride.

Testosterone and androstenedione are converted to estrogen in adipose tissue and Sertoli cells by enzyme aromatase.

Exogenous testosterone → inhibition of HPG axis → ↓ intratesticular testosterone → ↓ testicular size → azoospermia.

---

**Estrogen**

Source

Ovary (17β-estradiol), placenta (estriol), blood (aromatization).

Function
1. Development of genitalia and breast, female fat distribution
2. Growth of follicle, endometrial proliferation, ↑ myometrial excitability
3. Upregulation of estrogen, LH, and progesterone receptors; feedback inhibition of FSH and LH, then LH surge; stimulation of prolactin secretion (**but** blocks its action at breast)
4. ↑ transport of proteins, SHBG; ↑ HDL; ↓ LDL

Potency—estradiol > estrone > estriol.
Pregnancy:
50-fold ↑ in estradiol and estrone
1000-fold ↑ in estriol (indicator of fetal well-being)
Estrogen receptors expressed in the nuclei of cells.

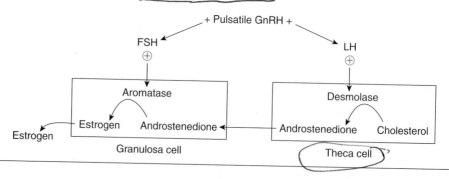

**Progesterone**

Source     Corpus luteum, placenta, adrenal cortex, testes.

Function
1. Stimulation of endometrial glandular secretions and spiral artery development
2. Maintenance of pregnancy
3. ↓ myometrial excitability
4. Production of thick cervical mucus, which inhibits sperm entry into the uterus
5. ↑ body temperature
6. Inhibition of gonadotropins (LH, FSH)
7. Uterine smooth muscle relaxation (preventing contractions)
8. ↓ estrogen receptor expressivity

Elevation of progesterone is indicative of ovulation.
**PROGEST**erone is **PRO-GEST**ation.

**Menstrual cycle**

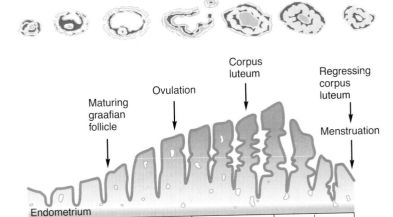

Corpus luteum

Ovulation

Regressing corpus luteum

Maturing graafian follicle

Menstruation

Endometrium

Proliferative phase (follicular)     Secretory phase (luteal)

Follicular growth is fastest during 2nd week of proliferative phase.

Estrogen stimulates endometrial proliferation.

Progesterone maintains endometrium to support implantation.

↓ progesterone leads to ↓ fertility.

Follicular phase can vary in length. Luteal phase is usually a constant 14 days. Ovulation day + 14 days = menstruation.

Oligomenorrhea: > 35-day cycle.

Polymenorrhea: < 21-day cycle.

Metrorrhagia: frequent but irregular menstruation.

Menometrorrhagia: heavy menstruation.

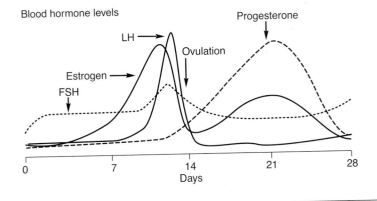

Blood hormone levels

Progesterone

LH

Ovulation

Estrogen

FSH

0     7     14     21     28

Days

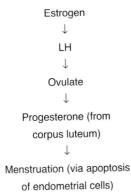

Estrogen
↓
LH
↓
Ovulate
↓
Progesterone (from corpus luteum)
↓
Menstruation (via apoptosis of endometrial cells)

**Ovulation**

↑ estrogen, ↑ GnRH receptors on anterior pituitary. Estrogen surge then stimulates LH release, causing ovulation (rupture of follicle).
↑ temperature (progesterone induced).

Mittelschmerz—blood from ruptured follicle causes peritoneal irritation that can mimic appendicitis.

**Oogenesis**

1° oocytes begin meiosis I during fetal life and complete meiosis I just prior to ovulation.
Meiosis I is arrested in pr**O**phase for years until **O**vulation (1° oocytes).
Meiosis II is arrested in **MET**aphase until fertilization (2° oocytes).
If fertilization does not occur, the 2° oocyte degenerates.

An egg **MET** a sperm.

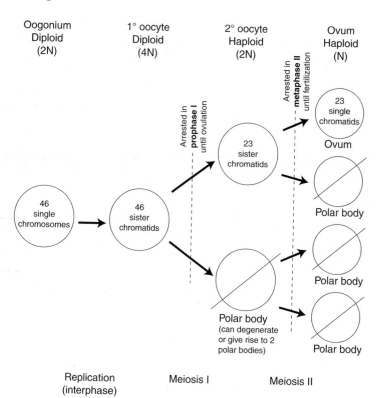

**Pregnancy**

Fertilization most commonly occurs in upper end of fallopian tube (the ampulla). Occurs within 1 day after ovulation.

Implantation within the wall of the uterus occurs 6 days after fertilization. Trophoblasts secrete β-hCG, which is detectable in blood 1 week after conception and on home test in urine 2 weeks after conception.

Lactation—after labor, the ↓ in maternal steroids induces lactation. Suckling is required to maintain milk production, since ↑ nerve stimulation ↑ oxytocin and prolactin.

Prolactin—induces and maintains lactation and ↓ reproductive function.

Oxytocin—appears to help with milk letdown and may be involved with uterine contractions (function not yet entirely known).

HIGH-YIELD SYSTEMS

REPRODUCTIVE

## hCG

**Source**
**Function**

Syncytiotrophoblast of placenta.
1. Maintains the corpus luteum (and thus progesterone) for the 1st trimester by acting like LH (otherwise no luteal cell stimulation, and abortion results). In the 2nd and 3rd trimester, the placenta synthesizes its own estriol and progesterone and the corpus luteum degenerates.
2. Used to detect pregnancy because it appears early in the urine (see above).
3. Elevated hCG in pathologic states (e.g., hydatidiform moles, choriocarcinoma, gestational trophoblastic tumors).

---

**Menopause**

↓ estrogen production due to age-linked decline in number of ovarian follicles. Average age of onset is 51 years (earlier in smokers).
Usually preceded by 4–5 years of abnormal menstrual cycles. Source of estrogen (estrone) after menopause becomes peripheral conversion of androgens. ↑ androgens cause hirsutism.

Hormonal changes:
↓ estrogen, ↑↑ FSH, ↑ LH (no surge), ↑ GnRH. ↑↑ FSH used as confirmatory test.
Menopause causes **HHAVOC**:
Hirsutism, Hot flashes, Atrophy of the Vagina, Osteoporosis, Coronary artery disease.
Early menopause can indicate premature ovarian failure.

---

▶ **REPRODUCTIVE—PATHOLOGY**

### Sex chromosome disorders

**Klinefelter's syndrome [male] (XXY), 1:850**

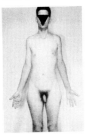

Testicular atrophy, eunuchoid body shape, tall, long extremities, gynecomastia, female hair distribution. May present with developmental delay. Presence of inactivated X chromosome (Barr body). Common cause of hypogonadism seen in infertility workup.

Dysgenesis of seminiferous tubules → ↓ inhibin → ↑ FSH.
Abnormal Leydig cell function → ↓ testosterone → ↑ LH → ↑ estrogen.

**Turner's syndrome**

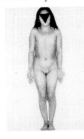

Short stature (if left untreated, < 5 feet), ovarian dysgenesis (streak ovary), shield chest, bicuspid aortic valve, webbing of neck (cystic hygroma), preductal coarctation of the aorta, most common cause of 1° amenorrhea. No Barr body.

"Hugs and kisses" (**XO**) from Tina **Turner** (female).
↓ estrogen leads to ↑ LH and FSH.

**Double Y males [male] (XYY), 1:1000**

Phenotypically normal, very tall, severe acne, antisocial behavior (seen in 1–2% of XYY males). Normal fertility.

**Diagnosing disorders of sex hormones**

| Testosterone levels | LH levels | Diagnosis |
|---|---|---|
| ↑ | ↑ | Defective androgen receptor |
| ↑ | ↓ | Testosterone-secreting tumor, exogenous steroids |
| ↓ | ↑ | 1° hypogonadism |
| ↓ | ↓ | Hypogonadotropic hypogonadism |

| | |
|---|---|
| **Pseudo-hermaphroditism** | Disagreement between the phenotypic (external genitalia) and gonadal (testes vs. ovaries) sex. |
| Female pseudo-hermaphrodite (XX) | Ovaries present, but external genitalia are virilized or ambiguous. Due to excessive and inappropriate exposure to androgenic steroids during early gestation (e.g., congenital adrenal hyperplasia or exogenous administration of androgens during pregnancy). |
| Male pseudo-hermaphrodite (XY) | Testes present, but external genitalia are female or ambiguous. Most common form is androgen insensitivity syndrome (testicular feminization). |
| **True hermaphrodite (46,XX or 47,XXY)** | Both ovary and testicular tissue present; ambiguous genitalia. Very rare. |
| **Androgen insensitivity syndrome (46,XY)** | Defect in androgen receptor resulting in normal-appearing female; female external genitalia with rudimentary vagina; uterus and uterine tubes generally absent; presents with no sexual hair; develops testes (often found in labia majora; surgically removed to prevent malignancy). ↑ **testosterone, estrogen, LH** (vs. sex chromosome disorders). |
| **5α-reductase deficiency** | Inability of males to convert testosterone to DHT. Ambiguous genitalia until puberty, when ↑ testosterone causes masculinization/↑ growth of external genitalia. Testosterone/estrogen levels are normal; LH is normal or ↑. "Penis at 12." Internal genitalia are normal. |

HIGH-YIELD SYSTEMS

REPRODUCTIVE

**Hydatidiform mole**  Cystic swelling of chorionic villi and proliferation of chorionic epithelium (trophoblast) that presents with abnormal vaginal bleeding. Most common precursor of choriocarcinoma. ↑ β-hCG. "Honeycombed uterus," "cluster of grapes" appearance, abnormally enlarged uterus (see Image 74). Complete moles classically have "snowstorm" appearance with no fetus during 1st sonogram. Moles can lead to uterine rupture. Treatment: dilatation and curettage and methotrexate. Monitor β-hCG.

|  | Complete Mole | Partial Mole |
|---|---|---|
| Karyotype | 46,XX (46,XY) | 69,XXY |
| hCG | ↑↑↑↑ | ↑ |
| Uterine size | ↑ | — |
| Convert to choriocarcinoma | 2% | Rare |
| Fetal parts | No | Yes (**partial** = fetal **parts**) |
| Components | 2 sperm + empty egg | 2 sperm + 1 egg |
| Risk of complications | 15-20% malignant trophoblastic disease | Low risk of malignancy (< 5%) |

**Common causes of recurrent miscarriages**
1st weeks—low progesterone levels (no response to β-hCG).
1st trimester—chromosomal abnormalities (e.g., robertsonian translocation).
2nd trimester—bicornuate uterus (incomplete fusion of paramesonephric ducts).

**Pregnancy-induced hypertension (preeclampsia-eclampsia)**
Preeclampsia—hypertension, proteinuria, and edema. Eclampsia—preeclampsia + seizures. Occurs in 7% of pregnant women from 20 weeks' gestation to 6 weeks postpartum (before 20 weeks suggests molar pregnancy). ↑ incidence in patients with preexisting hypertension, diabetes, chronic renal disease, and autoimmune disorders. Caused by **placental ischemia** due to impaired vasodilation of spiral arteries, resulting in ↑ vascular tone. Can be associated with **HELLP syndrome** (**H**emolysis, **E**levated **LF**Ts, **L**ow **P**latelets). Mortality due to cerebral hemorrhage and ARDS.

Clinical features
Headache, blurred vision, abdominal pain, edema of face and extremities, altered mentation, hyperreflexia; lab findings may include thrombocytopenia, hyperuricemia.

Treatment
Delivery of fetus as soon as viable. Otherwise bed rest, salt restriction, and monitoring and treatment of hypertension. Treatment: IV magnesium sulfate and diazepam to prevent and treat seizures of eclampsia.

**HIGH-YIELD SYSTEMS**

**REPRODUCTIVE**

| Pregnancy complications | | |
|---|---|---|
| | Abruptio placentae—premature detachment of placenta from implantation site. Fetal death. May be associated with DIC. ↑ risk with smoking, hypertension, cocaine use. | Painful bleeding in 3rd trimester. **Abrupt** detachment/death. |
| | Placenta accreta—defective decidual layer allows placenta to attach to myometrium. No separation of placenta after birth. Prior C-section, inflammation, and placenta previa predispose. | Massive bleeding after delivery. Accreta = "encased in" → encased in myometrium. |
| | Placenta previa—attachment of placenta to lower uterine segment. May occlude internal os. Multiparity and prior C-section predispose. | Painless bleeding in any trimester. |
| | Ectopic pregnancy—most often in fallopian tubes. Suspect with ↑ hCG and sudden lower abdominal pain; confirm with ultrasound. Often clinically mistaken for appendicitis. | Pain with or without bleeding. Risk factors: —History of infertility —Salpingitis (PID) —Ruptured appendix —Prior tubal surgery |
| | Retained placental tissue—may cause postpartum hemorrhage. | |

**Amniotic fluid abnormalities**

| | |
|---|---|
| Polyhydramnios | > 1.5–2 L of amniotic fluid; associated with esophageal/duodenal atresia, causing inability to swallow amniotic fluid, and with anencephaly. |
| Oligohydramnios | < 0.5 L of amniotic fluid; associated with placental insufficiency, bilateral renal agenesis, or posterior urethral valves (in males) and resultant inability to excrete urine. Can give rise to Potter's syndrome. |

**Cervical pathology**

| | | |
|---|---|---|
| Dysplasia and carcinoma in situ | Disordered epithelial growth; begins at basal layer of squamo-columnar junction and extends outward. Classified as CIN 1, CIN 2, or CIN 3 (carcinoma in situ), depending on extent of dysplasia. Associated with HPV **16, 18.** Vaccine available. May progress slowly to invasive carcinoma if left untreated. Risk factors: multiple sexual partners, smoking, early sexual intercourse, HIV infection. | Koilocytic change typical of HPV infection 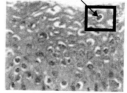 **HPV cell** (Reproduced, with permission, from Kantarjian HM et al. *MD Anderson Manual of Medical Oncology.* New York: McGraw-Hill, 2006, Fig. 24-4B.) |
| Invasive carcinoma | Often squamous cell carcinoma. Pap smear can catch cervical dysplasia (koilocytes) before it progresses to invasive carcinoma. Lateral invasion can block ureters, causing renal failure. | |

| | |
|---|---|
| **Endometriosis** | Non-neoplastic endometrial glands/stroma in abnormal locations outside the uterus. Characterized by **cyclic bleeding** (menstrual type) from ectopic endometrial tissue resulting in blood-filled **"chocolate cysts."** In ovary or on peritoneum. Manifests clinically as severe menstrual-related pain. Often results in infertility. Can be due to retrograde menstrual flow or ascending infection.<br>Adenomyosis—endometrium within the myometrium. |

### Endometrial proliferation

| | |
|---|---|
| Endometrial hyperplasia | Abnormal endometrial gland proliferation usually caused by excess estrogen stimulation. ↑ risk for endometrial carcinoma. Clinically manifests as postmenopausal vaginal bleeding. Risk factors include anovulatory cycles, hormone replacement therapy, polycystic ovarian syndrome, and granulosa cell tumor. |
| Endometrial carcinoma | **Most common gynecologic malignancy.** Peak occurrence at 55–65 years of age. Clinically presents with vaginal bleeding. Typically preceded by endometrial hyperplasia. Risk factors include prolonged use of estrogen without progestins, obesity, diabetes, hypertension, nulliparity, and late menopause. ↑ myometrial invasion → ↓ prognosis. |

### Myometrial tumors

| | |
|---|---|
| Leiomyoma (fibroid)<br>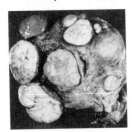 | **Most common of all tumors** in females. Often presents with multiple tumors with well-demarcated borders. ↑ incidence in blacks. Benign smooth muscle tumor; malignant transformation is rare. Estrogen sensitive—tumor size ↑ with pregnancy and ↓ with menopause. Peak occurrence at 20–40 years of age. May be asymptomatic, cause abnormal uterine bleeding, or result in miscarriage. Severe bleeding may lead to iron deficiency anemia. Does not progress to leiomyosarcoma. **Whorled pattern of smooth muscle bundles.** |
| Leiomyosarcoma | Bulky, irregularly shaped tumor with areas of necrosis and hemorrhage, typically arising de novo (not from leiomyoma). ↑ incidence in blacks. Highly aggressive tumor with tendency to recur. May protrude from cervix and bleed. Most commonly seen in middle-aged women. |

| | |
|---|---|
| **Gynecologic tumor epidemiology** | Incidence—endometrial > ovarian > cervical (data pertain to the United States; cervical cancer is most common worldwide).<br>Worst prognosis—ovarian > cervical > endometrial. |

| | | |
|---|---|---|
| **Premature ovarian failure** | Premature atresia of ovarian follicles in women of reproductive age. Patients present with signs of menopause after puberty but before age 40. | ↓ estrogen, ↑ LH, FSH. |

| | |
|---|---|
| **Most common causes of anovulation** | Polycystic ovarian syndrome, obesity, Asherman's syndrome (adhesions), HPO axis abnormalities, premature ovarian failure, hyperprolactinemia, thyroid disorders, eating disorders, Cushing's syndrome, adrenal insufficiency. |

**Polycystic ovarian syndrome**

↑ LH production leads to anovulation, hyperandrogenism due to deranged steroid synthesis by theca cells. Enlarged, bilateral cystic ovaries manifest clinically with amenorrhea, infertility, obesity, and hirsutism. Associated with insulin resistance. ↑ risk of endometrial cancer. Treatment: weight loss, OCPs, gonadotropin analogs, clomiphene, or surgery.

↑ LH, ↓ FSH, ↑ testosterone.

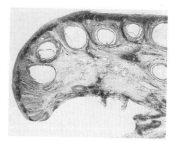

(Reproduced, with permission, from DeCherney AH, Nathan L. *Current Diagnosis & Treatment: Obstetrics & Gynecology,* 10th ed. New York, McGraw-Hill, 2007, Fig. 40-3.)

**Ovarian cysts**

| | |
|---|---|
| Follicular cyst | Distention of unruptured graafian follicle. May be associated with hyperestrinism and endometrial hyperplasia. |
| Corpus luteum cyst | Hemorrhage into persistent corpus luteum. Commonly regresses spontaneously. |
| Theca-lutein cyst | Often bilateral/multiple. Due to gonadotropin stimulation. Associated with choriocarcinoma and moles. |
| "Chocolate cyst" | Blood-containing cyst from ovarian endometriosis. Varies with menstrual cycle. |

**Ovarian germ cell tumors**  Most common in adolescents.

| Type | Characteristics | Tumor markers |
|---|---|---|
| Dysgerminoma | Malignant, equivalent to male seminoma but rarer (1% of germ cell tumors in females vs. 30% in males). Sheets of uniform cells. | hCG, LDH. |
| Choriocarcinoma | Rare but malignant; can develop during pregnancy in mother or baby. Large, hyperchromatic syncytiotrophoblastic cells. ↑ frequency of theca-lutein cysts. Along with moles, comprise spectrum of gestational trophoblastic neoplasia. | hCG. |
| Yolk sac (endodermal sinus) tumor | Aggressive malignancy in ovaries (testes in boys) and sacrococcygeal area of young children. Yellow, friable, solid masses. 50% have Schiller-Duval bodies (resemble glomeruli). | AFP. |
| Teratoma | 90% of ovarian germ cell tumors. Contain cells from 2 or 3 germ layers. Mature teratoma ("dermoid cyst")—most frequent benign ovarian tumor. Immature teratoma—aggressively malignant. Struma ovarii—contains functional thyroid tissue. Can present as hyperthyroidism. | |

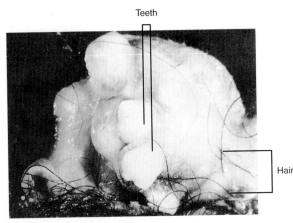

Teratoma of the ovary

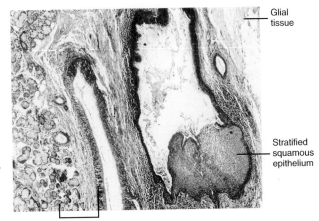

Respiratory epithelium and glands

### Ovarian non–germ cell tumors

| | | |
|---|---|---|
| Serous cystadenoma | 20% of ovarian tumors. Frequently bilateral, lined with fallopian tube–like epithelium. Benign. | ↑ CA-125 is general ovarian cancer marker. |
| Serous cystadenocarcinoma | 50% of ovarian tumors, malignant and frequently bilateral. | Risk factors—BRCA-1, HNPCC. Significant genetic |
| Mucinous cystadenoma | Multilocular cyst lined by mucus-secreting epithelium. Benign. Intestine-like tissue. | predisposition makes family history the most important |
| Mucinous cystadenocarcinoma | Malignant. Pseudomyxoma peritonei—intraperitoneal accumulation of mucinous material from ovarian or appendiceal tumor. | risk factor. |
| Brenner tumor | **B**enign. Looks like **B**ladder. | |
| Fibromas | Bundles of spindle-shaped fibroblasts. Meigs' syndrome—triad of ovarian fibroma, ascites, and hydrothorax. Pulling sensation in groin. | |
| Granulosa cell tumor | Secretes estrogen → precocious puberty (kids). Can cause endometrial hyperplasia or carcinoma in adults. Call-Exner bodies—small follicles filled with eosinophilic secretions. Abnormal uterine bleeding. | |
| Krukenberg tumor | GI malignancy that metastasizes to ovaries, causing a mucin-secreting signet cell adenocarcinoma. | |

| | |
|---|---|
| **Vaginal carcinoma** | 1. Squamous cell carcinoma (SCC)—2° to cervical SCC. |
| | 2. Clear cell adenocarcinoma—affects women who had exposure to DES in utero. |
| | 3. Sarcoma botryoides (rhabdomyosarcoma variant)—affects girls < 4 years of age; spindle-shaped tumor cells that are desmin positive. |
| | 4. Bartholin's gland cyst—rare; pain in labia majora; can result from previous infection. |

### Benign breast tumors

| Type | Characteristics | Epidemiology | Notes |
|---|---|---|---|
| Fibroadenoma | **Small**, mobile, firm mass with sharp edges. | Most common tumor in those < 25 years of age. | ↑ size and tenderness with ↑ estrogen (e.g., pregnancy, menstruation). Not a precursor to breast cancer. |
| Intraductal papilloma | Small tumor that grows in lactiferous ducts. Typically beneath areola. | | Serous or bloody nipple discharge. Slight (1.5–2 ×) ↑ in risk for carcinoma. |
| Phyllodes tumor | **Large** bulky mass of connective tissue and cysts. "Leaf-like" projections. | Most common in 6th decade. | Some may become malignant. |

**Malignant breast tumors**

Common postmenopause. Arise from mammary duct epithelium or lobular glands. Overexpression of estrogen/progesterone receptors or *erb*-B2 (HER-2, an EGF receptor) is common; affects therapy and prognosis. Axillary lymph node involvement is the single most important prognostic factor.

Risk factors: ↑ estrogen exposure, ↑ total number of menstrual cycles, older age at 1st live birth, obesity (adipose tissue serves as major source of estrogen in postmenopausal women by converting androstenedione to estrone; therefore, obesity is associated with ↑ estrogen exposure).

| Type | Characteristics | Notes |
|---|---|---|
| Ductal carcinoma in situ (DCIS) | Fills ductal lumen. Arises from ductal hyperplasia. | Early malignancy without basement membrane penetration. |
| Invasive ductal | Firm, fibrous, "rock-hard" mass with sharp margins and small, glandular, duct-like cells. | Worst and most invasive. Most common (76% breast cancer). |
| Invasive lobular | Orderly row of cells. | Often multiple. Bilateral. |
| Medullary | Fleshy, cellular, lymphatic infiltrate. | Good prognosis. |
| Comedocarcinoma | Ductal, caseous necrosis. Subtype of DCIS. | |
| Inflammatory | Dermal lymphatic invasion by breast carcinoma. Peau d'orange (breast skin resembles orange peel). | 50% survival at 5 years. |
| Paget's disease | Eczematous patches on nipple. Paget cells = large cells in epidermis with clear halo. | Suggests underlying carcinoma. Also seen on vulva. |

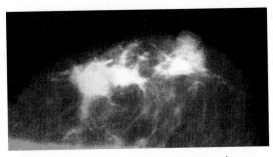

Breast cancer: mammogram displaying a dense, irregularly shaped mass.

(Reproduced, with permission, from the PEIR Digital Library.)

### Common breast conditions

| | |
|---|---|
| Fibrocystic disease | Most common cause of "breast lumps" from age 25 to menopause. Presents with premenstrual breast pain and multiple lesions, often bilateral. Fluctuation in size of mass. Usually does not indicate ↑ risk of carcinoma. Histologic types: |

    1. Fibrosis—hyperplasia of breast stroma.
    2. Cystic—fluid filled, blue dome. Ductal dilation.
    3. Sclerosing adenosis—↑ acini and intralobular fibrosis. Associated with calcifications.
    4. Epithelial hyperplasia—↑ in number of epithelial cell layers in terminal duct lobule. ↑ risk of carcinoma with atypical cells. Occurs in women > 30 years of age.

| | | |
|---|---|---|
| Acute mastitis | Breast abscess; during breast-feeding, ↑ risk of bacterial infection through cracks in the nipple; *S. aureus* is the most common pathogen. | |
| Fat necrosis | A benign painless lump; forms as a result of injury to breast tissue. Up to 50% of patients may not report trauma. | |
| Gynecomastia | Results from hyperestrogenism (cirrhosis, testicular tumor, puberty, old age), Klinefelter's syndrome, or drugs (estrogen, marijuana, heroin, psychoactive drugs, **S**pironolactone, **D**igitalis, **C**imetidine, **A**lcohol, **K**etoconazole). | **S**ome **D**rugs **C**reate **A**wesome **K**nockers. |

### Breast pathology

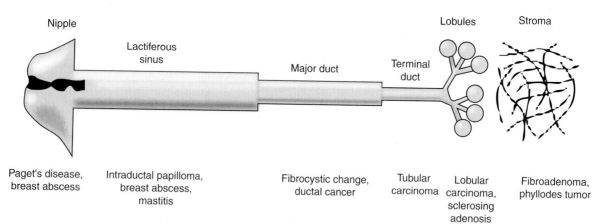

Nipple — Paget's disease, breast abscess

Lactiferous sinus / Major duct — Intraductal papilloma, breast abscess, mastitis

Terminal duct — Fibrocystic change, ductal cancer

Lobules — Tubular carcinoma; Lobular carcinoma, sclerosing adenosis

Stroma — Fibroadenoma, phyllodes tumor

### Prostate pathology

Prostatitis—dysuria, frequency, urgency, low back pain. Acute: bacterial (e.g., *E. coli*); chronic: bacterial or abacterial (most common).

| | |
|---|---|
| **Benign prostatic hyperplasia (BPH)** | Common in men > 50 years of age. Hyperplasia (**not** hypertrophy) of the prostate gland. May be due to an age-related ↑ in estradiol with possible sensitization of the prostate to the growth-promoting effects of DHT. Characterized by a nodular enlargement of the periurethral (lateral and middle) lobes, which compress the urethra into a vertical slit. Often presents with ↑ frequency of urination, nocturia, difficulty starting and stopping the stream of urine, and dysuria. May lead to distention and hypertrophy of the bladder, hydronephrosis, and UTIs. Not considered a premalignant lesion. ↑ **free prostate-specific antigen (PSA)**. Treatment: $\alpha_1$-antagonists (terazosin, tamsulosin), which cause relaxation of smooth muscle. |

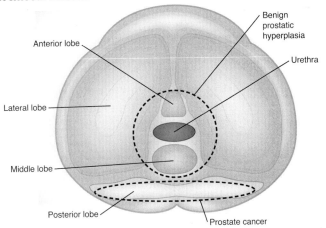

| | |
|---|---|
| **Prostatic adenocarcinoma** | Common in men > 50 years of age. Arises most often from the posterior lobe (peripheral zone) of the prostate gland and is most frequently diagnosed by digital rectal examination (hard nodule) and prostate biopsy. Prostatic acid phosphatase (PAP) and PSA are useful tumor markers (↑ total PSA, with ↓ **fraction of free PSA**). Osteoblastic metastases in bone may develop in late stages, as indicated by lower back pain and an ↑ in serum alkaline phosphatase and PSA. |

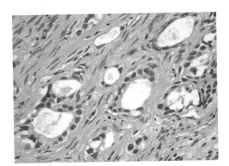

Prostatic adenocarcinoma: small infiltrating
glands with prominent nucleoli
(Reproduced, with permission, from USMLERx.com.)

| | |
|---|---|
| **Cryptorchidism** | Undescended testis (one or both); lack of spermatogenesis due to ↑ body temperature; associated with ↑ risk of germ cell tumors. Prematurity ↑ the risk of cryptorchidism. |

| | |
|---|---|
| **Testicular germ cell tumors** | ~95% of all testicular tumors. Can present as a mixed germ cell tumor. |
|   Seminoma | Malignant; painless, homogenous testicular enlargement; most common testicular tumor, mostly affecting males age 15–35. Large cells in lobules with watery cytoplasm and a "fried egg" appearance. Radiosensitive. Late metastasis, excellent prognosis. |
|   Embryonal carcinoma | Malignant; painful; worse prognosis than seminoma. Often glandular/papillary morphology. Can differentiate to other tumors. May be associated with ↑ AFP, hCG. |
|   Yolk sac (endodermal sinus) tumor | Yellow, mucinous. Analogous to ovarian yolk sac tumor. Schiller-Duval bodies resemble primitive glomeruli (↑ AFP). |
|   Choriocarcinoma | Malignant, ↑ hCG. Disordered syncytiotrophoblastic and cytotrophoblastic elements. Hematogenous metastases. |
|   Teratoma | Unlike in females, mature teratoma in males is most often malignant. |

| | |
|---|---|
| **Testicular non–germ cell tumors** | 5% of all testicular tumors. Mostly benign. |
|   Leydig cell | Contains Reinke crystals; usually androgen producing, gynecomastia in men, precocious puberty in boys. Golden brown color. |
|   Sertoli cell | Androblastoma from sex cord stroma. |
|   Testicular lymphoma | Most common testicular cancer in older men. |

| | |
|---|---|
| **Tunica vaginalis lesions** | Lesions in the serous covering of testis—present as testicular masses that can be transilluminated (vs. testicular tumors).<br>1. Varicocele—dilated vein in pampiniform plexus; can cause infertility; "bag of worms"<br>2. Hydrocele—↑ fluid 2° to incomplete fusion of processus vaginalis<br>3. Spermatocele—dilated epididymal duct |

| | |
|---|---|
| **Penile pathology** | |
|   **Carcinoma in situ** | |
|     Bowen's disease | Gray, solitary, crusty plaque, usually on the shaft of the penis or on the scrotum; peak incidence in 5th decade of life; progresses to invasive SCC in < 10% of cases. |
|     Erythroplasia of Queyrat | Red velvety plaques, usually involving the glans; otherwise similar to Bowen's disease. |
|     Bowenoid papulosis | Multiple papular lesions; affects younger age group than other subtypes; usually does not become invasive. |
|   **Squamous cell carcinoma (SCC)** | More common in Asia, Africa, and South America. Commonly associated with HPV, lack of circumcision. |
|   **Peyronie's disease** | Bent penis due to acquired fibrous tissue formation. |

## Control of reproductive hormones

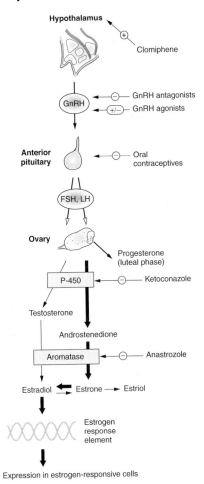

Control of female hormones

(Adapted, with permission, from Katzung BG. *Basic & Clinical Pharmacology,* 10th ed. New York: McGraw-Hill, 2006, Fig. 40-5.)

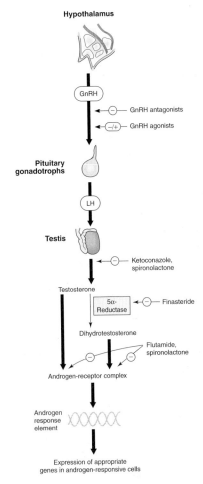

Control of androgen secretion

(Adapted, with permission, from Katzung BG. *Basic & Clinical Pharmacology,* 10th ed. New York: McGraw-Hill, 2006, Fig. 40-6.)

### Leuprolide

| | | |
|---|---|---|
| Mechanism | GnRH analog with agonist properties when used in pulsatile fashion; antagonist properties when used in continuous fashion. | **Leu**prolide can be used in **lieu** of GnRH. |
| Clinical use | Infertility (pulsatile), prostate cancer (continuous— use with flutamide), uterine fibroids. | |
| Toxicity | Antiandrogen, nausea, vomiting. | |

### Testosterone (methyltestosterone)

| | |
|---|---|
| Mechanism | Agonist at androgen receptors. |
| Clinical use | Treat hypogonadism and promote development of 2° sex characteristics; stimulation of anabolism to promote recovery after burn or injury; treat ER-positive breast cancer (exemestane). |
| Toxicity | Causes masculinization in females; reduces intratesticular testosterone in males by inhibiting release of LH (via negative feedback), leading to gonadal atrophy. Premature closure of epiphyseal plates. ↑ LDL, ↓ HDL. |

| | | |
|---|---|---|
| **Antiandrogens** | Testosterone $\xrightarrow{5\alpha\text{-reductase}}$ DHT (more potent). | |
| Finasteride (Propecia) | A 5α-reductase inhibitor (↓ conversion of testosterone to dihydrotestosterone). Useful in BPH. Also promotes hair growth—used to treat male-pattern baldness. | To prevent male-pattern hair loss, give a drug that will encourage female breast growth. |
| Flutamide | A nonsteroidal competitive inhibitor of androgens at the testosterone receptor. Used in prostate carcinoma. | Ketoconazole and spironolactone are used in the treatment of polycystic ovarian syndrome |
| Ketoconazole | Inhibits steroid synthesis (inhibits desmolase). | to prevent hirsutism. Both have side effects of |
| Spironolactone | Inhibits steroid binding. | gynecomastia and amenorrhea. |

**Estrogens (ethinyl estradiol, DES, mestranol)**

| | |
|---|---|
| Mechanism | Bind estrogen receptors. |
| Clinical use | Hypogonadism or ovarian failure, menstrual abnormalities, HRT in postmenopausal women; use in men with androgen-dependent prostate cancer. |
| Toxicity | ↑ risk of endometrial cancer, bleeding in postmenopausal women, clear cell adenocarcinoma of vagina in females exposed to DES in utero, ↑ risk of thrombi. Contraindications—ER-positive breast cancer, history of DVTs. |

**Estrogen partial agonists (selective estrogen receptor modulators—SERMs)**

| | |
|---|---|
| Clomiphene | Partial agonist at estrogen receptors in hypothalamus. Prevents normal feedback inhibition and ↑ release of LH and FSH from pituitary, which stimulates ovulation. Used to treat infertility and PCOS. May cause hot flashes, ovarian enlargement, multiple simultaneous pregnancies, and visual disturbances. |
| Tamoxifen | Antagonist on breast tissue; used to treat and prevent recurrence of ER-positive breast cancer. |
| Raloxifene | Agonist on bone; reduces resorption of bone; used to treat osteoporosis. |

| | |
|---|---|
| **Hormone replacement therapy (HRT)** | Used for relief or prevention of menopausal symptoms (e.g., hot flashes, vaginal atrophy) and osteoporosis (↑ estrogen, ↓ osteoclast activity). Unopposed estrogen replacement therapy (ERT) ↑ the risk of endometrial cancer, so progesterone is added. Possible ↑ CV risk. |

| | |
|---|---|
| **Anastrozole/ exemestane** | Aromatase inhibitors used in postmenopausal women with breast cancer. |

**Progestins**

| | |
|---|---|
| Mechanism | Bind progesterone receptors, reduce growth, and ↑ vascularization of endometrium. |
| Clinical use | Used in oral contraceptives and in the treatment of endometrial cancer and abnormal uterine bleeding. |

**Mifepristone (RU-486)**

| | |
|---|---|
| Mechanism | Competitive inhibitor of progestins at progesterone receptors. |
| Clinical use | Termination of pregnancy. Administered with misoprostol ($PGE_1$). |
| Toxicity | Heavy bleeding, GI effects (nausea, vomiting, anorexia), abdominal pain. |

HIGH-YIELD SYSTEMS

REPRODUCTIVE

| Oral contraception (synthetic progestins, estrogen) | Oral contraceptives prevent estrogen surge, LH surge does not occur → ovulation does not occur. | |
|---|---|---|
| | **Advantages** | **Disadvantages** |
| | Reliable (< 1% failure) | Taken daily |
| | ↓ risk of endometrial and ovarian cancer | No protection against STDs |
| | | ↑ triglycerides |
| | ↓ incidence of ectopic pregnancy | Depression, weight gain, nausea, hypertension |
| | ↓ pelvic infections | Hypercoagulable state |
| | Regulation of menses | |

| **Dinoprostone** | $PGE_2$ analog causing cervical dilation and uterine contraction, inducing labor. | |
|---|---|---|

| **Ritodrine/terbutaline** | $\beta_2$-agonists that relax the uterus; reduce premature uterine contractions. | **Ritodrine** allows the fetus to "**return to dreams**" by preventing early delivery. |
|---|---|---|

| **Tamsulosin** | $\alpha_1$-antagonist used to treat BPH by inhibiting smooth muscle contraction. Selective for $\alpha_{1A,D}$ receptors (found on prostate) vs. vascular $\alpha_{1B}$ receptors. | |
|---|---|---|

| **Sildenafil, vardenafil** | | |
|---|---|---|
| Mechanism | Inhibit cGMP phosphodiesterase, causing ↑ cGMP, smooth muscle relaxation in the corpus cavernosum, ↑ blood flow, and penile erection. | Silden**afil** and varden**afil** **fill** the penis. |
| Clinical use | Treatment of erectile dysfunction. | |
| Toxicity | Headache, flushing, dyspepsia, impaired blue-green color vision. Risk of life-threatening hypotension in patients taking nitrates. | "**H**ot and sweaty," but then **H**eadache, **H**eartburn, **H**ypotension. |

# Respiratory

*"There's so much pollution in the air now that if it weren't for our lungs, there'd be no place to put it all."*

—Robert Orben

*"Mars is essentially in the same orbit. Somewhat the same distance from the Sun, which is very important. We have seen pictures where there are canals, we believe, and water. If there is water, that means there is oxygen. If there is oxygen, that means we can breathe."*

—Former Vice President Dan Quayle

▷ Anatomy

▷ Physiology

▷ Pathology

▷ Pharmacology

**Respiratory tree**

Conducting zone — Consists of nose, pharynx, trachea, bronchi, bronchioles, and terminal bronchioles. Cartilage is present only in the trachea and bronchi. Brings air in and out. Warms, humidifies, filters air. Anatomic dead space. Walls of conducting airways contain smooth muscle.

Respiratory zone — Consists of respiratory bronchioles, alveolar ducts, and alveoli. Participates in gas exchange.

**Pneumocytes**

Pseudostratified ciliated columnar cells extend to the respiratory bronchioles (macrophages clear debris in alveoli); goblet cells extend only to the terminal bronchioles.

Type I cells (97% of alveolar surfaces) line the alveoli. Squamous; thin for optimal gas diffusion.

Type II cells (3%) secrete pulmonary surfactant (dipalmitoyl phosphatidylcholine), which ↓ the alveolar surface tension. Cuboidal and clustered. Also serve as precursors to type I cells and other type II cells. Type II cells proliferate during lung damage.

Clara cells—nonciliated; columnar with secretory granules. Secrete component of surfactant; degrade toxins; act as reserve cells.

Mucus secretions are swept out of the lungs toward the mouth by ciliated cells.

A lecithin-to-sphingomyelin ratio of > 2.0 in amniotic fluid is indicative of fetal lung maturity.

**Gas exchange barrier**

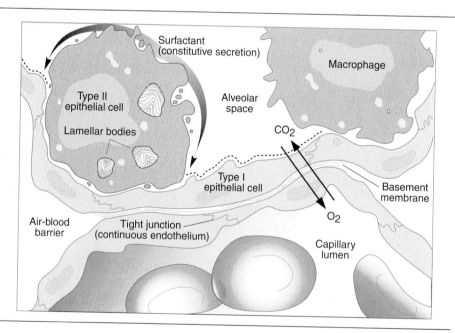

| | | |
|---|---|---|
| **Bronchopulmonary segments** | Each bronchopulmonary segment has a 3° (segmental) bronchus and 2 arteries (bronchial and pulmonary) in the center; veins and lymphatics drain along the borders.<br>Pulmonary arteries carry deoxygenated blood from the right side of the heart. Elastic walls maintain pulmonary arterial pressure at relatively constant levels throughout cardiac cycle. | Arteries run with Airways. |
| **Lung relations** | Right lung has 3 lobes; Left has 2 lobes and Lingula (homologue of right middle lobe). Right lung is more common site for inhaled foreign body because the right main stem bronchus is wider and more vertical than the left.<br>Aspirate a peanut:<br>  While upright—lower portion of right inferior lobe.<br>  While supine—superior portion of right inferior lobe. | Instead of a middle lobe, the left lung has a space occupied by the heart. The relation of the pulmonary artery to the bronchus at each lung hilus is described by RALS—Right Anterior; Left Superior. |

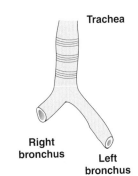
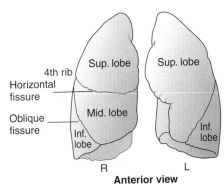
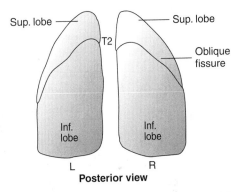

| | | |
|---|---|---|
| **Diaphragm structures** | Structures perforating diaphragm:<br>  At T8: IVC.<br>  At T10: esophagus, vagus (2 trunks).<br>  At T12: aorta (red), thoracic duct (white), azygous vein (blue).<br>Diaphragm is innervated by C3, 4, and 5 (phrenic nerve). Pain from the diaphragm can be referred to the shoulder. | Number of letters = T level:<br>  T8: vena cava<br>  T10: (o)esophagus<br>  T12: aortic hiatus<br>"I (IVC) ate (8) ten (10) eggs (esophagus) at (aorta) twelve (12)."<br>"C3, 4, 5 keeps the diaphragm alive." |

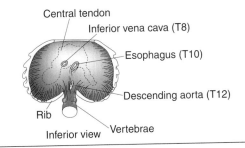

**Muscles of respiration**

Quiet breathing:
  Inspiration—diaphragm.
  Expiration—passive.
Exercise:
  InSpiration—external intercostals, Scalene muscles, Sternomastoids.
  Expiration—rectus abdominis, internal and external obliques, transversus abdominis, internal intercostals.

▶ RESPIRATORY—PHYSIOLOGY

**Important lung products**

1. Surfactant—produced by type II pneumocytes, ↓ alveolar surface tension, ↑ compliance, ↓ work of inspiration
2. Prostaglandins
3. Histamine ↑ bronchoconstriction
4. Angiotensin-converting enzyme (ACE)— angiotensin I → angiotensin II; inactivates bradykinin (ACE inhibitors ↑ bradykinin and cause cough, angioedema)
5. Kallikrein—activates bradykinin

**Surfactant**—dipalmitoyl phosphatidylcholine (lecithin) deficient in neonatal RDS.

Collapsing pressure =
$$\frac{2 \text{ (tension)}}{\text{radius}}$$

Tendency to collapse on expiration as radius ↓.

**Lung volumes**

1. Residual volume (RV)—air in lung after maximal expiration; cannot be measured on spirometry
2. Expiratory reserve volume (ERV)—air that can still be breathed out after normal expiration
3. Tidal volume (TV)—air that moves into lung with each quiet inspiration, typically 500 mL
4. Inspiratory reserve volume (IRV)—air in excess of tidal volume that moves into lung on maximum inspiration
5. Vital capacity (VC): TV + IRV + ERV
6. Functional residual capacity (FRC): RV + ERV (volume in lungs after normal expiration)
7. Inspiratory capacity (IC): IRV + TV
8. Total lung capacity: TLC = IRV + TV + ERV + RV

Vital capacity is everything but the residual volume.

A capacity is a sum of ≥ 2 volumes.

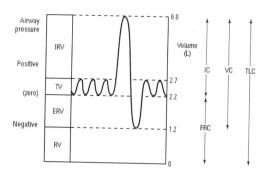

## Determination of physiologic dead space

$$V_D = V_T \times \frac{(PaCO_2 - PeCO_2)}{PaCO_2}$$

$V_D$ = physiologic dead space = anatomical dead space of conducting airways plus functional dead space in alveoli; apex of healthy lung is largest contributor of functional dead space. Volume of inspired air that does not take part in gas exchange.

$V_T$ = tidal volume.

$PaCO_2$ = arterial $PCO_2$, $PeCO_2$ = expired air $PCO_2$.

## Lung and chest wall

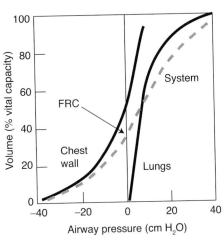

Relaxation pressure-volume curve

Tendency for lungs to collapse inward and chest wall to spring outward.

At FRC, inward pull of lung is balanced by outward pull of chest wall, and system pressure is atmospheric.

Elastic properties of both chest wall and lungs determine their combined volume.

## Hemoglobin

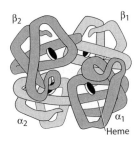

Hemoglobin is composed of 4 polypeptide subunits (2 α and 2 β) and exists in 2 forms:
1. T (taut) form has low affinity for $O_2$.
2. R (relaxed) form has high affinity for $O_2$ (300×). Hemoglobin exhibits positive cooperativity and negative allostery (accounts for the sigmoid-shaped $O_2$ dissociation curve for hemoglobin), unlike myoglobin.

↑ Cl⁻, H⁺, $CO_2$, 2,3-BPG, and temperature favor T form over **R** form (shifts dissociation curve to right, leading to ↑ $O_2$ unloading).

Fetal hemoglobin (2α and 2γ subunits) has lower affinity for 2,3-BPG than adult hemoglobin (HbA) and thus has higher affinity for $O_2$.

When you're **R**elaxed, you do your job better (carry $O_2$).

| **Hemoglobin modifications** | Lead to tissue hypoxia from ↓ $O_2$ saturation and ↓ $O_2$ content. | |
|---|---|---|
| Methemoglobin | Oxidized form of hemoglobin (ferric, $Fe^{3+}$) that does not bind $O_2$ as readily, but has ↑ affinity for $CN^-$.<br><br>Iron in hemoglobin is normally in a reduced state (ferrous, $Fe^{2+}$).<br><br>To treat cyanide poisoning, use nitrites to oxidize hemoglobin to methemoglobin, which binds cyanide, allowing cytochrome oxidase to function. Use thiosulfate to bind this cyanide, forming thiocyanate, which is renally excreted. | **METH**emoglobinemia can be treated with **METH**ylene blue. |
| Carboxyhemoglobin | Form of hemoglobin bound to CO in place of $O_2$. Causes ↓ oxygen-binding capacity with a left shift in the oxygen-hemoglobin dissociation curve. ↓ oxygen unloading in tissues. | CO has 200 × greater affinity than $O_2$ for hemoglobin. |

## Oxygen-hemoglobin dissociation curve

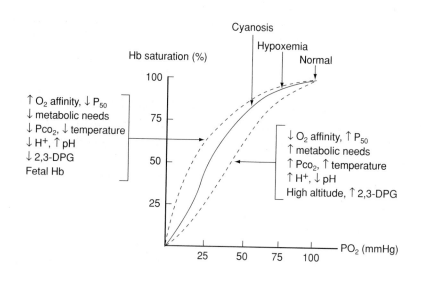

Sigmoidal shape due to positive cooperativity, i.e., hemoglobin can bind 4 oxygen molecules and has higher affinity for each subsequent oxygen molecule bound.

When curve shifts to the right, ↓ affinity of hemoglobin for $O_2$ (facilitates unloading of $O_2$ to tissue).

An ↑ in all factors (except pH) causes a shift of the curve to the right.

A ↓ in all factors (except pH) causes a shift of the curve to the left.

Fetal Hb has a higher affinity for oxygen than adult Hb, so its dissociation curve is shifted left.

**Right** shift—**CADET** face **right**:
$CO_2$
Acid/Altitude
DPG (2,3-DPG)
Exercise
Temperature

**V/Q mismatch**

Ideally, ventilation is matched to perfusion (i.e., V/Q = 1) in order for adequate gas exchange to occur.

Lung zones:
1. Apex of the lung—V/Q = 3 (wasted ventilation)
2. Base of the lung—V/Q = 0.6 (wasted perfusion)

Both ventilation and perfusion are greater at the base of the lung than at the apex of the lung.

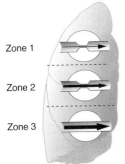

Zone 1

Zone 2

Zone 3

Apex: $P_A > P_a > P_v \rightarrow$ V/Q = 3 (wasted ventilation, ↑ dead space); NOTE: high alveolar pressure compresses capillaries

$P_a > P_A > P_v$

Base: $P_a > P_v > P_A \rightarrow$ V/Q = 0.6 (wasted perfusion); NOTE: both ventilation and perfusion are greater at the base of the lung than at the apex

With exercise (↑ cardiac output), there is vasodilation of apical capillaries, resulting in a V/Q ratio that approaches 1.

Certain organisms that thrive in high $O_2$ (e.g., TB) flourish in the apex.

V/Q → 0 = airway obstruction (shunt). In shunt, 100% $O_2$ does not improve $P_{O_2}$.

V/Q → ∞ = blood flow obstruction (physiologic dead space). Assuming < 100% dead space, 100% $O_2$ improves $P_{O_2}$.

---

**$CO_2$ transport**

Carbon dioxide is transported from tissues to the lungs in 3 forms:
1. **Bicarbonate (90%)**

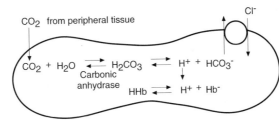

$CO_2$ from peripheral tissue

$CO_2 + H_2O \rightleftharpoons H_2CO_3 \rightleftharpoons H^+ + HCO_3^-$

Carbonic anhydrase

$HHb \rightleftharpoons H^+ + Hb^-$

$Cl^-$

(Figure modified, with permission, from Ganong WF. *Review of Medical Physiology,* 22nd ed. New York: McGraw-Hill, 2005: 670.)

2. Bound to hemoglobin at N terminus of globin (**not** heme) as carbaminohemoglobin (5%). $CO_2$ binding favors taut form ($O_2$ unloaded).
3. Dissolved $CO_2$ (5%).

In lungs, oxygenation of Hb promotes dissociation of $H^+$ from Hb. This shifts equilibrium toward $CO_2$ formation; therefore, $CO_2$ is released from RBCs (Haldane effect).

In peripheral tissue, ↑ $H^+$ from tissue metabolism shifts curve to right, unloading $O_2$ (Bohr effect).

---

**Response to high altitude**

1. Acute ↑ in ventilation
2. Chronic ↑ in ventilation
3. ↑ erythropoietin → ↑ hematocrit and hemoglobin (chronic hypoxia)
4. ↑ 2,3-DPG (binds to hemoglobin so that hemoglobin releases more $O_2$)
5. Cellular changes (↑ mitochondria)
6. ↑ renal excretion of bicarbonate (e.g., can augment by use of acetazolamide) to compensate for the respiratory alkalosis
7. Chronic hypoxic pulmonary vasoconstriction results in RVH

---

**Response to exercise**

1. ↑ $CO_2$ production
2. ↑ $O_2$ consumption
3. ↑ ventilation rate to meet $O_2$ demand
4. V/Q ratio from apex to base becomes more uniform
5. ↑ pulmonary blood flow due to ↑ cardiac output
6. ↓ pH during strenuous exercise (2° to lactic acidosis)
7. No change in $Pa_{O_2}$ and $Pa_{CO_2}$, but ↑ in venous $CO_2$ content

| | | |
|---|---|---|
| **Embolus types** | Fat, Air, Thrombus, Bacteria, Amniotic fluid, Tumor. Fat emboli are associated with long bone fractures and liposuction. Amniotic fluid emboli can lead to DIC, especially postpartum. Pulmonary embolus—chest pain, tachypnea, dyspnea. | An embolus moves like a **FAT BAT**. Approximately 95% of pulmonary emboli arise from deep leg veins. |
| **Deep venous thrombosis** | Predisposed by Virchow's triad: 1. Stasis 2. Hypercoagulability (e.g., defect in coagulative cascade proteins) 3. Endothelial damage (exposed collagen provides impetus for clotting cascade) | Can lead to pulmonary embolus. Homans' sign— dorsiflexion of foot → tender calf muscle. Prevent with heparin. |

**Obstructive lung disease (COPD)**

Obstruction of air flow resulting in air trapping in the lungs. Airways close prematurely at high lung volumes, resulting in ↑ RV and ↓ FVC. PFTs: ↓↓ $FEV_1$, ↓ FVC → ↓ $FEV_1$/FVC ratio (hallmark), V/Q mismatch.

| Type | Pathology | Other |
|---|---|---|
| Chronic **B**ronchitis ("**B**lue **B**loater") | Hypertrophy of mucus-secreting glands in the bronchioles → Reid index = gland depth / total thickness of bronchial wall; in COPD, Reid index > 50%. | Productive cough for > 3 consecutive months in ≥ 2 years. Disease of small airways. Findings: wheezing, crackles, cyanosis (early-onset hypoxemia due to shunting), late-onset dyspnea. |
| Emphysema ("pink puffer," barrel-shaped chest) | Enlargement of air spaces and ↓ recoil resulting from destruction of alveolar walls. Centriacinar—caused by smoking. Panacinar—$\alpha_1$-antitrypsin deficiency (also liver cirrhosis). Paraseptal emphysema—associated with bullae → can rupture → spontaneous pneumothorax; often in young, otherwise healthy males. | ↑ elastase activity. ↑ lung compliance due to loss of elastic fibers. Exhale through pursed lips to ↑ airway pressure and prevent airway collapse during exhalation. Findings: dyspnea, ↓ breath sounds, tachycardia, late-onset hypoxemia due to eventual loss of capillary beds (occurs with loss of alveolar walls), early-onset dyspnea. |
| Asthma | Bronchial hyperresponsiveness causes reversible bronchoconstriction. Smooth muscle hypertrophy and Curschmann's spirals (shed epithelium from mucous plugs). | Can be triggered by viral URIs, allergens, and stress. Findings: cough, wheezing, dyspnea, tachypnea, hypoxemia, ↓ I/E ratio, pulsus paradoxus, mucus plugging. |
| Bronchiectasis | Chronic necrotizing infection of bronchi → permanently dilated airways, purulent sputum, recurrent infections, hemoptysis. | Associated with bronchial obstruction, CF, poor ciliary motility, Kartagener's syndrome. Can develop aspergillosis. |

| **Restrictive lung disease** | Restricted lung expansion causes ↓ lung volumes (↓ FVC and TLC). PFTs—$FEV_1$/FVC ratio > 80%. |
|---|---|

Types:
1. Poor breathing mechanics (extrapulmonary, peripheral hypoventilation):
   a. Poor muscular effort—polio, myasthenia gravis
   b. Poor structural apparatus—scoliosis, morbid obesity
2. Interstitial lung diseases (pulmonary, lowered diffusing capacity):
   a. Acute respiratory distress syndrome (ARDS)
   b. Neonatal respiratory distress syndrome (hyaline membrane disease)
   c. Pneumoconioses (coal miner's, silicosis, asbestosis)
   d. Sarcoidosis
   e. Idiopathic pulmonary fibrosis (repeated cycles of lung injury and wound healing with ↑ collagen)
   f. Goodpasture's syndrome
   g. Wegener's granulomatosis
   h. Eosinophilic granuloma (histiocytosis X)
   i. Drug toxicity (bleomycin, busulfan, amiodarone)

**Pneumoconioses**

| | | |
|---|---|---|
| Coal miner's | Associated with coal mines. Can result in cor pulmonale, Caplan's syndrome. | Affects upper lobes. |
| Silicosis | Associated with foundries, sandblasting, and mines. Macrophages respond to silica and release fibrogenic factors, leading to fibrosis. It is thought that silica may disrupt phagolysosomes and impair macrophages, increasing susceptibility to TB. | Affects upper lobes. "Eggshell" calcification of hilar lymph nodes. |
| Asbestosis | Associated with shipbuilding, roofing, and plumbing. Results in "ivory white," calcified pleural plaques. Associated with an ↑ incidence of bronchogenic carcinoma and mesothelioma (see Image 42). | Affects lower lobes. Asbestos bodies are golden-brown fusiform rods resembling dumbbells, located inside macrophages. |

| **Neonatal respiratory distress syndrome** | Surfactant deficiency leading to ↑ surface tension, resulting in alveolar collapse. Surfactant is made by type II pneumocytes most abundantly after 35th week of gestation. The lecithin-to-sphingomyelin ratio in the amniotic fluid, a measure of lung maturity, is usually < 1.5 in neonatal respiratory distress syndrome. Persistently low $O_2$ tension → risk of PDA. Therapeutic supplemental $O_2$ can result in retinopathy of prematurity.<br><br>Surfactant—dipalmitoyl phosphatidylcholine.<br><br>Risk factors: prematurity, maternal diabetes (due to elevated insulin), cesarean delivery (↓ release of fetal glucocorticoids).<br><br>Treatment: maternal steroids before birth; artificial surfactant for infant; thyroxine. |
|---|---|

| **Acute respiratory distress syndrome (ARDS)** | May be caused by trauma, sepsis, shock, gastric aspiration, uremia, acute pancreatitis, or amniotic fluid embolism. Diffuse alveolar damage → ↑ alveolar capillary permeability → protein-rich leakage into alveoli. Results in formation of intra-alveolar hyaline membrane. Initial damage due to neutrophilic substances toxic to alveolar wall, activation of coagulation cascade, or oxygen-derived free radicals (see Image 39). |
|---|---|

### Obstructive vs. restrictive lung disease

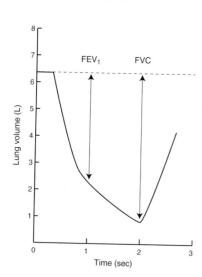

$\dfrac{FEV_1}{FVC} = 80\%$

**Normal**

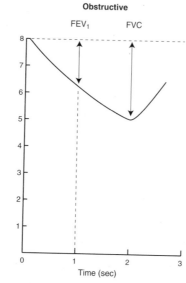

$\dfrac{FEV_1}{FVC} < 80\%$

**Obstructive**

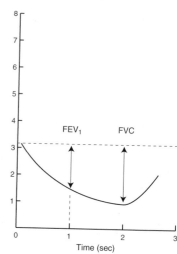

$\dfrac{FEV_1}{FVC} > 80\% \downarrow TLC$

**Restrictive**

Note: Obstructive lung volumes > normal ($\uparrow$ TLC, $\uparrow$ FRC, $\uparrow$ RV); restrictive lung volumes < normal. In both obstructive and restrictive, $FEV_1$ and FVC are reduced, but in obstructive, $FEV_1$ is more dramatically reduced, resulting in a $\downarrow FEV_1/FVC$ ratio.

| | |
|---|---|
| **Sleep apnea** | Person stops breathing for at least 10 seconds repeatedly during sleep.<br>**Central sleep apnea**—no respiratory effort.<br>**Obstructive sleep apnea**—respiratory effort against airway obstruction.<br>Associated with obesity, loud snoring, systemic/pulmonary hypertension, arrhythmias, and possibly sudden death.<br>Individuals may become chronically tired. |

Treatment: weight loss, CPAP, surgery.

### Lung—physical findings

| Abnormality | Breath Sounds | Resonance | Fremitus | Tracheal Deviation |
|---|---|---|---|---|
| Bronchial obstruction | Absent/$\downarrow$ over affected area | $\downarrow$ | $\downarrow$ | Toward side of lesion |
| Pleural effusion | $\downarrow$ over effusion | Dullness | $\downarrow$ | — |
| Pneumonia (lobar) | May have bronchial breath sounds over lesion | Dullness | $\uparrow$ | — |
| Tension pneumothorax | $\downarrow$ | Hyperresonant | Absent | Away from side of lesion (see Image 40) |

**Lung cancer**

Lung cancer is the leading cause of cancer death.

Presentation: cough, hemoptysis, bronchial obstruction, wheezing, pneumonic "coin" lesion on x-ray film.

Metastases to lung—most common; present with dyspnea.

Primary in lung—presents with cough.

**SPHERE** of complications:
**S**uperior vena cava syndrome
**P**ancoast's tumor
**H**orner's syndrome
**E**ndocrine (paraneoplastic)
**R**ecurrent laryngeal symptoms (hoarseness)
**E**ffusions (pleural or pericardial)

| Type | Location | Characteristics | Histology |
|---|---|---|---|
| Squamous cell carcinoma (Squamous Sentral Smoking) | Central | Hilar mass arising from bronchus; Cavitation; Clearly linked to Smoking; parathyroid-like activity → PTHrP. | Keratin pearls and intercellular bridges. |
| Adenocarcinoma: Bronchial<br><br>Bronchioloalveolar | Peripheral | Develops in site of prior pulmonary inflammation or injury (most common lung cancer in nonsmokers and females).<br>Not linked to smoking; grows along airways; can present like pneumonia.<br>Can result in hypertrophic osteoarthropathy. | Both types: Clara cells → type II pneumocytes; multiple densities on x-ray of chest. |
| Small cell (oat cell) carcinoma | Central | Undifferentiated → very aggressive; often associated with ectopic production of ACTH or ADH; may lead to Lambert-Eaton syndrome (autoantibodies against calcium channels). Responsive to chemotherapy. Inoperable. | Neoplasm of neuroendocrine Kulchitsky cells → small dark blue cells (see Image 37). |
| Large cell carcinoma | Peripheral | Highly anaplastic undifferentiated tumor; poor prognosis; less responsive to chemotherapy. Removed surgically. | Pleomorphic giant cells with leukocyte fragments in cytoplasm. |
| Carcinoid tumor | — | Secretes serotonin, can cause carcinoid syndrome (flushing, diarrhea, wheezing, salivation). | — |
| Mesothelioma | — | Malignancy of the pleura associated with asbestosis. Results in hemorrhagic pleural effusions and pleural thickening. | Psammoma bodies. |
| Metastases | — | Very common. Adrenals, brain (epilepsy), bone (pathologic fracture), and liver (jaundice, hepatomegaly). | — |

**Pancoast's tumor**

Carcinoma that occurs in apex of lung and may affect cervical sympathetic plexus, causing Horner's syndrome.

Horner's syndrome—ptosis, miosis, anhidrosis.

**Pneumonia**

| Type | Organism(s) | Characteristics |
|------|-------------|-----------------|
| Lobar | Pneumococcus most frequently, *Klebsiella* | Intra-alveolar exudate → consolidation; may involve entire lung |
| Bronchopneumonia | *S. aureus*, *H. flu*, *Klebsiella*, *S. pyogenes* | Acute inflammatory infiltrates from bronchioles into adjacent alveoli; patchy distribution involving ≥ 1 lobes (see Image 107). |
| Interstitial (atypical) pneumonia | Viruses (RSV, adenoviruses), *Mycoplasma*, *Legionella*, *Chlamydia* | Diffuse patchy inflammation localized to interstitial areas at alveolar walls; distribution involving ≥ 1 lobes. Generally follows a more indolent course than bronchopneumonia. |

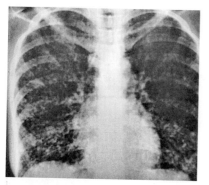

Interstitial pneumonia

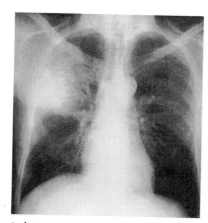

Lobar pneumonia

| | |
|---|---|
| **Lung abscess** | Localized collection of pus within parenchyma, usually resulting from bronchial obstruction (e.g., cancer) or aspiration of oropharyngeal contents (especially in patients predisposed to loss of consciousness, e.g., alcoholics or epileptics). Often due to *S. aureus* or anaerobes. |

**Pleural effusions**

| | |
|---|---|
| Transudate | ↓ protein content. Due to CHF, nephrotic syndrome, or hepatic cirrhosis. |
| Exudate | ↑ protein content, cloudy. Due to malignancy, pneumonia, collagen vascular disease, trauma (occurs in states of ↑ vascular permeability). Must be drained in light of risk of infection. |
| Lymphatic | Milky fluid; ↑ triglycerides. |

▶ RESPIRATORY–PHARMACOLOGY

| | |
|---|---|
| **H$_1$ blockers** | Reversible inhibitors of H$_1$ histamine receptors. |
| **1st generation** | Diphenhydramine, dimenhydrinate, chlorpheniramine. |
| Clinical uses | Allergy, motion sickness, sleep aid. |
| Toxicity | Sedation, antimuscarinic, anti-α-adrenergic. |
| **2nd generation** | Loratadine, fexofenadine, desloratadine, cetirizine. |
| Clinical uses | Allergy. |
| Toxicity | Far less sedating than 1st generation because of ↓ entry into CNS. |

HIGH-YIELD SYSTEMS

RESPIRATORY

| | |
|---|---|
| **Asthma drugs** | Bronchoconstriction is mediated by (1) inflammatory processes and (2) sympathetic tone; therapy is directed at these 2 pathways. |
| Nonspecific β-agonists β₂-agonists | **Isoproterenol**—relaxes bronchial smooth muscle ($\beta_2$). Adverse effect is tachycardia ($\beta_1$). **Albuterol**—relaxes bronchial smooth muscle ($\beta_2$). Use during acute exacerbation. **Salmeterol**—long-acting agent for prophylaxis. Adverse effects are tremor and arrhythmia. |
| Methylxanthines | **Theophylline**—likely causes bronchodilation by inhibiting phosphodiesterase, thereby ↓ cAMP hydrolysis. Usage is limited because of narrow therapeutic index (cardiotoxicity, neurotoxicity); metabolized by P-450. Blocks actions of adenosine. |
| Muscarinic antagonists | **Ipratropium**—competitive block of muscarinic receptors, preventing bronchoconstriction. Also used for COPD. |
| Cromolyn | Prevents release of mediators from mast cells. Effective only for the prophylaxis of asthma. Not effective during an acute asthmatic attack. Toxicity is rare. |
| Corticosteroids | **Beclomethasone, prednisone**—inhibit the synthesis of virtually all cytokines. Inactivate NF-κB, the transcription factor that induces the production of TNF-α, among other inflammatory agents. 1st-line therapy for chronic asthma. |
| Antileukotrienes | **Zileuton**—A 5-lipoxygenase pathway inhibitor. Blocks conversion of arachidonic acid to leukotrienes. **Zafirlukast, montelukast**—block leukotriene receptors. Especially good for aspirin-induced asthma. |

Treatment strategies in asthma

(Adapted, with permission, from Katzung BG, Trevor AJ. *Pharmacology: Examination & Board Review,* 5th ed. Stamford, CT: Appleton & Lange, 1998: 159 and 161.)

**Expectorants**

| | |
|---|---|
| Guaifenesin (Robitussin) | Removes excess sputum but large doses necessary; does not suppress cough reflex. |
| N-acetylcysteine | Mucolytic → can loosen mucous plugs in CF patients. Also used as an antidote for acetaminophen overdose. |

| | |
|---|---|
| **Bosentan** | Used to treat pulmonary hypertension. Competitively antagonizes endothelin-1 receptors, decreasing pulmonary vascular resistance. |

# Rapid Review

The following tables represent a collection of high-yield associations of diseases with their clinical findings and pathophysiology. They serve as a quick review before the exam to tune your senses to commonly tested cases and "buzzwords."

| Clinical presentation | Diagnosis/disease |
|---|---|
| Abdominal pain, ascites, hepatomegaly | Budd-Chiari syndrome (posthepatic venous thrombosis) |
| Achilles tendon xanthoma | Familial hypercholesterolemia |
| Adrenal hemorrhage, hypotension, DIC | Waterhouse-Friderichsen syndrome (meningococcemia) |
| Arachnodactyly, lens dislocation, aortic dissection, hyperflexible joints | Marfan's syndrome (fibrillin defect) |
| Back pain, fever, night sweats, weight loss | Pott's disease (vertebral tuberculosis) |
| Big toe extension/fanning upon plantar scrape | Babinski's sign (UMN lesion) |
| Bilateral hilar adenopathy, uveitis | Sarcoidosis (noncaseating granulomas) |
| Blue sclera | Osteogenesis imperfecta (collagen defect) |
| Bluish line on gingiva | Burton's line (lead poisoning) |
| Bone pain, bone enlargement, arthritis | Paget's disease of bone ($\uparrow$ osteoblastic and osteoclastic activity) |
| Café-au-lait spots, Lisch nodules (iris hamartoma) | Neurofibromatosis type I (+ bilateral acoustic neuromas = type II) |
| Calf pseudohypertrophy | Muscular dystrophy (most commonly Duchenne's) |
| "Cherry-red spot" on macula | Tay-Sachs (ganglioside accumulation) or Niemann-Pick (lysosomal storage disease) |
| Chest pain, pericardial effusion/friction rub, persistent fever following MI | Dressler's syndrome (autoimmune-mediated post-MI fibrinous pericarditis) |
| Child uses arms to stand up from squat | Gowers' sign (Duchenne muscular dystrophy: X-linked recessive deleted dystrophin gene) |
| Child with fever develops red rash on face that spreads to body | "Slapped cheeks" (erythema infectiosum/fifth disease: parvovirus B19) |
| Chorea, dementia, caudate degeneration | Huntington's disease (autosomal-dominant CAG repeat expansion) |
| Chronic exercise intolerance with myalgia, fatigue, painful cramps | McArdle's disease (muscle phosphorylase deficiency) |
| Cold intolerance | Hypothyroidism |
| Conjugate lateral gaze palsy, horizontal diplopia | Internuclear ophthalmoplegia (damage to MLF; bilateral [multiple sclerosis], unilateral [stroke]) |
| Continuous "machinery" heart murmur | PDA (close with indomethacin; open with misoprostol) |
| Cutaneous/dermal edema due to connective tissue deposition | Myxedema (hypothyroidism, Graves' disease) |
| Dark purple skin/mouth nodules | Kaposi's sarcoma (usually AIDS patients [gay men]: associated with HHV-8) |
| Deep, labored breathing/hyperventilation | Kussmaul breathing (diabetic ketoacidosis) |
| Dermatitis, dementia, diarrhea | Pellagra (niacin [vitamin B$_3$] deficiency) |

| | |
|---|---|
| Dilated cardiomyopathy, edema, polyneuropathy | Wet beriberi (thiamine [vitamin B$_1$] deficiency) |
| Dog or cat bite resulting in infection | *Pasteurella multocida* |
| Dry eyes, dry mouth, arthritis | Sjögren's syndrome (autoimmune destruction of exocrine glands) |
| Dysphagia (esophageal webs), glossitis, iron deficiency anemia | Plummer-Vinson syndrome (may progress to esophageal squamous cell carcinoma) |
| Elastic skin, hypermobility of joints | Ehlers-Danlos syndrome (collagen defect) |
| Enlarged, hard left supraclavicular node | Virchow's node (abdominal metastasis) |
| Erythroderma, lymphadenopathy, hepatosplenomegaly, atypical T cells | Sézary syndrome (cutaneous T-cell lymphoma) or mycosis fungoides |
| Facial muscle spasm upon tapping | Chvostek's sign (hypocalcemia) |
| Fat, female, forty, and fertile | Acute cholecystitis (bile duct blockage) |
| Fever, chills, headache, myalgia following antibiotic treatment for syphilis | Jarisch-Herxheimer reaction (rapid lysis of spirochetes results in toxin release) |
| Fever, cough, conjunctivitis, coryza, diffuse rash | Measles (Morbillivirus) |
| Fever, night sweats, weight loss | B symptoms (lymphoma) |
| Fibrous plaques in soft tissue of penis | Peyronie's disease (connective tissue disorder) |
| Gout, mental retardation, self-mutilating behavior in a boy | Lesch-Nyhan syndrome (HGPRT deficiency) |
| Green-yellow rings around peripheral cornea | Kayser-Fleischer rings (copper accumulation from Wilson's disease) |
| Hamartomatous GI polyps, hyperpigmentation of mouth/feet/hands | Peutz-Jeghers syndrome (genetic benign polyposis can cause bowel obstruction; ↑ cancer risk) |
| Hepatosplenomegaly, osteoporosis, neurologic symptoms | Gaucher's disease (glucocerebrosidase deficiency) |
| Hereditary nephritis, sensorineural hearing loss, cataracts | Alport's syndrome (collagen mutation) |
| Hypercoagulability (leading to migrating DVTs and vasculitis) | Trousseau's sign (adenocarcinoma of pancreas or lung) |
| Hyperphagia, hypersexuality, hyperorality, hyperdocility | Klüver-Bucy syndrome (bilateral amygdala lesion) |
| Hypertension, hypokalemia, metabolic acidosis | Conn's syndrome (1° hyperaldosteronism) |
| Hypoxemia, polycythemia, hypercapnia | "Blue bloater" (chronic bronchitis: hyperplasia of mucous cells) |
| Indurated, ulcerated genital lesion (nonpainful) | Chancre (1° syphilis: *Treponema pallidum*) |
| Infant with failure to thrive, hepatosplenomegaly, neurodegeneration | Niemann-Pick disease (genetic sphingomyelinase deficiency) |

| | |
|---|---|
| Infant with hypoglycemia, failure to thrive, and hepatomegaly | Cori's disease (debranching enzyme deficiency) |
| Infant with microcephaly, rocker-bottom feet, and structural heart defect | Edwards' syndrome (trisomy 18) |
| Jaundice, RUQ pain, fever | Charcot's triad 2 (ascending cholangitis) |
| Keratin pearls on a skin lesion | Squamous cell carcinoma |
| Large rash with bull's-eye appearance | Erythema chronicum migrans from tick bite (Lyme disease: *Borrelia*) |
| Lucid interval after traumatic brain injury | Epidural hematoma |
| Male child, recurrent infections, no mature B cells | Bruton's disease (X-linked agammaglobulinemia) |
| Mucosal bleeding and prolonged bleeding time | Glanzmann's thrombasthenia (defect in platelet aggregation due to lack of GpIIb/IIIa) |
| Multiple colon polyps, osteomas/soft tissue tumors, impacted/supernumerary teeth | Gardner's syndrome (genetic disorder, predisposes to colon cancer) |
| Necrotizing vasculitis (lungs) and necrotizing glomerulonephritis | Wegener's and Goodpasture's syndromes (hemoptysis and glomerular disease) |
| Neonate with arm paralysis following difficult birth | Erb-Duchenne palsy (superior trunk [C5–C6] brachial plexus injury: "waiter's tip") |
| No lactation postpartum, absent menstruation, cold intolerance | Sheehan's syndrome (pituitary infarction) |
| Nystagmus, intention tremor, scanning speech | Charcot's triad 1 (multiple sclerosis) |
| Oscillating slow/fast breathing | Cheyne-Stokes respirations (central apnea in CHF or ↑ intracranial pressure) |
| Painful blue fingers/toes, hemolytic anemia | Cold agglutinin disease (autoimmune hemolytic anemia caused by *Mycoplasma pneumoniae*, infectious mononucleosis) |
| Painful, pale, cold fingers/toes | Raynaud's syndrome (vasospasm in extremities) |
| Painful, raised red lesions on palms and soles | Osler's node (infective endocarditis) |
| Painless jaundice | Cancer of the pancreatic head obstructing bile duct |
| Palpable purpura, joint pain, abdominal pain (child) | Henoch-Schönlein purpura (IgA vasculitis affecting skin and kidneys) |
| Pancreatic, pituitary, parathyroid tumors | Wermer's syndrome (MEN 1) |
| Pink complexion, dyspnea, hyperventilation | "Pink puffer" (emphysema: centroacinar [smoking], panacinar [$\alpha_1$-antitrypsin deficiency]) |
| Polyostotic fibrous dysplasia, precocious puberty, café-au-lait spots, short stature in a young girl | McCune-Albright syndrome (mosaic G-protein signaling mutation) |

| | |
|---|---|
| Polyuria, acidosis, growth failure, electrolyte imbalances | Fanconi's syndrome (proximal tubular reabsorption defect) |
| Positive anterior "drawer sign" | Anterior cruciate ligament (ACL) injury |
| Ptosis, miosis, anhidrosis | Horner's syndrome (sympathetic chain lesion) |
| Pupil accommodates but doesn't react | Argyll Robertson pupil (neurosyphilis) |
| Rapidly progressive leg weakness that ascends (following GI/upper respiratory infection) | Guillain-Barré syndrome (autoimmune acute inflammatory demyelinating polyneuropathy) |
| Rash on palms and soles | 2° syphilis, Rocky Mountain spotted fever |
| Recurrent colds, unusual eczema, high serum IgE | Job's syndrome (hyper-IgE syndrome: neutrophil chemotaxis abnormality) |
| Red "currant jelly" sputum | *Klebsiella pneumoniae* |
| Red, itchy, swollen rash of nipple/areola | Paget's disease of the breast (represents underlying neoplasm) |
| Red urine in the morning | Paroxysmal nocturnal hemoglobinuria |
| Renal cell carcinoma, hemangioblastomas, angiomatosis, pheochromocytoma | von Hippel–Lindau disease (dominant tumor suppressor gene mutation) |
| Resting tremor, rigidity, akinesia, postural instability | Parkinson's disease (nigrostriatal dopamine depletion) |
| Restrictive cardiomyopathy (juvenile form: cardiomegaly), exercise intolerance | Pompe's disease (lysosomal glucosidase deficiency) |
| Retinal hemorrhages with pale centers | Roth's spots (bacterial endocarditis) |
| Severe jaundice in neonate | Crigler-Najjar syndrome (congenital unconjugated hyperbilirubinemia) |
| Severe RLQ pain with rebound tenderness | McBurney's sign (appendicitis) |
| Short stature, ↑ incidence of tumors/ leukemia, aplastic anemia | Fanconi's anemia (genetically inherited; often progresses to AML) |
| Single palm crease | Simian crease (Down syndrome) |
| Situs inversus, chronic sinusitis, bronchiectasis | Kartagener's syndrome (dynein defect affecting cilia) |
| Skin hyperpigmentation | Addison's disease (1° adrenocortical insufficiency of autoimmune or infectious etiology) |
| Slow, progressive muscle weakness in boys | Becker's muscular dystrophy (X-linked, defective dystrophin; less severe than Duchenne's) |
| Small, irregular red spots on buccal/ lingual mucosa with blue-white centers | Koplik spots (measles) |
| Small, nontender, erythematous lesions on palms/soles | Janeway lesions (infective endocarditis) |
| Smooth, flat, moist white lesions on genitals | Condylomata lata (2° syphilis) |
| Splinter hemorrhages in fingernails | Bacterial endocarditis |
| "Strawberry tongue" | Scarlet fever, Kawasaki disease, toxic shock syndrome |

| | |
|---|---|
| Streak ovaries, congenital heart disease, horseshoe kidney | Turner's syndrome (XO, short stature, webbed neck, lymphedema) |
| Sudden swollen/painful big toe joint, tophi | Gout/podagra (hyperuricemia) |
| Swollen gums, mucous bleeding, poor wound healing, spots on skin | Scurvy (vitamin C deficiency: can't hydroxylate proline/lysine for collagen synthesis) |
| Swollen, hard, painful finger joints | Osteoarthritis (osteophytes on PIP [Bouchard's nodes], DIP [Heberden's nodes]) |
| Systolic ejection murmur (crescendo-decrescendo) | Aortic valve stenosis |
| Thyroid, parathyroid, adrenal tumors | Sipple's syndrome (MEN 2A) |
| Ulcerated genital lesion with exudate (painful) | Chancroid (*Haemophilus ducreyi*) |
| Unilateral facial drooping | Bell's palsy (LMN CN VII palsy) |
| Urethritis, conjunctivitis, arthritis in a male | Reiter's syndrome (reactive arthritis associated with HLA-B27) |
| Vascular birthmark (port-wine stain) | Hemangioma (benign, but associated with Sturge-Weber syndrome) |
| Vasculitis from exposure to endotoxin causing glomerular thrombosis | Shwartzman reaction (following second exposure to endotoxin) |
| Vomiting blood following esophagogastric lacerations | Mallory-Weiss syndrome (alcoholics and eating disorders) |
| "Waxy" casts with very low urine flow | Chronic end-stage renal disease |
| WBC casts in urine | Acute pyelonephritis or cystitis |
| Weight loss, diarrhea, arthritis, fever, adenopathy | Whipple's disease (*Tropheryma whippelii*) |
| "Worst headache of my life" | Berry aneurysm (associated with adult polycystic kidney disease) |

| Lab/diagnostic finding | Diagnosis/disease |
|---|---|
| Anticentromere antibodies | Scleroderma (CREST) |
| Antidesmoglein (epithelial) antibodies | Pemphigus vulgaris (blistering) |
| Anti–glomerular basement membrane antibodies | Goodpasture's syndrome (glomerulonephritis and lung hemorrhage) |
| Antihistone antibodies | Drug-induced SLE |
| Anti-IgG antibodies | Rheumatoid arthritis (systemic inflammation, joint pannus, boutonnière deformity) |
| Antimitochondrial antibodies (AMAs) | 1° biliary cirrhosis (female, cholestasis, portal hypertension) |
| Antineutrophil cytoplasmic antibodies (ANCAs) | Vasculitis (Wegener's, microscopic polyangiitis, glomerulonephritis) |
| Antinuclear antibodies (ANAs: anti-Smith and anti-dsDNA) | SLE (type III hypersensitivity) |
| Antiplatelet antibodies | Idiopathic thrombocytopenic purpura (ITP) (bleeding diathesis) |
| Anti-topoisomerase antibodies | Diffuse systemic scleroderma |
| Anti-transglutaminase/antigliadin antibodies | Celiac disease (diarrhea, distention, weight loss) |
| Azurophilic granular needles in leukemic blasts | Auer rods (acute myelogenous leukemia: especially the promyelocytic type) |
| "Bamboo spine" on x-ray | Ankylosing spondylitis (chronic inflammatory arthritis: HLA-B27) |
| Basophilic nuclear remnants in RBCs | Howell-Jolly bodies (due to splenectomy or nonfunctional spleen) |
| Basophilic stippling of RBCs | Lead poisoning or sideroblastic anemia |
| Bloody tap on LP | Subarachnoid hemorrhage |
| "Boot-shaped" heart on x-ray | Tetralogy of Fallot, RVH |
| Branching gram-positive rods with sulfur granules | *Actinomyces israelii* |
| Bronchogenic apical lung tumor | Pancoast's tumor (can compress sympathetic ganglion and cause Horner's syndrome) |
| "Brown" tumor of bone | Hemorrhage (hemosiderin) causes brown color of osteolytic cysts. Due to:<br>1. Hyperparathyroidism<br>2. Osteitis fibrosa cystica (von Recklinghausen's disease of bone) |
| Cardiomegaly with apical atrophy | Chagas' disease (*Trypanosoma cruzi*) |
| Cellular crescents in Bowman's capsule | Rapidly progressive crescentic glomerulonephritis |
| "Chocolate cyst" of ovary | Endometriosis (frequently involves both ovaries) |
| Circular grouping of dark tumor cells surrounding pale neurofibrils | Homer Wright rosettes (neuroblastoma, medulloblastoma, retinoblastoma) |
| Colonies of mucoid *Pseudomonas* in lungs | Cystic fibrosis (CFTR mutation in Caucasians resulting in fat-soluble vitamin deficiency and mucous plugs) |

| | |
|---|---|
| Degeneration of dorsal column nerves | Tabes dorsalis (3° syphilis) |
| Depigmentation of neurons in substantia nigra | Parkinson's disease (basal ganglia disorder: rigidity, resting tremor, bradykinesia) |
| Desquamated epithelium casts in sputum | Curschmann's spirals (bronchial asthma; can result in whorled mucous plugs) |
| Disarrayed granulosa cells in eosinophilic fluid | Call-Exner bodies (granulosa-theca cell tumor of the ovary) |
| Dysplastic squamous cervical cells with nuclear enlargement and hyperchromasia | Koilocytes (HPV: predisposes to cervical cancer) |
| Enlarged cells with intranuclear inclusion bodies | "Owl's-eye" appearance of CMV |
| Enlarged thyroid cells with ground-glass nuclei | "Orphan Annie" eye nuclei (papillary carcinoma of the thyroid) |
| Eosinophilic cytoplasmic inclusion in liver cell | Mallory bodies (alcoholic liver disease) |
| Eosinophilic cytoplasmic inclusion in nerve cell | Lewy body (Parkinson's disease) |
| Eosinophilic globule in liver | Councilman body (toxic or viral hepatitis, often yellow fever) |
| Eosinophilic inclusion bodies in cytoplasm of hippocampal nerve cells | Rabies virus (Lyssavirus) |
| Extracellular amyloid deposition in gray matter of brain | Senile plaques (Alzheimer's disease) |
| Giant B cells with bilobed nuclei with prominent inclusions ("owl's eye") | Reed-Sternberg cells (Hodgkin's lymphoma) |
| Glomerulus-like structure surrounding vessel in germ cells | Schiller-Duval bodies (yolk sac tumor) |
| "Hair-on-end" (crew-cut) appearance on x-ray | $\beta$-thalassemia, sickle cell anemia (extramedullary hematopoiesis) |
| hCG elevated | Choriocarcinoma, hydatidiform mole (occurs with and without embryo) |
| Heart nodules (inflammatory) | Aschoff bodies (rheumatic fever) |
| Heterophile antibodies | Infectious mononucleosis (EBV) |
| Hexagonal, double-pointed, needle-like crystals in bronchial secretions | Bronchial asthma (Charcot-Leyden crystals: eosinophilic granules) |
| High level of D-dimers | DVT, pulmonary embolism, DIC |
| "Honeycomb lung" on x-ray | Interstitial fibrosis |
| Hypersegmented neutrophils | Megaloblastic anemia ($B_{12}$, folate deficiency) |
| Hypochromic, microcytic anemia | Iron deficiency anemia, lead poisoning, thalassemia (HbF sometimes present) |

| | |
|---|---|
| Increased α-fetoprotein in amniotic fluid/maternal serum | Anencephaly, spina bifida (neural tube defects) |
| Increased uric acid levels | Gout, Lesch-Nyhan syndrome, myeloproliferative disorders, loop and thiazide diuretics |
| Intranuclear eosinophilic droplet-like bodies | Cowdry type A bodies (HSV or yellow fever) |
| Iron-containing nodules in alveolar septum | Ferruginous bodies (asbestosis: ↑ chance of mesothelioma) |
| Large lysosomal vesicles in phagocytes, immunocompromised | Chédiak-Higashi disease (failure of phagolysosome formation) |
| Low serum ceruloplasmin | Wilson's disease (hepatolenticular degeneration) |
| "Lumpy-bumpy" appearance of glomeruli on immunofluorescence | Poststreptococcal glomerulonephritis |
| Lytic ("hole-punched") bone lesions on x-ray | Multiple myeloma |
| Mammary gland ("blue-domed") cyst | Fibrocystic change of the breast |
| Monoclonal antibody spike | 1. Multiple myeloma (called the M protein; usually IgG or IgA)<br>2. Monoclonal gammopathy of undetermined significance (MGUS)<br>3. Waldenström's (M protein = IgM) macroglobulinemia |
| Monoclonal globulin protein in blood/urine | Bence Jones proteins (multiple myeloma [kappa or lambda Ig light chains in urine]), Waldenström's macroglobulinemia (IgM) |
| Mucin-filled cell with peripheral nucleus | Signet ring (gastric carcinoma) |
| Narrowing of bowel lumen on barium radiograph | "String sign" (Crohn's disease) |
| Needle-shaped, negatively birefringent crystals | Gout (hyperuricemia) |
| Nodular hyaline deposits in glomeruli | Kimmelstiel-Wilson nodules (diabetic nephropathy) |
| "Nutmeg" appearance of liver | Chronic passive congestion of liver due to right heart failure |
| "Onion-skin" periosteal reaction | Ewing's sarcoma (malignant round-cell tumor) |
| Periosteum raised from bone, creating triangular area | Codman's triangle on x-ray (osteosarcoma, Ewing's sarcoma, pyogenic osteomyelitis) |
| Podocyte fusion on EM | Minimal change disease (child with nephrotic syndrome) |
| Polished, "ivory-like" appearance of bone at cartilage erosion | Eburnation (osteoarthritis resulting in bony sclerosis) |
| Protein aggregates in neurons from hyperphosphorylation of protein tau | Neurofibrillary tangles (Alzheimer's disease and CJD) |
| Pseudopalisade tumor cell arrangement | Glioblastoma multiforme |
| RBC casts in urine | Acute glomerulonephritis |
| Rectangular, crystal-like inclusions in Leydig cells | Reinke crystals (Leydig cell tumor) |

| | |
|---|---|
| Renal epithelial casts in urine | Acute toxic/viral nephrosis |
| Rhomboid crystals, positively birefringent | Pseudogout (calcium pyrophosphate dihydrate) |
| Rib notching | Coarctation of the aorta |
| Sheets of medium-sized lymphoid cells ("starry sky" appearance on histology) | Burkitt's lymphoma (t[8:14] c-myc activation, associated with EBV) |
| Silver-staining spherical aggregation of tau proteins in neurons | Pick bodies (Pick's disease: progressive dementia, similar to Alzheimer's) |
| Small granulomatous lesion in lungs (can calcify) | Ghon focus (1° TB: Mycobacterium bacilli) |
| Small, round RBC inclusions | Heinz bodies (G6PD deficiency, α-thalassemia, chronic liver disease) |
| "Soap bubble" on x-ray | Giant cell tumor of bone (generally benign) |
| "Spikes" on basement membrane, "dome-like" endothelial deposits | Membranous glomerulonephritis (may progress to nephrotic syndrome) |
| Stacks of red blood cells | Rouleaux formation (high ESR: multiple myeloma) |
| Stippled vaginal epithelial cells | "Clue cells" (Gardnerella vaginalis) |
| "Tennis-racket"-shaped cytoplasmic organelles (EM) in Langerhans cells | Birbeck granules (histiocytosis X: eosinophilic granuloma) |
| Thrombi made of white/red layers | Lines of Zahn (arterial thrombus, layers of platelets/RBCs) |
| "Thumb sign" on lateral x-ray | Epiglottitis (Haemophilus influenzae) |
| Thyroid-like appearance of kidney | Chronic bacterial pyelonephritis |
| "Tram-track" appearance on LM | Membranoproliferative glomerulonephritis |
| Triglyceride accumulation in liver cell vacuoles | Fatty liver disease (alcoholic or metabolic syndrome) |
| WBCs that look "smudged" | CLL (almost always B cell; affects the elderly) |
| "Wire loop" glomerular appearance on LM | Lupus nephropathy |
| Yellow CSF | Xanthochromia (subarachnoid hemorrhage) |

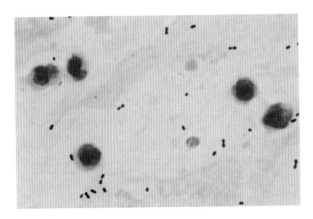

**Image 1. *Streptococcus pneumoniae.*** Sputum sample from a patient with pneumonia shows gram-positive diplococci.

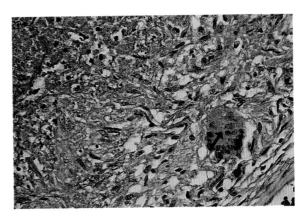

**Image 2A. *Mycobacterium tuberculosis*** is characterized by caseating granulomas containing Langhans' giant cells, which have a "horseshoe" pattern of nuclei (see arrow).*

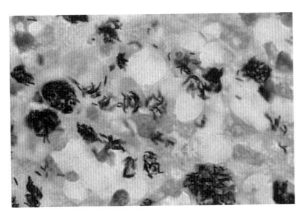

**Image 2B. *Mycobacterium tuberculosis*** organisms are identified by their red color on acid-fast staining ("red snappers").*

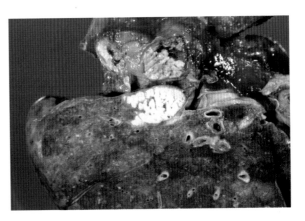

**Image 2C. Miliary tuberculosis** is seen here with large caseous lesions at the left medial upper lobe and miliary lesions in the surrounding hilar node. This life-threatening infection is caused by blood-borne dissemination of *Mycobacterium tuberculosis* to many organs from a quiescent site of infection.*

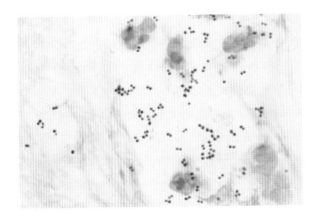

**Image 3. *Staphylococcus aureus.*** Sputum sample from another patient with pneumonia shows gram-positive cocci in clusters.

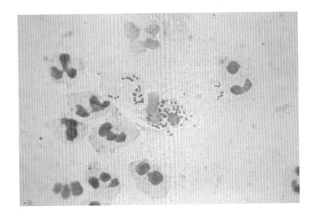

**Image 4. *Neisseria gonorrhoeae.*** Gram stain shows multiple gram-negative diplococci within polymorphonuclear leukocytes as well as in the extracellular areas of a smear from a urethral discharge. (Reproduced, with permission, from Wolff K et al. *Fitzpatrick's Color Atlas and Synopsis of Clinical Dermatology*, 5th ed. New York: McGraw-Hill, 2005: 906.)

*Images reproduced courtesy of the Pathology Education Instructional Resource Digital Library (http://peir.net) at the University of Alabama, Birmingham.

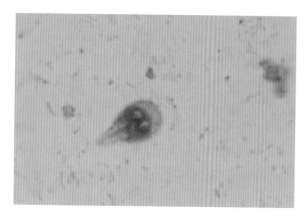

Image 5. *Giardia lamblia,* small intestine, microscopic. The trophozoite has a classic pear shape, with double nuclei giving an "owl's-eye" appearance.

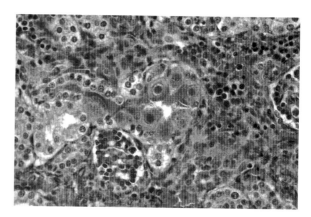

Image 6. **Cytomegalovirus (CMV).** Renal tubular cells in a neonate with congenital CMV infection show prominent Cowdry type A nuclear inclusions resembling owls' eyes. (Reproduced, with permission, from USMLERx.com.)

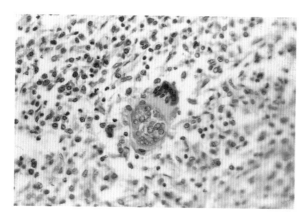

Image 7. **Coccidioidomycosis.** Endospores within a spherule in infected lung parenchyma. Initial infection usually resolves spontaneously, but when immunity is compromised, dissemination to almost any organ can occur. Endemic in the southwestern United States.

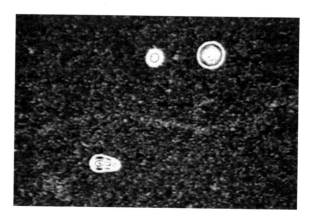

Image 8. *Cryptococcus neoformans.* The polysaccharide capsule is visible by India ink preparation in CSF from an AIDS patient with meningoencephalitis.*

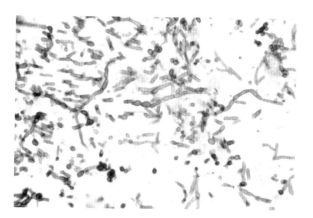

Image 9. *Candida albicans.* Silver stain preparation. Note the branched budding and pseudohyphae.*

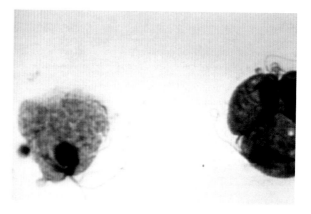

Image 10. *Trichomonas vaginalis* demonstrating trophozoites with flagellae.*

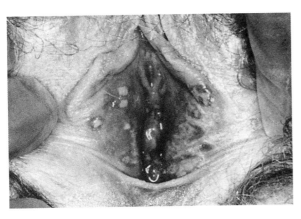

**Image 11. Herpes genitalis.** Ulcerating vesicles associated with HSV-2. (Reproduced, with permission, from De-Cherney AH. *Current Obstetric and Gynecologic Diagnosis and Treatment*, 9th ed. New York: McGraw-Hill, 2003: 664.)

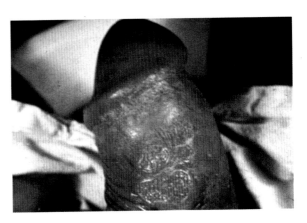

**Image 12A. Syphilis.** Chancre associated with primary syphilis. These ulcerative lesions are painless.*

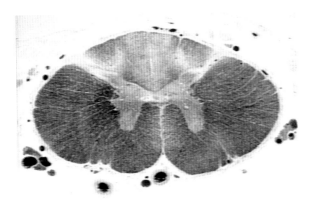

**Image 12B. Syphilis. Tabes dorsalis** resulting from progressive syphilis infection, thoracic spinal cord. Note degeneration of the dorsal columns and dorsal roots.*

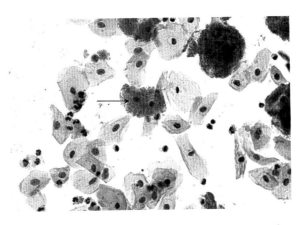

**Image 13. Bacterial vaginosis.** Arrow points to a clue cell. (Reproduced, with permission, from USMLERx.com.)

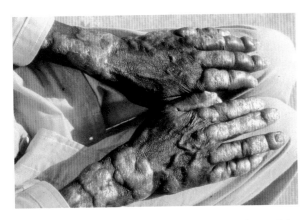

**Image 14. Leprosy, lepromatous type.** Note the nodules and thick plaques on the dorsa of the fingers, wrists, and forearms, with hypopigmentation of the overlying skin. Also note the symmetry of involvement and loss of tissue of several fingertips. (Reproduced, with permission, from Wolff K et al. *Fitzpatrick's Color Atlas and Synopsis of Clinical Dermatology*, 5th ed. New York: McGraw-Hill, Fig. 22-52.)

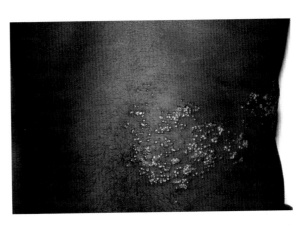

**Image 15. Herpes zoster.** Reactivation of virus spreads along the dermatomal distribution of infected nerves and can occur many years after initial infection. It is considered benign unless it affects an immunocompromised host or is a reinfection of the $V_1$ branch of the trigeminal nerve with eye/cornea involvement.*

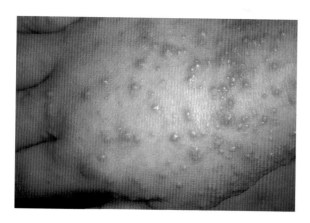

**Image 16. Coxsackie exanthem (hand-foot-mouth disease).** Diffuse eruptive vesiculopapules are seen on the hand of a three-year-old child. (Reproduced, with permission, from Hurwitz RM et al. *Pathology of the Skin: Atlas of Clinical-Pathological Correlation*, 2nd ed. Stamford, CT: Appleton & Lange, 1998.)

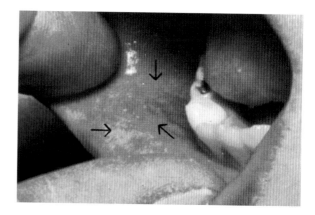

**Image 17. Koplik spots.** Pathognomonic for measles, Koplik spots appear as tiny white lesions with an erythematous halo, like "grains of sand." They precede the generalized rash by 1–2 days. (Reproduced, with permission, from Wolff K et al. *Fitzpatrick's Dermatology in General Medicine*, 7th ed. New York: McGraw-Hill, 2007, Fig. 192-1.)

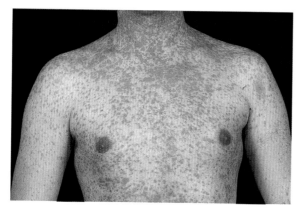

**Image 18A. Rash of measles.** Discrete erythematous lesions become confluent as the rash spreads downward. (Reproduced, with permission, from Fitzpatrick TB et al. *Fitzpatrick's Color Atlas and Synopsis of Clinical Dermatology*, 5th ed. New York: McGraw-Hill, 2001: 788.)

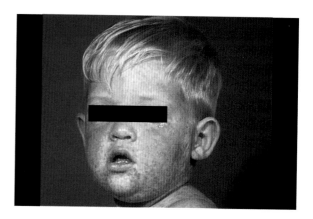

**Image 18B. Rash of measles.** In measles, rash often begins in the head and neck area.

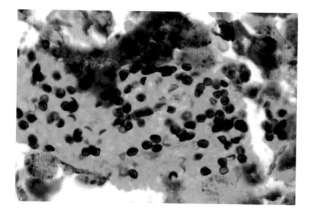

**Image 19A. *Pneumocystis jiroveci* (formerly *carinii*).** Special silver stain of lung epithelium shows numerous small, disk-shaped organisms. (Reproduced, with permission, from USMLERx.com.)

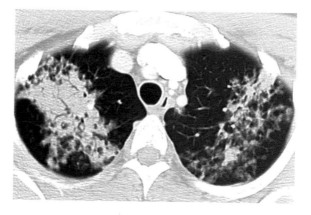

**Image 19B. *Pneumocystis* pulmonary infection** seen on CT chest image. Note the bilateral confluent air-space opacities in a central distribution.

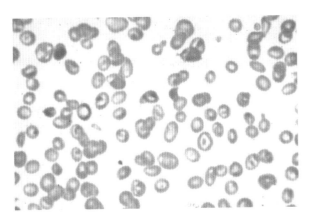

**Image 20A. Target cells.** Due to an increase in surface area–to-volume ratio from iron deficiency anemia (decreased cell volume) or in obstructive liver disease (increased cell membrane).*

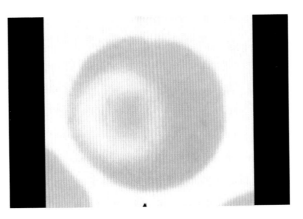

**Image 20B. Target cell, solitary.** Note the classic target-shaped appearance.

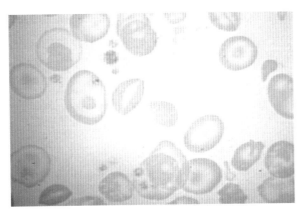

**Image 21. Thalassemia major.** A blood dyscrasia caused by a defect in β-chain synthesis in hemoglobin. Note the presence of target cells.*

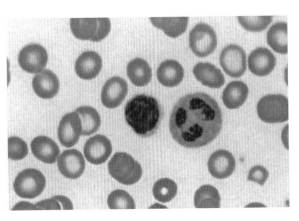

**Image 22. Iron deficiency anemia.** Microcytosis and hypochromia can be seen.

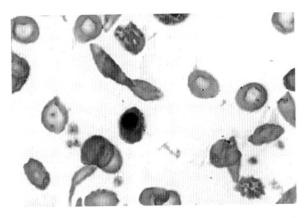

**Image 23A. Sickle cell anemia.** Sickle cell peripheral blood smear. Note the sickled cells as well as anisocytosis, poikilocytosis, and nucleated RBCs.*

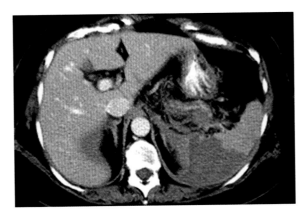

**Image 23B. Sickle cell anemia. Splenic infarction.** The splenic artery lacks collateral supply, making the spleen particularly susceptible to ischemic damage. Coagulative necrosis has occurred in a wedge shape. Individual sickle cells cause generalized splenic infarcts that result in autosplenectomy by adolescence.*

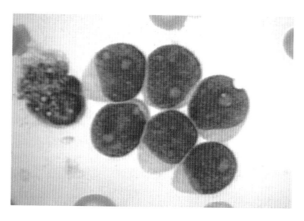

**Image 24A. Leukemia. Acute lymphocytic leukemia,** peripheral blood smear. Affects children less than 10 years of age.*

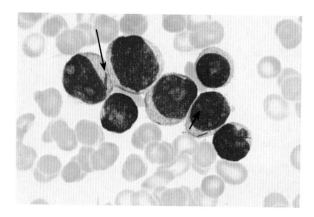

**Image 24B. Leukemia. Acute myelocytic leukemia** with Auer rods (long arrow), peripheral blood smear. Affects adolescents to young adults, but most commonly diagnosed in older adults.*

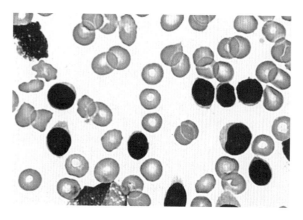

**Image 24C. Leukemia. Chronic lymphocytic leuke-mia,** peripheral blood smear. In CLL, the lymphocytes are excessively fragile. These lymphocytes are easily destroyed during slide preparation, forming "smudge cells." Affects individuals older than 60 years of age.*

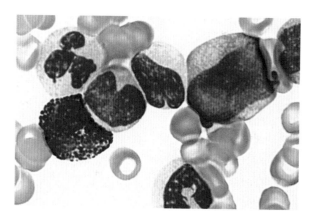

**Image 24D. Leukemia. Chronic myeloid leukemia,** peripheral blood smear. Promyelocytes and myelocytes are seen adjacent to a vascular structure. Affects individuals from 30 to 60 years of age.*

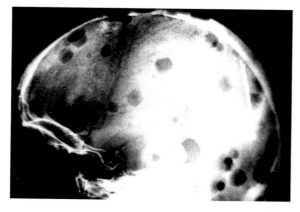

**Image 25A. Multiple myeloma.** Classic bone lytic lesions seen in multiple myeloma.*

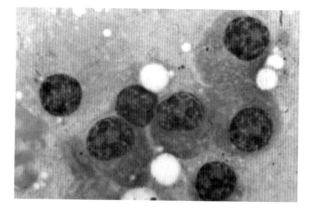

**Image 25B. Multiple myeloma.** Smears from a patient with multiple myeloma display an abundance of plasma cells. RBCs will often be seen in rouleaux formation, stacked like poker chips.*

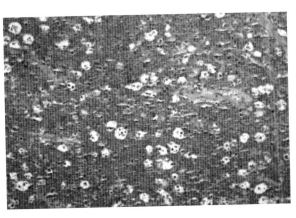

**Image 26A. Burkitt's lymphoma.** The classic "starry-sky" appearance from macrophage ingestion of tumor cells can be seen.*

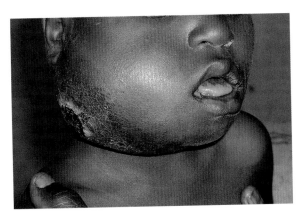

**Image 26B. Burkitt's lymphoma.** Young Nigerian boy with history of jaw swelling unresponsive to antibiotics.

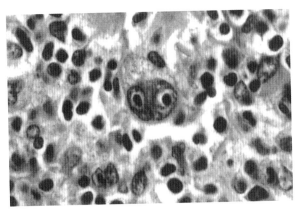

**Image 27. Hodgkin's disease (Reed-Sternberg cells).** Binucleate RS cells displaying prominent inclusion-like nucleoli surrounded by lymphocytes and other reacting inflammatory cells. The RS cell is a necessary but insufficient pathologic finding for the diagnosis of Hodgkin's disease.

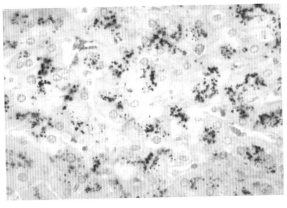

**Image 28. Hemochromatosis** with cirrhosis. Prussian blue iron stain shows hemosiderin in the liver parenchyma. Such deposition occurs throughout the body, causing organ damage and the characteristic darkening of the skin.*

**Image 29A. Fatty metamorphosis** (macrovesicular steatosis) of the liver, microscopic. Early reversible change associated with alcohol consumption can be seen; there are abundant fat-filled vacuoles, but as yet there is no inflammation due to fibrosis of more serious alcoholic liver damage.*

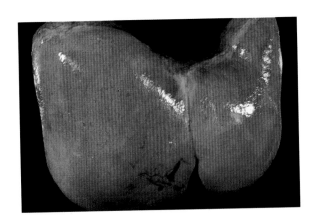

**Image 29B. Fatty liver.** Gross specimen showing enlarged yellow appearance.

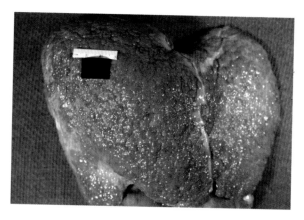

**Image 30A. Cirrhosis. Micronodular cirrhosis of the liver,** gross, from an alcoholic patient. The liver is approximately normal in size with a fine, granular appearance. Later stages of disease result in an irregularly shrunken liver with larger nodules, giving it a "hobnail" appearance.*

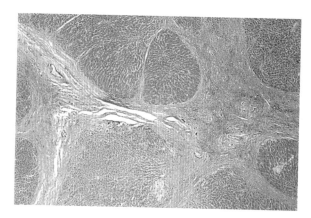

**Image 30B. Cirrhosis,** microscopic. Regenerative lesions are surrounded by fibrotic bands of collagen ("bridging fibrosis"), forming the characteristic nodularity.*

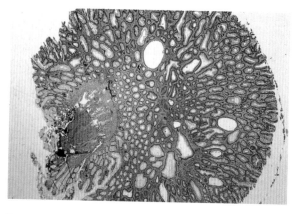

**Image 31A. Colonic polyps. Tubular adenomas** are smaller and rounded in morphology and have less malignant potential than do **villous adenomas.**

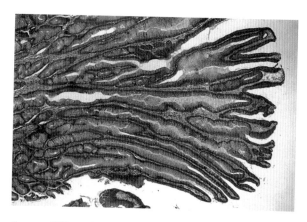

**Image 31B. Villous adenomas** are composed of long, fingerlike projections.

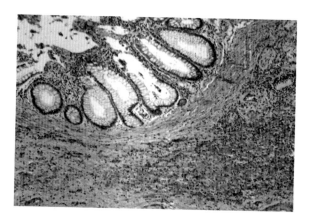

**Image 32. Diverticulitis.** Inflammation of the diverticula typically causes LLQ pain and can progress to perforation, peritonitis, abscess formation, or bowel stenosis. Note the presence of macrophages. Gut lumen is seen at the top of the photo.*

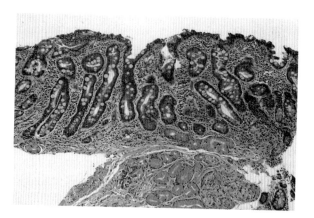

**Image 33. Celiac sprue** (gluten-sensitive enteropathy). Histology shows blunting of villi and crypt hyperplasia.

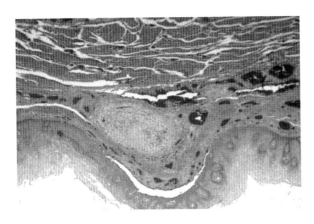

Image 34. Sclerosed **esophageal varix.** Overlying esophageal mucosa is generally normal.*

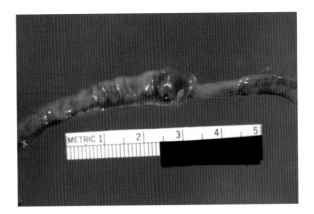

Image 35. **Intussusception** of infant gut, gross.*

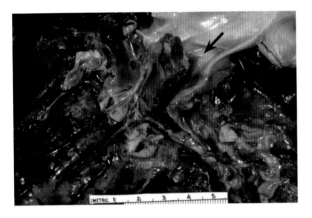

Image 36A. **Pulmonary emboli. Pulmonary thromboembolus (arrow),** gross. Most often arises from deep venous thrombosis.*

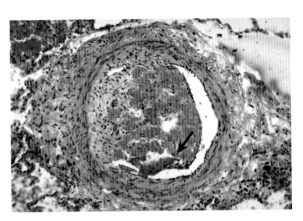

Image 36B. **Pulmonary thromboembolus** in a small muscular pulmonary artery. The interdigitating areas of pale pink and red within the organizing embolus form the "lines of Zahn" (arrow) characteristic of a thrombus. These lines represent layers of red cells, platelets, and fibrin that are laid down in the vessel as the thrombus forms.*

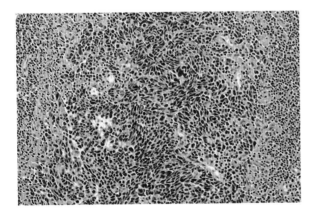

Image 37. **Small (oat) cell carcinoma** in a pulmonary hilar lymph node. Almost all of these tumors are related to tobacco smoking. They can arise anywhere in the lung, most often near the hilum, and quickly spread along the bronchi.*

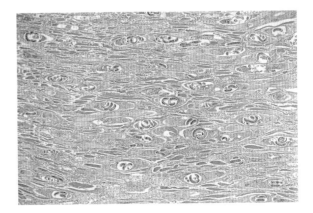

Image 38. *Taenia solium,* the pig tapeworm, infesting porcine myocardium. When humans ingest this meat, the larvae attach to the wall of the small intestine and mature to adult worms.

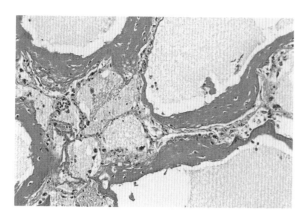

**Image 39. Acute respiratory distress syndrome (ARDS).** Persistent inflammation leads to poor pulmonary compliance and edema; note both alveolar fluid and hyaline membranes.

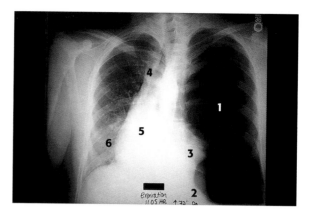

**Image 40. Tension pneumothorax.** Note these features: 1—Hyperlucent lung field; 2—Hyperexpansion lowers diaphragm; 3—Collapsed lung; 4—Deviation of trachea; 5—Mediastinal shift; 6—Compression of opposite lung.

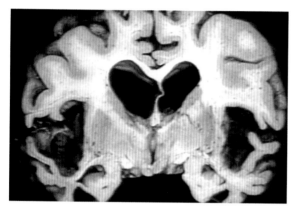

**Image 41A. Alzheimer's disease.** Key histologic features include "senile plaques" (not pictured); a coronal section showing atrophy, especially of the temporal lobes.*

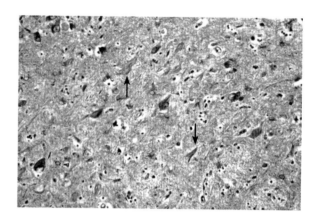

**Image 41B.** Focal masses of interwoven neuronal processes around an amyloid core; arrows mark neurofibrillary tangles).*

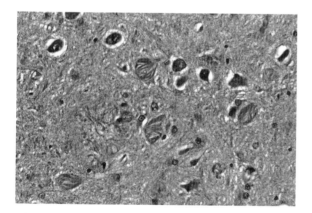

**Image 41C.** The remnants of neuronal degeneration are also associated with Alzheimer's disease, the most common cause of dementia in older persons.*

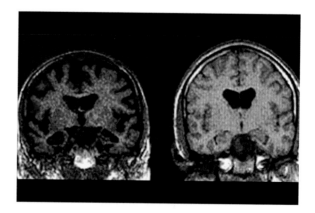

**Image 41D. Alzheimer's disease.** The T1-weighted coronal brain MRI image on the left demonstrates bilateral temporal lobe atrophy (arrows) as compared with normal appearance on the right.

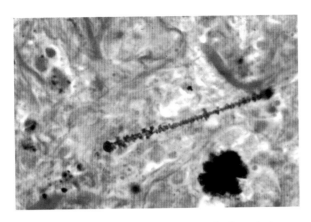

Image 42. **Asbestosis.** Ferruginous bodies (asbestos bodies with Prussian blue iron stain) in the lung, microscopic. Inhaled asbestos fibers are ingested by macrophages.*

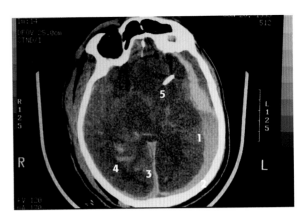

Image 43. **Subdural hemorrhage.** Note the hyperdense extra-axial blood on the left side. Concomitant subarachnoid hemorrhage. 1—subdural blood, layering; 2—skull; 3—falx; 4—subarachnoid blood; 5—shunt catheter; 6—frontal sinus.

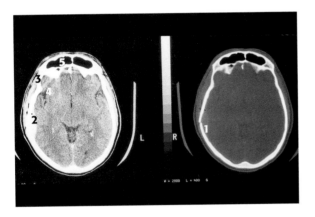

Image 44. **Epidural hematoma** from skull fracture. Note the lens-shaped (biconvex) dense blood next to the fracture. 1—skull fracture; 2—hematoma in epidural space; 3—temporalis muscle; 4—Sylvian fissure; 5—frontal sinus.

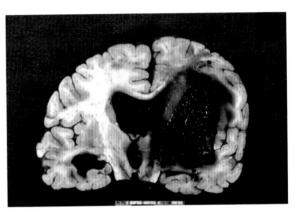

Image 45. Brain with **hypertensive hemorrhage** in the region of the left basal ganglia, gross.*

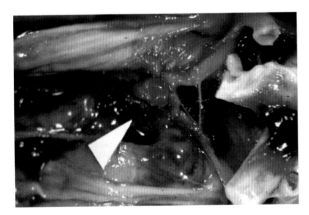

Image 46A. **Berry aneurysm** located on the anterior cerebral artery. The small, saclike structure can easily rupture during periods of hypertension or stress.*

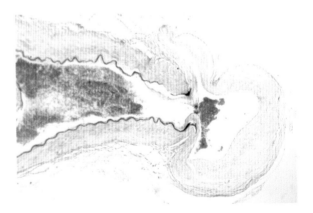

Image 46B. **Berry aneurysm** histologic section at the origin of the aneurysm shows lack of internal elastic lamina.*

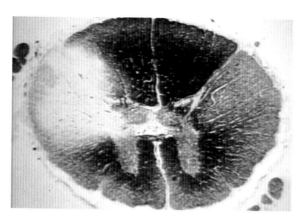

**Image 47A. Multiple sclerosis.** Lumbar spinal cord with mostly random and asymmetric white-matter lesions.*

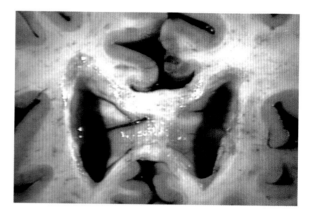

**Image 47B. Multiple sclerosis.** Brain with periventricular white-matter plaques of demyelination, gross. Demyelination occurs in a bilateral asymmetric distribution. Classic clinical findings are nystagmus, scanning speech, and intention tremor.*

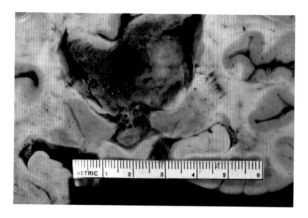

**Image 48A. Glioblastoma multiforme** extending across the midline of the cerebral cortex, gross.*

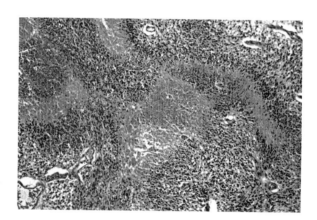

**Image 48B. Glioblastoma multiforme.** Histology shows necrosis with surrounding pseudopalisading of malignant tumor cells. (Reproduced, with permission, from USMLERx.com.)

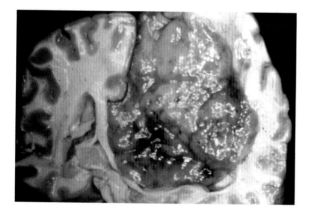

**Image 49A. Oligodendroglioma.** Gross natural-color coronal section of cerebral hemisphere with a large lesion of the left parieto-occipital white matter.*

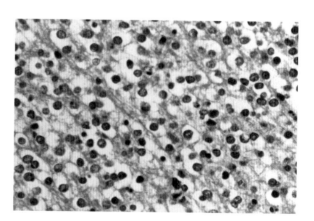

**Image 49B. Oligodendroglioma.** Classic "fried egg" appearance with perinuclear halos and "chicken-wire" capillary pattern.*

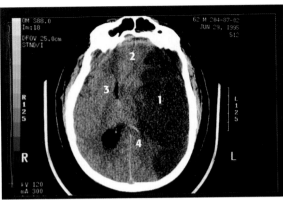

**Image 50. Left middle cerebral artery stroke.** Large left MCA territory stroke with edema and mass effect but no visible hemorrhage. The patient experienced deficits in speech and in the right side of the face and upper extremities. 1—ischemic brain parenchyma; 2—subtle midline shift to the right; 3—the right frontal horn of the lateral ventricle; 4—the left lateral ventricles obliterated by edema.

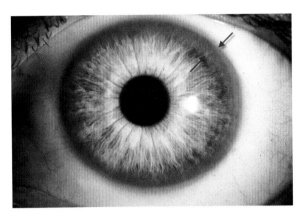

**Image 51. Kayser-Fleischer ring** in Wilson's disease. This corneal ring (between arrows) was golden brown and contrasted clearly against a gray-blue iris. Note that the darkness of the ring increases as the outer border (limbus) of the cornea is approached (right arrow).

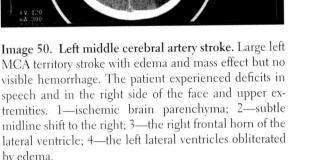

**Image 52. Acute systemic lupus erythematosus.** Bright red, sharply defined erythema is seen with slight edema and minimal scaling in a "butterfly pattern" on the face (the typical "malar rash"). Note also that the patient is female and young. (Reproduced, with permission, from Wolff K et al. *Fitzpatrick's Color Atlas and Synopsis of Clinical Dermatology*, 5th ed. New York: McGraw-Hill, 2005: 385.)

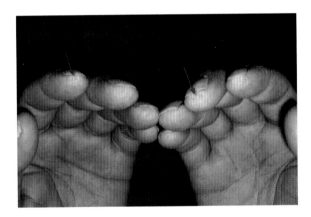

**Image 53. Scleroderma.** The progressive "tightening" of the skin has contracted the fingers. Also note ulceration of fingertips. Fibrosis is widespread and may also involve the esophagus (dysphagia), lung (restrictive disease), and small vessels of the kidney (hypertension).

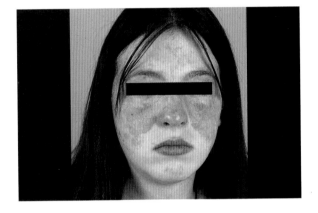

**Image 54A. Gout.** Tophi within joints consist of aggregates of urate crystals surrounded by an inflammatory reaction consisting of macrophages, lymphocytes, and giant cells. (Reproduced, with permission, from USMLERx.com.)

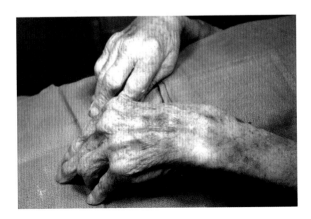

**Image 54B. Gout.** Tophi affect the proximal interphalangeal (PIP) joints, knees, and elbows, growing like tubers from the bones.*

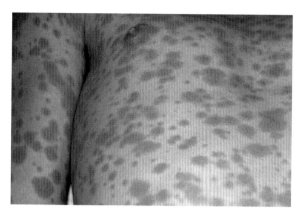

**Image 55. Erythema multiforme.** Erythematous macules and papules are seen. (Reproduced, with permission, from USMLERx.com.)

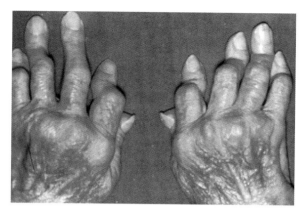

**Image 56. Rheumatoid arthritis.** Note the swan-neck deformities of the digits and severe, symmetric involvement of the PIP joints.

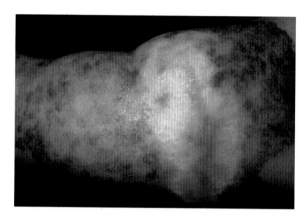

**Image 57. Arteriovenous malformation.** The markedly enlarged and distorted arm of a six-month-old boy with confluent erythematous papules and nodules. (Reproduced, with permission, from Hurwitz RM et al. *Pathology of the Skin: Atlas of Clinical-Pathological Correlation,* 2nd ed. Stamford, CT: Appleton & Lange, 1998.)

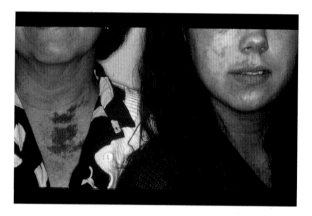

**Image 58. Capillary malformation, port-wine type.** Irregular purple patches and plaques are seen on the neck and chest of the mother, and pink patches are seen on the cheek, lip, chin, neck, and chest of the daughter. Both lesions were present at birth. (Reproduced, with permission, from Hurwitz RM et al. *Pathology of the Skin: Atlas of Clinical-Pathological Correlation,* 2nd ed. Stamford, CT: Appleton & Lange, 1998.)

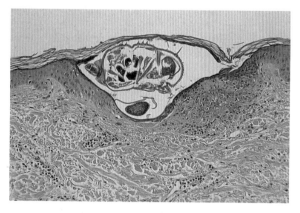

**Image 59. Scabies.** Adult female mite with egg containing embryo within the epidermis. (Reproduced, with permission, from Hurwitz RM et al. *Pathology of the Skin: Atlas of Clinical-Pathological Correlation,* 2nd ed. Stamford, CT: Appleton & Lange, 1998.)

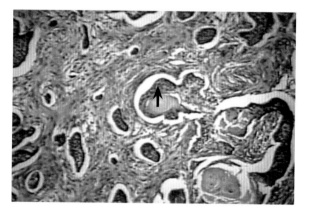

**Image 60. Squamous cell carcinoma.** Malignant skin tumor involving the epidermal skin layer. Note the presence of keratin pearls (arrows).*

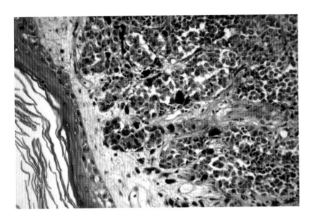

**Image 61A. Malignant melanoma.** Lesion just beneath the epidermis with pigmented and nonpigmented cells. The tumor cells are usually polyhedral but may be spindle shaped, dendritic, or ballooned or may resemble oat cells. Many but by no means all melanomas make melanin. Large nucleoli are common.*

**Image 61B. Malignant melanoma.** A multicolored tan, red, and dark brown irregular plaque. Note the "hazy," indefinite border and pigmentary variation. The depth of the lesion is a prognostic indicator.*

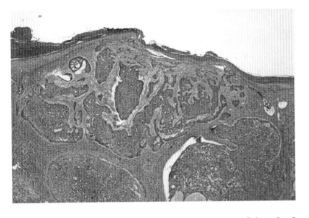

**Image 62A. Basal cell carcinoma.** Nests of basaloid cells are present within the dermis with peripheral palisading and prominent retraction artifacts. (Reproduced, with permission, from USMLERx.com.)

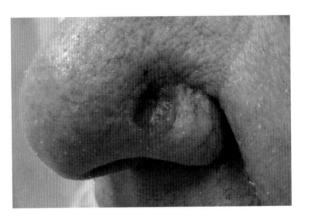

**Image 62B. Basal cell carcinoma.** Note the appearance of the small lesion on the nose.

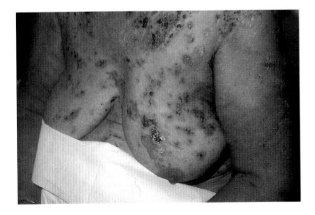

**Image 63A. Pemphigus vulgaris.** Numerous crusted, denuded, and weepy erythematous plaques are seen on the chest, breast, abdomen, and arms. (Reproduced, with permission, from Hurwitz RM et al. *Pathology of the Skin: Atlas of Clinical-Pathological Correlation*, 2nd ed. Stamford, CT: Appleton & Lange, 1998.)

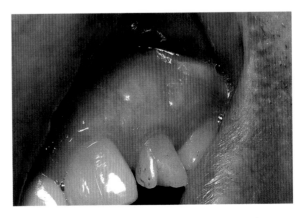

**Image 63B. Pemphigus vulgaris.** Vesicles on the gingiva. (Reproduced, with permission, from Hurwitz RM et al. *Pathology of the Skin: Atlas of Clinical-Pathological Correlation*, 2nd ed. Stamford, CT: Appleton & Lange, 1998.)

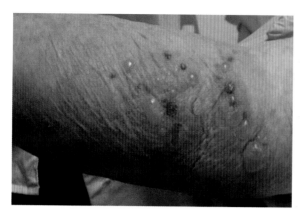

**Image 64. Bullous pemphigoid.** Note the tense bullae and urticarial plaques. (Reproduced, with permission, from USMLERx.com.)

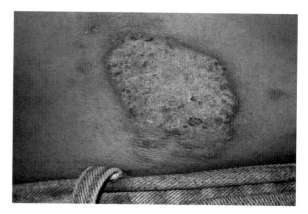

**Image 65. Psoriasis.** Note the well-demarcated, erythematous plaque with scale. (Reproduced, with permission, from USMLERx.com.)

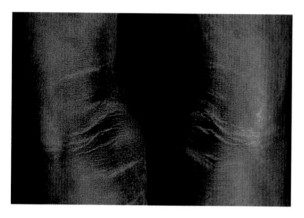

**Image 66A. Acanthosis nigricans.** Extensive hyperpigmented plaques on the arms in a patient with congenital lipodystrophy. This is an unusual distribution for acanthosis nigricans. (Reproduced, with permission, from Hurwitz RM et al. *Pathology of the Skin: Atlas of Clinical-Pathological Correlation*, 2nd ed. Stamford, CT: Appleton & Lange, 1998.)

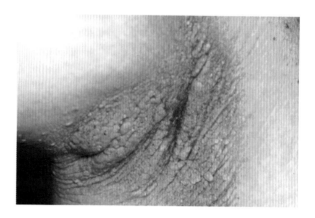

**Image 66B. Acanthosis nigricans.** Typical distribution at the underarm.

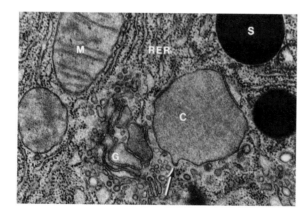

**Image 67A. Pancreas. Pancreatic acinar cell (EM).** A condensing vacuole (C) is receiving secretory product (arrow) from the Golgi complex (G). M—mitochondrion; RER—rough endoplasmic reticulum; S—mature condensed secretory zymogen granules.

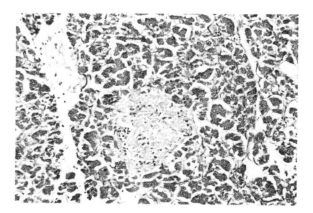

**Image 67B. Pancreas.** Pancreatic islet cells in **diabetes mellitus type 1.** In patients with diabetes mellitus type 1, autoantibodies against β cells cause a chronic inflammation until, over time, islet cells are entirely replaced by fibrosis.

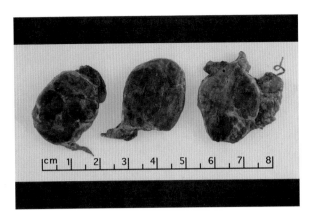

**Image 68. Adrenocortical adenoma,** gross. Cause of hypercortisolism (Cushing's syndrome) or hyperaldosteronism (Conn's syndrome).*

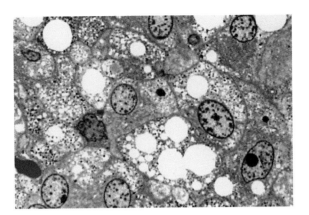

**Image 69. Pheochromocytoma.** The tumor cells have numerous vacuolar spaces within the cytoplasm (pseudoacini). Most of the punctate blue-black granules of variable density are dense-core neurosecretory granules.*

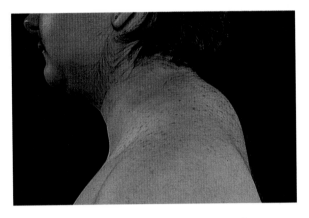

**Image 70A. Cushing's disease.** The clinical picture includes moon facies and buffalo hump.

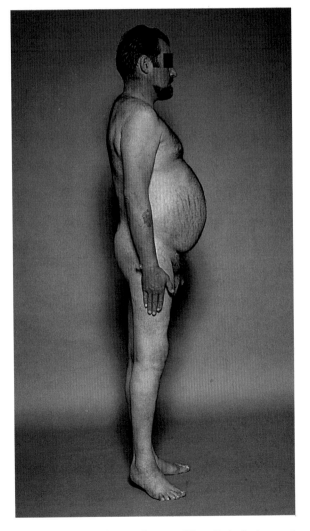

**Image 70B. Cushing's disease.** The clinical picture includes truncal obesity and abdominal striae.

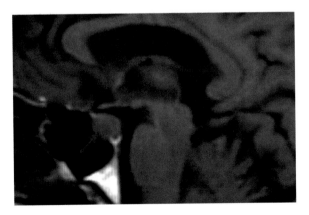

**Image 70C. Cushing's disease.** Sagittal T1-weighted MRI image showing a small pituitary mass (hormone-secreting). Note the accessibility to a transsphenoidal surgical approach.

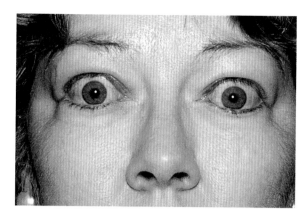

**Image 71A. Graves' disease.** Exophthalmos in a patient with proptosis and periorbital edema.*

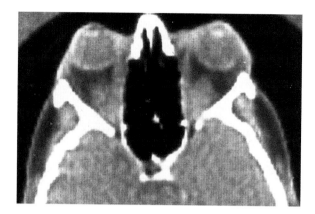

**Image 71B. Graves' disease.** CT shows extraocular muscle enlargement at the orbital apex.*

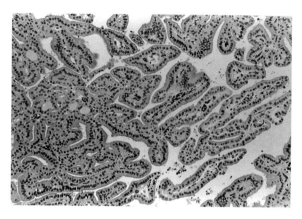

**Image 71C. Graves' disease.** Stimulation of follicular cells by autoantibodies that stimulate TSH receptors causes the normal uniform architecture to be replaced by hyperplastic papillary, involuted borders, and decreased colloid. Typical medical therapy is propylthiouracil, which inhibits the production of thyroid hormone as well as peripheral conversion of $T_4$ to $T_3$.*

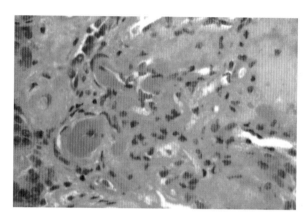

**Image 72. Arteriolar sclerosis** showing masses of hyaline material in glomerular afferent and efferent arterioles and in the glomerulus. From a type 1 diabetic patient.*

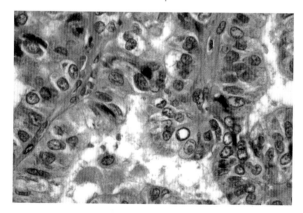

**Image 73A. Papillary carcinoma.** The image shows the papillary architecture and classic nuclear features that are key in making the diagnosis, including ground-glass or "Orphan Annie eye" chromatin, nuclear grooves, and intranuclear pseudoinclusions. Psammoma bodies are not seen here but are often present. (Reproduced, with permission, from USMLERx.com.)

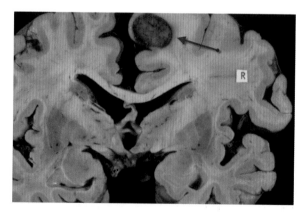

**Image 73B. Papillary carcinoma.** Metastatic solitary lesion seen on gross specimen in the coronal plane.

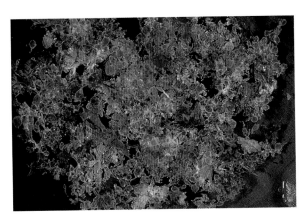

**Image 74. Hydatidiform mole.** The characteristic gross appearance is a "bunch of grapes." Hydatidiform moles are the most common precursors of choriocarcinoma. Complete moles usually display a 46,XX diploid pattern with all the chromosomes derived from the sperm. In partial moles, the karyotype is triploid or tetraploid, and fetal parts may be present.

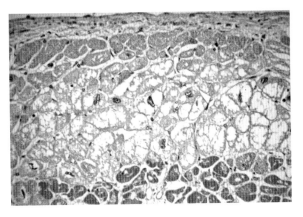

**Image 75. Endocardial chronic ischemia.** Microscopic example of myocytolysis and coagulation necrosis beneath the endocardium.*

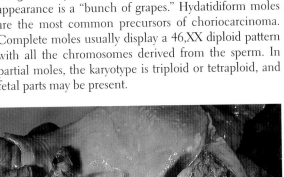

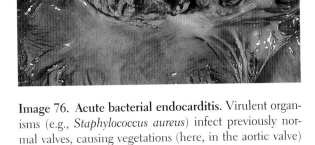

**Image 76. Acute bacterial endocarditis.** Virulent organisms (e.g., *Staphylococcus aureus*) infect previously normal valves, causing vegetations (here, in the aortic valve) and potentially giving rise to septic emboli.

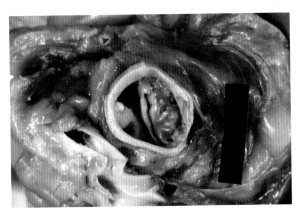

**Image 77.** Calcified **bicuspid aortic valve** showing false raphe. The abnormal architecture of the valve makes its leaflets susceptible to otherwise ordinary hemodynamic stresses, which ultimately leads to valvular thickening, calcification, increased rigidity, and stenosis.*

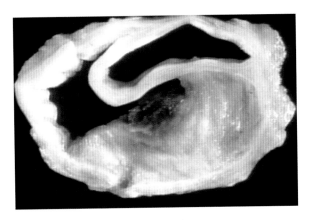

**Image 78. Aortic dissection** with a blood clot compressing the aortic lumen. A tear in the intima allowed blood to surge through the muscular layer to the adventitia (may lead to sudden death from hemothorax). Risk factors are hypertension, Marfan's syndrome, pregnancy, Ehlers-Danlos syndrome, and trauma.*

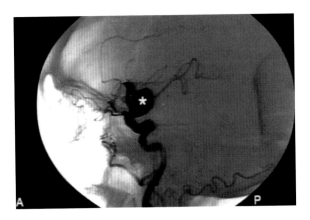

**Image 79. Carotid angiogram showing aneurysm.** Note the path of the internal carotid artery through the neck and its major branches (ophthalmic artery, anterior cerebral artery, middle cerebral artery). The aneurysm is inferior to the terminal branches in this angiogram.*

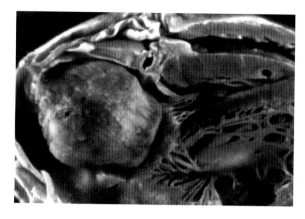

**Image 80A. Left atrial myxoma.** The most common primary cardiac tumor; known to produce VEGF (vascular endothelial growth factor).*

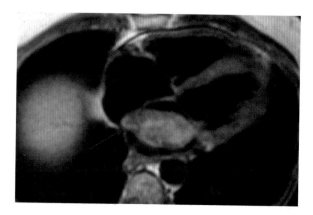

**Image 80B. Left atrial myxoma.** Axial T1-weighted cardiac MRI demonstrates ovoid mass attached to the interatrial septum.

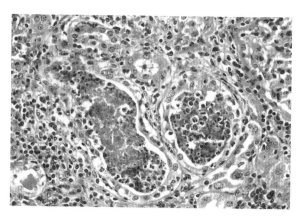

**Image 81A. Acute pyelonephritis** is characterized by neutrophilic infiltration and abscess formation within the renal interstitium. Abscesses may rupture, introducing collections of white cells to the tubular lumen.

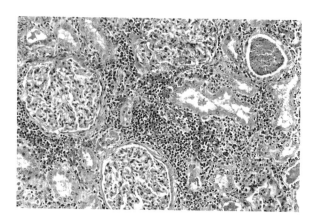

**Image 81B. Chronic pyelonephritis** has a lymphocytic invasion with fibrosis.

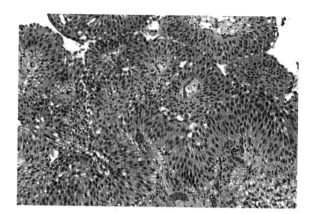

**Image 82. Transitional cell carcinoma.** The image shows a papillary growth lined by transitional epithelium with mild nuclear atypia and pleomorphism. (Reproduced, with permission, from USMLERx.com.)

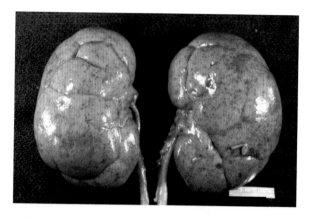

**Image 83. Lupus erythematosus, kidneys.** Enlarged, very pale kidneys with "flea bite" or ectasia from a patient with nephrotic syndrome or subacute glomerulonephritis as a result of lupus erythematosus.*

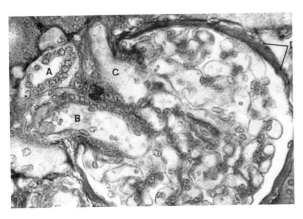

Image 84. Normal glomerulus, microscopic, with (A) macula densa and (B) afferent and (C) efferent arterioles.

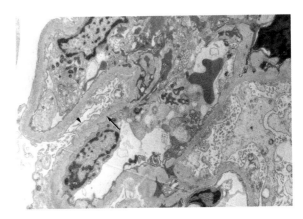

Image 85. Minimal change disease (lipoid nephrosis) shows normal glomeruli on light microscopy but effacement of foot processes on EM (arrowhead). The full arrow points to a normal foot process. Treatment consists of corticosteroids.

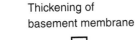
Thickening of basement membrane

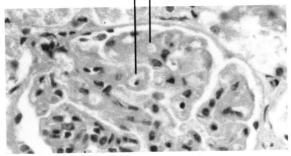

Image 86A. Systemic lupus erythematosus, kidney pathology. In the membranous glomerulonephritic pattern, "wire-loop" thickening occurs as a result of immune complex deposition. Associated with subendothelial deposits and mesangial hyercellularity.

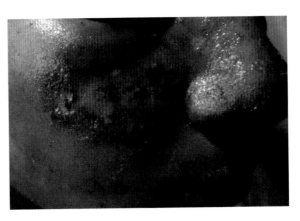

Image 86B. Systemic lupus erythematosus. Typical facial malar rash.

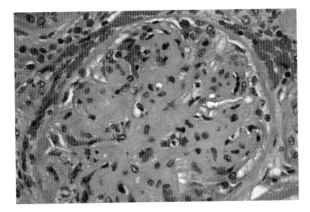

Image 87A. Diabetic glomerulosclerosis. Nodular diabetic glomerulosclerosis is also known as Kimmelstiel-Wilson syndrome and is characterized by acellular ovoid nodules in the periphery of the glomerulus. (Reproduced, with permission, from USMLERx.com.)

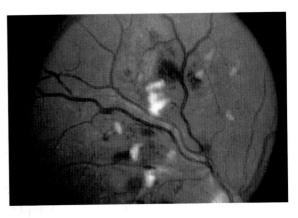

Image 87B. Diabetic retinopathy. Funduscopic image showing cotton wool spots and macular edema.

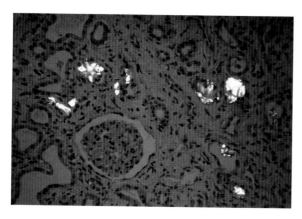

**Image 88A. Calcium oxalate crystals** in the kidney, viewed with partially crossed polarizers. Tubular failure in oxalate nephropathy can result from vitamin C or antifreeze abuse.*

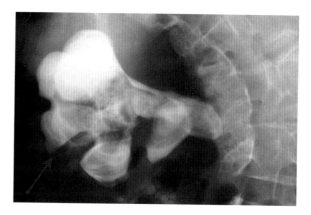

**Image 88B. Calcium oxalate** outlining a large right renal collecting system creating a "staghorn" calculus.

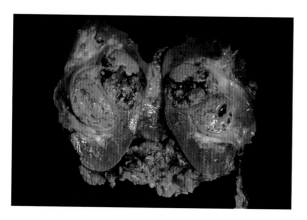

**Image 89A. Renal cell carcinoma.** Gross. The kidney has been bivalved, revealing a nodular, golden-yellow tumor in the midkidney with areas of hemorrhage and necrosis. (Reproduced, with permission, from USMLERx.com.)

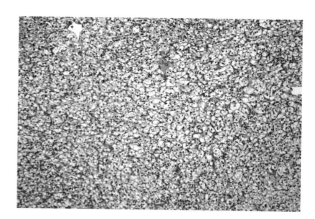

**Image 89B. Renal cell carcinoma.** Histology shows polygonal cells with small nuclei and abundant clear cytoplasm with a rich, delicate branching vasculature. (Reproduced, with permission, from USMLERx.com.)

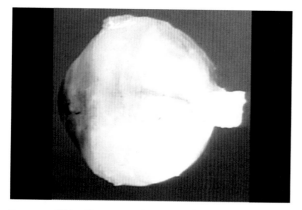

**Image 90A. Osteogenesis imperfecta.** Blue sclera caused by translucency of connective tissue over the choroid. The optic nerve is on the right side of the image.*

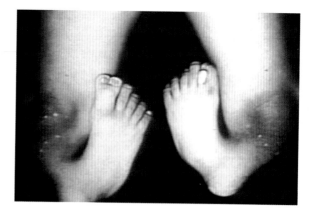

**Image 90B. Osteogenesis imperfecta.** Abnormal collagen synthesis results from a variety of gene mutations and causes brittle bones and connective tissue malformations.*

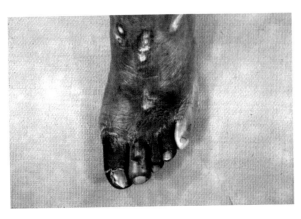

**Image 91. Foot gangrene.** The first four toes and adjacent skin are dry, shrunken, and blackened with superficial necrosis and peeling of the skin. A well-defined line of demarcation separates the black region from the viable skin.*

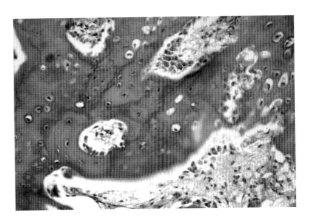

**Image 92. Bone fracture.** New bone formation with osteoblasts.*

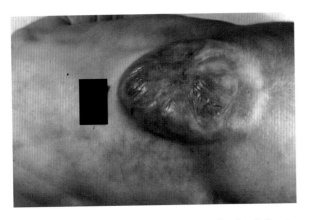

**Image 93. Meningomyelocele.** A neural tube defect in which the meninges and spinal cord herniate through the spinal canal; gross image of infant's lower back.*

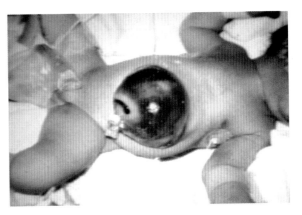

**Image 94. Omphalocele** in a newborn. Note that the defect is midline and is covered by peritoneum, as opposed to gastroschisis, which is not covered by peritoneum and is often not midline.*

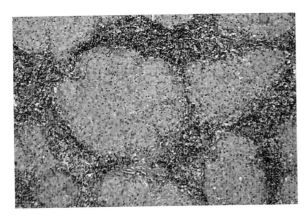

**Image 95. Sarcoidosis.** Numerous tightly formed granulomas are seen on histology of a lymph node in a patient with sarcoidosis. (Reproduced, with permission, from USMLERx.com.)

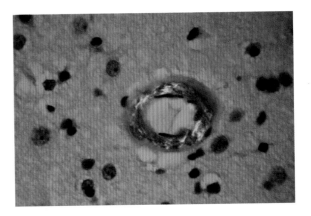

**Image 96. Amyloidosis.** Congo red stain demonstrates amyloid deposits in the artery wall that show apple-green birefringence under polarized light. (Reproduced, with permission, from USMLERx.com.)

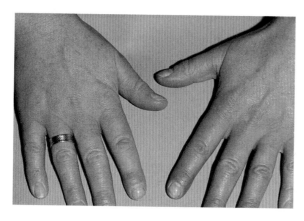

**Image 97A. Raynaud's disease.** The left hand exhibits a distal cyanosis compared to the right hand; it is seen especially well in the nail beds. Unilateral episodes such as this one may occur after contact with a cold object. (Reproduced, with permission, from Wolff K et al. *Fitzpatrick's Color Atlas and Synopsis of Clinical Dermatology,* 5th ed. New York: McGraw-Hill, 2005: 403.)

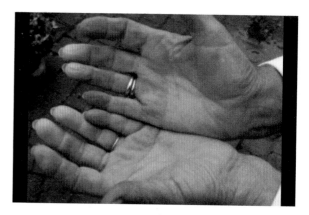

**Image 97B. Raynaud's disease.** Note the bilateral distal distribution of cyanosis.

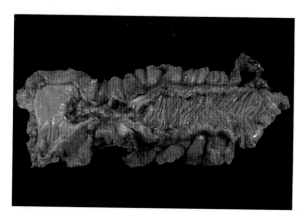

**Image 98A. Colon cancer.** Note the circumferential tumor with heaped-up edges and central ulceration. (Reproduced, with permission, from USMLERx.com.)

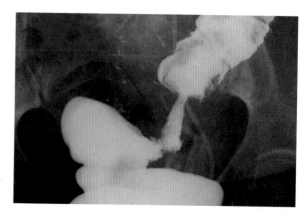

**Image 98B. Colon cancer.** Classic "apple-core" lesion of the sigmoid colon seen on barium enema. (Reproduced, with permission, from USMLERx.com.)

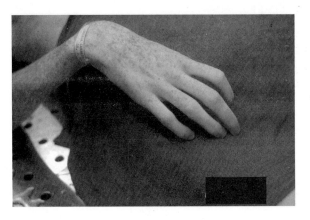

**Image 99. Marfan's syndrome.** Patients are tall with very long extremities. The joints are hyperextensible, with slim bone structure and wiry muscles.*

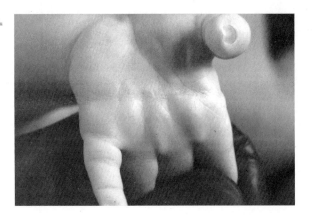

**Image 100. Simian crease.** A characteristic feature of Down syndrome (trisomy 21). The palm has a single transverse crease instead of the normal two creases.*

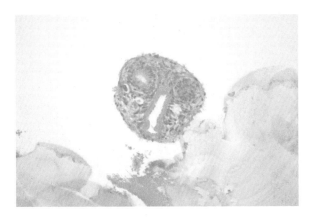

**Image 101. Hydatid cyst.** *Echinococcus* eggs develop into larvae in the intestine, penetrate the intestinal wall, and disseminate throughout the body. The larvae form hydatid cysts in the liver and, less commonly, in the lungs, kidney, and brain. (Reproduced, with permission, from USMLERx.com.)

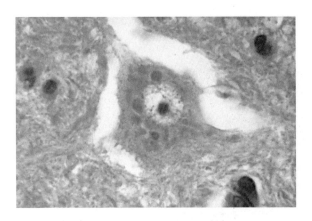

**Image 102. Negri bodies** are pathognomonic inclusions in the cytoplasm of neurons infected by the rabies virus. (Reproduced, with permission, from the Centers for Disease Control and Prevention, Atlanta, GA.)

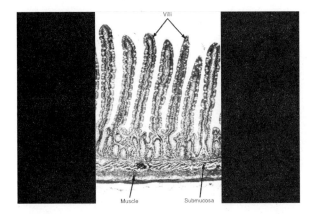

**Image 103.** Photomicrograph of the **small intestine.**

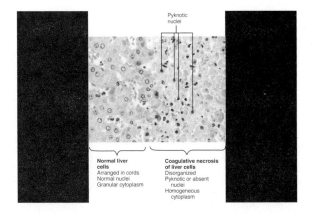

**Image 104. Coagulative necrosis** of hepatocytes.

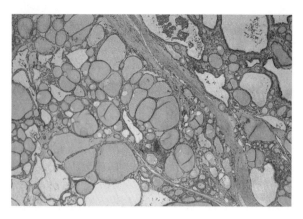

**Image 105. Multinodular goiter** with hyperplasia and subsequent involution of the thyroid gland. The image shows follicles distended with colloid and lined by a flattened epithelium with areas of fibrosis and hemorrhage. (Reproduced, with permission, from USMLERx.com.)

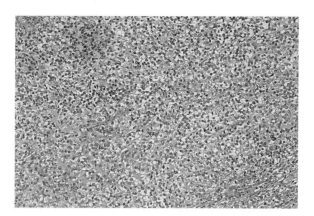

**Image 106. Ewing's sarcoma.** This malignant tumor of bone occurs in children and is characterized by the (11;22) translocation that results in the fusion gene EWS-FLI1. The tumor is composed of sheets of uniform small, round cells. (Reproduced, with permission, from USMLERx.com.)

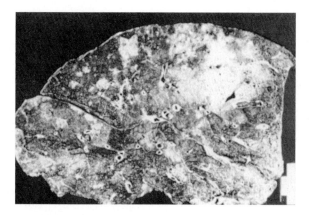

**Image 107A. Pneumonia.** Gross. Note the large area of consolidation at the base plus multiple small areas of consolidation (pale) involving bronchioles and surrounding alveolar sacs throughout the lung.

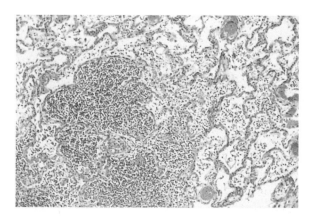

**Image 107B. Pneumonia.** "Bronchopneumonia" with neutrophils in alveolar spaces, microscopic.

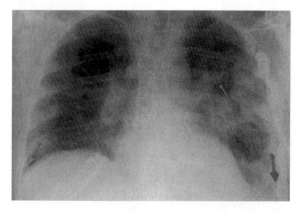

**Image 107C. Cavitary pneumonia.** Chest x-ray showing left-sided pneumonia with cavitation and bilateral pleural effusions. (Adapted, with permission, from A. Christaras.)

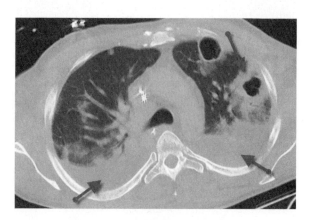

**Image 107D. Cavitary pneumonia.** Chest CT scan showing cavitary lesions with bilateral pleural effusions.

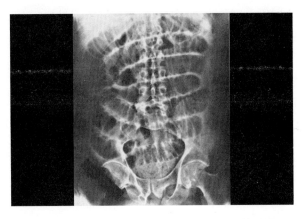

**Image 108A. Small bowel obstruction** on supine abdominal x-ray. Note dilated loops of small bowel in a ladder-like pattern. Air-fluid levels may be seen if an upright x-ray is done. (Reproduced, with permission, from Way L, Doherty G. *Current Surgical Diagnosis & Treatment*, 11th ed. New York: McGraw-Hill, 2003.)

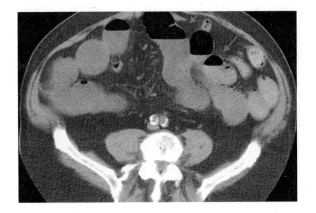

**Image 108B. Small bowel obstruction,** seen on abdominal CT scan showing multiple dilated loops of small bowel with air-fluid levels.

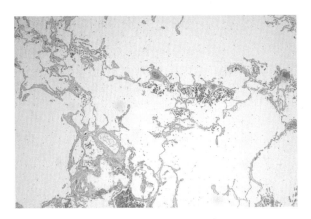

**Image 109A. Emphysema.** Note the abnormal permanent enlargement of the airspaces distal to the terminal bronchiole. On microscopy, enlarged alveoli are seen separated by thin septa, some of which appear to float within the alveolar spaces. (Reproduced, with permission, from USMLERx.com.)

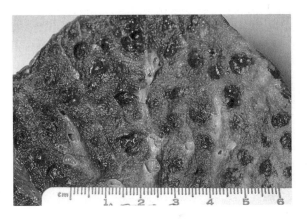

**Image 109B. Emphysema.** Gross specimen showing multiple cavities lined by heavy black carbon deposits, typical of smoking.

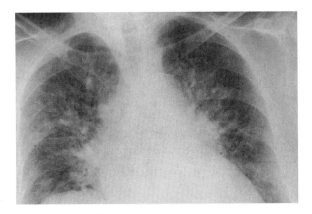

**Image 110. Pulmonary edema.** Posteroanterior chest x-ray in a man with acute pulmonary edema due to left ventricular failure. Note the bat's-wing density, cardiac enlargement, increased size of upper lobe vessels, and pulmonary venous congestion. (Reproduced, with permission, from McPhee SJ et al. *Pathophysiology of Disease: An Introduction to Clinical Medicine*, 4th ed. New York: McGraw-Hill, 2002.)

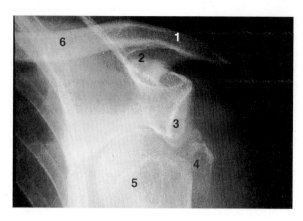

**Image 111A. Anterior shoulder dislocation.** Note the humeral head inferior and medial to the glenoid fossa and fracture fragments from the greater tuberosity. 1—Acromion; 2—Coracoid; 3—Glenoid fossa; 4—Fracture fragments; 5—Humeral head; 6—Clavicle

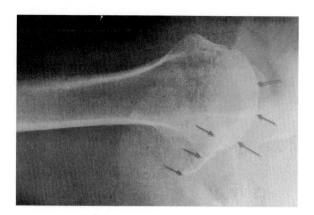

**Image 111B. Anterior shoulder dislocation.** Axillary view showing humeral head dislocated anteriorly with respect to the glenoid fossa.

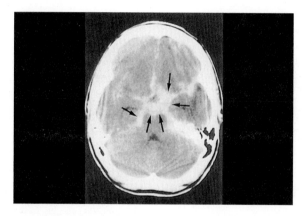

**Image 112A. Subarachnoid hemorrhage.** CT scan without contrast reveals blood in the subarachnoid space at the base of the brain.

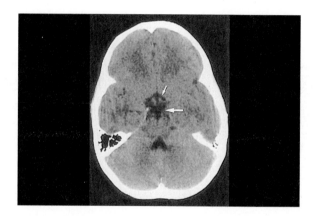

**Image 112B. Subarachnoid hemorrhage.** Normal comparison study at the same level.

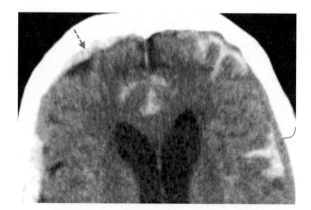

**Image 112C. Subarachnoid hemorrhage.** CT scan showing subarachnoid hemorrhage (straight arrow), acute subdural hemorrhage (dotted arrow), and chronic isodense subdural hemorrhage (curved arrow).

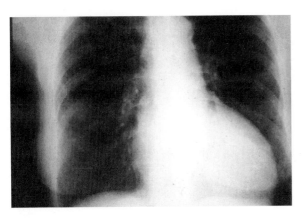

**Image 113. Left ventricular hypertrophy** (mediastinum wider than 50% of the width of the chest) from aortic valve stenosis, a borderline case.*

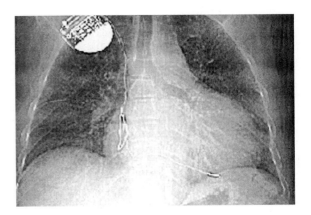

**Image 114. Amiodarone toxicity.** Diffuse interstitial bilateral pulmonary markings in a reticular nodular pattern, most prominent in the lung bases and posteriorly, are evidence of pulmonary fibrosis.*

HIGH-YIELD FACTS

HIGH-YIELD IMAGES

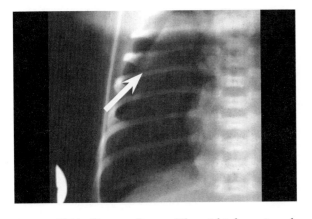

**Image 115A. Pneumothorax.** The right lung is collapsed; the apparent straight line off the rightmost edge of the pleural space indicated by the arrow shows the edge of the collapsed lung.*

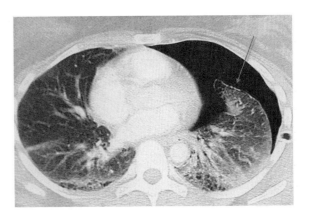

**Image 115B. Pneumothorax.** CT chest image showing collapsed left lung with ipsilateral increased density of the lung parenchyma.

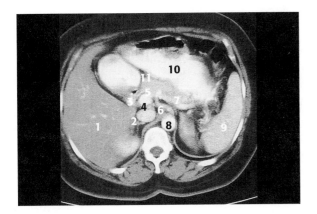

**Image 116. CT of the abdomen** with contrast—normal anatomy. 1—Liver; 2—IVC; 3—Portal vein; 4—Hepatic artery; 5—Gastroduodenal artery; 6—Celiac trunk; 7—Splenic vein; 8—Aorta; 9—Spleen; 10—Stomach; 11—Pancreas

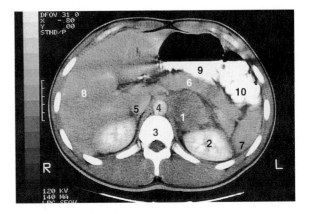

**Image 117. Left adrenal mass.** 1—Large left adrenal mass; 2—Kidney; 3—Vertebral body; 4—Aorta; 5—IVC; 6—Pancreas; 7—Spleen; 8—Liver; 9—Stomach with air and contrast; 10—Colon–splenic flexure

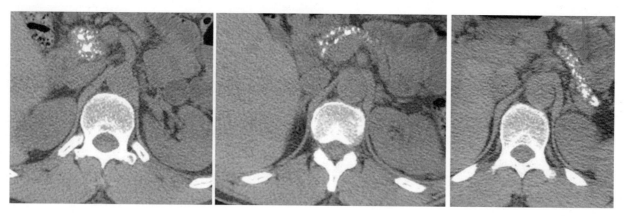

**Image 118. Chronic pancreatitis** seen on three consecutive non-contrast CT scan images showing punctate calcifications in the head, body, and tail of the pancreas.

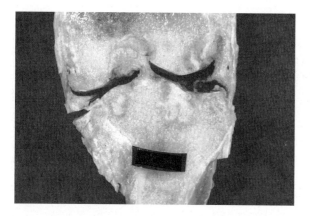

**Image 119A. Osteoarthritis.** Increased fibrosis of the joint and a decreased amount of cartilage are apparent. *

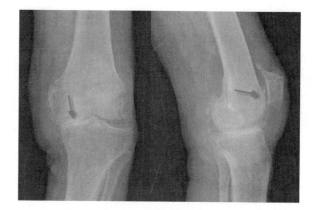

**Image 119B. Osteoarthritis.** X-ray of the knee, frontal and lateral views, showing medial and patello femoral join space narrowing and sclerosis.

| Disease/finding | Most common/important associations |
|---|---|
| Actinic (solar) keratosis | Squamous cell carcinoma |
| Acute gastric ulcer associated with CNS injury | Cushing's ulcer (↑ ICP stimulates vagal gastric secretion) |
| Acute gastric ulcer associated with severe burns | Curling's ulcer (greatly reduced plasma volume results in sloughing of gastric mucosa) |
| Alternating areas of transmural inflammation and normal colon | Skip lesions (Crohn's disease: autoimmune) |
| Aneurysm, dissecting | Hypertension |
| Aortic aneurysm, abdominal and descending aorta | Atherosclerosis |
| Aortic aneurysm, ascending | 3° syphilis |
| Atrophy of the mammillary bodies | Wernicke's encephalopathy (thiamine deficiency causing ataxia, ophthalmoplegia, and confusion) |
| Autosplenectomy (fibrosis and shrinkage) | Sickle cell anemia (HbS) |
| Bacteremia/pneumonia (IV drug user) | S. aureus |
| Bacteria associated with stomach cancer | H. pylori |
| Bacterial meningitis (adults and elderly) | Streptococcus pneumoniae |
| Bacterial meningitis (newborns and kids) | Group B streptococcus (newborns), S. pneumoniae/Neisseria meningitidis (kids) |
| Benign melanocytic nevus | Spitz nevus (most common in first two decades) |
| Bleeding disorder with GpIb deficiency | Bernard-Soulier disease (defect in platelet adhesion) |
| Brain tumor (adults) | Supratentorial: mets > astrocytoma (including glioblastoma multiforme) > meningioma > schwannoma |
| Brain tumor (kids) | Infratentorial: medulloblastoma (cerebellum) or supratentorial: craniopharyngioma (cerebrum) |
| Breast cancer | Infiltrating ductal carcinoma (in the United States, 1 in 9 women will develop breast cancer) |
| Breast mass | 1. Fibrocystic change<br>2. Carcinoma (in postmenopausal women) |
| Breast tumor (benign) | Fibroadenoma |
| Bug in debilitated, hospitalized pneumonia patient | Klebsiella |
| Cardiac 1° tumor (kids) | Rhabdomyoma |
| Cardiac manifestation of lupus | Libman-Sacks endocarditis (nonbacterial, affecting mitral) |
| Cardiac tumor (adults) | 1. Metastasis<br>2. 1° myxoma (4:1 left to right atrium; "ball and valve") |
| Cardiomyopathy | Dilated cardiomyopathy (40% are familial) |

| | |
|---|---|
| Cerebellar tonsillar herniation | Arnold-Chiari malformation (often causes hydrocephalus) |
| Chronic arrhythmia | Atrial fibrillation (associated with high risk of emboli) |
| Chronic atrophic gastritis (autoimmune) | Predisposition to gastric carcinoma (can also cause pernicious anemia) |
| Clear cell adenocarcinoma of the vagina | DES exposure in utero |
| Congenital adrenal hyperplasia | 21-hydroxylase deficiency |
| Congenital cardiac anomaly | VSD |
| Congenital conjugated hyperbilirubinemia (black liver) | Dubin-Johnson syndrome (inability of hepatocytes to secrete conjugated bilirubin into bile) |
| Constrictive pericarditis in developing world | Tuberculosis |
| Coronary artery involved in thrombosis | LAD > RCA > LCA |
| Cretinism | Iodine deficit/hypothyroidism |
| Cushing's syndrome | 1. Corticosteroid therapy<br>2. Excess ACTH secretion by pituitary |
| Cyanosis (early; less common) | Tetralogy of Fallot, transposition of great vessels, truncus arteriosus |
| Cyanosis (late; more common) | VSD, ASD, PDA |
| Death in CML | Blast crisis |
| Death in SLE | Lupus nephropathy |
| Dementia | 1. Alzheimer's disease<br>2. Multiple infarcts |
| Demyelinating disease | Multiple sclerosis |
| DIC | Gram-negative sepsis, obstetric complications, cancer, burn trauma |
| Dietary deficit | Iron |
| Diverticulum in pharynx | Zenker's diverticulum (diagnosed by barium swallow) |
| Ejection click | Aortic /pulmonic stenosis |
| Esophageal cancer | Squamous cell carcinoma |
| Food poisoning | *S. aureus* |
| Gene involved in cancer | *p53* tumor suppressor gene |
| Glomerulonephritis (adults) | Berger's disease (IgA nephropathy) |
| Gynecologic malignancy | Endometrial carcinoma |
| Heart murmur | Mitral valve prolapse |
| Heart valve in bacterial endocarditis | Mitral (rheumatic fever), tricuspid (IV drug abuse), aortic (2nd affected in rheumatic fever) |
| Helminth infection (U.S.) | 1. *Enterobius vermicularis*<br>2. *Ascaris lumbricoides* |

| | |
|---|---|
| Hematoma—epidural | Rupture of middle meningeal artery (arterial bleeding is fast) |
| Hematoma—subdural | Rupture of bridging veins (trauma; venous bleeding is slow) |
| Hemochromatosis | Multiple blood transfusions (can result in CHF and ↑ risk of hepatocellular carcinoma) |
| Hepatocellular carcinoma | Cirrhotic liver (often associated with hepatitis B and C) |
| Hereditary bleeding disorder | von Willebrand's disease |
| Hereditary harmless jaundice | Gilbert's syndrome (benign congenital unconjugated hyperbilirubinemia) |
| HLA-B27 | Ankylosing spondylitis, Reiter's syndrome, ulcerative colitis |
| HLA-DR3 or -DR4 | Diabetes mellitus type 1, rheumatoid arthritis, SLE |
| Holosystolic murmur | VSD, tricuspid regurgitation, mitral regurgitation |
| Hypercoagulability, endothelial damage, blood stasis | Virchow's triad (results in venous thrombosis) |
| Hypertension, 2° | Renal disease |
| Hypoparathyroidism | Thyroidectomy |
| Hypopituitarism | Adenoma |
| Infection in blood transfusion | Hepatitis C |
| Kidney stones | 1. Calcium = radiopaque<br>2. Struvite (ammonium) = radiopaque (formed by urease-positive organisms such as *Proteus vulgaris* or *Staphylococcus*)<br>3. Uric acid = radiolucent |
| Late cyanotic shunt (uncorrected L → R becomes R → L) | Eisenmenger's syndrome (caused by ASD, VSD, PDA; results in pulmonary hypertension/polycythemia) |
| Liver disease | Alcoholic liver disease |
| Lysosomal storage disease | Gaucher's disease |
| Male cancer | Prostatic carcinoma |
| Malignancy associated with noninfectious fever | Hodgkin's lymphoma |
| Malignant skin tumor | Basal cell carcinoma (rarely metastasizes) |
| Mental retardation | 1. Down syndrome<br>2. Fragile X syndrome |
| Mets to bone | Breast, lung, thyroid, testes, prostate, kidney |
| Mets to brain | Lung, breast, skin (melanoma), kidney (renal cell carcinoma), GI |
| Mets to liver | Colon, gastric, pancreatic, breast, and lung carcinomas |
| Mitral valve stenosis | Rheumatic heart disease |
| Motor neuron disease | ALS |
| Myocarditis | Coxsackie B |
| Neoplasm (kids) | 1. ALL<br>2. Cerebellar medulloblastoma |
| Nephrotic syndrome (adults) | Membranous glomerulonephritis |

| | |
|---|---|
| Nephrotic syndrome (kids) | Minimal change disease (associated with infections/vaccinations; treat with corticosteroids) |
| Obstruction of male urinary tract | BPH |
| Opening snap | Mitral stenosis |
| Opportunistic infection in AIDS | *Pneumocystis jiroveci* (formerly *carinii*) pneumonia |
| Organ receiving mets | Adrenal glands (due to rich blood supply) |
| Organ sending mets | Lung > breast, stomach |
| Osteomyelitis | *S. aureus* |
| Osteomyelitis in patients with sickle cell disease | *Salmonella* |
| Osteomyelitis with IV drug use | *Pseudomonas* |
| Ovarian metastasis from gastric carcinoma or breast cancer | Krukenberg tumor (mucin-secreting signet-ring cells) |
| Ovarian tumor (benign) | Serous cystadenoma |
| Ovarian tumor (malignant) | Serous cystadenocarcinoma |
| Pancreatic tumor | Adenocarcinoma (head of pancreas) |
| Pancreatitis (acute) | EtOH and gallstones |
| Pancreatitis (chronic) | EtOH (adults), cystic fibrosis (kids) |
| Patient with ALL /CLL /AML /CML | ALL: child, CLL: adult > 60, AML: adult > 60, CML: adult 35–50 |
| Patient with Hodgkin's disease | Young male (except nodular sclerosis type: female) |
| Pelvic inflammatory disease | *Neisseria gonorrhoeae* (monoarticular arthritis) |
| Philadelphia chromosome t(9;22) (*bcr-abl*) | CML (may sometimes be associated with ALL/AML) |
| Pituitary tumor | 1. Prolactinoma<br>2. Somatotropic "acidophilic" adenoma |
| Pneumonia, hospital acquired | *Klebsiella* |
| Primary amenorrhea | Turner's syndrome (XO) |
| Primary bone tumor (adults) | Multiple myeloma |
| Primary hyperaldosteronism | Adenoma of adrenal cortex |
| Primary hyperparathyroidism | 1. Adenomas<br>2. Hyperplasia<br>3. Carcinoma |
| Primary liver cancer | Hepatocellular carcinoma (also known as hepatoma) |
| Pulmonary hypertension | COPD |
| Recurrent inflammation/thrombosis of small/medium vessels in extremities | Buerger's disease (strongly associated with tobacco) |

| | |
|---|---|
| Renal tumor | Renal cell carcinoma: associated with von Hippel–Lindau and adult polycystic kidney disease; paraneoplastic syndromes (erythropoietin, renin, PTH, ACTH) |
| Right heart failure due to a pulmonary cause | Cor pulmonale |
| S3 (protodiastolic gallop) | $\uparrow$ ventricular filling (L $\rightarrow$ R shunt, mitral regurgitation, LV failure [CHF]) |
| S4 (presystolic gallop) | Stiff/hypertrophic ventricle (aortic stenosis, restrictive cardiomyopathy) |
| Secondary hyperparathyroidism | Hypocalcemia of chronic kidney disease |
| Sexually transmitted disease | Chlamydia |
| SIADH | Small cell carcinoma of the lung |
| Site of diverticula | Sigmoid colon |
| Site of metastasis | 1. Regional lymph nodes<br>2. Liver |
| Sites of atherosclerosis | Abdominal aorta > coronary > popliteal > carotid |
| Stomach cancer | Adenocarcinoma |
| Stomach ulcerations and high gastrin levels | Zollinger-Ellison syndrome (gastrinoma of duodenum or pancreas) |
| t(14;18) | Follicular lymphomas (*bcl*-2 activation) |
| t(8;14) | Burkitt's lymphoma (c-*myc* activation) |
| t(9;22) | Philadelphia chromosome, CML (*bcr-abl* hybrid) |
| Temporal arteritis | Risk of ipsilateral blindness due to thrombosis of ophthalmic artery |
| Testicular tumor | Seminoma |
| Thyroid cancer | Papillary carcinoma |
| Tumor in women | Leiomyoma (estrogen dependent) |
| Tumor of infancy | Hemangioma |
| Tumor of the adrenal medulla (adults) | Pheochromocytoma (usually benign) |
| Tumor of the adrenal medulla (kids) | Neuroblastoma (malignant) |
| Type of Hodgkin's | Nodular sclerosis (vs. mixed cellularity, lymphocytic predominance, lymphocytic depletion) |
| Type of non-Hodgkin's | Diffuse large cell |
| UTI | *E. coli, Staphylococcus saprophyticus* (young women) |
| Viral encephalitis | HSV |
| Vitamin deficiency (U.S.) | Folic acid (pregnant women are at high risk; body stores only 3- to 4-month supply) |

| Topic | Equation | Page |
|---|---|---|
| Sensitivity | Sensitivity $= TP / (TP + FN)$ | 53 |
| Specificity | Specificity $= TN / (TN + FP)$ | 53 |
| Positive predictive value | $PPV = TP / (TP + FP)$ | 53 |
| Negative predictive value | $NPV = TN / (TN + FN)$ | 53 |
| Relative risk | $RR = \dfrac{\left[\dfrac{a}{a+b}\right]}{\left[\dfrac{c}{c+d}\right]}$ | 54 |
| Attributable risk | $AR = \left[\dfrac{a}{a+b}\right] - \left[\dfrac{c}{c+d}\right]$ | 54 |
| Hardy-Weinberg equilibrium | $p^2 + 2pq + q^2 = 1$ <br> $p + q = 1$ | 84 |
| Henderson-Hasselbalch equation | $pH = pKa + \log \dfrac{[HCO_3^-]}{0.03\ P_{CO_2}}$ | 463 |
| Volume of distribution | $V_d = \dfrac{\text{amount of drug in the body}}{\text{plasma drug concentration}}$ | 228 |
| Clearance | $CL = \dfrac{\text{rate of elimination of drug}}{\text{plasma drug concentration}}$ | 228 |
| Half-life | $t_{\frac{1}{2}} = \dfrac{0.7 \times V_d}{CL}$ | 228 |
| Loading dose | $LD = C_p \times \dfrac{V_d}{F}$ | 229 |
| Maintenance dose | $MD = C_p \times \dfrac{CL}{F}$ | 229 |
| Cardiac output | $CO = \dfrac{\text{rate of } O_2 \text{ consumption}}{\text{arterial } O_2 \text{ content} - \text{venous } O_2 \text{ content}}$ | 250 |
| Cardiac output | $CO = \text{stroke volume} \times \text{heart rate}$ | 250 |
| Mean arterial pressure | $MAP = \text{cardiac output} \times \text{total peripheral resistance}$ | 250 |
| Mean arterial pressure | $MAP = \frac{1}{3} \text{ systolic} + \frac{2}{3} \text{ diastolic}$ | 250 |
| Stroke volume | $SV = \text{end diastolic volume} - \text{end systolic volume}$ | 250 |
| Ejection fraction | $EF = \dfrac{\text{stroke volume}}{\text{end diastolic volume}} \times 100$ | 251 |
| Resistance | $R = \dfrac{\text{driving pressure}}{\text{flow}} = \dfrac{8\eta \text{ (viscosity)} \times \text{length}}{\pi\ r^4}$ | 252 |
| Net filtration pressure | $P_{net} = \left[(P_c - P_i) - (\pi_c - \pi_i)\right]$ | 262 |

| | | |
|---|---|---|
| Glomerular filtration rate | $GFR = U_{inulin} \times \dfrac{V}{P_{inulin}} = C_{inulin}$ | 457 |
| Glomerular filtration rate | $GFR = K_f \left[ (P_{GC} - P_{BS}) - (\pi_{GC} - \pi_{BS}) \right]$ | 457 |
| Effective renal plasma flow | $ERPF = U_{PAH} \times \dfrac{V}{P_{PAH}} = C_{PAH}$ | 457 |
| Renal blood flow | $RBF = \dfrac{RPF}{1 - Hct}$ | 457 |
| Filtration fraction | $FF = \dfrac{GFR}{RPF}$ | 458 |
| Free water clearance | $C_{H_2O} = V - C_{osm}$ | 458 |
| Physiologic dead space | $V_D = V_T \times \dfrac{(Pa_{CO_2} - Pe_{CO_2})}{Pa_{CO_2}}$ | 503 |

# SECTION IV

# Top-Rated Review Resources

This section is a database of top-rated basic science review books, sample examination books, software, Web sites, and commercial review courses that have been marketed to medical students studying for the USMLE Step 1. At the end of the section is a list of publishers and independent bookstores with addresses and phone numbers. For each recommended resource, we list the **Title** of the book, the **First Author** (or editor), the **Series Name** (where applicable), the **Current Publisher**, the **Copyright Year**, the **Number of Pages**, the **ISBN Code**, the **Approximate List Price**, the **Format** of the resource, and the **Number of Test Questions**. The entries for most books also include **Summary Comments** that describe their style and overall utility for studying. Finally, each recommended resource receives a **Rating**. Within each section, books are arranged first by Rating and then alphabetically by First Author within each Rating group.

A letter rating scale with six different grades reflects the detailed student evaluations for **Rated Resources**. Each rated resource receives a rating as follows:

| | |
|---|---|
| A+ | Excellent for boards review. |
| A<br>A– | Very good for boards review; choose among the group. |
| B+<br>B | Good, but use only after exhausting better sources. |
| B– | Fair, but there are many better books in the discipline; or low-yield subject material. |

The Rating is meant to reflect the overall usefulness of the resource in helping medical students prepare for the USMLE Step 1 examination. This is based on a number of factors, including:

- The cost
- The readability of the text
- The appropriateness and accuracy of the material
- The quality and number of sample questions
- The quality of written answers to sample questions
- The quality and appropriateness of the illustrations (e.g., graphs, diagrams, photographs)
- The length of the text (longer is not necessarily better)
- The quality and number of other resources available in the same discipline
- The importance of the discipline for the USMLE Step 1 examination

Please note that ratings do not reflect the quality of the resources for purposes other than reviewing for the USMLE Step 1 examination. Many books with lower ratings are well written and informative but are not ideal for boards preparation. We have not listed or commented on general textbooks available in the basic sciences.

Evaluations are based on the cumulative results of formal and informal surveys of thousands of medical students at many medical schools across the country. The summary comments and overall ratings represent a consensus opinion, but there may have been a broad range of opinion or limited student feedback on any particular resource.

Please note that the data listed are subject to change in that:

- Publishers' prices change frequently.
- Bookstores often charge an additional markup.
- New editions come out frequently, and the quality of updating varies.
- The same book may be reissued through another publisher.

We actively encourage medical students and faculty to submit their opinions and ratings of these basic science review materials so that we may update our database. (See p. xvii, How to Contribute.) In addition, we ask that publishers and authors submit for evaluation review copies of basic science review books, including new editions and books not included in our database. We also solicit reviews of new books or suggestions for alternate modes of study that may be useful in preparing for the examination, such as flash cards, computer software, commercial review courses, and Web sites.

### Disclaimer/Conflict of Interest Statement

No material in this book, including the ratings, reflects the opinion or influence of the publisher. All errors and omissions will gladly be corrected if brought to the attention of the authors through our blog at www.firstaidteam.com. Please note that USMLERx and the entire First Aid for the USMLE series are publications by the senior authors of this book; their ratings are based solely on recommendations from the student authors of this book as well as data from the student survey and feedback forms.

**USMLEWorld Qbank**
USMLEWORLD
www.usmleworld.com

**$99 for 1 month;**
**$185 for 3 months**

Test/2000 q

An excellent bank of well-constructed questions that closely mirror those found on Step 1. Questions demand multistep reasoning and are often more difficult than those on the actual exam. Offers excellent, detailed explanations with figures and tables. Features a number of test customization and analysis options. Unfortunately, the program does not allow other application windows to be open for reference. Users can see cumulative results both over time and compared to other test takers.

**Kaplan Qbank**
KAPLAN
www.kaplanmedical.com

**$109 for 1 month;**
**$189 for 3 months**

Test/2400 q

A high-quality question bank tailored to boards preparation. Questions cover most content found on Step 1 but emphasize recall of overly specific details rather than the integrative problem-solving skills tested on the actual exam. Test content and performance feedback can be organized by both organ system and discipline. Includes well-written, detailed explanations of all answer choices with references to *First Aid*. Additional Qbanks for physiology and clinical vignettes are available. Users can see cumulative results both over time and compared to other test takers.

**USMLERx Qmax**
MEDIQ LEARNING
www.usmlerx.com

**$79 for 1 month;**
**$149 for 3 months**

Test/3000 q

A well-priced question bank that offers Step 1–style questions accompanied by thorough explanations. Some obscure material is omitted, making it more straightforward than other question banks. Each explanation includes high-yield facts and references from *First Aid*. However, the proportion of questions covering a given subject area does not always reflect the actual exam's relative emphasis. Question stems occasionally rely on "buzzwords." Provides detailed performance analyses.

REVIEW RESOURCES

QUESTION BANKS

**B+**

**USMLE Consult**                            **$79 for 1 month;**          Test/2500 q
Elsevier                                      **$149 for 3 months**

www.usmleconsult.com

A solid question bank that can be divided according to discipline and subject area. Question length, difficulty, and test interface (FRED) are similar to those of the actual exam. Offers concise explanations with links to Student Consult and First Consult content. Users can see cumulative results both over time and compared to other test takers. Student Consult also offers a Robbins Pathology Test Bank ($35 for 1 month, $49 for 3 months) featuring 500 USMLE-style questions as well as the Scorrelator ($35), a 3-hour, 150-question mock exam that predicts your USMLE Step 1 score. Limited student feedback on Student Consult products.

**B**

**USMLEasy**                                 **$79 for 1 month;**          Test/2000 q
McGraw-Hill                                   **$169 for 3 months**

www.usmleasy.com

A question bank based on the PreTest series. Many questions are shorter and more obscure than those on the actual Step 1 exam. Users can track questions completed as well as customize tests. Useful as a supplemental review after other resources have been exhausted.

**B+**

### Kaplan USMLE Step 1 Qbook
KAPLAN

$44.95    Test/850 q

Kaplan, 2008, 480 pages, ISBN 9781419553158

A resource consisting of seventeen 50-question exams organized by the traditional basic science disciplines. Similar to the Kaplan Qbank, and offers good USMLE-style questions with clear, detailed explanations; however, lacks the classic images typically seen on the exam. Also includes a guide on test-taking strategies.

**B+**

### First Aid Q&A for the USMLE Step 1
LE

$44.95    Test/1000 q

McGraw-Hill, 2009, 676 pages, ISBN 9780071597944

A great source of more than 1000 questions drawn from the USMLE Step 1 Qmax test bank, organized according to subject. Also features one full-length exam of 350 questions. Questions are slightly less complex than those found on Step 1 but provide representative coverage of the concepts typically tested. Includes brief but adequate explanations of both correct and incorrect answer choices.

**B**

### Blueprints Q&A Step 1
CLEMENT

$36.95    Test/350 q

Lippincott Williams & Wilkins, 2003, 184 pages,
ISBN 9781405103237

Contains one full-length exam of 350 questions written by students. Good for practicing the multistep questions common on Step 1, but questions are easier than those on the actual test.

**B**

### Lange Practice Tests: USMLE Step 1
GOLDBERG

$42.95    Test/650 q

McGraw-Hill, 2006, 191 pages, ISBN 9780071446150

A good resource for review questions consisting of 13 blocks of 50 questions with explanations. In general, questions are not as lengthy or challenging as those on the actual Step 1 exam. Includes explanations of correct answer choices only.

REVIEW RESOURCES

QUESTION BOOKS

### *Lange Q&A: USMLE Step 1*

KING

**McGraw-Hill, 2008, 520 pages, ISBN 9780071445788**

Offers many questions organized by subject area along with three comprehensive practice exams. Questions are often challenging but are not always representative of Step 1 style. Includes detailed explanations of both correct and incorrect answer choices.

*$44.95*   Test/1200 q

### *NMS Review for USMLE Step 1*

LAZO

**Lippincott Williams & Wilkins, 2005, 480 pages + CD-ROM, ISBN 9780781779210**

A text and CD-ROM that offers 17 practice exams with answers. Some questions are too picky or difficult. Annotated explanations are well written but are sometimes unnecessarily detailed. The six pages of color plates are helpful. The CD-ROM attempts to simulate the computer-based testing format but is disorganized.

*$48.95*   Test/850 q

### A
**WebPath: The Internet Pathology Laboratory**    **Free (online version);**    Review/Test/1000 q
http://library.med.utah.edu/WebPath/    **$60 for CD-ROM**

Features more than 1900 outstanding gross and microscopic images, clinical vignette questions, and case studies. Includes eight general pathology exams and 11 system-based exams with approximately 1000 questions. Also features 170 questions associated with images. Questions reflect boards format and difficulty but are typically shorter. A WebPath CD-ROM is available for $60 and features the online material supplemented with additional images, topics, tutorials, and radiology.

### B
**The Pathology Guy**    **Free**    Review
FRIEDLANDER
www.pathguy.com

A free Web site containing extensive but poorly organized information on a variety of fundamental concepts in pathology. A high-yield summary intended for USMLE review can be found at www.pathguy.com/meltdown.txt, but the information given is limited by a lack of images and frequent digressions.

### B
**Lippincott's 350-Question Practice Test for USMLE Step 1**    **Free**    Test/350 q
Lippincott Williams & Wilkins
www.lww.com/medstudent/usmle

A free, full-length, seven-block, 350-question practice exam in a format similar to that of the real Step 1. Questions are easier than those on the actual exam, and the explanations provided are sparse. Users can bookmark questions and can choose between taking the test all at once or by section.

### B⁻
**The Whole Brain Atlas**    **Free**    Review
JOHNSON
www.med.harvard.edu/AANLIB/home.html

A collection of high-quality brain MR and CT images with views of normal and diseased brains. The interface is technologically impressive but complex, and the subject matter is overly specific, limiting its use as a boards review study tool.

### B⁻
**Digital Anatomist Interactive Atlases**    **Free**    Review
UNIVERSITY OF WASHINGTON
www9.biostr.washington.edu/da.html

A good site containing an interactive neuroanatomy course along with a three-dimensional atlas of the brain, thorax, and knee. Atlases have computer-generated images and cadaver sections. Each atlas also has a quiz in which users identify structures in the slide images; however, questions do not focus on high-yield anatomy for Step 1.

**A**

### First Aid Cases for the USMLE Step 1

LE

$44.95     Review

McGraw-Hill, 2009, 497 pages, ISBN 9780071601351

A series of more than 400 high-yield cases divided into sections by organ system. Each case features a paragraph-long clinical vignette with relevant images, followed by questions and short explanations. Offers great coverage of many frequently tested concepts, and integrates subject matter in the discussion of a single vignette. A good source of questions to review material outlined in *First Aid for the USMLE Step 1*.

**A⁻**

### USMLE Step 1 Secrets

BROWN

$39.95     Review

Elsevier, 2008, 324 pages, ISBN 9780323054393

Clarifies difficult concepts in a concise, easy-to-read manner. Employs a case-based format and integrates information well. Complements other boards study resources, with a focus on understanding preclinical fundamentals rather than on rote memorization.

**A⁻**

### medEssentials for the USMLE Step 1

MANLEY

$49.95     Review

Kaplan, 2008, 544 pages, ISBN 9781607144823

A comprehensive review divided into general principles and organ systems, and organized using high-yield tables and figures. Excellent for visual learners, but can be overly detailed and time consuming. Also includes color images in the back along with a monthly subscription to online interactive exercises, although these are of limited value for Step 1 preparation.

**B⁺**

### Cases & Concepts Step 1: Basic Science Review

CAUGHEY

$39.95     Review

Lippincott Williams & Wilkins, 2009, 400 pages,
ISBN 9780781793919

One hundred sixteen clinical cases integrating basic science with clinical data, followed by USMLE-style questions with answers and rationales. Thumbnail and key-concept boxes highlight key facts. Limited student feedback.

REVIEW RESOURCES

COMPREHENSIVE

### Kaplan's USMLE Step 1 Home Study Program
KAPLAN

$499.00     Review

Kaplan, 2008, 1900 pages, ISBN 0X63410105

A resource consisting of two general principle and two organ system review books. All are highly comprehensive but can be overwhelmingly lengthy if they are not started very early. Although costly, the program can serve as an excellent reference for studying by virtue of its detail. Books can be purchased at www.kaptest.com.

### First Aid for the Basic Sciences: General Principles
LE

$69.95     Review

McGraw-Hill, 2008, 561 pages, ISBN 9780071545457

A comprehensive review of the basic sciences covered in year 1 of medical school. Organized by discipline, and includes hundreds of full-color images and tables. Can be started with coursework and then used as a review/reference during boards preparation. Limited student feedback.

### First Aid for the Basic Sciences: Organ Systems
LE

$89.95     Review

McGraw-Hill, 2008, 938 pages, ISBN 9780071545433

A comprehensive review of the basic sciences covered in year 2 of medical school. Organized by organ system, and includes hundreds of full-color images and tables. Can be started with coursework and then used as a review/reference during boards preparation. Limited student feedback.

### PreTest Clinical Vignettes for the USMLE Step 1
MCGRAW-HILL

$29.95     Test/350 q

McGraw-Hill, 2008, 323 pages, ISBN 9780071471848

Clinical vignette–style questions with detailed explanations, divided into seven blocks of 50 questions covering basic sciences. In general, questions are representative of the length and complexity of those on Step 1.

### Step-Up to USMLE Step 1
MEHTA

$44.95     Review

Lippincott Williams & Wilkins, 2009, 416 pages, ISBN 9781605474700

An organ system–based review text with clinical vignettes that is useful for integrating the basic sciences covered in Step 1. The text is composed primarily of outlines, charts, tables, and diagrams, making the depth of material covered somewhat limited. Includes access to a sample online question bank.

## B+

### Déjà Review: USMLE Step 1
NAHEEDY

$25.95    Review

McGraw-Hill, 2006, 192 pages, ISBN 9780071447904

A resource featuring questions and answers in a two-column, quiz-yourself format similar to that of the Recall series, divided according to discipline. Features a section of high-yield clinical vignettes along with useful mnemonics throughout. Contains a few mistakes, but remains a good alternative to flash cards as a last-minute review before the exam.

## B+

### USMLE Step 1 Recall: Buzzwords for the Boards
REINHEIMER

$42.95    Review

Lippincott Williams & Wilkins, 2008, 330 pages, ISBN 9780781770705

A review of core Step 1 topics presented in a two-column, quiz-yourself format. Best for a quick last-minute review before the exam. Covers many important subjects, but not comprehensive or tightly organized. Sometimes focuses on obscure details. Compare with the Déjà Review series. Includes all questions and answers in downloadable MP3 files so that files can be used on any digital audio playback device.

## B+

### Underground Clinical Vignettes: Step 1 Bundle
SWANSON

$169.95    Review

Lippincott Williams & Wilkins, 2007, 9 volumes, ISBN 9780781763622

A bundle that includes nine books. Designed for easy quizzing with a group. Case-based vignettes provide a good review supplement. Best when started early with coursework or when used in conjunction with another primary review resource.

## B

### USMLE Step 1 Made Ridiculously Simple
CARL

$29.95    Review

MedMaster, 2008, 376 pages, ISBN 9780940780712

A quick and easy read. Uses a table and chart format organized by subject, but some charts are poorly labeled. Consider as an adjunct to more comprehensive sources.

*Lange Outline Review: USMLE Step 1*                    *$39.95*     Review
GOLDBERG
McGraw-Hill, 2006, 367 pages, ISBN 9780071451918
A comprehensive outline review that begins with a short chapter on general principles. Each of the chapters that follow employs a bulleted format aimed at reviewing major disease processes by organ system. Coverage is at times low yield. Includes some black-and-white images of gross and microscopic pathology.

**A⁻**

### High-Yield Embryology
DUDEK
Lippincott Williams & Wilkins, 2006, 208 pages,
ISBN 9780781768726

A very good but lengthy review of a relatively low-yield subject. Offers
excellent organization with clinical correlations. Includes a high-yield
list of embryologic origins of tissues.

**$27.95**   Review

---

**A⁻**

### High-Yield Neuroanatomy
FIX
Lippincott Williams & Wilkins, 2008, 160 pages,
ISBN 9780781779463

An easy-to-read, straightforward format with excellent diagrams and illustrations. Features a useful atlas of brain section images, a glossary
of important terms, an appendicized table of neurologic lesions, and
an expanded index. Overall, a great resource, but more detailed than
what is required for Step 1.

**$28.95**   Review/Test/50
Q&A provided
online

---

**A⁻**

### Underground Clinical Vignettes: Anatomy
SWANSON
Lippincott Williams & Wilkins, 2007, 256 pages,
ISBN 9780781764759

Concise clinical cases illustrating approximately 100 frequently tested
diseases with an anatomic basis. Cardinal signs, symptoms, and buzzwords are highlighted. Also includes 20 additional boards-style questions. A useful source for isolating important anatomy concepts tested
on Step 1.

**$22.95**   Review/Test/20 q

---

**A⁻**

### USMLE Road Map: Gross Anatomy
WHITE
McGraw-Hill, 2006, 240 pages, ISBN 9780071445160

An overview of high-yield gross anatomy with clinical correlations
throughout. Also features numerous effective charts and clinical problems with explanations at the end of each chapter. Features good integration of facts, but may be overly detailed and offers few illustrations.
May require an anatomy reference text.

**$26.95**   Review/Test/150 q

---

REVIEW RESOURCES

ANATOMY AND EMBRYOLOGY

**High-Yield Gross Anatomy**
DUDEK
Lippincott Williams & Wilkins, 2007, 352 pages,
ISBN 9780781770156

$27.95     Review

A good review of gross anatomy with some clinical correlations. Contains well-labeled, high-yield radiographic images, but often goes into excessive detail that is beyond the scope of the boards.

**Clinical Anatomy Made Ridiculously Simple**
GOLDBERG
MedMaster, 2007, 187 pages, ISBN 9780940780798

$29.95     Review

An easy-to-read text offering simple diagrams along with numerous mnemonics and amusing associations. The humorous style has variable appeal for students, so browse before buying. Offers good coverage of selected topics. Best if used during coursework. Includes more detail than typically tested on Step 1.

**Clinical Neuroanatomy Made Ridiculously Simple**
GOLDBERG
MedMaster, 2007, 96 pages + CD-ROM, ISBN 9780940780576

$22.95     Review/Test/Few q

An easy-to-read, memorable, and simplified format with clever diagrams. Offers a quick, high-yield review of clinical neuroanatomy, but does not serve as a comprehensive resource for boards review. Places good emphasis on clinically relevant pathways, cranial nerves, and neurologic diseases. Includes a CD-ROM with CT and MR images as well as a tutorial on neurologic localization. Compare with *High-Yield Neuroanatomy.*

**Crash Course: Anatomy**
GRANGER
Elsevier, 2006, 264 pages, ISBN 9780323043199

$29.95     Review

Part of the Crash Course review series for basic sciences, integrating clinical topics. Offers two-color illustrations, handy study tools, and Step 1 review questions. Includes online access. Provides a solid review of anatomy for Step 1. Best if started early.

**Rapid Review: Gross and Developmental Anatomy**
MOORE
Elsevier, 2006, 400 pages, ISBN 9780323045513

$38.95     Review/Test/350 q

A detailed treatment of basic anatomy and embryology, presented in an outline format similar to that of other books in the series. At times more detailed than necessary for boards review. Contains high-yield charts and figures throughout, but has limited diagrams illustrating anatomic relationships. Includes two 50-question tests with extensive explanations, with an additional 250 questions available online.

### Case Files: Gross Anatomy

Toy

McGraw-Hill, 2008, 372 pages, ISBN 9780071489805

A case-based review of gross anatomy essentials. Each case includes a concise discussion, comprehension questions, and a short list of take-home pearls. Diagrams are sparse but high yield.

**$29.95** — Review/Test/150 q

### Déjà Review: Neuroscience

Tremblay

McGraw-Hill, 2007, 217 pages, ISBN 9780071474627

A resource that features questions and answers in a two-column, quiz-yourself format similar to that of the Recall series. Includes several useful diagrams and CT images. A perfect length for Step 1 neurophysiology and anatomy review.

**$25.95** — Review

### USMLE Road Map: Neuroscience

White

McGraw-Hill, 2008, 241 pages, ISBN 9780071496230

An outline review of basic neuroanatomy and physiology with clinical correlations throughout. Also features high-yield facts in boldface along with numerous charts and figures. Clinical problems with explanations are given at the end of each chapter. May be overly detailed for Step 1 review, but a good tool to use as a reference.

**$26.95** — Review/Test/300 q

### Elsevier's Integrated Anatomy and Embryology

Bogart

Elsevier, 2007, 448 pages, ISBN 9781416031659

Part of a new Integrated series that seeks to link basic science concepts across disciplines. Case-based and Step 1–style questions at the end of each chapter allow readers to gauge their comprehension of the material. Includes online access. Best if used during coursework. Limited student feedback.

**$39.95** — Review

### BRS Embryology

Dudek

Lippincott Williams & Wilkins, 2007, 304 pages,
ISBN 9780781771160

An outline-based review of embryology that is typical of the BRS series. Offers a good review, but has limited illustrations and includes much more detail than is required for Step 1 embryology. A discussion of congenital malformations is included at the end of each chapter along with relevant questions. The comprehensive exam at the end of the book is high yield.

**$37.95** — Review/Test/500 q

### PreTest Neuroscience

SIEGEL

McGraw-Hill, 2007, 370 pages, ISBN 9780071471800

A resource that features questions accompanied by detailed explanations. Similar to other titles in the PreTest series. The question format differs significantly from that typically found in Step 1. Black-and-white images are referenced to questions throughout. Includes a brief section of high-yield facts.

**$25.95**   Test/500 q

### BRS Gross Anatomy Flash Cards

SWANSON

Lippincott Williams & Wilkins, 2004, 254 pages,
ISBN 9780781756549

Clinical anatomy cases presented in flash-card format. Cases are too specific for boards preparation, and anatomy basics and radiographic images are generally excluded. Best suited to students who are already relatively well versed in anatomy.

**$34.95**   Flash cards

### Rapid Review: Neuroscience

WEYHENMEYER

Elsevier, 2006, 320 pages, ISBN 9780323022613

A detailed treatment of neuroscience, presented in an outline format similar to that of other books in the series. Should be started early given its extensive treatment of a relatively narrow topic. Contains high-yield charts and figures throughout. Includes two 50-question tests with extensive explanations as well as 250 additional questions online.

**$38.95**   Review

**A**

### High-Yield Behavioral Science
**$26.95**    Review

FADEM

Lippincott Williams & Wilkins, 2009, 126 pages,
ISBN 9780781782586

An extremely concise yet comprehensive review of behavioral science
for Step 1. Offers a logical presentation with charts, graphs, and tables, but lacks questions. Features brief but adequate coverage of statistics. Overall, an excellent, high-yield resource.

**A⁻**

### BRS Behavioral Science
**$37.95**    Review/Test/500 q

FADEM

Lippincott Williams & Wilkins, 2008, 320 pages,
ISBN 9780781782579

An easy-to-read outline-format review of behavioral science. Offers
good, detailed coverage of essential topics, but at a level of depth that
often exceeds what is tested on Step 1. Incorporates excellent tables
and charts as well as a short but complete statistics chapter. Features
high-quality review questions, including a 100-question comprehensive exam.

**A⁻**

### High-Yield Biostatistics
**$27.95**    Review

GLASER

Lippincott Williams & Wilkins, 2005, 128 pages,
ISBN 9780781796446

A well-written, easy-to-read text that offers extensive coverage of epidemiology and biostatistics. Includes good review questions and tables, but somewhat lengthy given the low-yield nature of the subject
matter on Step 1.

**A⁻**

### Underground Clinical Vignettes: Behavioral Science
**$22.95**    Review/Test/20 q

SWANSON

Lippincott Williams & Wilkins, 2007, 256 pages,
ISBN 9780781764643

Concise clinical cases illustrating commonly tested diseases in behavioral science. Cardinal signs, symptoms, and buzzwords are highlighted. Useful for picking out important points in this very broad subject, but requires supplementation from other review sources. Also
includes 20 Step 1–style questions.

REVIEW RESOURCES

BEHAVIORAL SCIENCE

**Platinum Vignettes: Behavioral Science & Biostatistics**
BROCHERT

**$29.95**      Review

Elsevier, 2003, 100 pages, ISBN 9781560535768

A series of cases followed by explanations and discussions on subsequent pages, presented in a format similar to that of other books in the Platinum Vignettes series. In contrast to *Underground Clinical Vignettes: Behavioral Science*, the Platinum Vignettes series includes vignettes for biostatistics; however, there are only half as many cases. Expensive for the amount of material.

**High-Yield Brain & Behavior**
FADEM

**$32.95**      Review

Lippincott Williams & Wilkins, 2007, 256 pages,
ISBN 9780781792288

Part of the new High-Yield Systems series that covers embryology, gross anatomy, radiology, histology, physiology, microbiology, and pharmacology as they relate to the nervous system. Written by the same author as the *High-Yield Behavioral Science* and *BRS Behavioral Science* texts. Overall, provides a good review of neuroscience and behavioral science.

**B**

**PreTest Behavioral Sciences**
EBERT

**$24.95**      Test/500 q

McGraw-Hill, 2001, 300 pages, ISBN 9780071374705

Contains good questions and detailed answers cross-referenced with other resources. Some questions test material beyond the scope of Step 1. Requires time commitment.

**B**

**Kaplan USMLE Medical Ethics**
FISCHER

**$39.00**      Review

Kaplan, 2006, 208 pages, ISBN 9781419542091

Includes 100 cases, each followed by a single question and a detailed explanation. Also offers guidelines on how Step 1 requires test takers to think about ethics and medicolegal questions. Unfortunately, a lengthy review for such a low-yield subject.

**B**

**Blueprints Notes & Cases: Behavioral Science
and Epidemiology**
NEUGROSCHL

**$32.95**      Review/Test/184 q

Lippincott Williams & Wilkins, 2003, 224 pages,
ISBN 9781405103558

A case-oriented approach to behavioral science. Each case includes a clinical history, a basic science review and discussion, key points, and questions. The 8.5″ × 11″ layout may feel overwhelming to some, but the font size is conducive to easy review. A good way to master the intangibles of behavioral science, but more detailed than necessary for Step 1 review.

### *Rapid Review: Behavioral Science*　　　　　*$38.95*　　Review/Test/350 q

STEVENS
Elsevier, 2006, 320 pages, ISBN 9780323045711

Similar in style to other books in the Rapid Review series. Provides a good but low-yield review of a broad subject. Includes 100 questions and explanations along with an additional 250 questions online. Limited student feedback.

### Lippincott's Illustrated Reviews: Biochemistry

CHAMPE

**$54.95**     Review/Test/250 q

Lippincott Williams & Wilkins, 2007, 528 pages,
ISBN 9780781769600

An excellent, integrative, comprehensive review of biochemistry that includes good clinical correlations and highly effective color diagrams. Extremely detailed and requires significant time commitment, so it should be started with coursework. The new edition features high-yield chapter summaries and a "big picture" chapter at the end of the book that highlights important concepts.

### Déjà Review: Biochemistry

MANZOUL

**$22.95**     Review

McGraw-Hill, 2007, 175 pages, ISBN 9780071474634

Features questions and answers in a two-column, quiz-yourself format similar to that of the Recall series. Includes a helpful chapter on molecular biology and many good diagrams. Some questions review more detail than is usually tested on Step 1.

### Rapid Review: Biochemistry

PELLEY

**$38.95**     Review/Test/350 q

Elsevier, 2006, 320 pages, ISBN 9780323044370

A review of basic topics in biochemistry. Presented in outline format, but often goes beyond the level of detail tested on Step 1. High-yield disease correlation boxes are especially useful. Excellent tables and helpful figures are included throughout the text. Offers two 50-question multiple-choice tests with explanations plus 250 questions online.

### BRS Biochemistry and Molecular Biology

SWANSON

**$38.95**     Review/Test/600 q

Lippincott Williams & Wilkins, 2007, 484 pages,
ISBN 9780781786249

A highly detailed review featuring many excellent figures and clinical correlations highlighted in colored boxes. The biochemistry portion includes much more detail than required for Step 1 but may be useful for students without a strong biochemistry background or as a reference text. The molecular biology section is more focused and high yield. Also offers a chapter on laboratory techniques and a comprehensive, 120-question exam. Questions are clinically oriented.

**Underground Clinical Vignettes: Biochemistry**
SWANSON
Lippincott Williams & Wilkins, 2007, 256 pages,
ISBN 9780781764728
Concise clinical cases illustrating approximately 100 frequently tested diseases with a biochemical basis. Cardinal signs, symptoms, and buzzwords are highlighted. Also includes 20 additional boards-style questions. A nice review of "take-home" points for biochemistry and a useful supplement to other sources of review.

$22.95    Review/Test/20 q

**USMLE Road Map: Biochemistry**
MacDONALD
McGraw-Hill, 2007, 223 pages, ISBN 9780071442053
A clear, readable outline review of biochemistry. High-yield references to important diseases of metabolism are scattered throughout, but coverage of clinical correlations is not comprehensive. Includes brief review questions at the end of each chapter. Lacks "big picture" integration of related pathways. Limited student feedback.

$26.95    Review

**Clinical Biochemistry Made Ridiculously Simple**
GOLDBERG
MedMaster, 2004, 93 pages + foldout, ISBN 9780940780309
A conceptual approach to clinical biochemistry, presented with humor. The casual style does not appeal to all students. Offers a good overview and integration of all metabolic pathways. Includes a 23-page clinical review that is very high yield and crammable. Also contains a unique foldout "road map" of metabolism. For students who already have a solid grasp of biochemistry.

$22.95    Review

**BRS Biochemistry and Molecular Biology Flash Cards**
SWANSON
Lippincott Williams & Wilkins, 2007, 512 pages,
ISBN 9780781779029
Quick-review flash cards covering a range of topics in biochemistry and molecular biology. Inadequate for learning purposes, as cards provide only snippets of isolated information and contain some inaccuracies.

$32.95    Flash cards

REVIEW RESOURCES

BIOCHEMISTRY

**High-Yield Biochemistry**                                   *$29.95*        Review

WILCOX

Lippincott Williams & Wilkins, 2009, 128 pages,
ISBN 9780781799249

A concise and crammable text in outline format with good clinical
correlations at the end of each chapter. Features many diagrams and
tables. Best used as a supplemental review, as explanations are scarce
and details are limited.

**PreTest Biochemistry and Genetics**                        *$26.95*        Test/500 q

WILSON

McGraw-Hill, 2007, 498 pages, ISBN 9780071471831

Difficult questions with detailed, referenced explanations. Best for
motivated students when used in combination with a review book.
Lacks clinical vignettes, but features a useful high-yield facts section
at the front of the book.

**A⁻**

### High-Yield Cell and Molecular Biology
DUDEK

Lippincott Williams & Wilkins, 2006, 254 pages,
ISBN 9780781768870

**$27.95**    Review

Cellular and molecular biology presented in an outline format, with good diagrams and clinical correlations. Includes subjects that other review resources do not cover in detail, such as laboratory techniques and second-messenger systems. Not all sections are equally useful; many students skim or read select chapters. Contains no questions or vignettes.

**B⁺**

### Rapid Review: Histology and Cell Biology
BURNS

Elsevier, 2006, 336 pages, ISBN 9780323044257

**$38.95**    Review/Test/350 q

A resource whose format is similar to that of other books in the Rapid Review series. Features an outline of basic concepts with numerous charts, but histology images are limited. Two 50-question multiple-choice tests are presented with explanations, along with 250 more questions online.

**B⁺**

### High-Yield Genetics
DUDEK

Lippincott Williams & Wilkins, 2008, 134 pages,
ISBN 9780781768771

**$28.95**    Review

A concise, clinically oriented summary of genetics in the popular outline format. Illustrated with schematic line drawings and photographs of the most clinically relevant diseases. Limited student feedback.

**B⁺**

### Déjà Review: Histology & Medical Cell Biology
GRISSON

McGraw-Hill, 2007, 274 pages, ISBN 9780071470490

**$22.95**    Review

Features questions and answers in a two-column, quiz-yourself format similar to that of the Recall series. Sections are divided by organ system and vary in quality. Histology images are few and are printed in black and white. Good for a quick review.

**B⁺**

### Crash Course: Cell Biology and Genetics
LAMB

Elsevier, 2006, 224 pages, ISBN 9780323044943

**$29.95**    Review

Part of the Crash Course review series for basic sciences, integrating clinical topics. Offers two-color illustrations, handy study tools, and Step 1 review questions. Includes online access. Too much coverage for a low-yield subject.

### Elsevier's Integrated Genetics

ADKISON

$39.95     Review

Elsevier, 2007, 336 pages, ISBN 9780323043298

Part of the new Integrated series that seeks to link basic science concepts across disciplines. Case-based and Step 1–style questions at the end of each chapter allow readers to gauge their comprehension of the material. Includes online access. Best if used during coursework. Limited student feedback.

### High-Yield Histology

DUDEK

$26.95     Review

Lippincott Williams & Wilkins, 2004, 288 pages, ISBN 9780781747639

A quick and easy review of a relatively low-yield subject. Tables include some high-yield information. Contains good pictures. The appendix features classic electron micrographs. Too lengthy for Step 1 review.

### BRS Cell Biology and Histology

GARTNER

$39.95     Review/Test/500 q

Lippincott Williams & Wilkins, 2006, 384 pages + CD-ROM, ISBN 9780781785778

Covers concepts in cell biology and histology in an outline format. Can be used alone for cell biology study, but does not include enough histology images to be considered comprehensive on that subject. Includes more detail than is required for Step 1, and information is less high yield than that of other books in the BRS series. Includes a CD-ROM with helpful review questions.

### PreTest Anatomy, Histology, and Cell Biology

KLEIN

$26.95     Test/500 q

McGraw-Hill, 2007, 576 pages, ISBN 9780071471855

A resource containing difficult questions with detailed answers as well as some illustrations. Requires extensive time commitment, and much of the material is beyond what is required for Step 1. The most useful part of the book is the high-yield facts section at the beginning, which is divided according to discipline.

### Wheater's Functional Histology

YOUNG

$76.95     Review

Elsevier, 2006, 448 pages, ISBN 9780443068508

A color atlas with illustrations of normal histology with image captions and accompanying text. Far too detailed to use for boards studying given the low-yield nature of the material, but useful as a coursework text or boards reference.

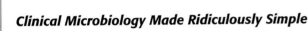

**A⁻**

### Déjà Review: Microbiology & Immunology
CHEN

McGraw-Hill, 2007, 373 pages, ISBN 9780071468664

Features questions and answers in a two-column, quiz-yourself format similar to that of the Recall series. Provides an excellent review of high-yield facts. Best used after study of a more comprehensive microbiology text.

**$22.95**       Review

---

**A⁻**

### Clinical Microbiology Made Ridiculously Simple
GLADWIN

MedMaster, 2007, 392 pages, ISBN 9780940780811

An excellent, easy-to-read, detailed review of microbiology that includes clever and memorable mnemonics. The style of the series does not appeal to everyone. The sections on bacterial disease are most high yield, whereas the pharmacology chapters lack sufficient detail. Many students find it most useful to read the text during their initial study of microbiology and just revisit the concise charts included at the end of each chapter during boards review. Requires a supplemental source for immunology.

**$32.95**       Review

---

**A⁻**

### Microcards Flash Cards
HARPAVAT

Lippincott Williams & Wilkins, 2007, 300 pages, ISBN 9780781769242

A well-organized and complete resource for students who like to use flash cards for review. Cards feature the clinical presentation, pathobiology, diagnosis, treatment, and high-yield facts for a particular organism. Some cards also include excellent flow charts organizing important classes of bacteria or viruses. Overall, a good review resource, but at times it is overly detailed, requiring a significant time commitment.

**$34.95**       Flash cards

---

**A⁻**

### High-Yield Microbiology and Infectious Diseases
HAWLEY

Lippincott Williams & Wilkins, 2007, 226 pages, ISBN 9780781760324

A very high yield review of central concepts and keywords, with chapters organized by microorganism. The last few sections contain brief questions and answers organized by organ system. Also offers a useful chapter on "microbial comparisons" that groups organisms by shared virulence factors, lab results, and the like.

**$27.95**       Review/Test/200 q

### High-Yield Immunology
JOHNSON
Lippincott Williams & Wilkins, 2006, 112 pages,
ISBN 9780781774697

Accurately covers high-yield immunology concepts, although at times it includes more detail than necessary for Step 1 preparation. Good for quick review. The newest edition includes many improvements.

**$27.95**      Review

### Review of Medical Microbiology
MURRAY
Elsevier, 2005, 176 pages, ISBN 9780323033251

A resource that features Step 1–style questions divided into bacteriology, virology, mycology, and parasitology. All questions are accompanied by detailed explanations, and some are paired with high-quality images. Questions are similar to those on Step 1 and provide a nice review. Supplements Murray's *Medical Microbiology*.

**$37.95**      Test/550 q

### Medical Microbiology and Immunology Flash Cards
ROSENTHAL
Elsevier, 2005, 414 pages, ISBN 9780323033923

Flash cards covering the microorganisms most commonly found on Step 1. Each card features full-color microscopic images and clinical presentations on one side and relevant bug information in conjunction with a short case on the other side. Also includes Student Consult online access for extra features. Overemphasizes "trigger words" related to each bug. Not a comprehensive resource.

**$34.95**      Flash cards

### Rapid Review: Microbiology and Immunology
ROSENTHAL
Elsevier, 2006, 368 pages, ISBN 9780323044264

A resource presented in a format similar to that of other books in the Rapid Review series. Contains many excellent tables and figures, but requires significant time commitment and is not as high yield as comparable review books. Two 50-question tests with extensive explanations complement the topics covered in the review, along with 250 questions online.

**$34.95**      Review/Test/350 q

### Underground Clinical Vignettes: Microbiology Vol. I: Virology, Immunology, Parasitology, Mycology

$22.95    Review/Test/20 q

SWANSON

Lippincott Williams & Wilkins, 2007, 256 pages,
ISBN 9780781764704

A resource containing 100 concise clinical cases that illustrate frequently tested diseases in microbiology and immunology. Cardinal signs, symptoms, and buzzwords are highlighted. Also includes 20 additional boards-style questions. Best if used as a supplement to other review resources.

### Underground Clinical Vignettes: Microbiology Vol. II: Bacteriology

$22.95    Review/Test/20 q

SWANSON

Lippincott Williams & Wilkins, 2007, 256 pages,
ISBN 9780781764711

A resource containing 100 concise clinical cases that illustrate frequently tested diseases in microbiology and immunology. Cardinal signs, symptoms, and buzzwords are highlighted. Also includes 20 additional boards-style questions. Best if used as a supplement to other review resources.

### Basic Immunology

$61.95    Review

ABBAS

Elsevier, 2006, 336 pages, ISBN 9781416029748

A useful text that offers clear explanations of complex topics in immunology. Best if used during the year in conjunction with coursework and later skimmed for quick Step 1 review. Includes colorful diagrams, images, tables, and a lengthy glossary for further study. Features online access.

### Elsevier's Integrated Immunology and Microbiology

$40.95    Review

ACTOR

Elsevier, 2006, 192 pages, ISBN 9780323033893

Part of the new Integrated series that seeks to link basic science concepts across disciplines. Case-based and Step 1–style questions at the end of each chapter allow users to gauge their comprehension of the material. Includes online access. Best if used during coursework. Limited student feedback.

### B+ Concise Medical Immunology
DOAN

$39.95    Review

Lippincott Williams & Wilkins, 2005, 256 pages,
ISBN 9780781757416

Lives up to its name as a concise text with useful diagrams, illustrations, and tables. Good for students who need extra immunology review or for those who wish to study the subject thoroughly for the boards. End-of-chapter multiple-choice questions help reinforce key concepts.

### B+ Case Studies in Immunology: Clinical Companion
GEHA

$49.95    Review

Garland Science, 2007, 344 pages, ISBN 9780815341451

A text that was originally designed as a clinical companion to *Janeway's Immunobiology*. Provides a great synopsis of the major disorders of immunity in a clinical vignette format. Integrates basic and clinical sciences. Features excellent images and illustrations from Janeway, as well as questions and discussions.

### B+ Review of Medical Microbiology and Immunology
LEVINSON

$44.95    Review/Test/654 q

McGraw-Hill, 2006, 580 pages, ISBN 9780071460316

A clear, comprehensive text with outstanding diagrams and tables. Includes an excellent immunology section. The "Summary of Medically Important Organisms" is highly crammable. Requires time commitment. Can be detailed and dense at points, so best if started early. Features comprehensive coverage of material. Includes excellent practice questions and a comprehensive exam, but does not provide explanations of answers. Compare with *Lippincott's Illustrated Reviews: Microbiology*.

### B+ Review of Immunology
LICHTMAN

$33.95    Test/500 q

Elsevier, 2005, 192 pages, ISBN 9780721603438

Complements Abbas's *Cellular and Molecular Immunology* and *Basic Immunology* textbooks. Contains 500 boards-style questions featuring full-color illustrations along with explanations of all answer choices. A good resource for questions in a lower-yield topic. Limited student feedback.

### B+ Crash Course: Immunology
NOVAK

$29.95    Review

Elsevier, 2006, 144 pages, ISBN 9781416030072

Part of the Crash Course review series for basic sciences, integrating clinical topics. Offers two-color illustrations, handy study tools, and Step 1 review questions. Includes online access. Good length and detail for boards review.

**BRS Microbiology Flash Cards**
SWANSON
Lippincott Williams & Wilkins, 2003, 500 pages,
ISBN 9780781744270
A concise series of flash cards featuring high-yield microbiology facts with an emphasis on virulence factors. A good last-second microbiology review after study of a more comprehensive text.

$32.95    Flash cards

**Case Files: Microbiology**
TOY
McGraw-Hill, 2008, 382 pages, ISBN 9780071492584
Fifty clinical microbiology cases reviewed in an interactive learning format. Each case is followed by a clinical correlation, a discussion with boldfaced buzzwords, and questions. Covers many important microorganisms, but lacks the high-yield charts and tables found in comparable review resources.

$29.95    Review

**Lippincott's Illustrated Reviews: Immunology**
DOAN
Lippincott Williams & Wilkins, 2008, 336 pages,
ISBN 9780781795432
A clearly written, highly detailed review of basic concepts in immunology. Features many useful tables and review questions at the end of each chapter. Offers abbreviated coverage of immune deficiencies and autoimmune disorders. Best if started with initial coursework and used as a reference during Step 1 study.

$46.95    Review/Test/Few q

**Blueprints Notes and Cases: Microbiology and Immunology**
GANDHI
Lippincott Williams & Wilkins, 2003, 224 pages,
ISBN 9781405103473
Fifty-eight succinct clinical cases covering Step 1–relevant microbiology and immunology facts. Charts, tables, illustrations, and useful "thumbnails" are included in the discussion section to facilitate rapid synthesis of key concepts. Best used during microbiology coursework. For students who are already comfortable with immunology concepts.

$29.95    Review

### Lippincott's Illustrated Reviews: Microbiology
HARVEY

$47.95    Review/Test/Few q

Lippincott Williams & Wilkins, 2006, 432 pages,
ISBN 9780781782159

A comprehensive, highly illustrated review of microbiology that is similar in style to other titles in the Illustrated Reviews series. Includes a 50-page color section with more than 150 clinical and laboratory photographs. Compare with Levinson's *Review of Medical Microbiology and Immunology*.

### Bugcards: The Complete Microbiology Review for Class, the Boards, and the Wards
LEVINE

$26.50    Flash cards

BL Publishing, 2004, 150 pages, ISBN 9780967165530

High-quality flash cards geared toward Step 1 material. Cards cover all medically relevant bacteria, viruses, fungi, and parasites. Includes important buzzwords, mnemonics, and clinical vignettes to aid recall. Unique "disease process cards" summarize all organisms for a particular disease (e.g., UTI, pneumonia).

### USMLE Road Map: Immunology
PARMELY

$26.95    Review

McGraw-Hill, 2006, 223 pages, ISBN 9780071452984

An outline review of immunology with a special focus on molecular mechanisms and laboratory techniques. Features abbreviated coverage of immunologic deficiency and autoimmune diseases that are emphasized on Step 1. Offers a collection of brief review questions at the end of each chapter. Limited student feedback.

### Clinical Microbiology Review
WARINNER

$36.95    Review

Wysteria, 2001, 146 pages, ISBN 9780967783932

A concise review in chart format with some clinical correlations. Each page covers a single organism with ample space for adding notes during class. Spatial organization, color coding, and bulleting of facts facilitate review. A great cross-reference section groups organisms by general characteristics. Includes color plates of significant microbes. Contains no immunology. Not comprehensive enough to use as a sole resource.

**A**

### Rapid Review: Pathology

**$38.95**   Review/Test/350 q

GOLJAN

Elsevier, 2006, 768 pages, ISBN 9780323044141

The best of the Rapid Review series. A comprehensive source for key concepts in pathology, presented in a bulleted outline format with many tables and figures. Features detailed explanations of disease mechanisms. Integrates concepts across disciplines with a strong clinical orientation. Offers excellent color images of both gross and microscopic pathology. Much longer than other books in this series, but very high yield. Best if started early with coursework. Includes access to additional online resources.

**A**

### BRS Pathology

**$39.95**   Review/Test/450 q

SCHNEIDER

Lippincott Williams & Wilkins, 2009, 464 pages,
ISBN 9780781779418

An excellent, concise review with appropriate content emphasis. Chapters are organized by organ system and feature an outline format with boldfacing of key facts. Includes good questions with explanations at the end of each chapter plus a comprehensive exam at the end of the book. Offers well-organized tables and diagrams as well as photographs representative of classic pathology. Contains a chapter on laboratory testing and "key associations" with each disease. The new edition contains excellent color images and access to an online test and interactive question bank. Most effective if started early in conjunction with coursework, as it does not discuss detailed mechanisms of disease pathology.

**A⁻**

### Pathophysiology for the Boards and Wards

**$36.95**   Review/Test/75 q

AYALA

Lippincott Williams & Wilkins, 2003, 352 pages, ISBN
9781405103428

A systems-based outline with a focus on pathology. Well organized with glossy color plates of relevant pathology and excellent, concise tables. The appendix includes a helpful overview of neurology, immunology, unusual "zebra" syndromes, and high-yield pearls. Features good integration of Step 1–relevant material from various subject areas. Compare with *Rapid Review: Pathology.*

REVIEW RESOURCES

PATHOLOGY

### Lange Pathology Flash Cards

BARON

$34.95   Flash cards

McGraw-Hill, 2009, 277 flash cards, ISBN 9780071613057

Pathology flash cards with information on one disease per card. Each card includes a clinical vignette with pathophysiology, clinical manifestations, treatment, and relevant color images. Most effective when started during coursework. A useful resource for quick, high-yield pathology review.

### Lippincott's Review of Pathology: Illustrated, Interactive Q & A

FENDERSON

$44.95   Review/Test/1100 q

Lippincott Williams & Wilkins, 2006, 336 pages, ISBN 9780781795807

A review book featuring more than 1100 multiple-choice questions that follow the Step 1 template. Questions frequently require multi-step reasoning, probing the student's ability to integrate basic science knowledge in a clinical situation. Detailed rationales are linked to clinical vignettes and address incorrect answer choices. More than 300 full-color images link clinical and pathologic findings, with normal lab values provided for reference. Questions are presented both online and in print. Students can work through the online questions either in "quiz mode," which provides instant feedback, or in "test mode," which simulates the Step 1 experience. Overall, a resource that is similar in quality to *Robbins and Cotran Review of Pathology*.

### Déjà Review: Pathology

GALFIONE

$25.95   Review

McGraw-Hill, 2007, 380 pages, ISBN 9780071474955

Features questions and answers in a two-column, quiz-yourself format similar to that of the Recall series. A great review that integrates pathophysiology and pathology. Includes many vignette-style questions. Limited student feedback.

### Robbins and Cotran Review of Pathology

KLATT

$48.95   Review/Test/1000 q

Elsevier, 2009, 464 pages, ISBN 9781416049302

A review question book that follows the main Robbins textbooks. Questions are more detailed and difficult than those on the actual Step 1 exam, but the text offers a great review of pathology integrated with images. Thorough answer explanations reinforce key points. Requires significant time commitment, so best if started early.

REVIEW RESOURCES

PATHOLOGY

**Underground Clinical Vignettes: Pathophysiology Vol. I: Pulmonary, Ob/Gyn, ENT, Hem/Onc**

SWANSON

Lippincott Williams & Wilkins, 2007, 228 pages,
ISBN 9780781764650

Concise clinical cases illustrating 100 frequently tested pathology and physiology concepts. Cardinal signs, symptoms, and buzzwords are highlighted. Also includes 20 additional boards-style questions. Best if used as a supplement to other sources of review.

$24.95    Review/Test/20 q

**Underground Clinical Vignettes: Pathophysiology Vol. II: GI, Neurology, Rheumatology, Endocrinology**

SWANSON

Lippincott Williams & Wilkins, 2007, 256 pages,
ISBN 9780781764667

Concise clinical cases illustrating 100 frequently tested pathology and physiology concepts. Cardinal signs, symptoms, and buzzwords are highlighted. Also includes 20 additional boards-style questions. Best if used as a supplement to other sources of review.

$24.95    Review/Test/20 q

**Underground Clinical Vignettes: Pathophysiology Vol. III: CV, Dermatology, GU, Orthopedics, General Surgery, Peds**

SWANSON

Lippincott Williams & Wilkins, 2007, 256 pages,
ISBN 9780781764681

Concise clinical cases illustrating 100 frequently tested pathology and physiology concepts. Cardinal signs, symptoms, and buzzwords are highlighted. Also includes 20 additional boards-style questions. Best if used as a supplement to other sources of review.

$24.95    Review/Test/20 q

**MedMaps for Pathophysiology**

AGOSTI

Lippincott Williams & Wilkins, 2007, 259 pages,
ISBN 9780781777551

A rapid review that contains 102 concept maps of disease processes and mechanisms organized by organ system, as well as classic diseases. Useful for both coursework and Step 1 preparation. Ample room is provided for notes. A good resource for looking up specific mechanisms, especially when used in conjunction with other primary review sources.

$32.95    Review

### Cases & Concepts Step 1: Pathophysiology Review
CAUGHEY

$39.95    Review/Test/150 q

Lippincott Williams & Wilkins, 2009, 400 pages,
ISBN 9780781782548

Eighty-eight clinical cases integrating basic science concepts with clinical data, followed by USMLE-style questions with answers and rationales. Thumbnail and key-concept boxes highlight key facts. Limited student feedback.

### PreTest Pathology
BROWN

$27.95    Test/500 q

McGraw-Hill, 2007, 592 pages, ISBN 9780071471824

Difficult questions with detailed, complete answers. Questions are shorter than those found on Step 1 and primarily test recall rather than multistep reasoning. Features high-quality black-and-white photographs but no color illustrations. Can be used as a supplement to other review books. Thirty-nine pages of high-yield facts are useful for concept summaries.

### Appleton & Lange Review: General Pathology
CATALANO

$39.95    Test/850 q

McGraw-Hill, 2002, 344 pages, ISBN 9780071389952

Short text sections followed by numerous questions with answers. Some useful high-yield tables are included at the beginning of each section. Features good photomicrographs. Covers both general and organ-based pathology. Can be used as a supplement to more detailed texts. A good review when time is short.

### Blueprints Notes & Cases—Pathophysiology: Renal, Hematology, and Oncology
CAUGHEY

$29.95    Review

Lippincott Williams & Wilkins, 2003, 208 pages,
ISBN 9781405103527

A review book that follows the format of the Blueprints series, in which each case takes the form of a discussion followed by key points and a series of questions. The pathophysiology volumes would be a good companion to organ-based teaching modules, but the content is not always representative of what will be tested on the boards.

### Colour Atlas of Anatomical Pathology
COOKE

$95.95    Review

Elsevier, 2003, 300 pages, ISBN 9780443073601

An impressive color atlas of gross pathology. Photographs are clinically relevant and have concise captions that include relevant pathologic details. Limited student feedback.

### Color Atlas of Physiology
DESPOPOULOS                                                $39.95    Review
Thieme, 2003, 432 pages, ISBN 9781588900616

A text containing more than 180 high-quality illustrations of disturbed physiologic processes that lead to dysfunction. An alternative to standard texts, but not high yield for boards review.

### High-Yield Histopathology
DUDEK                                                      $27.95    Review
Lippincott Williams & Wilkins, 2007, 336 pages,
ISBN 9780781769594

A new book that reviews the relationship of basic histology to the pathology, physiology, and pharmacology of clinical conditions that are tested on Step 1. Includes case studies, numerous light and electron micrographs, and pathology photographs. Given its considerable length, should be started with coursework. Limited student feedback.

### Crash Course: Pathology
FISHBACK                                                   $29.95    Review
Elsevier, 2005, 368 pages, ISBN 9780323033084

Part of the Crash Course review series for basic sciences, integrating clinical topics. Offers two-color illustrations, handy study tools, and Step 1 review questions. Includes online access. Best if started during coursework.

### Blueprints Notes & Cases—Pathophysiology: Cardiovascular, Endocrine, and Reproduction
LEUNG                                                      $32.00    Review
Lippincott Williams & Wilkins, 2003, 208 pages,
ISBN 9781405103503

A review book that follows the format of the Blueprints series, in which each case takes the form of a discussion followed by key points and a series of questions. The pathophysiology volumes would be a good companion to organ-based teaching modules, but the content is not always representative of what will be tested on the boards.

### Pathcards
MARCUCCI                                                   $36.95    Flash cards
Lippincott Williams & Wilkins, 2003, 553 pages,
ISBN 9780781743990

Flash cards that offer comprehensive and detailed information instead of a bulleted, high-yield facts format. Appropriate level of depth for Step 1 pathology. Lacks clinical vignettes and color images found in other review resources. Compare with *Lange Flash Cards*.

### Pathophysiology of Disease: Introduction to Clinical Medicine

McPHEE

**$59.95**  Review/Test/Few q

McGraw-Hill, 2005, 784 pages, ISBN 9780071441599

An interdisciplinary text useful for understanding the pathophysiology of clinical symptoms. Effectively integrates the basic sciences with mechanisms of disease. Features great graphs, diagrams, and tables. In view of its length, most useful if started during coursework. Includes a few non-boards-style questions. The text's clinical emphasis nicely complements *BRS Pathology*.

### Haematology at a Glance

MEHTA

**$36.95**  Review

Blackwell Science, 2005, 117 pages, ISBN 9781405126663

A resource that covers common hematologic issues. Includes color illustrations. Presented in a logical sequence that is easy to read. Good for use with coursework.

### Pocket Companion to Robbins and Cotran Pathologic Basis of Disease

MITCHELL

**$39.95**  Review

Elsevier, 2006, 816 pages, ISBN 9780721602653

A resource that is good for reviewing keywords associated with most important diseases. Presented in a highly condensed format, but the text is complete and easy to understand. Contains no photographs or illustrations. Useful as a quick reference.

### PreTest Pathophysiology

MUFSON

**$27.95**  Test/500 q

McGraw-Hill, 2004, 480 pages, ISBN 9780071434928

Includes 500 questions and answers with explanations. Questions are often overly specific, and explanations vary in quality. Features a brief section of high-yield topics. Good economic value.

### BRS Pathology Flash Cards

SWANSON

**$32.95**  Flash cards

Lippincott Williams & Wilkins, 2002, 250 flash cards,
ISBN 9780781737104

A series of 250 pathology flash cards categorized by organ system. Effective when used in combination with the *BRS Pathology* textbook or another pathology review text, but not comprehensive enough when used alone.

### Lange Pharmacology Flash Cards

**$34.95**   Flash cards

BARON

McGraw-Hill, 2009, 189 flash cards, ISBN 9780071622417

One hundred eighty-nine pocket-sized flash cards featuring clinical vignettes involving relevant drugs, with high-yield information highlighted in bold. Limited student feedback.

### Lippincott's Illustrated Reviews: Pharmacology

**$54.95**   Review/Test/200 q

HARVEY

Lippincott Williams & Wilkins, 2009, 564 pages, ISBN 9780781771559

A resource presented in outline format with practice questions, many excellent illustrations, and comparison tables. Effectively integrates pharmacology and pathophysiology. The new edition has been updated to cover recent changes in pharmacotherapy. Best started with coursework, as it is highly detailed and requires significant time commitment.

### BRS Pharmacology Flash Cards

**$32.95**   Flash cards

KIM

Lippincott Williams & Wilkins, 2004, 640 pages, ISBN 9780781747967

A series of flash cards that facilitate memorization of the appropriate clinical use of drugs rather than describing mechanisms and toxicities in detail. Not a comprehensive review resource, but may be useful for those who find other pharm cards overwhelming. Considered by many to be an excellent resource for quick, last-minute review.

### Katzung & Trevor's Pharmacology: Examination and Board Review

**$44.95**   Review/Test/1000 q

TREVOR

McGraw-Hill, 2008, 645 pages, ISBN 9780071488693

A well-organized text in narrative format with concise explanations. Features good charts and tables; the crammable list of "top boards drugs" is especially high yield. Also good for drug interactions and toxicities. Offers two practice exams with questions and detailed answers. Includes some low-yield/obscure drugs. Compare with *Lippincott's Illustrated Reviews: Pharmacology*.

### Déjà Review: Pharmacology
YOUNG

**$22.95**     Review

McGraw-Hill, 2007, 186 pages, ISBN 9780071474610

Features questions and answers in a two-column, quiz-yourself format similar to that of the Recall series. Covers basic high-yield facts, but many questions review particular agents in more detail than typically tested in Step 1 pharmacology questions.

### Pharmacology for the Boards and Wards
AYALA

**$36.95**     Review/Test/150 q

Lippincott Williams & Wilkins, 2006, 256 pages, ISBN 9781405105118

Like other books in the Boards and Wards series, the pharmacology volume is presented primarily in tabular format with bulleted key points. Review questions are in Step 1 style. At times can be too dense, but does a great job of focusing on the clinical aspects of drugs.

### Crash Course: Pharmacology
BARNES

**$29.95**     Review

Elsevier, 2006, 248 pages, ISBN 9781416029595

Part of the Crash Course review series for basic sciences, integrating clinical topics. Offers two-color illustrations, handy study tools, and Step 1–style review questions. Includes online access. Gives a solid, easy-to-follow overview of pharmacology. Limited student feedback.

### Pharmacology Flash Cards
BRENNER

**$34.95**     Flash cards

Elsevier, 2006, 576 pages, ISBN 9781416031864

Flash cards for more than 200 of the most commonly tested drugs. Cards include the name of the drug (both generic and brand) on the front and basic drug information on the back. Divided and color coded by class, and comes with a compact carrying case. Lacks figures and clinical vignettes.

### Pharm Cards: Review Cards for Medical Students
JOHANNSEN

**$39.95**     Flash cards

Lippincott Williams & Wilkins, 2006, 512 pages, ISBN 9780781766081

A series of flash cards that cover the mechanisms and side effects of major drugs and drug classes. Good for class review, but the level of detail is beyond what is necessary for Step 1. Lacks pharmacokinetics, but features good charts and diagrams. Well liked by students who enjoy flash card–based review. Compare with BRS Pharmacology Flash Cards.

### Elsevier's Integrated Pharmacology

KESTER

$39.95   Review

Elsevier, 2007, 336 pages, ISBN 9780323034081

Part of the new Integrated series that seeks to link basic science concepts across disciplines. Case-based and Step 1–style questions at the end of each chapter allow readers to gauge their comprehension of the material. Includes online access. Best if used during coursework. Limited student feedback.

### Rapid Review: Pharmacology

PAZDERNIK

$38.95   Review

Elsevier, 2006, 368 pages, ISBN 9780323045506

A detailed treatment of pharmacology, presented in an outline format similar to that of other books in the series. At times more detailed than necessary for Step 1 review. Contains high-yield charts and figures. Two 50-question tests with extensive explanations are included, and 250 additional questions can be found online.

### Lange Smart Charts: Pharmacology

PELLETIER

$40.95   Review

McGraw-Hill, 2003, 386 pages, ISBN 9780071388788

Pharmacology concepts organized in a tabular format. Most useful when used as a secondary source for organization when reviewing material. Limited student feedback.

### Pharmacology Recall: Print & Audio Package

RAMACHANDRAN

$39.95   Review

Lippincott Williams & Wilkins, 2008, 592 pages + audio,
ISBN 9780781787307

A resource presented in the two-column, question-and-answer format typical of the Recall series. At times questions delve into more clinical detail than required for Step 1, but overall the breadth of coverage is appropriate. Includes a high-yield drug summary. Good for last-minute cramming. Includes questions and answers that are recorded in MP3 format so that they can be used on any audio player.

### Underground Clinical Vignettes Step 1: Pharmacology

SWANSON

$22.95   Review/Test/20 q

Lippincott Williams & Wilkins, 2007, 256 pages,
ISBN 9780781764858

Concise clinical cases illustrating approximately 100 frequently tested pharmacology concepts. Cardinal signs, symptoms, and buzzwords are highlighted. Also includes 20 additional boards-style questions. Omits some important drugs and lacks detail on mechanisms, so best used as a supplement to other sources of review.

### USMLE Road Map: Pharmacology
KATZUNG

**$26.95**   Review

McGraw-Hill, 2006, 178 pages, ISBN 9780071445818

An outline review of pharmacology divided either by organ system or by disease process. Includes a collection of brief review questions at the end of each chapter. The appendix has a useful table of common side effects. Does not contain enough detail to serve as a comprehensive review. Limited student feedback.

### BRS Pharmacology
ROSENFELD

**$39.95**   Review/Test/200 q

Lippincott Williams & Wilkins, 2009, 368 pages, ISBN 9780781789134

Features two-color tables and figures that summarize essential information for quick recall. A list of drugs organized by drug family is included in each chapter. Too detailed for boards review; best used as a reference. Also offers end-of-chapter review tests with Step 1–style questions and a comprehensive exam with explanations of answers. An additional question bank is available online.

### PreTest Pharmacology
SHLAFER

**$26.95**   Test/500 q

McGraw-Hill, 2007, 460 pages, ISBN 9780071471817

Good questions divided into sections by organ system and accompanied by detailed answers. Sections on general principles and autonomics are especially useful. Best used as a resource for additional questions after other sources have been exhausted.

### Case Files: Pharmacology
TOY

**$29.95**   Review/Test/150 q

McGraw-Hill, 2008, 440 pages, ISBN 9780071488587

A case-based review of pharmacology. Each case includes a concise discussion, comprehension questions, and a short list of take-home pearls. An appealing text for students who prefer problem-based learning, but lacks the level of detail typically tested on Step 1.

### High-Yield Pharmacology
WEISS

**$27.95**   Review

Lippincott Williams & Wilkins, 2003, 160 pages, ISBN 9780781792738

A succinct pharmacology review presented in an easy-to-follow outline format. Features a drug index, key points in bold, and summary tables of high-yield facts. Lacks details on mechanisms or drug specifics, so best used with a more comprehensive resource.

### BRS Physiology

$38.95    Review/Test/400 q

COSTANZO

Lippincott Williams & Wilkins, 2006, 352 pages,
ISBN 9780781773119

A clear, concise review of physiology that is both comprehensive and efficient, making for fast, easy reading. Includes excellent high-yield charts and tables, but lacks some figures from Costanzo's *Physiology*. Features high-quality practice questions with explanations in each chapter along with a clinically oriented final exam. An excellent boards review resource, but best if started early in combination with coursework. Respiratory and acid-base sections are comparatively weak.

### Physiology

$58.95    Text

COSTANZO

Elsevier, 2006, 512 pages, ISBN 9781416023203

A comprehensive, clearly written text that covers concepts outlined in *BRS Physiology* in greater detail. Offers excellent color diagrams and charts. Each systems-based chapter features a detailed summary of objectives and a Step 1–relevant clinical case. Includes access to online interactive extras. Requires time commitment; best started with coursework.

### Rapid Review: Physiology

$38.95    Review

BROWN

Elsevier, 2006, 272 pages, ISBN 9780323019910

A resource that offers a good review of physiology in a format typical of the Rapid Review series. Features 100 questions with explanations. Includes online access to an additional 250 questions along with other extras. Limited student feedback.

### BRS Physiology Cases and Problems

$37.95    Review/Test/Many q

COSTANZO

Lippincott Williams & Wilkins, 2008, 352 pages,
ISBN 9780781788717

Sixty classic cases presented in vignette format with several questions per case. Includes exceptionally detailed explanations of answers. For students interested in an in-depth discussion of physiology concepts. May be useful for group review.

REVIEW RESOURCES

PHYSIOLOGY

### High-Yield Physiology
DUDEK

Lippincott Williams & Wilkins, 2008, 240 pages,
ISBN 9780781745871

An outline review of major concepts written at an appropriate level of
depth for Step 1; includes especially detailed coverage of cardiovascular, respiratory, and renal physiology. Features many excellent diagrams and boxes highlighting important equations. Large blocks of
dense text make it a slow and disorienting read at times. Limited student feedback.

**$27.95**    Review

### High-Yield Acid-Base Review
LONGENECKER

Lippincott Williams & Wilkins, 2006, 128 pages,
ISBN 9780781796552

A concise and well-written description of acid-base disorders. Includes
chapters discussing differential diagnoses and 12 clinical cases. Intro-
duces a multistep approach to the material. A bookmark with useful
factoids is included with the text. No index or questions.

**$26.95**    Review

### USMLE Road Map: Physiology
PASLEY

McGraw-Hill, 2006, 219 pages, ISBN 9780071445177

A text in outline format incorporating useful comparison charts and
clear diagrams. Provides a concise approach to physiology. Clinical
correlations are referenced to the text. Questions build on basic concepts and include detailed explanations. Limited student feedback.

**$26.95**    Review/Test/50 q

### Appleton & Lange Review: Physiology
PENNEY

McGraw-Hill, 2003, 278 pages, ISBN 9780071377263

Step 1–style questions divided into subcategories under physiology.
Good if subject-specific questions are desired, but may be too detailed
for many students. Some diagrams are used to explain answers. A
good way to test knowledge after coursework.

**$39.95**    Test/700 q

### Elsevier's Integrated Physiology
CARROLL

Elsevier, 2006, 256 pages, ISBN 9780323043182

Part of the new Integrated series that seeks to link basic science concepts across disciplines. A good text for initial coursework, but too
long for Step 1 review. Case-based and Step 1–style questions are included at the end of each chapter. Limited student feedback.

**$39.95**    Review

**Déjà Review: Physiology**
LIN
McGraw-Hill, 2007, 212 pages, ISBN 9780071475105
Features questions and answers in a two-column, quiz-yourself format similar to that of the Recall series. Includes helpful graphs and diagrams. Limited student feedback.

$26.95    Review

**PreTest Physiology**
METTING
McGraw-Hill, 2008, 365 pages, ISBN 9780071476638
Contains questions with detailed, well-written explanations. One of the best of the PreTest series. Best for use by the motivated student after extensive review of other sources. Includes a high-yield facts section with useful diagrams.

$25.95    Test/500 q

**Acid-Base, Fluids, and Electrolytes Made Ridiculously Simple**
PRESTON
MedMaster, 2002, 156 pages, ISBN 9780940780316
A resource that covers major acid-base and renal physiology concepts. Provides information beyond the scope of Step 1, but remains a useful companion for studying kidney function, electrolyte disturbances, and fluid management. Includes scattered diagrams and questions at the end of each chapter. Consider using after exhausting more high-yield physiology review resources.

$18.95    Review

**Case Files: Physiology**
TOY
McGraw-Hill, 2009, 456 pages, ISBN 9780071493741
A review text divided into 51 clinical cases followed by clinical correlations, a discussion, and take-home pearls, presented in a format similar to that of other texts in the Case Files series. A few questions accompany each case. Too lengthy for rapid review; best for students who enjoy problem-based learning.

$32.95    Review

**Pulmonary Pathophysiology: The Essentials**
WEST
Lippincott Williams & Wilkins, 2008, 199 pages,
ISBN 9780781764148
A volume offering comprehensive coverage of respiratory physiology. Clearly organized with useful charts and diagrams. Review questions at the end of each chapter have letter answers only and no explanations. Best used as a course supplement.

$39.95    Review/Test/50 q

### Clinical Physiology Made Ridiculously Simple
GOLDBERG

$19.95    Review

MedMaster, 2007, 160 pages, ISBN 9780940780217

An easy-to-read text with many amusing associations and memorable mnemonics. The style does not work for everyone. Not as well illustrated as the rest of the series, and lacks some important concepts. Best used as a supplement to other review books.

# SECTION IV

# Commercial Review Courses

- ▶ Falcon Physician Reviews
- ▶ Kaplan Medical
- ▶ Northwestern Medical Review
- ▶ The Princeton Review
- ▶ Doctor Youel's™ Prep, Inc.

Commercial preparation courses can be helpful for some students, but such courses are expensive and may leave limited time for independent study. They are usually an effective tool for students who feel overwhelmed by the volume of material they must review in preparation for the boards. Also note that while some commercial courses are designed for first-time test takers, others are geared toward students who are repeating the examination. Still other courses have been created for IMGs who want to take all three Steps in a limited amount of time. Finally, student experience and satisfaction with review courses are highly variable, and course content and structure can evolve rapidly. We thus suggest that you discuss options with recent graduates of review courses you are considering. Some student opinions can be found in discussion groups on the World Wide Web.

### Falcon Physician Reviews

Established in 2002, Falcon Physician Reviews provides intensive and comprehensive live reviews for students preparing for the USMLE and COMLEX. The seven-week Step 1 reviews are held throughout the year with small class sizes in order to increase student involvement and instructor accessibility. Falcon Physician Reviews uses an active learning system that focuses on comprehension, retention, and application of concepts. Falcon Online program components include:

- A full set of color Falcon textbooks
- Hundreds of hours of lectures optimized into high-yield streaming video
- On-screen PowerPoint slides
- Available 24/7, anywhere with high-speed Internet

Falcon Live programs are currently offered in Dallas, Texas; Pittsburgh, Pennsylvania; Blacksburg, Virginia; and New York City, New York. The fee is $4950. The all-inclusive program tuition fee includes:

- Lodging
- Complimentary daily breakfast and lunch
- A full set of color Falcon textbooks
- Daily clinical vignettes
- Daily tutoring
- High-speed Internet service
- Local hotel shuttle service

For more information, contact:

Falcon Physician Reviews
440 Wrangler Drive, Suite 100
Coppell, TX 75019
Phone: (888) 516-9991
Fax: (214) 292-8568
info@falconreviews.com
URL: www.falconreviews.com

## Kaplan Medical

Kaplan Medical offers a wide range of options for USMLE preparation, including live lectures, center-based study, and online products. All of its courses and products focus on providing the most exam-relevant information available.

**Live Lectures.** Kaplan's LivePrep offers a highly structured, interactive live lecture series led by expert faculty as 7-, 14-, or 16-week courses. This course's advantages include interaction with faculty and peers.

Kaplan also offers LivePrep Retreat, a 7-week course during which students stay and study in high-end hotel accommodations.

**Center Study.** Kaplan's CenterPrep, a center-based lecture course, is designed for medical students seeking flexibility. Essentially an independent study course, it is offered at more than 150 Kaplan Centers across the United States in 3-, 6-, or 9-month periods. Students have access to more than 160 hours of video lecture review. CenterPrep features seven volumes of lecture notes; a question book that includes 850 practice questions with answers and explanations; and a full-length simulated exam with a complete performance analysis and detailed explanations. The course also includes a Personalized Learning System (PLS), which allows students to create a customized study schedule and track their performance.

**Online Resources.** Kaplan Medical provides online content- and question-based review. WebPrep offers 80 hours of audio-streamed lectures, seven volumes of lecture notes, a full online Step 1 simulated exam, and access to Kaplan Medical's popular online question bank, Qbank, which contains more than 2150 USMLE-style practice questions with detailed explanations. WebPrep is designed to provide students with the most flexible content- and question-based review available.

Kaplan's popular Qbank allows students to create practice tests by discipline and organ system, receive instant on-screen feedback, and track their cumulative performance. Kaplan also offers Integrated Vignettes Qbank (IV Qbank), an online clinical-case question bank that allows users to practice answering case-based, USMLE-style vignettes that are organized by symptom. Each vignette contains multidisciplinary questions covering different ways the underlying basic science concepts could be tested.

Kaplan's most comprehensive question practice option is Qreview, which contains more than 3750 questions and provides six months of access to both Step 1 Qbank and IV Qbank. Qreview provides students with collective reporting of their results across both Qbanks and includes an online simulated exam. Qbank demos are available at www.kaplanmedical. com.

More information can be obtained at (800) 533-8850 or by visiting www.kaplanmedical.com.

## Northwestern Medical Review

Northwestern Medical Review offers live-lecture review courses, videotaped lectures, and home-study plans in preparation for both the COMLEX Level I and USMLE Step 1 examinations. Four review plans are available for each exam: NBI 100, a three-day course; NBI 150, a four-day course; NBI 200, a five-day course; and NBI 300, from 8 to 21 days. All courses are in live-lecture format, and most are taught by the authors of the Northwestern Review Books. In addition to organized lecture notes and books for each subject, courses include Web-based question bank access, audio CDs, and a large pool of practice questions and simulated exams. All plans are available in a customized, onsite format for groups of second-year students from individual U.S. medical schools. Additionally, public sites are frequently offered in East Lansing, Detroit, Philadelphia, San Antonio, Los Angeles, Chicago, New York City, Las Vegas, and San Juan. Live courses and Center preparations are also globally available in India, China, the Persian Gulf area, Eastern Europe, and select Caribbean islands.

Tuition ranges from $390 for the 3-day to $1780 for the 15-day course. Tuition includes all study materials and Web usage services, and it is based on group size, program duration, and early-enrollment discounts. Home-study materials, CBT question-bank access, and DVD materials are also available for purchase independent of the live-lecture plans. Northwestern offers a retake option as well as a liberal cancellation policy.

For more information, contact:

Northwestern Medical Review
P.O. Box 22174
Lansing, MI 48909-2174
Phone: (866) MedPass
Fax: (517) 347-7005
E-mail: contactus@northwesternmedicalreview.com
URL: www.northwesternmedicalreview.com

## The Princeton Review

The Princeton Review offers three flexible preparation options for the USMLE Step 1: the USMLE Online Course, the USMLE Classroom Course, and the USMLE Online Workout. In selected cities, The Princeton Review also offers a more intensive preparation course for IMGs.

**USMLE Step 1 Classroom Courses for Medical Students.** The USMLE Classroom Courses offer comprehensive preparation that includes the following:

- Seventy-five hours of online review, including lessons, vignettes, and drills
- Three full-length diagnostic tests with detailed score reports
- Seven comprehensive review manuals consisting of more than 1500 pages
- Seven minitests to gauge students' knowledge in each subject
- Twenty-four-hour e-mail support from Princeton Review Online instructors
- Three months of online access

**USMLE Online Workout.** The USMLE Online Workout offers the following:

- Two thousand USMLE-style questions presented in the CBT format
- Three full-length diagnostic exams
- Seven minitests covering Anatomy, Behavioral Science, Biochemistry, Microbiology and Immunology, Pathology, Pharmacology, and Physiology
- More than 40 subject-specific drills
- A high-yield slide review for Anatomy and Pathology
- Complete explanations of all questions and answers
- Three months of access

**USMLE Online Courses.** The USMLE Online Courses offer the following:

- Seventy-five hours of online review, including lessons, vignettes, and drills
- Complete review of all USMLE Step 1 subjects
- Three full-length CBTs
- Seven one-hour subject-based tests

- Complete set of print materials
- E-mail support from expert instructors
- 24/7 real-time support from the Princeton Review Online Coach
- Three months of access to tests, drills, and lessons

More information can be found on The Princeton Review's Web site at www.princetonreview.com.

## Doctor Youel's™ Prep, Inc.

Doctor Youel's™ Prep, Inc., has specialized in medical board preparation for 30 years. The company provides DVDs, audiotapes, videotapes, a CD (Pre-Prep™, Quick Start™), books (*Seven Steps to Board Success, Youel's Rules: Test-Taking Skills, Taming the Basic Science Beast,* and *Youel's Jewels I & II* and *Case Studies*), live lectures, and tutorials for small groups as well as for individuals (TutorialPrep™). All DVDs, videotapes, audiotapes, live lectures, and tutorials are correlated with a three-book set of Prep Notes© consisting of two textbooks, *Youel's Jewels I*© and *Youel's Jewels II*© (984 pages), and *Case Studies*©, a question-and-answer book (1854 questions, answers, and explanations).

The Comprehensive DVD program consists of 56 hours of lectures by the systems with a three-book set: *Youel's Jewels I and II* and *Case Studies*. Integrated with these programs are pre-tests and post-tests.

All Doctor Youel's Prep courses are taught and written by physicians, reflecting the clinical slant of the boards. All programs are systems based. In addition, all programs are updated continuously. Accordingly, books are not printed until the order is received.

Delivery in the United States or overseas is usually within one week. Optional express delivery is also available. Doctor Youel's Prep Home Study Program™ allows students to own their materials and to use them for repetitive study in the convenience of their homes. Purchasers of any of Doctor Youel's Prep materials, programs, or services are enrolled as members of the Doctor Youel's Prep Family of Students™, which affords them access to free telephone tutoring at (800) 645-3985. Students may call 24/7. Doctor Youel's Prep live lectures are held at select medical schools at the invitation of the school and students.

Programs are custom-designed for content, number of hours, and scheduling to fit students' needs. First-year students are urged to call early to arrange live-lecture programs at their schools for next year.

For more information, contact:

Youel's Prep, Inc.
P.O. Box 31479
Palm Beach Gardens, FL 33420
Phone: (800) 645-3985
Fax: (561) 622-4858
E-mail: info@youelsprep.com
www.youelsprep.net

# Publisher Contacts

ASM Press
P.O. Box 605
Herndon, VA 20172
(800) 546-2416
Fax: (703) 661-1501
asmmail@presswarehouse.com
www.asmpress.org

Biotest Publishing Company, Inc.
5850 Thille Street, Suite 103
Ventura, CA 93003
SkeletonDude@BiotestOnline.com
www.biotestonline.com

Churchill Livingstone
(see Elsevier Science)

Elsevier Science
Order Fulfillment
11830 Westline Industrial Drive
St. Louis, MO 63146
(800) 545-2522
Fax: (800) 535-9935
www.us.elsevierhealth.com

Exam Master
500 Ethel Court
Middletown, DE 19709-9410
(800) 572-3627
Fax: (302) 378-1153
customer_service@exammaster.com
www.exammaster.com

Garland Science Publishing
Taylor & Francis Group Ltd
2 Park Square
Milton Park, Abingdon
Oxford
OX14 4RN
UK
Tel: +44 (0) 20 7017 6000
Fax: +44 (0) 20 7017 6699
www.garlandscience.co.uk

Gold Standard Board Prep
2619 West Loughlin Drive
Chandler, AZ 85224
Fax: (480) 219-9070
www.boardprep.net

Icon Learning Systems
(see Elsevier Science)

John Wiley & Sons
10475 Crosspoint Blvd.
Indianapolis, IN 46256
(877) 762-2974
Fax: (800) 597-3299
consumers@wiley.com
www.wiley.com

Kaplan, Inc.
888 Seventh Avenue
New York, NY 10106
(212) 492-5800
www.kaplan.com

Lippincott Williams & Wilkins
P.O. Box 1600
Hagerstown, MD 21740
(800) 638-3030
Fax: (301) 223-2400
orders@lww.com
www.lww.com

MedMaster, Inc.
P.O. Box 640028
Miami, FL 33164
(800) 335-3480
Fax: (954) 962-4508
mmbks@aol.com
www.medmaster.net

McGraw-Hill Companies
Order Services
P.O. Box 182604
Columbus, OH 43272-3031
(877) 833-5524
Fax: (614) 759-3749
customer.service@mcgraw-hill.com
www.mhprofessional.com

Mosby-Year Book
(see Elsevier Science)

Parthenon Publishing/CRC Press
Taylor & Francis Group
6000 Broken Sound Parkway, NW, Suite 300
Boca Raton, FL 33487
(800) 272-7737
Fax: (800) 374-3401
orders@crcpress.com
www.crcpress.com

Princeton Review
2315 Broadway
New York, NY 10024
(212) 874-8282
Fax: (212) 874-0775
www.princetonreview.com

Thieme New York
333 Seventh Avenue
New York, NY 10001
(800) 782-3488
Fax: (212) 947-1112
www.thieme.com
customerservice@thieme.com

W. B. Saunders
(see Elsevier Science)

Wysteria Publishing
(888) 997-8300
www.wysteria.com

# APPENDIX

# Abbreviations and Symbols

| Abbreviation | Meaning |
|---|---|
| 1° | primary |
| 2° | secondary |
| 3° | tertiary |
| AA | amino acid |
| AAMC | Association of American Medical Colleges |
| aa-tRNA | aminoacyl-tRNA |
| Ab | antibody |
| ABP | androgen-binding protein |
| AC | air conduction |
| ACA | anterior cerebral artery |
| ACC | acetyl-CoA carboxylase |
| Ac-CoA | acetylcoenzyme A |
| ACD | anemia of chronic disease |
| ACE | angiotensin-converting enzyme |
| ACh | acetylcholine |
| AChE | acetylcholinesterase |
| AChR | acetylcholine receptor |
| ACL | anterior cruciate ligament |
| ACTH | adrenocorticotropic hormone |
| ADA | adenosine deaminase, Americans with Disabilities Act |
| ADH | antidiuretic hormone |
| ADHD | attention-deficit hyperactivity disorder |
| ADP | adenosine diphosphate |
| ADPKD | autosomal-dominant polycystic kidney disease |
| AFP | α-fetoprotein |
| Ag | antigen |
| AICA | anterior inferior cerebellar artery |
| AIDS | acquired immunodeficiency syndrome |
| AL | amyloidosis |
| ALA | aminolevulinic acid |
| ALL | acute lymphocytic leukemia |
| ALP | alkaline phosphatase |
| ALS | amyotrophic lateral sclerosis |
| ALT | alanine transaminase |
| AMA | antimitochondrial antibody |
| AML | acute myelocytic leukemia |
| AMP | adenosine monophosphate |
| ANA | antinuclear antibody |
| ANCA | antineutrophil cytoplasmic antibody |

| Abbreviation | Meaning |
|---|---|
| ANOVA | analysis of variance |
| ANP | atrial natriuretic peptide |
| ANS | autonomic nervous system |
| AOA | American Osteopathic Association |
| AP | action potential |
| APC | antigen-presenting cell |
| APP | amyloid precursor protein |
| APRT | adenine phosphoribosyltransferase |
| APSAC | anistreplase |
| aPTT | activated partial thromboplastin time |
| AR | autosomal recessive |
| ARB | angiotensin receptor blocker |
| ARC | Appalachian Regional Commission |
| ARDS | acute respiratory distress syndrome |
| Arg | arginine |
| ARMD | age-related macular degeneration |
| ARPKD | autosomal-recessive polycystic kidney disease |
| ASA | acetylsalicylic acid, anterior spinal artery |
| ASD | atrial septal defect |
| ASO | antistreptolysin O |
| Asp | aspartic acid |
| AST | aspartate transaminase |
| AT | angiotensin, antithrombin |
| ATCase | aspartate transcarbamoylase |
| ATP | adenosine triphosphate |
| ATPase | adenosine triphosphatase |
| AV | atrioventricular, azygous vein |
| AVM | arteriovenous malformation |
| AZT | azidothymidine |
| BAL | British anti-Lewisite [dimercaprol] |
| BC | bone conduction |
| BCG | bacille Calmette-Guérin |
| BIMS | Biometric Identity Management System |
| BM | basement membrane |
| BMI | body-mass index |
| BMR | basal metabolic rate |
| BP | bisphosphate, blood pressure |
| BPG | bisphosphoglycerate |
| BPH | benign prostatic hyperplasia |

| Abbreviation | Meaning |
|---|---|
| BUN | blood urea nitrogen |
| CAD | coronary artery disease |
| CALLA | common acute lymphoblastic leukemia antigen |
| cAMP | cyclic adenosine monophosphate |
| c-ANCA | cytoplasmic antineutrophil cytoplasmic antibody |
| CBG | corticosteroid-binding globulin |
| Cbl | cobalamin |
| CBSSA | Comprehensive Basic Science Self-Assessment |
| CBT | computer-based test, cognitive-behavioral therapy |
| CCK | cholecystokinin |
| $CCl_4$ | carbon tetrachloride |
| CCS | computer-based case simulation |
| CCT | cortical collecting tubule |
| CD | cluster of differentiation |
| CDK | cyclin-dependent kinase |
| CE | cholesterol ester |
| CEA | carcinoembryonic antigen |
| CETP | cholesterol-ester transfer protein |
| CF | cystic fibrosis |
| CFTR | cystic fibrosis transmembrane conductance regulator |
| CFX | circumflex [artery] |
| CGD | chronic granulomatous disease |
| cGMP | cyclic guanosine monophosphate |
| CGN | cis-Golgi network |
| CGRP | calcitonin gene–related peptide |
| ChAT | choline acetyltransferase |
| CHF | congestive heart failure |
| CHIP | Children's Health Insurance Program |
| CI | confidence interval |
| CIN | candidate identification number, cervical intraepithelial neoplasia |
| CIS | Communication and Interpersonal Skills |
| CJD | Creutzfeldt-Jakob disease |
| CK | clinical knowledge |
| CK-MB | creatine kinase, MB fraction |
| CL | clearance |
| CLL | chronic lymphocytic leukemia |
| CML | chronic myeloid leukemia |
| CMV | cytomegalovirus |
| CN | cranial nerve, cyanide |
| CNS | central nervous system |
| CO | cardiac output |
| CoA | coenzyme A |
| COMLEX | Comprehensive Osteopathic Medical Licensing Examination |
| COMSAE | Comprehensive Osteopathic Medical Self-Assessment Examination |
| COMT | catechol-O-methyltransferase |
| COP | coat protein |

| Abbreviation | Meaning |
|---|---|
| COPD | chronic obstructive pulmonary disease |
| CoQ | coenzyme Q |
| COX | cyclooxygenase |
| $C_p$ | plasma concentration |
| CPAP | continuous positive airway pressure |
| CPK | creatine phosphokinase |
| CRC | colorectal cancer |
| CRH | corticotropin-releasing hormone |
| CRP | C-reactive protein |
| CS | clinical skills |
| CSF | cerebrospinal fluid, colony-stimulating factor |
| CT | computed tomography |
| CTL | cytotoxic T lymphocyte |
| CTP | cytidine triphosphate |
| CV | cardiovascular |
| CVA | cerebrovascular accident, costovertebral angle |
| CVID | common variable immune deficiency |
| Cx | complication |
| CXR | chest x-ray |
| Cys | cysteine |
| d4T | didehydrodeoxythymidine [stavudine] |
| DAF | decay-accelerating factor |
| DAG | diacylglycerol |
| dATP | deoxyadenosine triphosphate |
| DCIS | ductal carcinoma in situ |
| DCT | distal convoluted tubule |
| ddC | dideoxycytidine [zalcitabine] |
| ddI | didanosine |
| DES | diethylstilbestrol |
| DHAP | dihydroxyacetone phosphate |
| DHB | dihydrobiopterin |
| DHEA | dehydroepiandrosterone |
| DHF | dihydrofolic acid |
| DHS | Department of Homeland Security |
| DHT | dihydrotestosterone |
| DI | diabetes insipidus |
| DIC | disseminated intravascular coagulation |
| DIP | distal interphalangeal [joint] |
| DIT | diiodotyrosine |
| DKA | diabetic ketoacidosis |
| DM | diabetes mellitus |
| DNA | deoxyribonucleic acid |
| 2,4-DNP | 2,4-dinitrophenol |
| DO | doctor of osteopathy |
| 2,3-DPG | 2,3-diphosphoglycerate |
| DPM | doctor of podiatric medicine |
| DS | double stranded |
| dsDNA | double-stranded deoxyribonucleic acid |
| dsRNA | double-stranded ribonucleic acid |
| dTMP | deoxythymidine monophosphate |
| DTR | deep tendon reflex |
| DTs | delirium tremens |

| Abbreviation | Meaning |
|---|---|
| dUDP | deoxyuridine diphosphate |
| dUMP | deoxyuridine monophosphate |
| DVT | deep venous thrombosis |
| EBV | Epstein-Barr virus |
| EC | ejection click |
| $EC_{50}$ | median effective concentration |
| ECF | extracellular fluid |
| ECFMG | Educational Commission for Foreign Medical Graduates |
| ECG | electrocardiogram |
| ECL | enterochromaffin-like [cell] |
| ECM | extracellular matrix |
| ECT | electroconvulsive therapy |
| $ED_{50}$ | median effective dose |
| EDRF | endothelium-derived relaxing factor |
| EDTA | ethylenediamine tetra-acetic acid |
| EDV | end-diastolic volume |
| EEG | electroencephalogram |
| EF | ejection fraction, elongation factor |
| EGF | epidermal growth factor |
| eIF | eukaryotic initiation factor |
| ELISA | enzyme-linked immunosorbent assay |
| EM | electron micrograph, electron microscopic, electron microscopy |
| EMB | eosin–methylene blue |
| EOM | extraocular muscle |
| epi | epinephrine |
| EPO | erythropoietin |
| EPS | extrapyramidal system |
| ER | endoplasmic reticulum, estrogen receptor |
| ERAS | Electronic Residency Application Service |
| ERCP | endoscopic retrograde cholangiopancreatography |
| ERP | effective refractory period |
| ERPF | effective renal plasma flow |
| ERT | estrogen replacement therapy |
| ERV | expiratory reserve volume |
| ESR | erythrocyte sedimentation rate |
| ESV | end-systolic volume |
| EtOH | ethyl alcohol |
| EV | esophageal vein |
| F1,6BP | fructose-1,6-bisphosphate |
| F2,6BP | fructose-2,6-bisphosphate |
| F6P | fructose-6-phosphate |
| FA | fatty acid |
| FAD | oxidized flavin adenine dinucleotide |
| $FADH_2$ | reduced flavin adenine dinucleotide |
| FAP | familial adenomatous polyposis |
| FBPase | fructose bisphosphatase |
| FcR | Fc receptor |
| 5f-dUMP | 5-fluorodeoxyuridine monophosphate |
| $Fe_{Na}$ | excreted fraction of filtered sodium |
| $FEV_1$ | forced expiratory volume in 1 second |
| FF | filtration fraction |

| Abbreviation | Meaning |
|---|---|
| FFA | free fatty acid |
| FGF | fibroblast growth factor |
| FGFR | fibroblast growth factor receptor |
| FISH | fluorescence in situ hybridization |
| f-met | formylmethionine |
| FMG | foreign medical graduate |
| FMN | flavin mononucleotide |
| FN | false negative |
| FP | false positive |
| FRC | functional residual capacity |
| FSH | follicle-stimulating hormone |
| FSMB | Federation of State Medical Boards |
| FTA-ABS | fluorescent treponemal antibody—absorbed |
| 5-FU | 5-fluorouracil |
| FVC | forced vital capacity |
| G3P | glucose-3-phosphate |
| G6P | glucose-6-phosphate |
| G6PD | glucose-6-phospate dehydrogenase |
| GABA | $\gamma$-aminobutyric acid |
| GBM | glomerular basement membrane |
| G-CSF | granulocyte colony-stimulating factor |
| GDP | guanosine diphosphate |
| GE | gastroesophageal |
| GERD | gastroesophageal reflux disease |
| GFAP | glial fibrillary acid protein |
| GFR | glomerular filtration rate |
| GGT | $\gamma$-glutamyl transpeptidase |
| GH | growth hormone |
| GHRH | growth hormone–releasing hormone |
| GI | gastrointestinal |
| GIP | gastric inhibitory peptide |
| GIST | gastrointestinal stromal tumor |
| Glu | glutamic acid |
| GLUT | glucose transporter |
| GM-CSF | granulocyte-macrophage colony-stimulating factor |
| GMP | guanosine monophosphate |
| GN | glomerulonephritis |
| GnRH | gonadotropin-releasing hormone |
| GP | glycogen phosphorylase, glycoprotein |
| GPe | globus pallidus externa |
| GPi | globus pallidus interna |
| GPI | glycosyl phosphatidylinositol |
| GPP | glycogen phosphorylase phosphatase |
| GRP | gastrin-releasing peptide |
| GS | glycogen synthase |
| GSH | reduced glutathione |
| GS-P | glycogen synthase phosphatase |
| GSSG | oxidized glutathione |
| GTP | guanosine triphosphate |
| GU | genitourinary |
| HAART | highly active antiretroviral therapy |
| HAV | hepatitis A virus |
| HAVAb | hepatitis A antibody |
| Hb | hemoglobin |

| Abbreviation | Meaning |
|---|---|
| HBcAb | hepatitis B core antibody |
| HBcAg | hepatitis B core antigen |
| HBeAb | hepatitis B early antibody |
| HBeAg | hepatitis B early antigen |
| HBsAb | hepatitis B surface antibody |
| HBsAg | hepatitis B surface antigen |
| HBV | hepatitis B virus |
| hCG | human chorionic gonadotropin |
| Hct | hematocrit |
| HCV | hepatitis C virus |
| HDL | high-density lipoprotein |
| HDV | hepatitis D virus |
| H&E | hematoxylin and eosin |
| HEV | hepatitis E virus |
| HGPRT | hypoxanthine-guanine phosphoribosyltransferase |
| HHS | [Department of] Health and Human Services |
| HHV | human herpesvirus |
| 5-HIAA | 5-hydroxyindoleacetic acid |
| His | histidine |
| HIT | heparin-induced thrombocytopenia |
| HIV | human immunodeficiency virus |
| HL | hepatic lipase |
| HLA | human leukocyte antigen |
| HMG-CoA | hydroxymethylglutaryl-coenzyme A |
| HMP | hexose monophosphate |
| HMSN | hereditary motor and sensory neuropathy |
| HMWK | high-molecular-weight kininogen |
| HNPCC | hereditary nonpolyposis colorectal cancer |
| hnRNA | heterogeneous nuclear ribonucleic acid |
| HPA | hypothalamic-pituitary-adrenal [axis] |
| HPG | hypothalamic-pituitary-gonadal [axis] |
| HPO | hypothalamic-pituitary-ovarian [axis] |
| HPSA | Health Professional Shortage Area |
| HPV | human papillomavirus |
| HR | heart rate |
| HRT | hormone replacement therapy |
| HSV | herpes simplex virus |
| HSV-1 | herpes simplex virus 1 |
| HSV-2 | herpes simplex virus 2 |
| 5-HT | 5-hydroxytryptamine (serotonin) |
| HTLV | human T-cell leukemia virus |
| HUS | hemolytic-uremic syndrome |
| HVA | homovanillic acid |
| IBD | inflammatory bowel disease |
| IBS | irritable bowel syndrome |
| IC | inspiratory capacity, immune complex |
| ICA | internal carotid artery |
| ICAM | intracellular adhesion molecule |
| ICE | Integrated Clinical Encounter |
| ICF | intracellular fluid |
| ICP | intracranial pressure, inferior cerebellar peduncle |

| Abbreviation | Meaning |
|---|---|
| IDDM | insulin-dependent diabetes mellitus |
| IDL | intermediate-density lipoprotein |
| I/E | inspiratory/expiratory [ratio] |
| IEV | inferior epigastric vein |
| IF | immunofluorescence |
| IFN | interferon |
| Ig | immunoglobulin |
| IGF | insulin-like growth factor |
| IL | interleukin |
| Ile | isoleucine |
| IMA | inferior mesenteric artery |
| IMED | International Medical Education Directory |
| IMG | international medical graduate |
| IMP | inosine monophosphate |
| IMV | inferior mesenteric vein |
| INH | isonicotine hydrazine [isoniazid] |
| INR | International Normalized Ratio |
| IO | inferior orbital [muscle] |
| $IP_3$ | inositol triphosphate |
| IPV | inactivated polio vaccine |
| IR | inferior rectus [muscle] |
| IRV | inferior rectal vein, inspiratory reserve volume |
| ITP | idiopathic thrombocytopenic purpura |
| IUGR | intrauterine growth retardation |
| IV | intravenous |
| IVC | inferior vena cava |
| JG | juxtaglomerular [cells] |
| JGA | juxtaglomerular apparatus |
| JVD | jugular venous distention |
| JVP | jugular venous pulse |
| $K_f$ | filtration constant |
| KOH | potassium hydroxide |
| KSHV | Kaposi's sarcoma–associated herpesvirus |
| LA | left atrial, left atrium |
| LAD | left anterior descending [artery] |
| LAF | left anterior fascicle |
| LCA | left coronary artery |
| LCAT | lecithin-cholesterol acyltransferase |
| LCFA | long-chain fatty acid |
| LCL | lateral collateral ligament |
| LCME | Liaison Committee on Medical Education |
| LCMV | lymphocytic choriomeningitis virus |
| $LD_{50}$ | median toxic dose |
| LDH | lactate dehydrogenase |
| LDL | low-density lipoprotein |
| LES | lower esophageal sphincter |
| Leu | leucine |
| LFA-1 | leukocyte function–associated antigen 1 |
| LFT | liver function test |
| LGN | lateral geniculate nucleus |
| LGV | left gastric vein |

| Abbreviation | Meaning |
|---|---|
| LH | luteinizing hormone |
| LLQ | left lower quadrant |
| LM | light microscopy |
| LMN | lower motor neuron |
| LP | lumbar puncture |
| LPL | lipoprotein lipase |
| LPS | lipopolysaccharide |
| LR | lateral rectus [muscle] |
| LSE | Libman-Sacks endocarditis |
| LT | leukotriene |
| LV | left ventricle, left ventricular |
| Lys | lysine |
| MAC | membrane attack complex, minimal alveolar concentration |
| MALT | mucosa-associated lymphoid tissue |
| MAO | monoamine oxidase |
| MAOI | monoamine oxidase inhibitor |
| MAP | mean arterial pressure |
| MC | midsystolic click |
| MCA | middle cerebral artery |
| MCHC | mean corpuscular hemoglobin concentration |
| MCL | medial collateral ligament |
| MCP | metacarpophalangeal [joint], middle cerebellar peduncle |
| MCV | mean corpuscular volume |
| MD | macula densa |
| MEN | multiple endocrine neoplasia |
| MEOS | microsomal ethanol oxidizing system |
| Met | methionine |
| MGN | medial geniculate nucleus |
| MGUS | monoclonal gammopathy of undetermined significance |
| MHC | major histocompatibility complex |
| MHPSA | Mental Health Professional Shortage Area |
| MI | myocardial infarction |
| MIF | müllerian inhibiting factor |
| MIT | monoiodotyrosine |
| MLCK | myosin light-chain kinase |
| MLF | medial longitudinal fasciculus |
| MMC | migrating motor complex |
| MMR | measles, mumps, rubella [vaccine] |
| 6-MP | 6-mercaptopurine |
| MPGN | membranoproliferative glomerulonephritis |
| MPO | myeloperoxidase |
| MPTP | 1-methyl-4-phenyl-1,2,3,6-tetrahydropyridine |
| MR | medial rectus [muscle], mental retardation, mitral regurgitation |
| MRI | magnetic resonance imaging |
| mRNA | messenger ribonucleic acid |
| MRSA | methicillin-resistant S. aureus |
| MS | multiple sclerosis |
| MSH | melanocyte-stimulating hormone |

| Abbreviation | Meaning |
|---|---|
| mtDNA | mitochondrial DNA |
| mTOR | mammalian target of rapamycin |
| MTP | metatarsophalangeal [joint] |
| MTX | methotrexate |
| MUA/P | Medically Underserved Area and Population |
| $MVO_2$ | myocardial oxygen consumption |
| $NAD^+$ | oxidized nicotinamide adenine dinucleotide |
| NADH | reduced nicotinamide adenine dinucleotide |
| $NADP^+$ | oxidized nicotinamide adenine dinucleotide phosphate |
| NADPH | reduced nicotinamide adenine dinucleotide phosphate |
| NBME | National Board of Medical Examiners |
| NBOME | National Board of Osteopathic Medical Examiners |
| NBPME | National Board of Podiatric Medical Examiners |
| NC | no change |
| NE | norepinephrine |
| NEG | nonenzymatic glycosylation |
| NF | neurofibromatosis |
| $NH_3$ | ammonia |
| NHL | non-Hodgkin's lymphoma |
| NIDDM | non-insulin-dependent diabetes mellitus |
| NK | natural killer [cells] |
| NMDA | N-methyl D-aspartate |
| NMJ | neuromuscular junction |
| NMS | neuroleptic malignant syndrome |
| NO | nitric oxide |
| NPV | negative predictive value |
| NSAID | nonsteroidal anti-inflammatory drug |
| OAA | oxaloacetic acid |
| OCD | obsessive-compulsive disorder |
| OCP | oral contraceptive pill |
| OMT | osteopathic manipulative technique |
| OPV | oral polio vaccine |
| OR | odds ratio |
| OS | opening snap |
| OTC | ornithine transcarbamoylase |
| OVLT | organum vasculosum of the lamina terminalis |
| PA | posteroanterior |
| PABA | para-aminobenzoic acid |
| PAH | para-aminohippuric acid |
| PALS | periarterial lymphatic sheath |
| PAN | polyarteritis nodosa |
| p-ANCA | perinuclear antineutrophil cytoplasmic antibody |
| PAP | prostatic acid phosphatase |
| PAS | periodic acid Schiff |
| PBP | penicillin-binding protein |

| Abbreviation | Meaning |
|---|---|
| $P_c$ | capillary pressure |
| PC | pyruvate carboxylase |
| PCL | posterior cruciate ligament |
| $P_{CO_2}$ | partial pressure of carbon dioxide |
| PCOS | polycystic ovarian syndrome |
| PCP | phencyclidine hydrochloride, *Pneumocystis carinii* (now *jiroveci*) pneumonia |
| PCR | polymerase chain reaction |
| PCT | proximal convoluted tubule |
| PCWP | pulmonary capillary wedge pressure |
| PD | posterior descending [artery] |
| PDA | patent ductus arteriosus |
| PDE | phosphodiesterase |
| PDGF | platelet-derived growth factor |
| PDH | pyruvate dehydrogenase |
| PE | pulmonary embolism |
| PECAM | platelet–endothelial cell adhesion molecule |
| PEP | phosphoenolpyruvate |
| PF | platelet factor |
| PFK | phosphofructokinase |
| PFT | pulmonary function test |
| PG | phosphoglycerate, prostaglandin |
| Phe | phenylalanine |
| $P_i$ | interstitial fluid pressure, inorganic phosphate |
| PICA | posterior inferior cerebellar artery |
| PID | pelvic inflammatory disease |
| PIP | proximal interphalangeal [joint] |
| $PIP_2$ | phosphatidylinositol 4,5-bisphosphate |
| PK | pyruvate kinase |
| PKD | polycystic kidney disease |
| PKU | phenylketonuria |
| PLP | pyridoxal phosphate |
| PML | progressive multifocal leukoencephalopathy |
| PMN | polymorphonuclear [leukocyte] |
| $P_{net}$ | net filtration pressure |
| PNET | primitive neuroectodermal tumor |
| PNH | paroxysmal nocturnal hemoglobinuria |
| PNS | peripheral nervous system |
| $P_{O_2}$ | partial pressure of oxygen |
| POMC | pro-opiomelanocortin |
| PPD | purified protein derivative |
| PPI | proton pump inhibitor |
| PPRF | paramedian pontine reticular formation |
| PPV | positive predictive value |
| PrP | prion protein |
| PRPP | phosphoribosylpyrophosphate |
| PSA | prostate-specific antigen |
| PSS | progressive systemic sclerosis |
| PT | prothrombin time |
| PTH | parathyroid hormone |
| PTHrP | parathyroid hormone–related protein |

| Abbreviation | Meaning |
|---|---|
| PTSD | post-traumatic stress disorder |
| PTT | partial thromboplastin time |
| PUV | paraumbilical vein |
| PV | plasma volume, portal vein |
| RA | rheumatoid arthritis, right atrium |
| RAAS | renin-angiotensin-aldosterone system |
| RBC | red blood cell |
| RBF | renal blood flow |
| RCA | right coronary artery |
| RDS | respiratory distress syndrome |
| REM | rapid eye movement |
| RER | rough endoplasmic reticulum |
| RNA | ribonucleic acid |
| RNP | ribonucleoprotein |
| ROI | reactive oxygen intermediate |
| RPF | renal plasma flow |
| RPR | rapid plasma reagin |
| RR | relative risk, respiratory rate |
| rRNA | ribosomal ribonucleic acid |
| RS | Reed-Sternberg [cells] |
| RSV | respiratory syncytial virus |
| RTA | renal tubular acidosis |
| RUQ | right upper quadrant |
| RV | renal vein, residual volume, right ventricle, right ventricular |
| RVH | right ventricular hypertrophy |
| SA | sinoatrial, subarachnoid |
| SAA | serum amyloid–associated [protein] |
| SAM | S-adenosylmethionine |
| SARS | severe acute respiratory syndrome |
| SC | subcutaneous |
| SCC | squamous cell carcinoma |
| SCID | severe combined immunodeficiency disease |
| SCJ | squamocolumnar junction |
| SCN | suprachiasmatic nucleus |
| SCP | superior cerebellar peduncle |
| SD | standard deviation, subdural |
| SEM | standard error of the mean |
| SEP | Spoken English Proficiency |
| SER | smooth endoplasmic reticulum |
| SEV | superficial epigastric vein |
| SEVIS | Student and Exchange Visitor Information System |
| SEVP | Student and Exchange Visitor Program |
| SGOT | serum glutamic oxaloacetic transaminase |
| SGPT | serum glutamic pyruvate transaminase |
| SHBG | sex hormone–binding globulin |
| SIADH | syndrome of inappropriate [secretion of] antidiuretic hormone |
| SLE | systemic lupus erythematosus |
| SLL | small lymphocytic lymphoma |
| SMA | superior mesenteric artery |
| SMV | superior mesenteric vein |

| Abbreviation | Meaning |
|---|---|
| SMX | sulfamethoxazole |
| SNc | substantia nigra compacta |
| SNP | single nucleotide polymorphism |
| SNr | substantia nigra pars reticulata |
| SNRI | selective norepinephrine receptor inhibitor |
| snRMP | small nuclear ribonucleoprotein |
| SO | superior oblique [muscle] |
| SOD | superoxide dismutase |
| SR | sarcoplasmic reticulum, superior rectus [muscle] |
| SRP | sponsoring residency program |
| SRV | superior rectal vein |
| SS | single stranded |
| SSB | single-stranded binding |
| ssDNA | single-stranded deoxyribonucleic acid |
| SSPE | subacute sclerosing panencephalitis |
| SSRI | selective serotonin reuptake inhibitor |
| ssRNA | single-stranded ribonucleic acid |
| SSSS | staphylococcal scalded-skin syndrome |
| STD | sexually transmitted disease |
| STN | subthalamic nucleus |
| SV | sinus venosus, splenic vein, stroke volume |
| SVC | superior vena cava |
| SVT | supraventricular tachycardia |
| $t_{1/2}$ | half-life |
| $T_3$ | triiodothyronine |
| $T_4$ | thyroxine |
| TA | truncus arteriosus |
| TAPVR | total anomalous pulmonary venous return |
| TB | tuberculosis |
| TBG | thyroxine-binding globulin |
| TBW | total body weight |
| 3TC | dideoxythiacytidine [lamivudine] |
| TCA | tricarboxylic acid [cycle], tricyclic antidepressant |
| Tc cell | cytotoxic T cell |
| TCR | T-cell receptor |
| TdT | terminal deoxynucleotidyl transferase |
| TFT | thyroid function test |
| 6-TG | 6-thioguanine |
| TG | triglyceride |
| TGA | trans-Golgi apparatus |
| TGF | transforming growth factor |
| THB | tetrahydrobiopterin |
| Th cell | helper T cell |
| THF | tetrahydrofolate |
| Thr | threonine |
| TI | therapeutic index |
| TIA | transient ischemic attack |
| TIBC | total iron-binding capacity |
| TLC | total lung capacity |
| TMP-SMX | trimethoprim-sulfamethoxazole |
| TN | true negative |

| Abbreviation | Meaning |
|---|---|
| TNF | tumor necrosis factor |
| TNM | tumor, node, metastases [staging] |
| TOEFL | Test of English as a Foreign Language |
| TP | true positive |
| tPA | tissue plasminogen activator |
| TPP | thiamine pyrophosphate |
| TPR | total peripheral resistance |
| TR | tricuspid regurgitation |
| TRAP | tartrate-resistant acid phosphatase |
| TRH | thyrotropin-releasing hormone |
| tRNA | transfer ribonucleic acid |
| Trp | tryptophan |
| TSH | thyroid-stimulating hormone |
| TSI | thyroid-stimulating immunoglobulin |
| TSS | toxic shock syndrome |
| TSST | toxic shock syndrome toxin |
| TTP | thrombotic thrombocytopenic purpura |
| TV | tidal volume |
| TxA | thromboxane |
| UA | urinalysis |
| UCB | unconjugated bilirubin |
| UCV | Underground Clinical Vignettes |
| UDP | uridine diphosphate |
| UMN | upper motor neuron |
| UMP | uridine monophosphate |
| URI | upper respiratory infection |
| USDA | United States Department of Agriculture |
| USIA | United States Information Agency |
| USMLE | United States Medical Licensing Examination |
| UTI | urinary tract infection |
| UV | ultraviolet |
| VA | ventral anterior [nucleus], Veterans Administration |
| Val | valine |
| VC | vital capacity |
| $V_d$ | volume of distribution |
| VDRL | Venereal Disease Research Laboratory |
| VF | ventricular fibrillation |
| VHL | von Hippel–Lindau [disease] |
| VIP | vasoactive intestinal peptide |
| VIPoma | vasoactive intestinal polypeptide-secreting tumor |
| VL | ventral lateral [nucleus] |
| VLDL | very low density lipoprotein |
| VMA | vanillylmandelic acid |
| VPL | ventral posterior nucleus, lateral |
| VPM | ventral posterior nucleus, medial |
| VPN | ventral posterior nucleus |
| V/Q | ventilation/perfusion [ratio] |
| VRE | vancomycin-resistant enterococcus |
| VSD | ventricular septal defect |

| Abbreviation | Meaning |
|---|---|
| vWF | von Willebrand factor |
| VZV | varicella-zoster virus |
| WAIS | Wechsler Adult Intelligence Scale |
| WBC | white blood cell |

| Abbreviation | Meaning |
|---|---|
| WISC | Wechsler Intelligence Scale for Children |
| XR | X-linked recessive |
| ZDV | zidovudine [formerly AZT] |

# Index

Page numbers preceded by *I-* refer to High-Yield Images.

Albuminuria, 457
Albuterol, 236, 513
**Alcohol**
  abuse, signs and symptoms of, 448
  and cirrhosis, 324
  and liver disease, 325
  and pancreatitis, 329
  as risk factor for esophageal cancer, 317
  **toxicity, 242**
**Alcoholic liver disease, 325**
**Alcoholism, 449**
Aldose reductase, 104
Aldosterone, 460, 461, 462
Alkaline phosphatase, 325
**Alkalosis, 463**
**Alkaptonuria (ochronosis), 108**
**Alkylating agents, 361**
Allantois, 125
Allopurinol, 388
α-agonists, 427
α-blockers, 237, 276
α-fetoprotein, 223, 325, 489, 523
α toxin, 143, 149
**Alport's syndrome, 80, 466, 517**
Alprazolam, 430
ALS. *See* Amyotrophic lateral sclerosis
ALT, 173, 325
Alternative hypothesis, 56
Altruism, 218
Aluminum hydroxide, 332
**Alveolar gas equation, 506**
**Alzheimer's disease, 393, 422, 440, 522, 523, 526, I-10**
  **drugs, 433**
**Amantadine, 193, 194, 432**
Amastigotes, 162
**Amblyopia, 419**
Amebiasis, 161
Amenorrhea, primary, 528
Amiloride, 474
α-Aminitin, 72
**Amino acids, 104**
  **clearance, 458**
  **derivatives, 106**
Aminoacyl-tRNA, 188
  synthetase, 74
**Aminoglycosides, 75, 141, 184, 187, 196**
Aminotransferases, 325
Amiodarone, 281
Amitriptyline, 452
Ammonia intoxication, 105

Ammonium, transport of by alanine and glutamine, 105
**Amnesia, 399, 441**
  anterograde, 399, 441
  dissociative, 441
  Korsakoff's, 441
  retrograde, 441
**Amniotic fluid abnormalities, 486**
Amniotic fluid embolism, 509
Amnionitis, 149
Amoxapine, 452
**Amoxicillin, 185, 332**
Amphetamines, 236, 440
  abuse, signs and symptoms of, 448
**Amphotericin, 192**
  **B, 158, 192**
**Ampicillin, 149, 185**
Ampulla of Vater, 308
Amygdala, 399
α-Amylase, 313, 314, 325
Amylin, 219
β-Amyloid, 219, 422, I-10
Amyloid angiopathy, 402
**Amyloidosis, 219, 269, 353, 465, 467, I-23**
**Amyotrophic lateral sclerosis (ALS), 407, 527**
**Anaclitic depression (hospitalism), 439**
**Analgesics (OTC), comparison of, 388**
Anaplasia, 221
**Anastrozole, 496**
Anatomical dead space, 503
**ANCA-positive vasculitides, 274**
*Ancylostoma*, 164
*Ancylostoma duodenale*, 163
Androgen-binding protein, 478
**Androgen insensitivity syndrome, 484**
**Androgens, 480**
Androstenedione, 480
Anemia, 222, 324, **343–347**, 353
  aplastic, 188, 344, 519
  Fanconi's, 345, 519
  **hemolytic, 98, 102, 240**
    autoimmune, 347, 518
    **extrinsic, 344, 347**
    **intrinsic, 344, 346**
  iron deficiency, 316, 343, 347, 517, 522, I-5
  **lab values in, 347**
    chronic disease, 347

    hemochromatosis, 347
    iron deficiency, 347
    pregnancy/OCP use, 347
  lead poisoning, 343
  **macrocytic, 344**
    nonmegaloblastic, 344
    megaloblastic, 195, 240, 342, 522
      caused by B$_{12}$ deficiency, 344, 522
      caused by folate deficiency, 344, 522
    microangiopathic, 347
  **microcytic, hypochromic, 343, 522**
  **normocytic, normochromic, 344**
    **nonhemolytic, 344, 345**
  pernicious, 222, 344
  sickle cell, 87, 342, 344, 346
  sideroblastic, 343, 521
  α-thalassemia, 343
Anencephaly, 127, 523
**Anergy, 207**
**Anesthetics**
  **general principles, 430**
  **inhaled, 430**
  **intravenous, 431**
  **local, 431**
**Aneurysms, 401, I-19**
  aortic, 525
  dissecting, 525
Angelman's syndrome, 83, 84
Angina, 266
Angiodysplasia, 322
Angiogenesis, 220
Angiomatosis, 519
  bacillary, 276
Angiomyolipoma, 222
Angiosarcoma, 221, 276
Angiotensin-converting enzyme (ACE), 502
Angiotensin II, 461, 462
Angiotensinogen, 460
Aniline dyes, 154
Anion gap, 463
Anisocytosis, 336
Anitschkow's cells, 272
Ankylosing spondylitis, 320, 381, 521, 527
*Anopheles*, 162
Anorexia, 329
Anorexia nervosa, 447
**ANOVA, 57**
**Anovulation, most common causes of, 487**

ANP. *See* Atrial natriuretic peptide
Antabuse (disulfiram), 94
**Antacids, 331, 332**
Antagonists
   competitive, 230
   noncompetetive, 230
Anterior cruciate ligament (ACL),
   366, 519
**Anthrax, 149**
**Antiandrogens, 496**
**Antianginal therapy, 277**
**Antiarrhythmics, 280–282**
**Antibiotics, 184, 361**
   antitumor, 361
   to avoid in pregnancy, 196
   bactericidal, 184
   bacteriostatic, 184
   resistance mechanisms for, 191
**Antibody structure and function,**
   **203**
Anticentromere antibodies, 521
Anticipation, 83
Anticoagulants, 188
**Antidepressants, 452, 453**
   atypical, 453
   tricyclic, 452
Antidesmoglein antibodies, 521
Anti-dig Fab fragments, 279
**Antidotes, specific, 239**
Antifreeze, *I-22*
**Antifungal therapy, 192**
**Antigen**
   **type and memory, 204**
   **variation, 207**
Antigen-presenting cell (APC), 337
Antigenic shifts, 170
Antigliadin antibodies, 318
Anti–glomerular basement
   membrane antibodies, 521
Antihistone antibodies, 521
**Antihypertensive therapy, 276**
Anti-IgG antibodies, 521
**Antimetabolites, 360**
**Antimicrobial prophylaxis,**
   **nonsurgical, 191**
**Antimicrobial therapy, 184**
Antimitochondrial antibodies, 521
Antimycin A, 100
**Antimycobacterial drugs, 190**
**Antineoplastics, 359**
Antineutrophil cytoplasmic
   antibodies, 521
**Antinuclear antibodies, 521**
   **positive, 381**
Antiphospholipid antibodies, 381

Antiplatelet antibodies, 521
**Antiplatelet interaction,**
   **mechanism of, 358**
**Antipseudomonals, 185**
**Antipsychotics (neuroleptics), 451**
   **atypical, 451**
Antisocial personality disorder, 440,
   446
**Anti-TB drugs, 190**
Antithrombin III, 339, 350
   deficiency, 350
Anti-topoisomerase antibodies, 521
Anti-transglutaminase/antigliadin
   antibodies, 521
Anxiety, 440
$\alpha_1$-**Antitrypsin, 80**
   **deficiency, 325, 326**
**Antiviral chemotherapy, 193**
Anxiety, 393
**Aorta, 305**
   **abdominal, and its branches,**
     **305**
   retroperitoneal, 302
**Aortic arch derivatives, 126**
**Aortic dissection, 265, 516,** *I-19*
Aortic hiatus, 501
Aortic regurgitation, 254, 255
Aortic stenosis, 254, 255, 520, 526,
   529
Aortic valve sclerosis, 254
APC gene, 323
**Apgar score, 61**
**Aphasia, 400**
   Broca's, 400
   Wernicke's, 400
**Apolipoproteins, major, 114**
**Apoptosis, 216**
**Appendicitis, 321,** 519
"Apple core" lesion, 323, *I-24*
Apple green birefringence, *I-23*
**Aqueous humor pathway, 417**
**Arachidonic acid,** 113
   **products, 387**
Arachnodactyly, 516
**Arbovirus, 169, 170, 171**
Arcuate fasciculus, 398
ARDS. *See* Acute respiratory
   distress syndome
Area postrema, 394
Arenaviruses, 169
Arginine, 106
**Argyll Robertson pupil, 155,** 181,
   408, 519
Aripiprazole, 451
Armadillos, 151

Arnold-Chiari malformation, 526
Aromatase, 480
Aromatization, 480
ARPKD, 87, 471
Arrhythmia, chronic, 526
Arsenic, 99
Arteries
   acute marginal, 250
   carotid, common, 126, 250
   celiac, 305
   circumflex (CFX), 250
   **coronary, 250**
     left main (LCA), 250
   epigastric, inferior, 310
   femoral, 309
   gastric
     right, 306
   gastroepiploic
     left, 306
     right, 306
     short, 306
   gastroduodenal, 306
   hepatic, 308
     common, 306
     left, 306
     right, 306
   mesenteric
     inferior (IMA), 305
     superior (SMA), 305
   maxillary, 126
   posterior
     descending/interventricular
     (PD), 250
   right coronary (RCA), 250
   splenic, 306
   stapedial, 126
   pancreaticoduodenal, superior,
     306
Arterioles, 252
   afferent, *I-21*
   efferent, *I-21*
Arteriolosclerosis, 265
**Arteriosclerosis, 265,** *I-18*
Arteriovenous malformation, *I-14*
Arteriovenous shunts, 376
Arteritis, 424
Artery of Adamkiewicz, 407
**Arthritis, 516,** 517, 520
   **infectious, 380**
   monoarticular, 528
   psoriatic, 381
   reactive, 157, 381
   **rheumatoid, 332, 379,** 521, 527,
     *I-14*
   septic, 152

Arthropods, 171
Arthus reaction, 208
Arylcyclohexylamines, 431
Arylsulfatase, 337
Arylsulfatase A, 111
Asbestos, 224
Asbestosis, 509, 523, *I-11*
*Ascaris lumbricoides*, 163, 526
Aschoff bodies, 272, 522
Ascites, 324, 325, 326, 516
**Ascorbic acid (vitamin C), 93**
  deficiency, 520
Asherman's syndrome, 487
ASO antibody, 143, 148
Aspartate, 67
Asperger's disorder, 440
Aspergilloma, 159
Aspergillosis, 508
  allergic bronchopulmonary, 159
  invasive, 182, 193
*Aspergillus*, 183
*Aspergillus fumigatus*, 159, 182
**Aspirin (ASA),** 100, 325, 341, **359,**
  387
Asplenia, 342
AST, 173, 325
Asterixis, 324, 327
Asthma, 272, 336, 508, 522
  drugs, 513
Astrocytes, 392, 392
Astrocytoma, 222, 425, 525
  pilocytic, 425
Ataxia-telangiectasia, 212
Atenolol, 281
Atheromas, 265
**Atherosclerosis, 265, 266,** 403,
  525, 529
**Athetosis, 397**
ATIII deficiency, 350
Atorvastatin, 278
ATP, 97
Atrial fibrillation, 259, 526
Atrial flutter, 259
Atrial myxoma, *I-20*
Atrial natriuretic peptide (ANP),
  261, 460, 462
Atrial septal defect (ASD), 254,
  263, 526
Atrium, left, 250
**Atropine, 235,** 312
Attention-deficit hyperactivity
  disorder (ADHD), 440
Attributable risk, 530
Auditory meatus, internal, 413
Autistic disorder, 440

**Auer bodies (rods),** 354, **355,** 521,
  *I-6*
Auerbach's plexus, 304, 316, 322
**Auscultation of the heart, 254**
**Autoantibodies, 210**
**Autonomic drugs, 233**
Autonomy, 59
**Autoregulation of blood flow, 262**
**Autosomal-dominant diseases, 86**
Autosomal-dominant polycystic
  kidney disease (ADPKD), 86
**Autosomal-recessive diseases, 87**
**Autosomal trisomies, 88**
Autosplenectomy, 525
AV block, 259
  first degree, 259
  second degree
    Mobitz type I (Wenckebach),
    260
    Mobitz type II, 260
  third degree (complete), 260
Avoidant personality disorder, 446
**Azathioprine, 214**
**Azoles, 192**
AZT. *See* Zidovudine
**Aztreonam, 186**
Azurophilic granular needles in
  leukemic blasts, 521
Azygous vein, 307

# B

B cells, 336
  **activation, 202**
  class switching, 202
  lymphoma, diffuse large, 352
  **major functions of, 201**
**B lymphocyte, 338**
*Babesia*, 154, 162
Babesiosis, 162
Babinski sign, 406, 516
Bacillary angiomatosis, 276
*Bacillus*, 139, 140, 146
*Bacillus anthracis*, 143, 148, 149
*Bacillus cereus*, 148, 176
Bacitracin, 146
Bacteremia, 525
**Bacteria**
  α-hemolytic, 146, 147
  β-hemolytic, 146
  encapsulated, 141
  enteric, lactose-fermenting, 151
  **highly resistant, treatment of,**
    191
  intracellular, 141

  pigment-producing, 141
  **with unusual cell**
    **membranes/walls, 139**
  urease-positive, 141
  zoonotic, 155
  **Bacterial endocarditis, 271**
    subacute, 147, 271
  **Bacterial genetics, 145**
  **Bacterial growth curve, 144**
  Bacterial structures, 138
  Bacterial superinfection, 170
  **Bacterial taxonomy, 139**
  **Bacterial toxins, effects of, 201**
  Bacterial vaginosis, 181
  **Bacterial virulence factors, 141**
  *Bacteroides*, 139, 141
  Bacteriophage, 142
  "Bamboo spine," 521
  **Barbiturates, 429, 431**
    abuse, signs and symptoms of,
    448
  Baroreceptors, 261
  **Barrett's esophagus, 222, 317**
  *Bartonella*, 139, 155, 217
  *Bartonella henselae*, 182, 276
  Basal cell carcinoma, 222, 386,
    527, *I-15*
  **Basal ganglia, 396,** 399
  Basal nucleus of Meynert, 393
  Basal plate, 118
  Base excision repair, 71
  Basement membrane, 220, 456
  Basilar artery, 401
  Basophilic nuclear remnants in
    RBCs, 521
  Basophilic stippling of RBCs, 521
  **Basophils, 336, 337**
  Becker's muscular dystrophy, 87,
    519
  Beclomethasone, 513
  Behavioral science, high-yield
    principles in, 51–64
    development, 61–63
    epidemiology/biostatistics, 52–58
    ethics, 59–61
    physiology, 63–64
  Bell's palsy, 154, 183, 382, 415, 520
  Bence Jones protein, 353, 523
  Beneficence, 59
  **Benign prostatic hyperplasia**
    **(BPH), 493,** 528
  Benzodiazepines, 428, 429, 430,
    431
    abuse, signs and symptoms of,
    448

FTA-ABS, 155
F2,6BP, regulation by, 98
Fungal infections, opportunistic, 159
Furosemide, 189, 473
Fusion inhibitors, 195

## G

G cells, 311, 312
G-protein-linked 2nd messengers, 232
GABA, 393
Gabapentin, 428, 429
Gag reflex, 412
Gage, Phineas, 398
Galactocerebrosidase, 111
Galactose metabolism, disorders of, 103
   galactokinase deficiency, 103
   galactosemia, 103
Galactose-1-phosphate uridyltransferase, 96
α-Galactosidase A, 111
Gallbladder, 308
Gallstones (cholelithiasis), 164, 329, 528
Gamma loop, 410
Ganciclovir, 194
Gangrene, I-23
Gap junction, 366
γ-globulins, 193
γ-glutamyl transferase, 325
γ-glutamyl transpeptidase, 325
Gardnerella, 139
Gardnerella vaginalis, 156, 181, 524
Gardner's syndrome, 323, 377, 518
Gas exchange barrier, 500
Gas gangrene, 149, 177
Gastric acid, 312
Gastric adenocarcinoma, 154, 523, 526
Gastric aspiration, 509
Gastric inhibitory peptide, 312
Gastric ulcer, 319, 525
Gastrin, 312
Gastrin-releasing peptide, 312
Gastrinoma, 312
Gastritis, 154, 318, 331
   acute (erosive), 318
   chronic (nonerosive), 318
     atrophic, 526
     type A (fundus/body), 318
     type B (antrum), 318

Gastrocolic ligament, 303
Gastroenteritis, 170
Gastroesophageal reflux disease (GERD), 316, 317
Gastrohepatic ligament, 303
Gastrointestinal stromal tumor (GIST), 222
Gastrointestinal system, 301–333
   anatomy, 302–310
   pathology, 315–330
   pharmacology, 331–333
   physiology, 311–315
Gastroparesis, 333
Gastroschisis, 132
Gastrosplenic ligament, 303
Gastrulation, 118
Gaucher's disease, 111, 517, 527
Gemfibrozil, 278
Gender identity disorder, 447
Generalized anxiety disorder, 445
Genes
   expression, regulation of, 72
   functional organization of, 72
Genetic code features, 69
Genetic drift, 170
Genetic shift, 170
Genetic terms, 83
Genital embryology, 134
Genital homologues, male/female, 135
Genital tubercle, 135
German measles (rubella), 169, 180
GFAP, 78, 392, 425
GGT (γ-glutamyl transpeptidase), 325
Ghon complex, 150
Ghon focus, 150, 524
Ghrelin, 311
Giemsa stain, 140
GI blood supply and innervation, 305
GI embryology, 132
GI hormones, 311
GI ligaments, important, 303
GI pathology, enzyme markers of, 325
GI polyps, hamartomatous, 517
GI secretory cells, locations of, 312
GI secretory products, 312
GI therapy, 331
Giant cell arteritis (temporal arteritis), 275
Giant cell tumor of bone, 524

Giardia, 177
Giardia lamblia, 161, I-2
Gilbert's syndrome, 327, 527
Gingiva, bluish line on, 516
Gingival hyperplasia, 241
Gingivostomatitis, 168
Glans clitoris, 135
Glanzmann's thrombasthenia, 349, 518
Glaucoma, 418
   closed/narrow angle, 418
   drugs, 427
   open/wide angle, 418
Gleevec (imatinib), 363
Gliadin, 318
Glioblastoma multiforme, 425, 523, 525, I-12
Gliosis, reactive, 392
Globose nuclei, 395
Globus pallidus externus, 396
Globus pallidus internus, 396
Glomerular disorders, 465
Glomerular dynamics, changes in, 458
Glomerular filtration barrier, 457
Glomerular filtration rate, 457, 530
Glomerular histopathology, 467
Glomerular structure, 456
Glomerulonephritis, 148, 271, 274, 521, 523, 526
   membranoproliferative, 524
   membranous, 465, 524, 527, I-21
   pauci-immune crescentic, 274
   poststreptococcal, 523
Glomerulosclerosis, diabetic, I-21
Glomerulus, 456, I-21
Glomus tumor, 276
Glossitis, 316, 517
Glossopharyngeal nerve, 261, 412
Glucagon, 284
β-Glucan, 193
β-Glucocerebrosidase, 111
   deficiency, 517
Glucocorticoids, 299
Glucokinase, 96, 97
Gluconeogenesis, 95, 96, 98, 99, 101
   enzymes, irreversible, 101
Glucose clearance, 458
Glucose-dependent insulinotropic peptide (GIP), 311
Glucose-6-phosphatase, 101, 110

Glucose-6-phosphate
   dehydrogenase (G6PD),
   87, 95, 96, 97, 101, **102**
   deficiency, 87, **102**, 189, 342,
      344, 346, 524
Glucosuria, 458
Glutamate, 106, 149
Glutamine, 67, 105
Glutamine-PRPP
   amidotransferase, 95
Glutathione, 101, 102, 106
Glycine, 67, 106
**Glycosides, cardiac, 279**
Glycogen phosphorylase, 110
**Glycogen storage diseases, 87, 110**
Glycogen synthase, 95, 109
**Glycogen, 109**
   **regulation by insulin and**
      **glucagon/epinephrine, 109**
   **synthesis, 9, 110**
Glycogenolysis, 95, 109, 110
**Glycolysis, 95, 96, 97**
   anaerobic, 99
   **regulation, key enzymes, 98**
**Glycolytic enzyme deficiency, 98**
**Glycoproteins, 196**
   IIb, 359
   IIIa, 359
   **T-cell, 201**
GM-CSF, 195
Goiter, toxic multinodular, 293, *I-26*
**Golgi apparatus, 77**
Golgi tendon, 410
**Gonadal drainage, 476**
Gonadal vein, 476
Gonorrhea, 181
**Good Samaritan law, 60**
Goodpasture's syndrome, 465, 466,
   509, 518, 521
**Gout, 224, 241, 380, 517, 520,**
   523, *I-13*
   drugs, 388
Gowers' maneuver, 87, 516
Gp1b receptor, 341
gp41, 174, 195
gp120, 174
Graft-versus-host disease, 213
**Grafts, 213**
**Gram-negative bacilli, penicillin**
   **and, 151**
**Gram-negative lab algorithm, 151**
**Gram-positive cocci, 147**
   identification of, 146
**Gram-positive lab algorithm, 146**

Gram stain limitations, 140
Granulocytes, 336
Granuloma, 217
**Granulomatous diseases, 207**
   chronic, 102
Granulation tissue, 217
Granulomas, 320
Granulosa cell, 480
   tumor, 490
Graves' disease, 293, 516, *I-18*
Gray baby syndrome, 188, 196,
   240
**Grief, 63**
   **Kübler-Ross stages of, 63**
Griseofulvin, 78, 192, **193**, 196
Ground-glass appearance, *I-18*
Guaifenesin (Robitussin), 514
Guanine, 67
   nucleotides, 194
Gubernaculum, 476
**Guillain-Barré syndrome, 392,**
   **423, 519**
Gummas, 155
**Gynecologic tumor epidemiology,**
   487
Gynecomastia, 192, 240, 324, 331,
   474, 492


**H**

**H$_1$ blockers, 512**
**H$_2$ blockers, 331**
HAART (highly active
   antiretroviral therapy), 195
Habituation, 436
*Haemophilus*, 139
*Haemophilus ducreyi*, 181, 520
*Haemophilus influenzae*, 140,
   141, 151, **152**, 177, 183,
   512, 524
Hageman factor, 144
Hair cells, 416
Hairy leukoplakia, oral, 175, 182,
   384
Haldane effect, 507
Half-life (t$_{1/2}$), 228, 530
**Hallucinations, 64, 441**
   types, **442**
      hypnagogic, 64, 442
      hypnopompic, 64, 442
Haloperidol, 451
Halothane, 430
Hamartomas, 424
**Hand, distortions of, 371**
**Hand muscles, 372**

Hand-Schüller-Christian disease,
   355
Hand-foot-mouth disease, 180, *I-4*
**Hansen's disease (leprosy), 151, *I-3***
   lepromatous, 151, *I-3*
   tuberculoid, 151
Hantavirus, 169
Hardy-Weinberg equilibrium, 530
**Hardy-Weinberg population**
   **genetics, 84**
**Hartnup disease, 91, 108**
Hashimoto's thyroiditis, 222, 293
Hawthorne effect, 55
HbC defect, 346
HbC disease, 342
**hCG, 223, 482, 483, 489**
   elevated, 522
HCO$_3^-$, 312
HDL. *See* High-density lipoprotein
**Headache, 333, 424**
   cluster, 424
   migraine, 424
   tension, 424
**Health care payment, 58**
Hearing loss, 416
   conductive, 416
   sensorineural, 416, 517
**Heart, auscultation of, 254**
**Heart disease**
   **congenital, 263, 520**
   holosystolic, 527
   **ischemic, 266**
      chronic, 266
   **rheumatic, 272**
   **syphilitic, 272**
**Heart embryology, 123**
Heart murmur, 526
   continuous "machinery," 516
Heart rate, 250
Heinz bodies, 102, 343, 524
Helicase, 70
*Helicobacter*, 139
*Helicobacter pylori*, **154**, 190, 318,
   319, 332, 525
Helmet cell, 342
**Helminths, medically important,**
   163–164
Hemagglutinin, 170
Hemangioblastoma, 424, 425, 519
Hemangioma, 221, 520, 529
Hematemesis, 324
Hematocrit, 252
Hematology and oncology,
   335–363
   anatomy, 336–338

Ketogenesis, 95
α-Ketoglutarate, 91, 99
α-Ketoglutarate dehydrogenase, 96, 100
**Ketone bodies, 112**, 113
**Kidney, 302**
   **anatomy, 456**
   **cysts, 471**
   disease, adult polycystic, 401, 520
   **embryology, 133**
   **endocrine functions, 461**
   **hormones acting on, 462**
   horseshoe, 520
   **stones, 468**, 527
Kimmelstiel-Wilson nodules, 295, 523
Kimmelstiel-Wilson syndrome, I-21
Kinase, 76, 95
   cyclin-dependent, 76
Kinesin, 78
*Klebsiella*, 139, 151, **153**, 177, 178, 183, 512, 525, 528
*Klebsiella pneumoniae*, 141, 179, 519
Klinefelter's syndrome, 483
**KLM sounds, 415**
**Klumpke's palsy, 371**
Klüver-Bucy syndrome, 517
**Knee injury, 366**
Koilocytes, 522
Koplik spots, 171, 183, 519, *I-4*
Korsakoff's amnesia, 441
Krabbe's disease, 111
*K-RAS* mutation, 324
Krebs cycle. *See* TCA cycle
Krukenberg tumor, 318, 490, 528
**Kübler-Ross grief stages, 63**
Kulchitsky cells, 511
Kupffer cell, 308
Kuru, 176
Kussmaul respirations, 296, 516
Kussmaul's pulse, 272
Kussmaul's sign, 273
**Kwashiorkor, 94**


L

Laboratory techniques, 81–82
Lacrimation reflex, 412
β-Lactam ring, 191
Lactase deficiency, 104
Lactation, 482
Lactic acidosis, 195

**Lactose-fermenting enteric bacteria, 151**
Ladder-like pattern, *I-27*
Lag, 144
Lambert-Eaton syndrome, 224, 382, 511
Lamellar bodies, 501
Lamellar bone, 375
Laminin, 220
Lamivudine (3TC), 195
Lamotrigine, 428, 429
Lancefield group D, 148
**Langerhans cell histiocytoses (histiocytosis X), 355**
Langhans' giant cells, *I-1*
Lanosterol, 192
Lansoprazole, 331
Large cell carcinoma of the lung, 511
Latanoprost, 427
Late-look bias, 55
Lateral geniculate nucleus (LGN), 395
Lateral striate arteries, 401
Lateral ventricle, 404
Latissimus dorsi, 302
LDL. *See* Low-density lipoprotein
**L-dopa, 432**
Lead-time bias, 55
**Leading causes of death in the United States by age, 58**
"Lead pipe," 320
**Lead poisoning, 239**, 343, **348, 349**, 516, 521, 522
**Learning**
   **simple, 436**
   **social, 437**
Leber's hereditary optic neuropathy, 85
Lecithin, 329
Lecithin-cholesterol acyltransferase (LCAT), 114
Lecithinase, 149
Left atrium, 250
Left main coronary artery (LCA), 250
Left ventricular hypertrophy, *I-29*
*Legionella*, 139, 140, 141, 177, 181, 512
*Legionella pneumophila*, 140, **152**
Legionnaires' disease, 152
Leiomyoma, 221, 487, 529
Leiomyosarcoma, 221, 487
*Leishmania donovani*, 162

Leishmaniasis, visceral, 162
Lens, 417
   dislocation, 516
**Lepirudin, 356**
**Leprosy (Hansen's disease), 151**, 217, *I-3*
   lepromatous, 151, *I-3*
   tuberculoid, 151
Leptomeningeal angiomatosis, 274
*Leptospira*, 139, 154
***Leptospira interrogans*, 154**
Leptospirosis, icterohemorrhagic (Weil's disease), 154
Lesch-Nyhan syndrome, 69, 87, 380, 517, 523
Letterer-Siwe disease, 355
Leucine, 99
**Leukemia, 221**, 350, **354–355**, *I-6*
   acute lymphoblastic (ALL), 222, 354, 355, 527, 528, *I-6*
   acute myelogenous (AML), 222, 354, 355, 521, 528, *I-6*
   M3 type, 355
   chronic lymphocytic (CLL), 354, 355, 524, 528, *I-6*
   chronic myelogenous (CML), 222, 354, 355, 356, 528
   death in, 526
   hairy cell, 354
   **vs. lymphoma, 350**
   small lymphocytic (SLL), 354
Leukemic patients, 159
**Leukemoid reaction, 355**
**Leukocyte, 336**
Leukocyte adhesion deficiency (type 1), 212
Leukocyte esterase, 179
**Leukocyte extravasation, 218**
Leukocytes, 196
Leukodystrophy, metachromatic, 111, 423
Leukotrienes, 336, 387
**Leuprolide, 495**
Levetiracetam, 428
**Levothyroxine, 299**
Lewy bodies, 397, 522
Lewy body dementia, 422
Leydig cell tumor, 494, 523
Leydig cells, 478, 523
Li-Fraumeni syndrome, 223
**Libman-Sacks endocarditis, 271**, 525
Lichen planus, 385
Lidocaine, 279, 280, 431
**Limbic system, 395**

snRNPs, 73
"Soap bubble," 524
Social phobia, 444
**Sodium pump, 79**
**Soft tissue tumors, 383**
Somatic (O) antigen, 153
Somatization disorder, 445
**Somatoform disorders, 445**
Somatostatin, 284, 299, 311, 331
Somatotropic "acidophilic"
    adenoma, 528
Sonic hedgehog gene, 118
**Sorbitol, 104**
Sotalol, 281
Southern blot, 81
Space of Disse, 308
"Spaghetti and meatballs," 159
Specific gravity, 217
Specificity, 53, 530
**Sperm parts, derivation of, 477**
Spermatid, 477, 479
Spermatocele, 494
Spermatocytes
    primary, 478, 479
    secondary, 479
**Spermatogenesis**
    **(spermiogenesis), 477, 478,**
      **479, 480**
    **regulation of, 479**
Spermatogonia, 478, 479
Spermatozoa, 477, 478, 479
Spherocytes, 342
Spherocytosis, hereditary, 86, 252,
    342, 344, 346
Sphincter of Oddi, 308
Sphingomyelinase, 111
    deficiency, genetic, 517
Sphingolipidoses, 87
Spider nevi, 324
Spinal arteries
    anterior, 405
    posterior, 405
Spina bifida occulta, 127, 523
**Spinal cord**
    **and associated tracts, 405**
    **lesions, 407**
    **lower extent, 405**
**Spinal nerves, 404**
**Spinal tract anatomy and**
    **functions, 406**
**Spindle muscle control, 410**
Spinothalamic tract, 405, 406
Spiral artery, 481
**Spirochetes, 154**
Spironolactone, 474

Spitz nevus, 525
**Spleen**
    dysfunction, 199
    **embryology, 133**
    **sinusoids of, 199**
Splenic infarction, *I-5*
Splenic vein, 307
Splenomegaly, 324
Splenorenal ligament, 303
Splicing, 73
Splinter hemorrhages, 271
**Splitting (cardiac), 254**
Splitting (ego defense), 218
**Spondyloarthropathies,**
    **seronegative, 381**
Spontaneous abortion, 149
**Spores**
    **bacterial, 148**
    **fungal, 158**
*Sporothrix schenckii,* 160
Sporotrichosis, 160
Squalene, 192
Squalene epoxidase, 193
Squamous cell carcinoma, 182,
    222, 518, 525, 526
    of the bladder, 164
    of the lung, 511
    of the penis, 494
    of the skin, 386, 518, *I-14*
SSPE, 171
**SSRIs, 452**
St. Louis encephalitis, 169
ST depression, 268
ST elevation, 268
ST toxin, 177
St. Vitus' dance, 272
Stab (band) cell, 336
**Stains, 140**
**Standard deviation vs. standard**
    **error, 56**
Standard error of the mean, 56
Stanford-Binet intelligence scale,
    436
Stapedial artery, 126
Stapes, 129
Staphylococcal scalded skin
    syndrome (SSSS), 384
*Staphylococcus,* 139, 146
*Staphylococcus aureus,* 87, 141,
    143, 146, **147,** 178, 183,
    201, 271, 512, 525, 526,
    528, *I-1*
    in bacterial endocarditis, 271
    methicillin-resistant (MRSA),
      147, 191

*Staphylococcus epidermidis,* 146,
    147, 178, 271
*Staphylococcus saprophyticus,* 146,
    178, 179, 529
**Starling curve, 251**
Starling forces, 262
"Starry sky" appearance, 524, *I-7*
Starvation, 113
**Start and stop codons, 72**
**Statistical distribution, 55**
**Statistical hypotheses, 56**
Stavudine (d4T), 195
Steatorrhea, 317, 318, 329
Stem cells, 336
Sternomastoid muscles, 502
**Steroid/thyroid hormone**
    **mechanism, 290**
**Steroids, 329**
    **adrenal, 287**
Stevens-Johnson syndrome, 241,
    385, 429
**Stomach, 304**
    **cancer, 318,** 525, 529
**Strabismus, 419**
Stranger anxiety, 62
Strawberry hemangioma, 276, 385
"Strawberry tongue," 275, 519
*Streptococcus,* 139, 146
    group A, 148
    group B, 148, 179, 183, 525
    group D, 148
    viridans, 146, 271
*Streptococcus agalactiae,* 146,
    148, 179
*Streptococcus bovis,* 148, 271
*Streptococcus pneumoniae,* 141,
    146, **147,** 177, 525, *I-1*
*Streptococcus pyogenes,* 143, 146,
    148, 180, 201, 512
Streptogramins, 191
Streptolysin O, 143
Streptozocin, 361
**Stress effects, 63**
Striatum (caudate and putamen),
    396
"String sign," 320, 523
Stroke, 516, *I-13*
Stroke volume, 250, 530
*Strongyloides stercoralis,* 163
**Structural theory of the mind,**
    **Freud's, 437**
Struma ovarii, 489
**Studies, types of, 52**
    adoption study, 52
    case-control study, 52

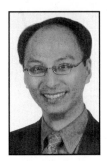

Tao Le, MD, MHS

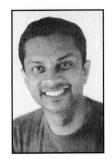

Vikas Bhushan, MD

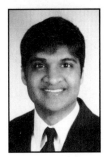

Neil Vasan

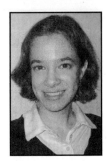

Juliana Tolles

**Tao Le, MD, MHS**

Tao has pursued his passion for medical education for the past 18 years. As senior editor, he has led the expansion of *First Aid* into a global educational series. In addition, he is the founder of the *USMLERx* on-line learning system as well as a cofounder of the *Underground Clinical Vignettes* series. As a medical student, he was editor-in-chief of the University of California, San Francisco *Synapse,* a university newspaper with a weekly circulation of 9000. Tao earned his medical degree from the University of California, San Francisco in 1996 and completed his residency training in internal medicine at Yale University and allergy and immunology fellowship training at Johns Hopkins University. At Yale, he was a regular guest lecturer on the USMLE review courses and an adviser to the Yale University School of Medicine curriculum committee. Tao subsequently went on to cofound Medsn and served as its chief medical officer. He is currently section chief of adult allergy and immunology at the University of Louisville. He enjoys travel, movies, good food, and spending time with his family.

**Vikas Bhushan, MD**

Vikas is an author, editor, entrepreneur, and roaming teleradiologist who divides his days between Los Angeles, Maui, and balmy remote locales with abundant bandwidth. In 1992 he conceived and authored the original *First Aid for the USMLE Step 1*, and in 1998 he originated and coauthored the *Underground Clinical Vignettes* series. His entrepreneurial adventures include a successful software company; a medical publishing enterprise (S2S); an e-learning company (Medsn); and, most recently, an ER teleradiology venture (24/7 Radiology). His eclectic interests include medical informatics, independent film, humanism, Urdu poetry, world music, South Asian diasporic culture, and avoiding a day job. He has also coproduced a music documentary on qawwali; coproduced and edited *Shabash 2.0: The Hip Guide to All Things South Asian in North America;* and is now completing a CD/book project on Sufi poetry translated into four languages. Vikas completed a bachelor's degree in biochemistry from the University of California, Berkeley; an MD with thesis from the University of California, San Francisco; and a radiology residency from the University of California, Los Angeles.

**Neil Vasan**

Neil is a fifth-year MD-PhD student at the Yale University School of Medicine, and this is his third year on the *First Aid* team. Originally from Vienna, West Virginia, Neil completed a dual bachelor's and master's degree in chemistry and chemical biology from Harvard University in 2005. Having recently been awarded an NIH F30 NRSA fellowship, Neil is currently working toward a PhD in cell biology, studying the structural biology of membrane trafficking in the laboratory of Karin Reinisch, PhD. Outside of school, Neil enjoys choral singing, cooking, and reading the *New York Times.* Like most people reading this book, he has no idea what he will specialize in.

**Juliana Tolles**

Juliana is a fifth-year medical student at the Yale University School of Medicine, and this is her second year on the *First Aid* team. Raised in Edina, Minnesota, she graduated from Harvard University in 2005 with a degree in biochemical sciences. At Harvard, she was an editor for the *Let's Go* travel guide series. After a year conducting research in the application of statistical models to tumor markers, she will graduate in 2011 with a dual degree in medicine and master's of health science. In her free time, she enjoys running and hiking in New England's beautiful parks.

# ABOUT THE AUTHORS

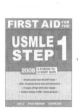
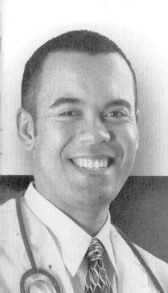